THE 21ST CENTURY PHARMACY TECHNICIAN

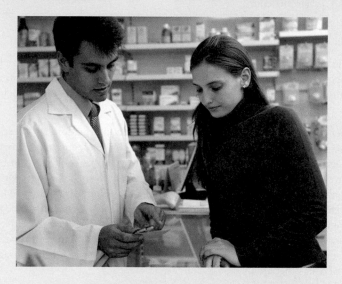

Brinda Shah, PharmD
President
Advanced Knowledge Concepts, Inc.

Jennifer L. Gibson, PharmD
President
Excalibur Scientific, LLC
Marietta, Georgia

Nick L. Tex, DM, MBA, RPh
Professor
Carrington College
Phoenix, Arizona

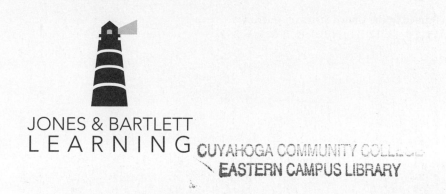

JONES & BARTLETT
LEARNING

World Headquarters
Jones & Bartlett Learning
5 Wall Street
Burlington, MA 01803
978-443-5000
info@jblearning.com
www.jblearning.com

Jones & Bartlett Learning books and products are available through most bookstores and online booksellers. To contact Jones & Bartlett Learning directly, call 800-832-0034, fax 978-443-8000, or visit our website, www.jblearning.com.

Substantial discounts on bulk quantities of Jones & Bartlett Learning publications are available to corporations, professional associations, and other qualified organizations. For details and specific discount information, contact the special sales department at Jones & Bartlett Learning via the above contact information or send an email to specialsales@jblearning.com.

The authors, editor, and publisher have made every effort to provide accurate information. However, they are not responsible for errors, omissions, or for any outcomes related to the use of the contents of this book and take no responsibility for the use of the products and procedures described. Treatments and side effects described in this book may not be applicable to all people; likewise, some people may require a dose or experience a side effect that is not described herein. Drugs and medical devices are discussed that may have limited availability controlled by the Food and Drug Administration (FDA) for use only in a research study or clinical trial. Research, clinical practice, and government regulations often change the accepted standard in this field. When consideration is being given to use of any drug in the clinical setting, the health care provider or reader is responsible for determining FDA status of the drug, reading the package insert, and reviewing prescribing information for the most up-to-date recommendations on dose, precautions, and contraindications, and determining the appropriate usage for the product. This is especially important in the case of drugs that are new or seldom used.

Production Credits

Chief Executive Officer: Ty Field
President: James Homer
SVP, Chief Operating Officer: Don Jones, Jr.
SVP, Chief Technology Officer: Dean Fossella
SVP, Chief Marketing Officer: Alison M. Pendergast
SVP, Curriculum Solutions: Christopher Will
VP, Business Development: Todd Giorza
VP, Design and Production: Anne Spencer
VP, Manufacturing and Inventory Control: Therese Connell
Publisher: David D. Cella
Editorial Management: High Stakes Writing, LLC, Editor and Publisher: Lawrence J. Goodrich
Managing Editor: Ruth Wallker
Editor: Kate Shoup

Technical Editor: Leslie Anne Hausser, PharmD, Medical Education and Environmental Management Solutions, Inc.
Managing Editor: Maro Gartside
Senior Production Editor: Susan Schultz
Production Assistant: Kristen Rogers
Marketing Manager: Grace Richards
Manufacturing and Inventory Control Supervisor: Amy Bacus
Rights and Photo Research Manager: Katherine Crighton
Composition: Publishers' Design and Production Services, Inc.
Cover Design: Scott Moden
Cover Image: © mangostock/ShutterStock, Inc.
Printing and Binding: Courier Kendallville
Cover Printing: Courier Kendallville

ISBN: 978-1-4496-3226-7

Library of Congress Cataloging in Publication Data unavailable at time of printing

6048

Printed in the United States of America
15 14 13 12 11   10 9 8 7 6 5 4 3 2

Contents

Introduction

To reach your career goal of becoming a pharmacy technician, you will travel through an obstacle course of classes, skills practice labs, online training, and an externship. *The 21st Century Pharmacy Technician* is designed to help you through it all with practical study tips that will make you confident and successful—as well as a valuable member of the pharmacy team—by helping you understand the rules of the game and the skills and strategies needed to win it.

How This Book Is Organized

The 21st Century Pharmacy Technician is designed to be enjoyable to read, as well as highly informative. The book is divided into three units:

- **Unit One: Foundation**—introduces you to the basic principles of pharmacy and the role of the pharmacy technician, while providing a solid foundation for entry into the profession.
- **Unit Two: Basic Principles**—guides you through the world of the community pharmacy, including dispensing and non-sterile compounding.
- **Unit Three: Advanced Principles**—leads you through the more advanced techniques in pharmacy practice, including institutional pharmacy and sterile compounding.

Special Features

What Would You Do? These scenarios show you how to apply the content to real-life situations in the classroom and in practice.

Tech Math Practice allows you to work through sample problems to provide you with additional practice in performing pharmaceutical calculations.

Drug Insights begin in chapter 6 and acquaint you with each category of medication, common drugs, and their uses in that category.

In addition, each chapter in *The 21st Century Pharmacy Technician* includes Key Terms, Chapter Summary, and Learning Assessment Questions.

Additional Resources

Additional educational materials are available to accompany *The 21st Century Pharmacy Technician*. To purchase additional products, visit *http://go.jblearning.com/PharmTech*. Teaching materials to accompany *The 21st Century Pharmacy Technician* are available to instructors online, visit: *http://go.jblearning.com/21stCenturyPharmTech* for more information. Additional resources include:

- **Online Resources**—glossary, review scenarios, top 200 drugs, Web links, review lessons, review activities, discussion boards, assignments, and quizzes.

- **Pocket Guide for Brand and Generic Drugs**—a handy pocket guide that provides the most common medications in alphabetical order by brand name with the corresponding generic name as well as by generic name with the corresponding brand name.
- **Instructor Resources**—learning assessment keys, Microsoft PowerPoint presentations, quiz questions, and assignments.

In summary, this textbook contains an organized approach to learning the roles and responsibilities of the pharmacy technician. It encompasses all areas of pharmacy practice from the very basic to the most complicated, with the intention of guiding you, the student technician, to mastery of all concepts. All those involved in the production of this book wish you success in your studies and new career.

Acknowledgments

To ensure the accuracy of the material presented throughout the textbook, an extensive review and development process was used. This included evaluation by a variety of knowledgeable healthcare professionals. We are deeply grateful to the numerous people who have shared their comments and suggestions. The quality of this body of work is a testament to the feedback we have received.

Reviewing a book or supplement takes an incredible amount of energy, time, and attention, and we recognize the sacrifices our colleagues made to help ensure the validity and appropriateness of content in this edition. The reviewers provided us with additional viewpoints and opinions to combine to make this text an incredible learning tool.

We wish to thank the following editorial and technical review team:

Reviewers

Dana Bernard, RN, MS
President, Boston Reed

John E. Fox, BS, RPhT, CPhT
Instructor, Pharmacy Technician

Reviewer & Contributor

James A. Lamberti, CPhT
Instructor, Pharmacy Technician

One

Foundation

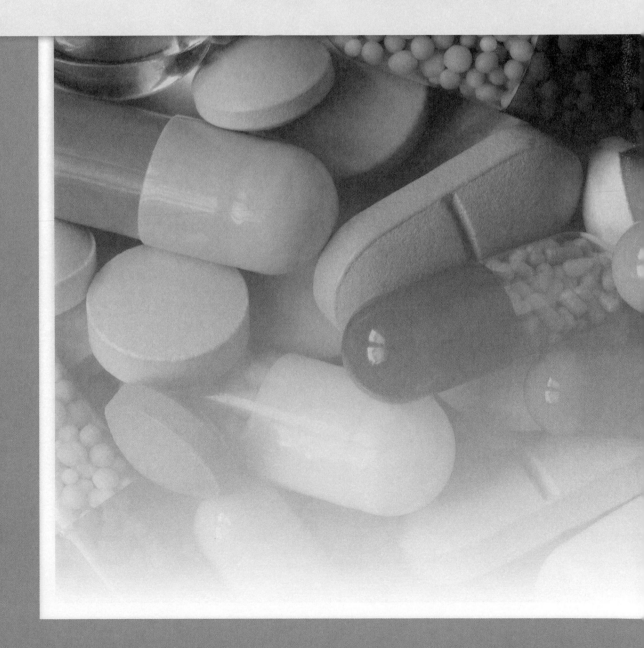

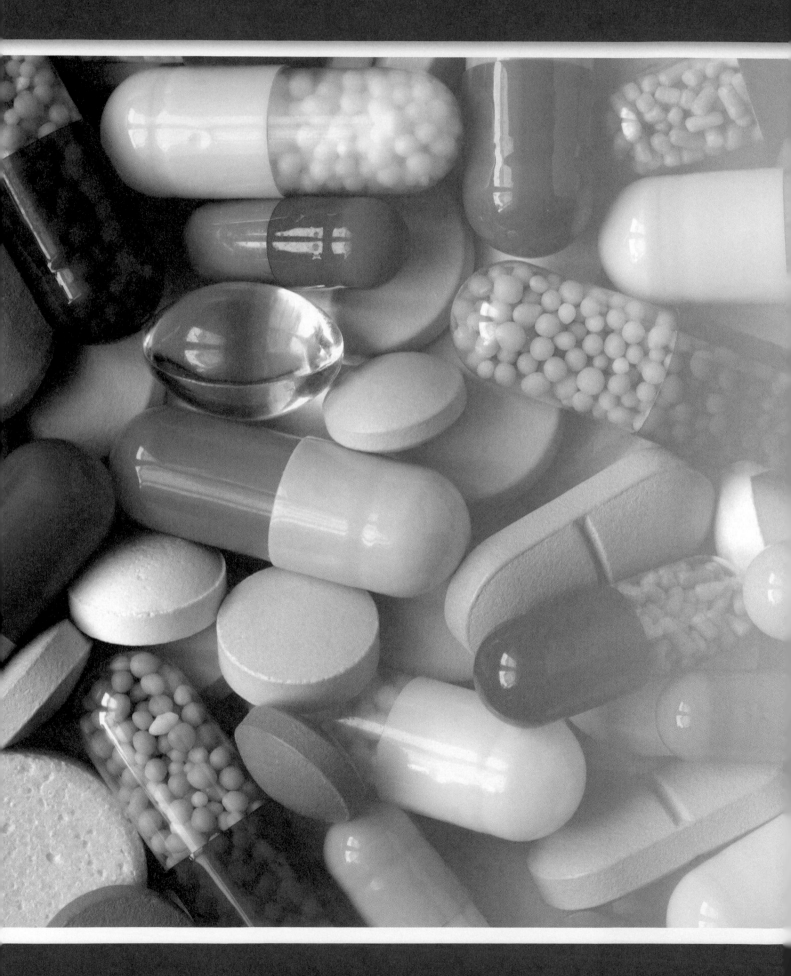

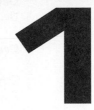

Pharmacy Profession, Law, Regulations, and Standards

OBJECTIVES

After reading this chapter, you will be able to:

* Outline the origins of pharmacy
* Differentiate between the various kinds of pharmacy practices
* Identify the four stages of development of the pharmacy profession in the 20th century
* Summarize the functions of a pharmacist
* Discuss the education curriculum for today's pharmacy student
* Explain the licensing requirements for pharmacists
* Explain the functions and work environments of the pharmacy technician
* Describe laws, regulations, professional standards, and ethics that affect the practice of pharmacy
* Outline the major pieces of statutory federal drug law in the 20th century
* Compare and contrast the roles of the Food and Drug Administration, the Drug Enforcement Administration, the Occupational Safety and Health Administration, and the national and state boards of pharmacy
* Review the functions that may legally be performed by pharmacy technicians in most states
* Discuss the potential for tort actions under the common law related to negligence and other forms of malpractice
* Understand the importance of drug and professional standards

KEY TERMS

Alchemy	Battery	Chain pharmacy
Apothecary	Brand name	Chemical name
Assault	Broken contract	Child-resistant container

Compounding pharmacy
Controlled substance
Defendant
Drug Enforcement
    Administration (DEA)
Drug-utilization review
    (DUR)
Ethics
Food and Drug
    Administration (FDA)
Formulary
Franchise pharmacy
Generic name
Health-maintenance
    organization (HMO)
Home health care
Home infusion pharmacy
Hospital pharmacy
Independent pharmacy
Institutional pharmacy

Law
Legend drugs
Libel
Long-term care facility
Long-term care
    pharmacy
Mail-order pharmacy
Malpractice
Managed-care
    organizations
National Association of
    Boards of Pharmacy
    (NABP)
Negligence
Nuclear pharmacy
Over-the-counter (OTC)
    drugs
Parenteral
Pharmacist
Pharmacognosy

Pharmacology
Pharmacy technician
Plaintiff
Point-of-service (POS)
    plan
Preferred provider
    organization (PPO)
Primary care physician
Professional standard
Regulation
Retail pharmacy
Slander
Standard of care
State boards of
    pharmacy
Tort
United States
    Pharmacopeia (USP)
USP-NF

Chapter Overview

Over the years, the practice of pharmacy has evolved into a scientific and knowledge-based profession. The role of the **pharmacist** has expanded from one who compounds and dispenses medications to one who also provides information and patient counseling regarding the safe use of medications.

Pharmacy in the United States is a heavily regulated profession, and knowledge of both federal and state law is necessary to practice pharmacy. Laws, regulations, and professional standards have been put in place to ensure public safety and the safe dispensing of medications. Regulatory bodies assist in the administration and enforcement of laws for the safe use of drugs. These agencies follow written rules or established guidelines to carry out federal or state laws.

The Origins of Pharmacy

Medicine has been practiced for thousands of years. Archeological discoveries have shown that early civilizations documented the use of animals, plants, and minerals to cure the sick. Over time, the practice of pharmacy has evolved into a more scientific approach to treating illness and disease. Learning about the history of pharmacy will help the pharmacy technician understand how the roles of a pharmacist and a pharmacy technician have evolved over time.

Pharmacy in Early Civilization

The history of pharmacy can be traced back thousands of years to early civilization, when disease was thought to be caused by evil forces, gods, or demons. Religious leaders, sorcerers, or medicinal healers would first identify the evil spirit before determining the medicinal remedy. These medicinal remedies were controlled primarily by religious leaders, who frequently mixed drug preparations with prayers, chants, rituals, and "magic."

Archaeologists found the earliest documentation (18th century B.C.E., or before the common era) of medicinal preparations on clay tablets in ancient Mesopotamia. These tablets identify drugs or medicinal preparations from various sources, including animals, plants, spices, and minerals. The people of ancient Egypt made several major medical discoveries and began treating diseases in a more rational physical manner along with using the older spiritual techniques.

Although much of the advancement in medicine was a result of trial and error or spiritual ceremonies, the effect on the knowledge and development of medicine was large. The ancient Egyptians compiled drugs or medicinal recipes in lists known largely as formularies or pharmacopeias. The most notable collection of medicinal recipes from natural ingredients, written in about 1534 B.C.E. and used for centuries in Egypt, is a 110-page document called the *Ebers papyrus*. Knowledge of the healing properties of these natural substances slowly evolved into a scientific endeavor that involved the compounding and dispensing of medications.

Clay tablets found in 18th century B.C.E. identified drugs or medicinal preparations from natural sources.

The history of plant usage for medicinal purposes can also be traced back to China, where plants and other naturally occurring substances were used in a similar fashion. More than 2,000 years ago, a Chinese named Li Che Ten wrote a plant book entitled *Peng T'Sao* that listed more than 1,000 plants and nearly 8,000 recipes for their use. Still today, much of Asia relies heavily on natural herbs to treat common illnesses.

The foundations of much of modern Western medicine come from ancient Greece. From about 800 B.C.E. to about 200 C.E., Greek medicine moved from the divine and spiritual toward scientific observation and logical reasoning. The word *pharmacy* is derived from the ancient Greek word *pharmako*, meaning *drug* or *poison*. The Greek physician Hippocrates (c. 460–377 B.C.E.), also known as "the Father of Medicine" was the first to believe that illness was not the result of superstitions, evil spirits, or punishment from God, but instead had a natural cause or physical and rational explanation. He based his practice on medical and scientific observations and recording, and on the study of the human body. Hippocrates also believed that the body must be treated as a whole and not just a series of parts. Hippocrates is perhaps best known for the Hippocratic Oath, an oath by which physicians pledge to uphold a number of professional ethical standards and "to do no harm."

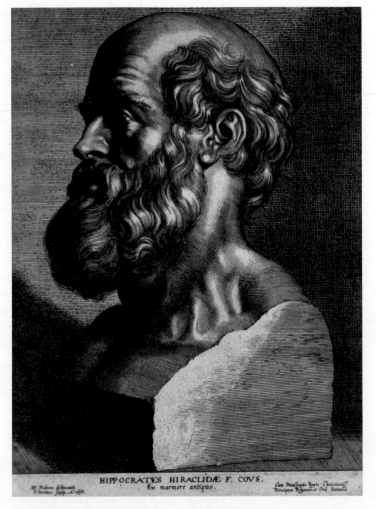

HIPPOCRATES HIRACLIDÆ F. COVS.
Ex marmore antiquo.

Hippocrates is known as the "Father of Medicine."

The word *pharmacy* comes from the Greek word *pharmako*.

Another Greek physician, Galen (130–200 C.E.), is often considered the most important contributor to modern-day medicine, apart from Hippocrates. Galen is credited with the discovery of blood in human arteries and for his dissection of the human cranial nerves, which supply key areas of the head, face, and upper chest. Galen dissected animals to further his knowledge of the human body and recorded his observations. The foundation of Galen's treatment methods was his belief that disease resulted from an imbalance in one of the four "humors"—blood, yellow bile, black bile, and phlegm—and that the diseases were cured with compounds of opposing qualities—moist, dry, cold, or warm. Galen believed that a disease-causing imbalance could be located within an organ. Treatments devised by Galen were more precise because he believed that disease primarily affected one organ or region of the body. He also produced a systemic classification of drugs for the treatment of various illnesses and described the process of creating extracts from plants. Although Galen was a physician, he is considered the "Father of Pharmacy."

Galen is considered to be the "Father of Pharmacy."

Dioscorides, a Greek physician, traveled extensively seeking medicinal substances. Between 50 and 70 C.E., he compiled a series of five books, collectively titled *De Materia Medica*, that included the properties, preparation, usage, dosages, storage, and testing of drugs. His text became the standard for pharmaceutical knowledge until the 16th century.

The *De Materia Medica* was the standard for pharmaceutical knowledge until the 16th century.

Pharmacy in the Middle Ages

Throughout Europe during the Middle Ages and Renaissance, physicians prescribed medications or herbal remedies to their patients, which were filled at **apothecary** shops. Along with the apothecary concept came the development of professional guilds, which controlled the training and length of apprenticeship for physicians (and other professionals).

The ancient pharmacy practices of the Greeks and Romans were questioned during the Renaissance. During this period, alchemy was prevalent. The goal of **alchemy** was to combine elements of chemistry, metallurgy, physics, and medicine with astrology and spiritualism to turn metals into gold. Exploration in the New World expanded the availability of medicinal agents in the form of new drugs and exotic spices. Pharmacies and hospitals run by religious orders also emerged during this period. These pharmacies and hospitals are the origin of pharmacies, healthcare clinics, and hospitals that we know today. It was also during this period that the works of Galen were challenged. Near the end of the Middle Ages, the *Nuovo Receptario* was published as the official pharmacopeia to be followed by all apothecaries.

The *Nuovo Receptario* was the first official pharmacopeia.

Pharmacy in the Modern Era

During the 17th and 18th centuries C.E., a more scientific approach to medicine emerged. Doctors began to question traditional ideas. More formal research and testing to determine the efficacy of natural ingredients was initiated, and several advances in pharmacy and medicine were made. Professional societies were formed in major

European cities. Scientists began to share their research by publishing their work in journals. During this time, William Harvey discovered how blood circulated through the body and Edward Jenner invented a vaccination for smallpox after discovering the relationship between cowpox and smallpox. Each major capital city in Europe published a list of commonly used drugs. The most notable of these is the one created in Great Britain, *Martindale's Pharmacopoeia*. It was also during this time that pharmacists began to be recognized as healthcare providers.

In North America, during the colonial period (from the 1600s to the 1700s), as new immigrants brought their families from other parts of the world, disease followed. Early colonists had few medical personnel and had to rely on home or natural remedies. The first pharmacists, known as druggists, were doctors until pharmacy became a specialty. As the colonies grew, more physicians came, bringing with them supplies from Britain. With the American Revolution and separation from Britain, colonists were forced to make their own preparations and chemical ingredients. It was during this time that the United States also developed its own pharmacopeia. After the Civil War, apothecaries began to emerge in towns across the country. Manufacturing plants were built, and people were trained to prepare medications accurately. As the physician's role changed from dispensing medication to diagnosing disease, the role of the pharmacist emerged, and the separation of duties between the pharmacist and physician was established.

During the 20th century, many new categories of medicine such as antiseptics, antimicrobials, and antibiotics, including penicillin, were discovered. Over time, pharmacology has evolved into a science based on systematic research to determine the effects that drugs have on the body.

Evolution of the Pharmacy Profession in the 20th Century

The evolution of the pharmacy profession in the 20th century can be categorized into four stages.

- Traditional era (1920s)—During this era, the pharmacy profession focused on preparing, compounding, and dispensing drugs from natural sources such as plants. A pharmacist in the traditional era not only sold drugs, but also often compounded and dispensed medicines made from botanicals. **Pharmacognosy**, the study of the medicinal properties of natural products from plant and animal sources and minerals, was emphasized during this period.
- Scientific era (1940s and 1950s)—During this era, the pharmacy profession focused on the development and testing of drugs and their effects on the human body. In the scientific era, pharmaceutical manufacturers developed ways to mass-produce new drugs consistently and economically. With the development of new drugs and dosage forms, **pharmacology**, the scientific study of drugs and their mechanisms of actions became important.
- Clinical era (1960s)—During this era, the pharmacy profession focused not only on the traditional roles of compounding and dispensing, but also provided drug information to patients and physicians. During the clinical area, pharmacy shifted from a product-focused profession to one that is patient focused.
- Pharmaceutical care era (from the 1990s to the present)—This era expanded the role of the pharmacist to include responsibility for appropriate medication use.

Pharmacy Practice Settings

The goal of the profession of pharmacy is to ensure the safe and effective use of medication. The scope of pharmacy practice includes traditional roles such as compounding and dispensing medications. It also includes modern roles related to patient care such as reviewing medications for safety and efficacy and providing drug information.

Pharmacists and pharmacy technicians can be employed in many different settings, including retail pharmacies (drug stores) and institutional pharmacies such as hospital pharmacies and pharmacies in assisted-living and long-term–care facilities, pharmaceutical manufacturing facilities, and insurance companies. They can also work in nuclear pharmacies, mail-order pharmacies, and home healthcare pharmacies.

Pharmacy technicians are employed in most of the same settings as pharmacists. Pharmacists and pharmacy technicians work in clean, organized, well-lit, and well-ventilated areas, and spend much of their day on their feet. Pharmacy technicians typically work the same hours as a pharmacist. Depending on where they work, this may include evenings, weekends, and holidays, particularly in pharmacies that are open 24 hours.

The mission of pharmacy is to protect the public's health and safety.

The U.S. Department of Labor's Bureau of Labor and Statistics reports that in 2008, pharmacy technicians and aides held approximately 381,200 jobs. Of these, about 326,300 were pharmacy technicians and roughly 54,900 were pharmacy aides. Approximately 75 percent of these jobs were in a retail setting, while about 16 percent were in hospitals. Pharmacy technicians also work in numerous other pharmacy settings and specialty pharmacy practices.

Retail Pharmacies

A **retail pharmacy**, also called a community pharmacy or drug store, is usually divided into two areas. One area, the front area, typically offers over-the-counter drugs, dietary aids, medical supplies, nutritionals, and other miscellaneous merchandise. A second area, the back area, usually contains the pharmacy. Most prescriptions filled in the United States are filled in retail pharmacies, and approximately 65 percent of all pharmacists work in a retail pharmacy setting. Retail pharmacies include the following:

- Chain pharmacies—A **chain pharmacy** is a pharmacy that has multiple outlets located regionally or nationally, and is usually owned by a corporation. These pharmacies may be found in grocery stores, department stores, or drug stores. Most chain pharmacies are located in high-traffic areas to allow for large-volume dispensing. Chain pharmacies typically employ a large number of pharmacists and pharmacy technicians. Administrative decisions in chain pharmacies are usually made at the corporate level. In some cases, prescriptions can be filled at central locations and then shipped to the customer or store.

- Independent pharmacies—An **independent pharmacy** is a pharmacy that is owned and operated by a private owner or owners. The number of independent pharmacies has decreased in recent years because they have difficulty competing with high-volume chain pharmacies.

- Compounding pharmacies—A **compounding pharmacy** is a specialized pharmacy wherein the pharmacist and/or pharmacy technician compounds or prepares medication mixtures that are customized specifically for the unique healthcare needs of the patient.

- Franchise pharmacies—A **franchise pharmacy** is a combination of a retail chain and an independent pharmacy. A franchise is a right granted to an individual or group (franchisee) to use the name of the company and market a company's goods or services within a certain territory or location.

- Mail-order pharmacies—A **mail-order pharmacy** is a closed-door, centralized pharmacy operation that dispenses a large number of prescriptions, which are mailed directly to the patient.

- Home infusion pharmacies—A **home infusion pharmacy** is one that specializes in **parenteral** mixtures (that is, mixtures administered by a needle or catheter into one or more layers of the skin), such as chemotherapy, antibiotics, nutrition and feeding supplies.

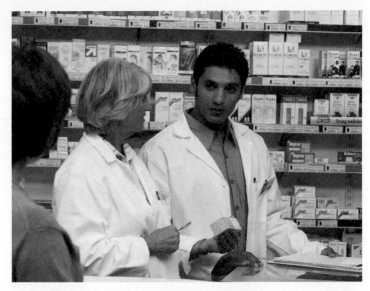

A customer talks to two pharmacists at the counter.

Institutional Pharmacies

An **institutional pharmacy** can broadly be defined as a facility that provides pharmaceutical-care services to patients in an institutional facility or organized healthcare system. Traditionally, this referred to a hospital pharmacy, but the definition has expanded to include long-term–care facilities, managed-care organizations, and nuclear pharmacies. As society's healthcare needs have changed, there has been an increased emphasis on providing care through organized healthcare settings. As a result, an increased number of pharmacists practice in institutional settings. As members of healthcare teams, pharmacists have an opportunity to be directly involved in patient care.

Hospital Pharmacies

A **hospital pharmacy** is an institutional pharmacy that provides services to patients and healthcare professionals in the hospital. Hospital pharmacies are responsible for maintaining patient records, and for ordering, stocking, compounding, and dispensing medications and other supplies.

Hospital pharmacy practice is composed of a number of highly specialized areas, including intravenous therapy, nuclear pharmacy, and drug information. In addition, a hospital may also provide clinical services in areas such as adult medicine, pediatrics, psychiatry, oncology, and infectious disease. The nature and size of the hospital helps determine the extent to which these services are needed. Hospitals provide services 24 hours per day, seven days a week. Pharmacists, pharmacy technicians,

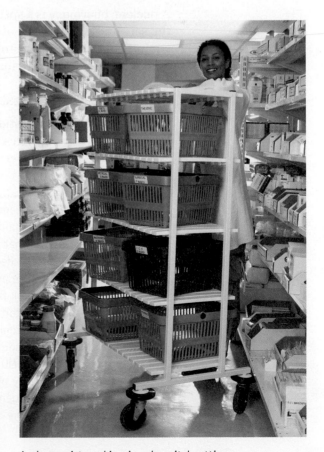

A pharmacist working in a hospital setting.

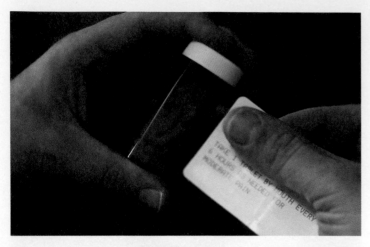

A pharmacist applies a label to a prescription medication bottle.

and hospital administrators with advanced degrees may work in a hospital pharmacy.

Long-Term–Care Facilities

A **long-term–care facility** provides a broad range of services for patients requiring a longer length of stay. These facilities may include nursing homes or assisted-living facilities. A **long-term–care pharmacy** dispenses medications, sterile intravenous preparations, and nutritional products to patients in nursing homes, assisted-living facilities, and hospice programs. Long-term–care pharmacies address the special needs of nursing homes, providing packaging for controlled administration (called *unit of use* or *bubble packs*), and special services that are more extensive than those provided by retail pharmacies. These special services include quality assurance checks, emergency drug kits and medication carts, regular and emergency (24-hours-a-day) delivery services, and in-service training programs for nursing assistants, nurses, and other professional nursing facility staff. Long-term–care pharmacies employ consultant pharmacists who conduct monthly drug-regimen reviews for each resident to assess the safety, efficacy, and appropriateness of drug therapies.

Nuclear Pharmacies

A **nuclear pharmacy** is a specialty practice of pharmacy that promotes health through the safe and effective use of radioactive drugs for diagnosis and therapy. Specialized equipment and training programs and certifications in radiotherapy are required to practice in a nuclear pharmacy.

Managed-Care Organizations

A **managed-care organization** is an organization that controls the financing and delivery of healthcare services for those who are involved in a specific healthcare plan. Managed-care plans deliver high-quality, medically necessary care while controlling cost. There are three types of managed-care plans:

There are three types of managed-care health plans: HMO, PPO, and POS.

- Health-maintenance organization (HMO) plan—A **health-maintenance organization (HMO)** provides care that is focused on keeping patients healthy or managing chronic diseases in an effort to decrease hospitalizations and emergency-room visits. HMOs encourage patients to take an active role in their health care by scheduling routine annual checkups, modifying risk factors, getting immunizations, and screening for diseases. HMOs have their own staff physicians. If patients would like to see a specialist, they need to get a referral from their primary care physician. A **primary care physician** is a "gatekeeper" who controls access to health care and costs. Some HMOs have an on-site pharmacy. An HMO has a **formulary**, which is a list of drugs that have been recommended for use by physicians and pharmacists. They may also have a tiered drug-pricing plan so that patients pay one price for a generic-name drug, a higher price for a "preferred" brand-name drug, and an even higher price for a "non-preferred" brand-name drug.

- Preferred provider organization (PPO) plan—A **preferred provider organization (PPO)** is similar to an HMO in that it has a preferred provider network, but patients do not need to see a primary care physician for a referral to a specialist. PPOs generally offer financial incentives to use network providers.
- Point-of-service (POS) plan—A **point-of-service (POS) plan** is a hybrid of an HMO and a PPO. It is called a point-of-service plan because each time a member seeks medical care, he or she must decide which option—HMO or PPO—to choose. This plan encourages the use of a primary care physician for referrals to specialists and offers financial incentives for using a primary care provider. It also allows the member to use out-of-network providers, but at a higher cost

Role of a Pharmacist

The educational background, knowledge, and clinical skills that the contemporary pharmacist possesses make this individual a source of drug information for physicians, nurses, and patients. Pharmacists still compound and dispense prescription drugs to individual patients, but they also advise patients, physicians, and other healthcare professionals on the selection, dosages, interactions, and side effects of the medications. The specific role of a pharmacist will vary depending on the type of pharmacy. The pharmacist's role may include the following:

- Obtaining a patient history, including a medical history, prescription and over-the-counter medication usage history, and allergy history
- Verifying dosage, strength, and formulation of the medication
- Counseling patients on the use of prescription and over-the-counter medications
- Monitoring and screening for drug interactions, duplications of therapy, response to therapy, and the safe usage of controlled substances
- Making recommendations and providing advice regarding usage of over-the-counter medications and devices
- Advising patients, physicians, and other healthcare professionals on the selection, dosages, interactions, side effects, and adverse reactions of the medications

The pharmacist possesses the education, knowledge, and clinical skills necessary to be a health and drug information expert.

Licensing Requirements for Today's Pharmacist

A license to practice pharmacy is required in all 50 States and the District of Columbia, as well as in Guam, Puerto Rico, and the U.S. Virgin Islands. To obtain a license, a pharmacy student must obtain a Pharm.D. degree from a college of pharmacy that has been approved by the Accreditation Council for Pharmacy Education (ACPE). The pharmacist candidate must then pass the North American Pharma-

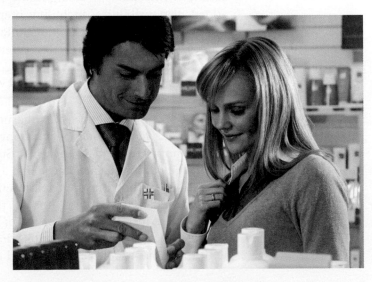

A pharmacist talks with a patient about a medication.

cist Licensure Exam (NAPLEX), which tests knowledge and pharmacy skills. Some states also require the Multistate Pharmacy Jurisprudence Exam (MPJE), which tests knowledge of pharmacy law. Both exams are administered by the **National Association of Boards of Pharmacy (NABP)**. Some states and territories that do not require the MJPE have their own pharmacy law exam. All state boards of pharmacy also require a specified number of hours of training in a practice setting before a license is awarded. In most states, pharmacists must also meet continuing-education requirements to renew their licenses. State boards of pharmacies oversee licensing requirements.

A license to practice pharmacy is required in all 50 states.

To obtain a license to practice pharmacy, one must have a Pharm.D. degree, a passing grade on the NAPLEX, training, and in some states a passing grade on the MPJE.

The Role of a Pharmacy Technician

The primary role of a pharmacy technician, also called a pharmacy tech, is to receive and fill prescriptions. These prescriptions can come from hospitals, physicians, nurses, the patient, or the patient's caregiver. A pharmacy technician can assist in all daily activities that do not require the professional judgment of a pharmacist. The work of a pharmacy technician must be overseen by a licensed pharmacist. Many states limit the number of pharmacy technicians by specifying a ratio of technicians to pharmacists.

A pharmacy technician must work under the direct supervision of a licensed pharmacist. A pharmacy technician can assist in all activities that do not require the professional judgment of a pharmacist.

Without pharmacy technicians, pharmacists would not have enough time to perform the clinical tasks necessary to ensure the safe use of medications. Pharmacy technicians help reduce the risk of preventable and costly medication errors.

The duties of a pharmacy technician will vary depending on the pharmacy practice setting. In hospitals, nursing homes, and assisted-living facilities, technicians have added responsibilities, including preparing sterile solutions and delivering medications to nurses or physicians. Technicians may also record the information about the prescribed medication onto the patient's profile.

The duties of a pharmacy technician will vary depending on the work environment.

The scope of practice for a pharmacy technician is a list of responsibilities that a technician is legally qualified and approved to perform in the workplace. From a broad list of competencies included in the State Pharmacy Practice Act, each practice setting will specify those that are considered a technician's responsibilities. These responsibilities will be outlined in the departmental policy and procedure handbook and/or the technician's job description. It is the professional responsibility of each technician to know the scope of practice for his or her practice setting and abide by it in the performance of daily technician duties. Each technician must perform all responsibilities with the utmost professionalism and concern for care of the patient.

In pharmacy practice, there is a definite difference between the professional judgment of the pharmacist and that of a technician. The pharmacist has the knowledge to evaluate the medication regimen of a patient and assist in clinical decision-making to improve the health of the patient. The technician must obtain the knowledge to evaluate information on a written prescription, be alert for drug interactions and drug-disease contraindications with other prescriptions or over-the-counter medications, accurately fill prescriptions, and communicate effectively with the patient to ascertain when he or she may need pharmacist counseling. In a busy pharmacy, the technician often must be the eyes and ears of the pharmacist and use professional judgment to alert the pharmacist about situations that may require pharmacist intervention.

> **What Would You Do?**
>
> *Question:* A customer comes into the pharmacy and asks the pharmacy technician to recommend an over-the-counter cough syrup for her one-year-old daughter. What should the technician do?
> *Answer:* Given the situation, the technician should ask the customer to wait and notify the pharmacist to speak with the customer.

The ultimate responsibility for a pharmacy technician's work rests with the supervising licensed pharmacist.

Education and Licensing Requirements of a Pharmacy Technician

Currently, there are no nationally standardized training requirements for pharmacy technicians. Some states require a high-school diploma or its equivalent. Other states require licensure or registration of pharmacy technicians with the state board of pharmacy. Still others require passing a certification exam. Several professional organizations offer a nationally recognized certification. The most common are the Pharmacy Technician Certification Board (PTCB) and the National Healthcareer Association (NHA). Although most pharmacy technicians receive informal on-the-job training, programs have been developed to better train pharmacy technicians.

There are no nationally standardized training requirements for pharmacy technicians.

Formal technician training programs are available through a variety of organizations, including community colleges, vocational schools, hospitals, and the military. These programs range from six months to two years and include classroom and laboratory work. They cover a variety of subject areas, such as medical and pharmaceutical terminology, pharmaceutical calculations, pharmacy recordkeeping, pharmaceutical techniques, and pharmacy law and ethics. In addition, they are designed to prepare the student to pass a certification exam. Technicians also are required to learn the names, actions, uses, and doses of the medications they work with. Many training programs include internships or externships, in which students gain hands-on experience in actual pharmacies.

After completion of a training program, students receive a diploma, a certificate, or an associate's degree, depending on the curriculum. In many states, pharmacy technicians are required to keep their knowledge current by attending educational seminars necessary for continued certification. In some states, pharmacy technicians are also required to obtain a certain number of continuing-education credits to maintain such certification.

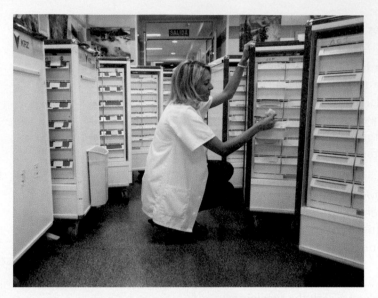

A pharmacy technician filling a hospital medication cart.

Depending on the area of practice, additional training and certifications may be required. To receive certification as a nuclear pharmacy technician, for example, students must complete an online self-study course and supervised instruction in addition to an internship under a nuclear pharmacist. Additional training may also be required by hospitals for pharmacy technicians who will perform sterile and non-sterile compounding.

Hospital

In addition to direct patient-care involvement, pharmacy technicians in hospitals are responsible for systems that control drug distribution. These systems are designed to ensure that each patient receives the appropriate medication, in the correct form and dosage, at the correct time. Hospital pharmacy technicians fill medications for stock on hospital units, fill orders for checking by the pharmacist, interpret medication orders, and, depending on state law, may enter them in the computer system pending a pharmacist's verification. These specialty pharmacy technicians also work in the IV room making sterile preparations. In addition, they work closely with other hospital personnel, including nurses and nurse's aides. They also fill medication carts, inventory medications, and compound various prescriptions. Hospital pharmacists maintain records on each patient, using them not only to fill medication orders but also to screen for drug allergies and adverse drug effects. The hospital pharmacist also prepares or supervises the distribution of a 24–72 hour supply of medication for each patient (unit dosage system). Pharmacists also advise the medical staff on the selection and side effects of drugs. They may make sterile solutions to be administered intravenously. They may counsel hospitalized patients on the use of drugs before the patients are discharged. In larger academic hospitals, pharmacists may accompany physicians on rounds. Hospital pharmacists may also be responsible for formulary development, managing drug product recalls, managing floor stock, dispensing investigational or hazardous drugs, and managing medication storage areas, drug delivery systems, and automated dispensing machines.

The hospital pharmacist ensures that each patient receives the right drug at the right time.

A pharmacy technician in the hospital setting, under the supervision of a licensed pharmacist, may also perform some of the aforementioned duties. In addition, they may also do the following:

- Package and label medications.
- Fill a 24–72-hour unit-dose cart.
- Maintain records and gather information for the pharmacist's use.
- Check the work of another pharmacy technician in the preparation of medication carts.
- Prepare IV medications.
- Deliver medications.
- Stock medications in the pharmacy and satellite locations.
- Inspect nursing stations for expired medications.

- Obtain laboratory results for pharmacists.
- Fill drug boxes or trays for emergency use.
- Operate manual or computerized robotic dispensing machines.

Retail

Pharmacists serve patients and the community by providing information and advice on health, providing medications and associated services, and by referring patients to other sources of help and care, such as physicians, when necessary. Pharmacists in retail pharmacies dispense medications, counsel patients on the use of prescription and over-the-counter medications, and advise physicians about

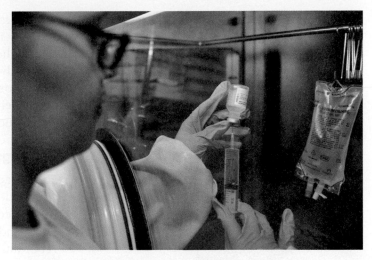
A pharmacy technician filling a syringe to the proper dose

medication therapy. Those who own or manage community pharmacies may sell non–health-related merchandise, hire and supervise personnel, and oversee the general operation of the pharmacy. Some retail pharmacists provide specialized services to help patients with conditions such as diabetes, asthma, smoking cessation, or high blood pressure. Some pharmacists are also trained to administer vaccinations.

In the retail setting, the duties that can be carried out by a technician (depending on state law) may include the following:

- Retrieving written prescription orders
- Accepting requests for prescription refills
- Retrieving medications from the shelf
- Verifying the information on the prescription for completeness
- Entering prescription orders into the computer
- Counting, pouring, weighing, and measuring medications
- Reconstituting medications
- Prepackaging bulk medications
- Filling and recording the prescription
- Selecting the appropriate prescription container
- Creating prescription labels
- Entering patient and prescription information
- Transferring prescriptions

Advances in the use of computers in pharmacy practice now allow pharmacists to spend more time educating patients and maintaining and monitoring patient records. As a result, patients have come to depend on the pharmacist as a health care and information resource. Pharmacists must be knowledgeable about the composition of drugs, their chemical and physical properties, and their manufacture

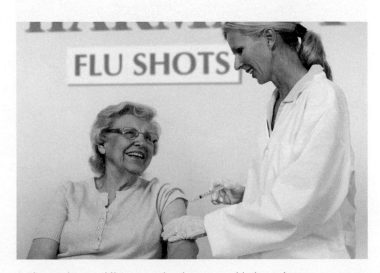
A pharmacist providing a vaccination to an elderly patient.

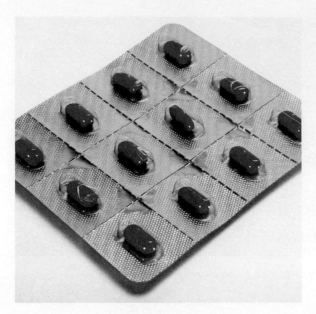

A blister card.

and uses, as well as how products are tested for purity and strength. Additionally, a pharmacist needs to understand the activity of a drug and how it will work within the body. More and more prescribers rely on pharmacists for information about various drugs, their availability, and their activity, just as consumers do when they ask about nonprescription medications.

Managed Care

Pharmacists and technicians are employed in various capacities within managed-care organizations (MCOs). Managed care is a system designed to optimize patient care and outcomes and foster quality through greater coordination of medical services. MCOs strive to improve access to primary and preventive care, and ensure the most appropriate and effective use of medical services in the most cost-effective manner. Besides dispensing medications and making sure that patients receive the right therapy conveniently and cost effectively, pharmacists may be involved in monitoring drugs used in chronic diseases.

Home Health Care Pharmacies

The pharmacist or technician who works in a **home health care** setting may prepare IV medications such as IV nutritionals, antibiotics, chemotherapy, and fluids for use at home. Pharmacists are also responsible for maintaining patient records, counseling patients and their caregivers, and monitoring the safe use of these medications at home.

Long-Term–Care Pharmacies

Long-term–care pharmacies employ consultant pharmacists to review the medication profiles of each resident monthly to assess the appropriateness and efficacy of drug therapies. They monitor the distribution and administration of medications and ensure that the medications administered have not expired. They also educate medical staff and family members regarding drug therapies. They may also provide medications to residents who are planning a leave from the facility. These pharmacies also prepare unit-dose packaging and specialized dispensing systems, which are patient-specific medication packages that are easy to administer. They also design their dispensing systems with multiple checkpoints to prevent potentially adverse drug interactions or patient reactions, and maintain customized medication-administration records for their client facilities.

In addition to the duties performed by a technician in a hospital or retail setting, a pharmacy technician working in a long-

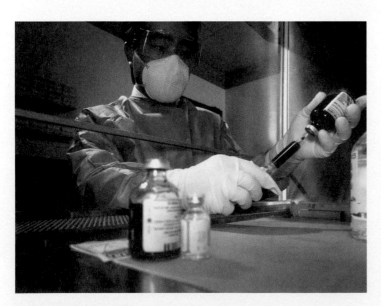

A pharmacist working in a nuclear pharmacy.

term–care facility, under the supervision of a licensed pharmacist, may also perform the following tasks:

- Fill and maintain drug boxes or emergency kits.
- Deliver medications to a nursing home.
- Prepare unit doses of medications.
- Conduct inspections in nursing homes to remove expired or recalled medications.

Nuclear Pharmacies

Nuclear pharmacy is a specialized area of pharmacy practice. A pharmacist practicing in a nuclear pharmacy specializes in the procurement, compounding, quality assurance, dispensing, packaging, distribution, and development of radiopharmaceuticals. In addition, the nuclear pharmacist monitors patient outcomes and provides information and consultation regarding health and safety issues.

Other Duties

In addition to the duties mentioned thus far, a pharmacy technician's role in various pharmacy practice settings may also involve the following:

- Preparing insurance claim forms
- Maintaining medication profiles
- Answering phones
- Stocking shelves and maintaining inventory
- Ordering medications
- Cleaning equipment
- Pricing prescriptions
- Operating the pharmacy cash register

Pharmacy Laws, Regulations, Professional Standards, and Ethics

Pharmacy is a highly regulated profession. A complex set of laws, regulations, and standards have been put in place to ensure public safety and the safe dispensing of medications. An understanding of these laws is necessary for pharmacists to pass the North American Pharmacist Licensure Exam (NAPLEX) and for pharmacy technicians to pass a certification examination, and more importantly to know the responsibilities of a pharmacist and pharmacy technician when working in a pharmacy.

Pharmacy laws, regulations, and standards have been designed to ensure public safety.

Laws

A **law** is a rule that represents the minimum level of acceptable standards. Laws are passed and enforced to protect the public. Laws are developed from a multitude of sources. In the United States, laws can be divided into four categories:

- Constitutional law—Constitutional law is derived from the Constitution and the Bill of Rights.

- Legislative law—Legislative law is drawn from the U.S. Congress and state legislatures.
- Administrative law—Administrative law is derived from the president or state governor.
- Common law—Common law is drawn from the judicial branch of the government.
- All these together govern the practice of pharmacy. Violations in laws may result in fines, probation, disciplinary action, suspension or loss of licensure, and even incarceration.

> Violation of a law may result in a fine, probation, disciplinary action, or incarceration.

Regulations

A **regulation** is a written rule or established guideline that exists to carry out a federal or state law. Regulatory bodies assist in the administration and enforcement of laws. For example, each state has its own board of pharmacy. These boards establish state-specific regulations for practicing pharmacy that must be followed within that state. They are also responsible for the licensing and/or certification of pharmacy personnel. The board is also responsible for disciplinary action against personnel who work in pharmacies.

The National Association of the Boards of Pharmacy (NABP) assists the boards of pharmacy in each state by implementing standards that reduce the likelihood of mistakes. The Drug Enforcement Administration (DEA) is a federal regulatory body that, in addition to its many other functions, has published regulations for enforcing the acquisition, storage, dispensing, and documentation of controlled substances. The DEA works with local and state agencies to ensure compliance of these regulations. The Food and Drug Administration (FDA) was established to protect public health by regulating the safety and efficacy of food, dietary supplements, drugs, medical devices, and biologics. It is also the governing body responsible for ensuring that only safe and effective drugs reach the consumer. The FDA also has regulations for generic drug substitution and patient counseling, and a system called MedWatch for reporting adverse events or product problems.

> MedWatch is a system utilized by the FDA to receive information about adverse events or product problems.

Professional Standards

A **professional standard** is a code of conduct or practice that professionals in a discipline would follow or carry out in a given circumstance. It can measure the quality of a product or the performance of a professional, comparing it against the norm. The Joint Commission is an agency that accredits and certifies healthcare organizations. It maintains higher standards for accreditation and works to improve the safety and quality of health care.

Ethics

Ethics are a system of moral standards of conduct and behavior for a person, group, or a profession. Ethics are the basis for reflection and analysis when a course of action is unclear. Codes of ethics regarding professional behavior provide language to aid in the decision-making process. Professional employees are held to high standards of conduct. Paraprofessionals such as pharmacy technicians are also held to high standards of conduct. The American Association of Pharmacy Technicians (AAPT) has a code of ethics that guides technicians in their associations with patients and other healthcare professionals.

History of United States Federal Pharmacy Law

Federal laws set the standards for the practice of pharmacy. These laws were established to protect the public from the unregulated manufacturing, distribution, and dispensing of unsafe drugs.

Pure Food and Drug Act (1906)

The Pure Food and Drug Act was the first federal law regulating drugs. It prevented the manufacture, sale, or distribution of inaccurately labeled food and drugs across state lines. It also required that labels not contain false information of a drug's strength and purity.

Food, Drug, and Cosmetic Act (1938)

The Federal Food, Drug, and Cosmetic Act (FD&C) was passed after a legally marketed elixir containing antifreeze killed 107 patients. This act called for the creation of the Food and Drug Administration (FDA) and required all drug manufacturers to file a New Drug Application (NDA) to provide evidence of a drug's safety before any drug could be approved for the market. Manufacturers had to ensure the purity, safety, packaging, and strength of the medication. It also gave the FDA the authority to approve or deny NDAs and conduct inspections of manufacturing facilities to ensure compliance with regulations. Pharmaceutical manufacturers were also required to conduct animal studies and human clinical trials and submit the results of these studies before approval of a new drug would be granted.

This act also clarified and extended the definitions of adulterated and misbranded drugs and defined the United States Pharmacopeia (USP) and the National Formulary (NF) as official compendia.

> The FD&C Act defined the USP and the NF as the official compendia.

Durham-Humphrey Amendment (1951)

This amendment to the Food, Drug, and Cosmetic Act established clear criteria for the classification of prescription or nonprescription over-the-counter medications. It prohibited the dispensing of legend "prescription" drugs without a prescription. **Legend drugs** are drugs that are not considered safe for use without medical supervision. **Over-the-counter (OTC) drugs** can be legally obtained without a prescription and are generally safe for use without medical supervision. Each prescription medication would be required to bear the legend "Caution: Federal Law Prohibits Dispensing Without a Prescription." It also authorized the taking of verbal prescriptions and the refilling of prescriptions.

> A legend drug cannot be dispensed without a prescription. Over-the-counter drugs can be obtained without a prescription.

Kefauver-Harris Amendment (1963)

This amendment required that all medications be pure, safe, and effective for use in humans. It also required all drug manufacturers to file an investigation new drug application (INDA) before starting a clinical trial in humans. After the drug has been proven safe and effective in clinical trials, the manufacturer can submit a new drug application to request approval for marketing. This amendment was enacted in response to the thalidomide tragedy, in which the use of thalidomide by pregnant women caused severe birth defects.

Comprehensive Drug Abuse Prevention and Control Act (1970)

This act, also known as the Controlled Substances Act (CSA), required the pharmaceutical industry to keep records and implement security measures for certain medications. It was created to prevent and control drug abuse. This act divided controlled substances into five schedules, or classes, based on their potential for abuse (see **TABLE 1.1**). Schedule I drugs have the highest abuse potential, while Schedule V drugs have the least. A **controlled substance** is defined as a drug with a potential for abuse or addiction. This act set limits on the number of refills allowed for each schedule. Schedule II drugs are not allowed any refills. Schedule III–IV drugs are allowed five refills, and

Table 1.1   The Five Schedules Under the Controlled Substances Act

Schedule of Drug	Manufacturer's Label	About These Drugs	Examples of Drugs
I	C-I	Drugs have no accepted medical use in the U.S.; highest abuse potential.	LSD, heroin
II	C-II	Drugs have an accepted medical use; high abuse potential, with severe psychological or physical dependence liability; no refill allowed.	Amphetamines, methadone, opium, codeine, morphine, oxycodone
III	C-III	Drugs have an accepted medical use; moderate abuse potential (less than those in Schedules I and II); five refills allowed.	Combination narcotics such as codeine/acetaminophen, hydrocodone/acetaminophen and anabolic steroids
IV	C-IV	Drugs have an accepted medical use; low abuse potential (less than those in Schedule III); five refills allowed.	Benzodiazepines, barbiturates
V	C-V	Drugs have an accepted medical use; lowest abuse potential (less than those in Schedule IV); some drugs may be dispensed OTC if over 18 years of age in some states.	Liquid cough preparations with codeine
Kilo	K	one thousand times	Base unit $\times 10^3$

the prescription is valid for six months after the date of issue. The Drug Enforcement Agency (DEA) regulates all matters relating to controlled substances.

> The DEA is responsible for all regulations pertaining to the acquisition, storage, dispensing, and documentation of controlled substances.

> The CSA placed legal limits on the number of refills allowed for controlled substances. Schedule II drugs are not refillable. Schedule III–IV drugs are allowed five refills and the prescription is valid for six months from the date of issue.

> There are five schedules for controlled substances.

Poison Prevention Packaging Act (PPPA) (1970)

This act established standards for child-resistant packaging to prevent accidental childhood poisonings. It required that some OTC medications and almost all legend drugs be packaged in child-resistant containers. A **child-resistant container** cannot be opened by 80 percent of children younger than five years old, but can be opened by 90 percent of adults. A patient or prescriber can request that a drug be dispensed in a non–child-resistant container.

Common examples of medications that do not need to be dispensed in a child-resistant container include the following:

- Sublingual nitroglycerin tablets
- Inhalation aerosols
- Oral contraceptives (available in blister packs)
- Potassium supplements in unit-dosage form
- Some corticosteroid tablets

Drug Listing Act (1972)

This act assigns a unique drug code to each medication known as the National Drug Code (NDC). This code consists of 11 characters that identify the manufacturer, medication and dosage form, and size and type of packaging. The first five digits identify the manufacturer or distributor of the drug. The next four digits identify the product, strength, and dosage form of the medication. The last two digits identify the packaging size and type. This act also allows the FDA to compile a list of currently marketed drugs (see Chapter 2 for more information).

> Each medication is assigned a unique code known as the National Drug Code.

Orphan Drug Act (1983)

This was enacted to stimulate the development of drugs for rare diseases. A rare disease is a disease that affects fewer than 200,000 people in the United States. Prior to this act, pharmaceutical companies had little incentive to invest money for the development of treatments for a small number of people because they were often not cost effective to develop and market. This law provides seven-year marketing exclusivity on the drug's patent, a tax credit of 50 percent of the cost of clinical trials in humans, and research grants for clinical testing of new therapies to treat orphan diseases. Many economists who focus on the pharmaceutical industry believe that these drugs will replace the "blockbuster" drugs of the 1990s in terms of drug manufacturer profits, as these medications are usually inordinately expensive.

The Orphan Drug Act deals with drugs used to treat rare diseases.

Waxman-Hatch Act (1984)

Also known as the Drug Price Competition and Patent-Term Restoration Act, this act ensured that brand-name drug manufacturers would have patent protection and a period of marketing exclusivity to enable them to recoup their investments in the development of valuable new drugs, as well as provide an incentive for new drugs to reach the marketplace. The act ensured that when the patent protection and marketing exclusivity for these new drugs expired, however, consumers would benefit from the rapid availability of lower-priced generic versions of brand-name drugs. It also created a generic drug-approval process and established the abbreviated new drug application (ANDA) approval process, which permits generic versions of previously approved innovator drugs to be approved without submitting a full new drug application (NDA).

One drug can have several names, including a brand, generic, and chemical name. A **brand name** is a name given by the manufacturer. A **generic name** is the non-proprietary name. The **chemical name** describes a drug's chemical composition and is the official name of a drug that describes the exact chemical formula of the drug. Generic drugs are equivalent to their brand-name counterparts in safety, efficacy, strength, dosage, route of administration, and intended use. A generic drug can be substituted for the brand-name drug if the drug is A/B rated by the FDA and the prescription does not state "dispense as written." (See Chapter 2.)

A brand name is the name the drug manufacturer gives the drug. A generic drug is equivalent to the brand-name drug in safety and efficacy.

Prescription Drug Marketing Act (PDMA) (1987)

This act was designed to increase safeguards to prevent the introduction and retail sale of substandard, ineffective, and counterfeit drugs in the U.S. supply chain. It also states that prescription drugs manufactured in the United States and exported can no longer be reimported, except by the product's manufacturer. Finally, it prohibits the sale or trading of drug samples to others than for whom they were intended or the distribution to persons other than licensed physicians.

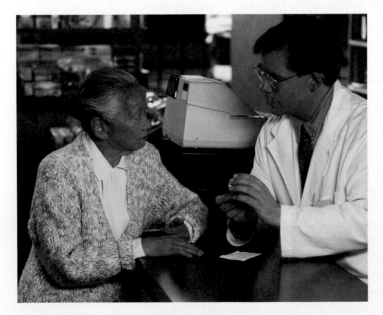

An elderly woman talks with a pharmacist.

Anabolic Steroid Control Act (1990)

Anabolic steroids are synthetic substances that promote human muscle growth and are often used illegally by athletes. Use of these medications have serious health consequences and can permanently damage the body when they are abused. Many of these drugs are manufactured illegally and sold on the black market. This act classified anabolic steroids as Schedule III controlled substances, increasing the penalty for the illegal distribution of these drugs. Prescriptions for Schedule III drugs can be refilled for up to six months or no more than five times, whichever comes first.

Omnibus Budget Reconciliation Act (OBRA) (1990)

This act requires that pharmacies that fill prescriptions for Medicaid obtain, record, and maintain basic patient information. It also says that each state must require its pharmacists to offer counseling on all aspects of drug therapy to patients, as well as perform a drug-utilization review (DUR). A **drug-utilization review (DUR)** is a review of a patient profile to ensure that medications dispensed to a patient in the past were correct. It also requires that the patient profile be reviewed prior to the filling of each prescription. Patients may refuse counseling; documentation of this refusal, either a patient signature or a notation in the computer, should be maintained.

Health Insurance Portability and Accountability Act (HIPAA) (1996)

This act was implemented to improve continuity and portability when transferring health-insurance coverage from one employer to another. It also sought to improve the effectiveness of Medicare and Medicaid by placing safeguards to protect patient confidentiality, including medical and prescription records. Privacy regulations established patients' rights, including rights to access their records, disclosures, and communication of health information. It also set standards for protection of identity and health information and ensured privacy while transmitting claims. Pharmacy staff must acknowledge and agree to abide by HIPAA standards for each patient. This can be maintained electronically or in a records book. Pharmacists and pharmacy technicians must not reveal any information about a patient outside the pharmacy, except to other healthcare providers with a "need to know" to provide care.

Pharmacists and pharmacy technicians must respect a patient's right to privacy.

Food and Drug Administration Modernization Act (1997)

This act focused on reforming the regulation of food, medical products, and cosmetics. It modified the process for getting approval for clinical studies, testing subjects, and having new drugs approved for human use. It also changed the labeling requirements of all legend or prescription medication from "Caution: Federal Law Prohibits Dispensing Without a Prescription" to an "Rx only" symbol. It also required further testing of all products containing mercury in the United States. This law also authorized pharmacy manufacturers submitting new drug applications (NDAs) to provide additional resources to help the FDA speed up the approval process.

Medicare Prescription Drug, Improvement, and Modernization Act (2003)

This act gives all people who receive Medicare benefits the option for prescription-drug coverage under the Medicare Part D plan. Participation in this program is voluntary. In order to receive benefits, patients are required to enroll with a third-party vendor and pay an

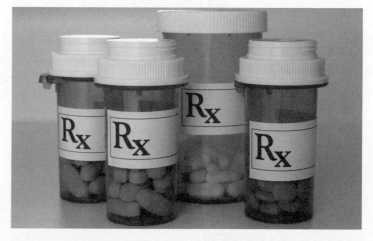

A group of prescription bottles containing pills with Rx on the labels.

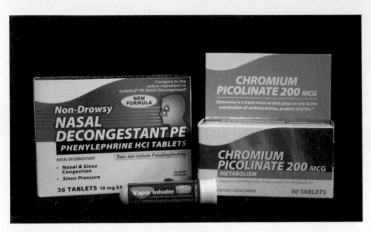

There is a legal limit to the quantity of nasal decongestants containing pseudoephedrine that can be purchased during a 30-day period.

additional premium. The act was designed to help alleviate the pressures of medical costs.

It also allowed for the reimbursement of medication management therapy services (MMTS) in those patients with certain health conditions or those on high-cost medications. MMTS provides a yearly review of a patient's profile to ensure that patients on expensive medications or with certain health conditions are not experiencing adverse reactions, drugs interactions, or paying high costs for unnecessary therapies.

This act also created health savings accounts (HSAs) as a health insurance option for patients under the age of 65. A health savings account is a medical savings account for those patients who have a high-deductible health plan (HDHP). Individuals pay high deductibles in return for lower negotiated medical expenses and tax-deductible premiums. Funds deposited into this account are not subject to federal tax and can be withdrawn for medical expenses. The funds that are not used in one calendar year can be rolled over to the next year without a penalty.

Combat Methamphetamine Epidemic Act (2005)

This was enacted to reduce the availability of drugs used to illegally produce methamphetamine and to stop the use of methamphetamine. It reclassified all products containing pseudoephedrine, phenylpropanolamine, and ephedrine, and set a limit on the quantity that can be purchased during a 30-day period (3.6g in one day, or 7.5g per 30 days). Both phenylpropoanolamine and ephedrine have since been taken off the market, meaning that this act now pertains only to pseudoephedrine. It also requires that the product be placed behind the counter or in a locked cabinet not accessible to the consumer. The purchaser must provide identification, and the seller must maintain a written bound book or electronic log book of all pseudoephedrine sales.

Regulatory Agencies

Regulatory agencies assist in the administration and enforcement of laws for the safe use of drugs. These agencies follow written rules or established guidelines to carry out federal or state laws.

Food and Drug Administration (FDA)

The **Food and Drug Administration (FDA)** is a federal agency that was established to protect public health by regulating the safety and efficacy of food, dietary supplements, drugs, medical devices, biologics, tobacco products, and cosmetics. It is responsible for ensuring that any drug or food approved for marketing is safe when used as directed. The FDA does not develop new therapies or conduct clinical trials to demonstrate safety and effectiveness. FDA members evaluate data and perform inspections of clinical-trial study sites to protect the rights of participants and verify the quality and integrity of the data. The FDA does not regulate the practice of pharmacy within each

A patient comes into the pharmacy and asks you for a 60-day supply of pseudoephedrine. Given the situation, you would inform the patient of the legal limit on the quantity that can be purchased and call the pharmacist.

state. The FDA is under the Department of Health and Human Services (HHS) and is divided into six product centers, one research center, and two offices.

The FDA requires that all manufacturers submit applications for investigational studies and approval for new drugs. A drug will not be approved for marketing by the FDA unless it has been deemed safe and effective for human use. The FDA also oversees all aspects of drug development and distribution, including packaging and marketing. A manufacturer may not make or advertise a false claim, and must fully disclose all side effects, adverse reactions, and contraindications.

The FDA also publishes a reference that identifies all drugs approved by the FDA and is used to make sure that generic drugs can be safely substituted for the brand-name product. The *Approved Drug Products with Therapeutic Equivalence Evaluations*, also known as the *FDA Orange Book*, is published annually.

> The FDA Orange Book contains information on which generic drugs can safely be substituted for the brand-name drug.

Drug Enforcement Administration (DEA)

The **Drug Enforcement Administration (DEA)** is a federal regulatory body that operates under the judicial branch of government. It is responsible for enforcing laws relating to the acquisition, storage, dispensing, and documentation of controlled substances. The DEA works closely with local and state agencies to ensure compliance of these regulations. The DEA inspects all medical facilities, including pharmacies, where suspicious or illegal activity has been detected, and monitors prescribers who prescribe controlled substances. The Controlled Substances Act requires that all institutions, pharmacies, or individuals involved in any activity relating to controlled substances be registered with the DEA. The DEA also issues a license to individual pharmacies so they can order scheduled drugs from wholesalers, and a license to physicians so they can write prescriptions for controlled substances.

Occupational Safety and Health Administration (OSHA)

The Occupational Safety and Health Administration is the main federal agency responsible for the enforcement of regulations relating to the safety and health of workers. It is under the Department of Labor. It provides training and education, and encourages continual improvement in workplace safety and health.

National Association of the Boards of Pharmacy

The **National Association of the Boards of Pharmacy (NABP)** is a professional pharmacy organization that represents the state boards of pharmacy in all 50 United States, the District of Columbia, Guam, Puerto Rico, the Virgin Islands, eight Canadian provinces, and New Zealand. It assists its member boards of pharmacy by developing, implementing, and enforcing uniform standards that protect public health by reducing the likelihood of mistakes. Although it has no regulatory authority, it is responsible for developing a national pharmacist licensure examination (NAPLEX), which is administered by local state boards of pharmacy. It also coordinates the administrative process of licensure reciprocation of pharmacists practicing in different states. In addition to working with each state board of pharmacy to meet the needs of their state, they provide several accreditation programs. The Verified Internet Pharmacy Practice Sites (VIPPS) provide an ongoing evaluation of an Internet pharmacy's practice. In order to be VIPPS-accredited, a pharmacy must comply with the licensing requirements of each state to which it dispenses medications.

Because many states have differing laws regarding the practice of pharmacy, the NABP developed the Model State Pharmacy Practice Act (MSPPA). It gives individual states a model on which to base their regulations and individualize them according to their state's needs.

State Boards of Pharmacy

Each state has its own board of pharmacy. These **state boards of pharmacy** establish state-specific regulations for practicing pharmacy that must be followed within that state. They are also responsible for the licensing and/or certification of pharmacy personnel, and for disciplinary action of personnel who work in a pharmacy. Each state board is also responsible for developing and administering a law exam necessary for licensure or reciprocity from another state.

> The state board of pharmacy has the authority to seek disciplinary action against a pharmacist or pharmacy technician.

Each state board may also provide regulations on the filling and refilling of prescription medications and controlled substances. Typically, most nonscheduled prescriptions are refillable for one year from the date of issuance. Controlled substances that are Schedule III, IV, or V can be refilled a maximum of five times or six months from the date of issuance, whichever comes first. The board may also regulate the sale of over-the-counter medications.

Each state board may also have specific requirements for the ratio of pharmacy technicians to pharmacists in various practice settings. They also regulate the activities of a technician and may have minimum educational and training requirements necessary to practice as a pharmacy technician.

> Licensing and professional oversight of pharmacists and pharmacy technicians is carried out by the state boards of pharmacy.

Violations of Laws

Violations of laws can occur at the local, state, or federal level, and the legal action taken as a result will depend upon the law that was violated. Civil law is a type of law that covers acts committed against individuals rather than against the local, state, or federal government, and suits are brought about by private citizens. Occasionally, the crimes committed may involve a violation of a state or federal law, in which case the responsible party can be prosecuted.

Torts

A **tort** is defined as causing personal injury intentionally or because of negligence. It is a civil case that one citizen brings against another. In a tort, the injured party sues the party they believe caused the injury. In a tort action, the person or party filing the case (**plaintiff**) must establish that the party being sued (**defendant**) was under a legal duty to act in a particular way. They must also demonstrate that the party being sued failed to act accordingly. Third, they must prove that the filing party, the plaintiff, suffered an injury or loss as a direct result of the party being sued. The law of torts seeks to compensate victims for injuries suffered by action or inaction of others. It also seeks to shift the cost of such injuries to the person or persons who are legally responsible for inflicting them. Third, it seeks to discourage injurious, careless, and risky behavior in the future.

Examples of torts include the following:

- Broken contracts—**Broken contracts** are the simplest form of torts. A broken contract is a broken promise to do or not do an act.
- Negligence—**Negligence** is conduct that falls below the standards of behavior established by law.
- Slander—**Slander** is verbal communication of false statements against another individual.
- Libel—**Libel** is written communication of false statements against another individual.
- Malpractice—**Malpractice** is negligence in meeting the standard of care.
- Assault—**Assault** is an unlawful threat to do bodily harm.
- Battery—**Battery** is causing physical harm to another person.

The most common tort against healthcare practitioners is negligence. Negligence is when a person unintentionally performs or fails to perform an act that a reasonable person would or would not have done in a similar situation. To prove negligence, you must prove that a person's conduct falls below the normal standard of care established by law. **Standard of care** is the level of performance that is expected of a healthcare worker in carrying out his or her professional duties. The standard of care takes into account the educational background and training of the healthcare provider, the normal practices within the geographic area of the healthcare provider's workplace, and compliance of local, state, and federal laws and regulations.

A pharmacist can be sued for negligence if he or she fails to meet a minimum standard of care.

In the case of a negligence or malpractice suit, the prosecutor or plaintiff must provide evidence that the party committed the four Ds of negligence: duty, derelict, direct cause, and damages. The plaintiff must prove that the defendant had a duty and that the provider of care breached this duty, resulting directly in injury to the patient. The plaintiff must prove his or her case by what is termed "preponderance of the evidence." Preponderance of the evidence is the level of proof that must be shown in a civil case to sway the judge or jury one way or another in a lawsuit.

Drug and Professional Standards

Laws and regulations from local, state, and federal agencies govern the practice of pharmacy. In addition to these laws, national standards for drugs and professional guidelines for behavior and performance have been established by professional organizations.

United States Pharmacopeia

United States Pharmacopeia (USP) is a non-governmental, independent scientific organization that sets standards for all over-the-counter and prescription medications and other healthcare products manufactured or sold in the United States. USP sets scientifically developed standards that help ensure the identity, quality, purity, strength, and consistency of medicines. The mission of the USP is to set standards and create programs that improve the health of people around the world by ensuring quality, safety, and benefits of food. The USP also publishes an unbiased reference, the **USP-NF** that contains standards for specific drugs and ingredients, dosage forms, medical devices, and dietary supplements. Pharmaceutical manufacturers must comply with these standards for their drugs to be approved by the FDA. The USP-NF also includes other standards designed for pharmacists covering key topics such as maintaining a physical environment in their pharmacies that promotes safe medication use, quality assurance in compounding, and sterile compounding practices.

Professional Organizations

Many national professional pharmacy organizations have set standards that are higher than the established guidelines for practice. Some examples of professional organizations include the following:

- The American Pharmacists Association (APhA)
- The American Society of Health-System Pharmacists (ASHP)
- The American Society of Consultant Pharmacists (ASCP)

The mission of each of these organizations varies, but all provide for a standard of care that is above those required by federal and state laws.

Professional organizations also exist for pharmacy technicians. The National Pharmacy Technician Association (NPTA) (http://www.pharmacytechnician.org/) is an organization created to meet the needs of all pharmacy technicians working in various practice settings. Another organization, The American Association of Pharmacy Technicians (AAPT) (http://www.pharmacytechnician.com), promotes the safe, efficacious, and cost-effective dispensing, distribution, and use of medications. It also provides continuing-education programs and services to help technicians update and maintain their skills.

The Pharmacy Technician Certification Board (PTCB) is one organization that develops, maintains, and administers certification and recertification programs for pharmacy technicians. Five organizations (the American Pharmacists Association, the American Society of Health-System Pharmacists, the Illinois Council of Health-System Pharmacists, the Michigan Pharmacists Association, and the National Association Boards of Pharmacy) joined in 1995 to oversee the PTCB and to maintain a national certification program. The PTCB develops standards and acts as the credentialing board. Pharmacy technicians must be recertified every two years.

PTCB is a national organization that develops standards for pharmacy technicians.

WRAP UP

Chapter Summary

- The history of pharmacy can be traced back thousands of years to early civilization, when medicinal remedies were largely controlled by religious leaders who frequently combined drug preparations with prayers, chants, rituals, and "magic."

- Today's pharmacist has a broader scope of practice. A pharmacist not only compounds and dispenses medication, but is also responsible for ensuring positive outcomes for drug therapy.

- Pharmacists are highly educated and trained professionals who can practice in a variety of settings.

- Pharmacists serve as resources for patients and healthcare professionals on all matters relating to drug therapy.

- The pharmacy technician is a paraprofessional who can assist in all daily activities that do not require the professional judgment of a pharmacist. The work of a pharmacy technician must be overseen by a licensed pharmacist.

- Pharmacy is a heavily regulated profession. Laws, regulations, and standards have been put in place to ensure public safety and the safe dispensing of medications.

- Statutory federal drug laws and amendments have shaped the practice of pharmacy by ensuring the safety and efficacy of drugs brought to the market.

- State boards of pharmacy have regulations to license pharmacists and technicians. They also have the authority to take disciplinary action for violations against their laws and regulations.

- The most common tort against healthcare practitioners is negligence.

- Standards for the practice of pharmacy are set by professional organizations, regulatory bodies, and state boards of pharmacy.

Learning Assessment Questions

1. The prescription label of a legend drug container will usually have two names on it: the generic and the trade or brand name. What is the trade or brand name?
   A. The chemical name of the drug
   B. The proprietary name of the drug given by the manufacturer
   C. The abbreviated generic name of the drug
   D. The common name

2. A technician takes a phone call from a patient who wants to know what the side effects are for her new medication. What should the technician do?
   A. Tell the patient what the side effects are.
   B. Tell the patient to hold on while he or she looks up the answer in a reference book.
   C. Put the patient on hold and notify the pharmacist.
   D. Tell the patient to stop taking her medication.

3. What do the last two digits in the NDC number identify?
   A. Product
   B. Strength
   C. Package size
   D. Formulation

4. The practice of pharmacy is regulated by federal and state law. Which of the following federal laws mandates the use of safety caps?
   A. OSHA
   B. HIPAA
   C. PPPA
   D. CSA

5. The Omnibus Budget Reconciliation Act (OBRA) required pharmacists to do which of the following?
   A. Use pharmacy technicians.
   B. Counsel patients.
   C. Limit the use of controlled substances.
   D. Bill third-party payers.

6. To what did the Health Insurance Portability and Accountability Act establish a patient's right?

   A. Protection of identity and health information

   B. Mortality

   C. Free health insurance

   D. Free prescription medications

7. A patient would like information concerning a good pain reliever that is available over the counter. What should you do?

   A. Show the patient where the pain relievers are in the pharmacy.

   B. Recommend a pain reliever.

   C. Inform the patient that he or she should speak with the pharmacist.

   D. Recommend several options and let the patient choose.

8. What is the system utilized by the FDA to receive information about adverse events or product problems?

   A. OSHA

   B. MedWatch

   C. Product recall

   D. DEA

9. Which act reclassified all products containing pseudoephedrine, and set a limit on the quantity that can be purchased during a 30-day period?

   A. DEA

   B. FD&C

   C. Food and Drug Administration Modernization Act

   D. Combat Methamphetamine Epidemic Act

10. According to CSA, a Schedule II drug is allowed how many refills?

    A. One refill

    B. Five refills, as long as they are within six months from the date of issue

    C. No refills are allowed

    D. eleven refills in one year

11. Questions involving controlled substances should be directed to which regulatory agency?

    A. The FDA

    B. The state board of pharmacy

    C. The DEA

    D. The National Association of the Boards of Pharmacy

12. Which regulatory agency is responsible for the licensure or registration of pharmacy personnel?

    A. The state board of pharmacy

    B. The FDA

    C. OSHA

    D. The National Association of Boards of Pharmacy

13. The Orphan Drug Act deals with drugs that are _____.

    A. Expired

    B. Controlled substances

    C. Used to treat rare diseases

    D. No longer marketed

14. Another name for a retail pharmacy is a _____.

    A. Hospital pharmacy

    B. Long-term–care facility

    C. Community pharmacy

    D. Nuclear pharmacy

15. A pharmacy technician can do all of the following except _____.

    A. Counsel patients

    B. Aid the pharmacist in filling prescriptions

    C. Maintain computerized patient records

    D. Maintain drug boxes or trays for emergencies

16. Which amendment established clear criteria for the classification of prescription and nonprescription over-the-counter medications?

    A. FD&C

    B. The Durham-Humphrey Amendment

    C. The Kefauver-Harris Amendment

    D. Food and Drug Administration Modernization Act

17. If a pharmacist fails to meet the minimum standard of care, he or she may be sued for _____.

    A. Slander
    B. Negligence
    C. Malpractice
    D. Libel

18. Which source would you use to determine whether a generic drug is interchangeable with a brand name drug?

    A. USP-NF
    B. The FDA Orange Book
    C. *Martindale's Pharmacopeia*
    D. USP

19. Which agency is responsible for ensuring the safety and efficacy of all marketed drugs?

    A. DEA
    B. FDA
    C. OSHA
    D. Joint Commission

20. The Comprehensive Drug Abuse Prevention and Control Act of 1970 designated how many schedules of controlled substances?

    A. Four
    B. Five
    C. None
    D. Six

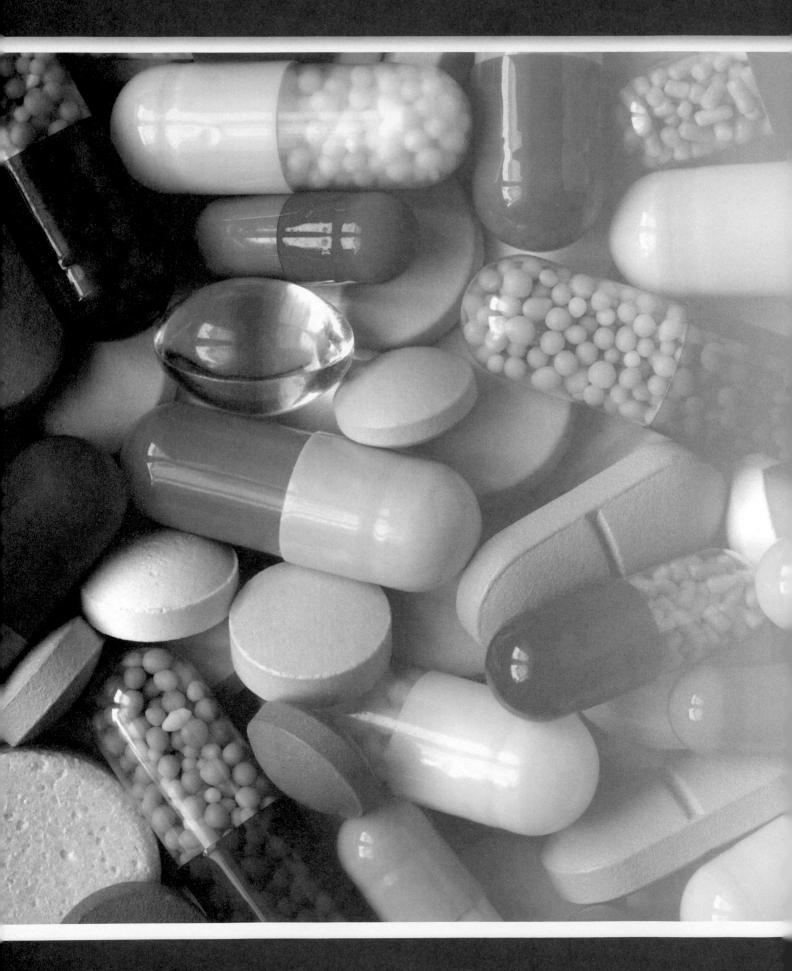

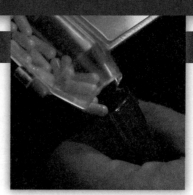

Basic Concepts of Pharmacology

OBJECTIVES

After reading this chapter, you will be able to:

- Discern the meaning of pharmacology
- Identify drugs, their sources, and how they work
- Identify federal laws that regulate drugs and the agencies that administer those laws
- Understand the procedure for getting a new drug to market
- Understand the term "drug"
- Understand the difference between active and inert ingredients
- Identify several medications that have improved quality of life and increased life expectancy
- Identify natural, synthetic, synthesized, and semi-synthetic drugs
- Identify therapeutic, pharmacodynamic, diagnostic, prophylactic, and destructive agents
- Understand the use of National Drug Code (NDC) numbers
- Identify various commonly used pharmaceutical reference texts
- Identify receptors and their function in mechanisms of drug action
- Understand the general principles of pharmacokinetics and the importance of those principles in developing and testing drugs
- Identify the beneficial and harmful effects of drugs
- Identify common terms used to describe drug interactions

KEY TERMS

Absorption	Adulteration	Allergic reaction
Active ingredient	Affinity	Anaphylactic reaction
Addiction	Agonist	Antagonist

Antibody	Efficacy	Monograph
Antigen	Elimination	Pharmacodynamic agent
Antineoplastic drug	Enzymes	Pharmacodynamics
Bioavailability	First-pass effect	Physical dependence
Bioequivalent	Half-life	Placebo
Biopharmaceutical	Histamine	Prophylactic agent
Black-box warning	Homeostasis	Prophylaxis
Ceiling effect	Idiosyncratic reaction	Psychological
Contraindication	Indication	dependence
Control group	Induction	Receptor
Deoxyribonucleic acid	Inert ingredient	Semi-synthetic drug
(DNA)	Inhibition	Side effect
Destructive agent	Investigational New Drug	Specificity
Diagnostic agent	(IND) application	Synthesized drug
Disintegration	Isotope	Synthetic drug
Dissolution	Loading dose	Systemic effect
Dose-response curve	Local effect	Therapeutic agent
Double-blind trial	Maintenance dose	Therapeutic effect
Drug	Metabolic pathway	Therapeutic window
Drug abuse	Metabolism	Tolerance
Drug dependence	Metabolite	Vaccine
Duration of action	Misbranding	Volume of distribution

Chapter Overview

Technological advances made in the field of pharmacy have allowed for advances in the delivery of health care. Early practices of compounding to more recent, large-scale pharmaceutical-manufacturing operations have improved the synthesis and delivery of pharmaceuticals. Earlier scientific-research discoveries provided the foundations of these medical advances. As new drugs were developed, laws and regulations were put in place to protect the public. As the number of drugs available continues to grow, so does the information available to use them safely and properly. How and where to find this information and the drug references used by pharmacists and pharmacy technicians in the workplace will be explained.

Pharmacology

During the 19th century, Claude Bernard, a French physiologist, used the laboratory to determine the relationship between drugs and their sites of action within the body. He established pharmacology—the study of drugs and their properties and how they interact with the body—as a discipline of study.

Pharmacology is the study of drugs and their properties and how they interact with the body.

The **active ingredient** of a drug is responsible for the drug's therapeutic effect. The active ingredient is the ingredient that produces the desired or intended effect. A drug may contain more than one active ingredient. Most drugs contain an active ingredient and one or several inert ingredients. An **inert ingredient**, also called an inactive ingredient, has little or no therapeutic value. These inert ingredients are generally used to stabilize the active ingredient or to serve as a vehicle when making a solution, suspension, or topical preparation.

The active ingredient is responsible for a drug's therapeutic effect.

An inert ingredient has little or no therapeutic value.

Drugs and Their Sources

A **drug** is any substance used for the diagnosis, cure, treatment, or prevention of a disease or is intended to affect the structure or function of any living system. Drugs can be made from a variety of sources. They can be derived from sources such as plants, animals, minerals, or chemicals. Drugs can also be produced by recombinant DNA technology. A drug that is produced from recombinant DNA technology is referred to as a **biopharmaceutical**. Drugs that are derived from animals, plants, or minerals are classified as natural substances. Examples of drugs derived from plants include opium from the opium poppy, digoxin from foxglove, and colchicine from the cinchona tree. Drugs derived from animal sources include conjugated estrogen tablets and thryoxine. Drugs derived from minerals include iron salts, used to treat anemia.

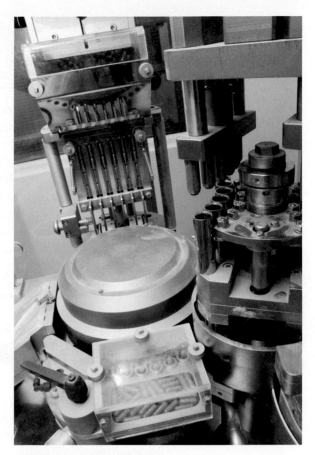

The pharmaceutical manufacturing process.

Drugs can be made from plant, animal, mineral, or chemical sources.

Drugs produced by recombinant DNA technology are called biopharmaceuticals.

Drugs derived from animals, plants, or minerals are classified as natural substances.

Most drugs available on the market today are synthesized from naturally occurring chemicals. Drugs derived from these chemicals can be further categorized into synthetic, synthesized, or semi-synthetic drugs. A **synthetic drug** is a drug that is created artificially and that has a specific mechanism of action that results in a specific pharmacologic effect. Penicillin and the sulfa drugs are examples of synthetic drugs. Synthetic drugs are not created to mimic a naturally occurring drug. A **synthesized drug** is a drug created in the laboratory to mimic the pharmacologic actions of a naturally occurring drug. Methamphetamine is an example of a synthesized drug. A **semi-synthetic drug** is one that contains a combination of artificially created molecules and natural molecules. Amoxicillin and ampicillin are examples of semi-synthetic drugs.

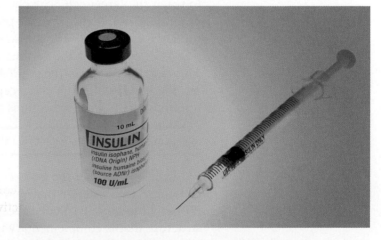

Biogenetically engineered drugs can treat many illnesses. Human insulin is a biogenetically engineered drug used to treat a type of diabetes.

These drugs are generally created to improve the properties of the naturally occurring substances or drugs.

Drugs that are derived from chemicals are synthetic, synthesized, or semi-synthetic.

Biogenetically engineered drugs are synthetic drugs with specific therapeutic effects that have been genetically engineered using recombinant **deoxyribonucleic acid (DNA)** technology. DNA is a complex, helically shaped molecule that carries the genetic code for each individual. DNA technology uses biology, chemistry, and immunology to create drugs that can alter the DNA code to prevent or treat diseases.

The classification of a drug is important because it places the drug into proper categories. Drugs can be classified according to their source, chemical structure, mechanism of action, or function.

Drugs can be classified according to their source, chemical structure, mechanism of action, or function.

Drug Actions

Drugs exert various actions on body organs and systems. Often, the quantity of a drug or how well it binds to the target cell receptor will determine the action of a drug. A drug's mechanism of action also determines how and where it works in the body. How the body affects a drug over a period of time is also crucial to understanding drug actions and disease management with medications.

Receptors

The human body maintains homeostasis by a system of control and feedback mechanisms. **Homeostasis** is the balance of the body with respect to fluid levels, pH, osmotic pressure, and concentrations of various substances. When the body's own system of control and feedback mechanisms cannot maintain balance, drugs can be used to help the body restore and maintain homeostasis.

For the body to maintain homeostasis, cells must be able to communicate with each other. They do this primarily through the action of chemical messengers. These cells produce chemical substances that then diffuse throughout the extracellular fluid to reach the target cell. The chemical messenger recognizes the target cell and communicates with it via a specific protein molecule called a **receptor**, located on or near the surface of the cell. The messenger molecule binds to the receptor in much the same way as a key fits into a lock, thus allowing absorption to take place in a cell **FIGURE 2.1**. This reaction produces the desired effect. These reactions take place naturally throughout the body. Only after the receptor makes a connection with the messenger will a reaction take place. Medications often mimic this natural mechanism.

Cells communicate with each other through chemical messengers to maintain homeostasis.

Different cells in the body contain different types of receptors, and only certain cells have the receptor that is the right fit for a particular chemical messenger. To properly bind to a particular receptor, the chemical messenger must have a chemical structure that is complementary to the receptor. This is referred to as **specificity**. The strength, or how tightly a drug binds to its receptor, is referred to as **affinity**.

Mechanisms of Action

A drug is administered to elicit a response in the body, either to prevent or manage a disease or to prevent or manage symptoms of a disease. The actions of the body on a drug over a period of time are described through pharmacokinetics. The effects a drug has on the body are described through **pharmacodynamics**. Drugs can act like chemical messengers and stimulate certain receptors, causing the human body to react in a specific way. Once the receptors are activated, they either trigger a particular response directly on the body or they trigger the release of hormones and/or other endogenous drugs in the body to stimulate a particular response.

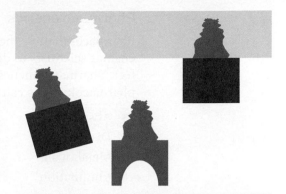

FIGURE 2.1 The messenger molecule binds to the receptor in much the same way as a key fits into a lock.

Some drugs will bind to a particular receptor to elicit the same response as the body's own chemical messenger. This type of drug is called an **agonist** because it stimulates and activates the receptors and enhances the natural reactions of the body.

> A drug that binds to receptors to elicit the same response as the body's own chemical messenger is called an agonist.

Other drugs block the action of the natural chemical messengers found in the body. This type of drug is called an **antagonist**. Antagonists have a similar affinity to the receptor sites and compete with the natural messenger for available receptor sites. When an antagonist binds to the receptor site, it prevents the naturally occurring chemical messenger from binding there, thus blocking the natural reaction of the body to the messenger.

> A drug that competes for receptor sites and blocks the action of natural chemical messengers is called an antagonist.

> Not all drugs are agonists and antagonists.

Some drugs do not interact with receptors, but instead produce their effects by combining with specific molecules such as **enzymes**, which are substances that act as biochemical catalysts. Others produce their effects by embedding themselves in cell membranes.

Understanding How an Agonist Works

Imagine for a moment the typical school custodian, carrying keys to fit the classroom and office locks for an entire high school. When the chemistry teacher locks himself out of his classroom, the custodian may try a number of keys before he finds the one that unlocks the door. Some keys will not fit in the lock, some may fit but not turn, but only one will fit in the lock and open the door. In this analogy, the keys represent an array of drugs. The lock on the door represents a specific drug receptor. The key that fits into the lock and opens the door represents an agonist. Keys that fit into the lock but do not open the door are like antagonists; not only will the keys not open the door, they also block other keys from entering the lock, thereby blocking an effective response. Keys that will not even fit in the lock represent drugs with no affinity for the specific receptor.

Pharmacokinetics

Pharmacokinetics, the study of how the body affects a drug over a period of time, enables scientists to develop dosage forms that are designed to produce a desired effect. Pharmacokinetics describes the effects that the body has on a drug. Each drug's pharmacokinetics can be described by the following processes in the body:

- Absorption
- Distribution
- Metabolism
- Elimination

Understanding these processes and their effects on drugs is critical to the drug-development process and the understanding of drug actions in the body. They are often learned by using the mnemonic ADME, for Absorption, Distribution, Metabolism, and Elimination.

> Pharmacokinetics describes the effect that the body has on a drug. It can be described by four processes: absorption, distribution, metabolism, and elimination.

Absorption

Absorption is the process by which a drug enters or passes through natural body barriers such as the skin, intestines, stomach, and blood-brain barrier and enters the bloodstream. How well the drug passes through these barriers depends on its route of administration, its solubility in blood or other bodily fluids, and other physical and chemical properties. It is one factor that determines how much of the drug is absorbed and, ultimately, its **efficacy**, or ability of the drug to produce a predictable effect in controlling or curing an illness in the body.

The route of administration can affect the rate and extent of absorption. Drugs administered in liquid solution are already dissolved, so they are absorbed more rapidly than those in solid dosage forms. Drugs administered intravenously do not require absorption because they are injected directly into the bloodstream. Drugs administered in solid dosage forms (tablets and capsules) require **disintegration** of the tablet or capsule and **dissolution** of the drug in the gastrointestinal tract, thereby slowing the rate of its absorption. Semi-solid dosage forms are also available for oral, vaginal, and rectal routes of administration. (You'll learn more about these routes of administration later on.) Disintegration and dissolution depend on the physical properties of the dosage form and the physical and chemical properties of the drugs.

The majority of oral drugs are absorbed in the small intestine because of its large sur-

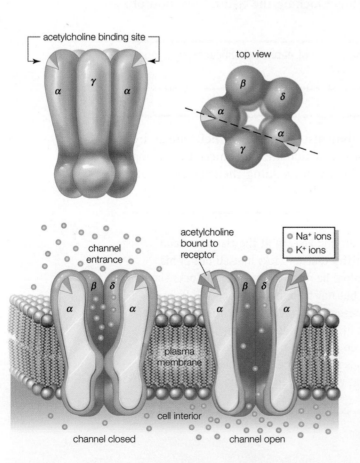

A lock-and-key mechanism allows absorption to take place in a cell.

face area. The degree of movement of a drug within the gastrointestinal tract also affects absorption. The faster a drug gets to the small intestine, the quicker it is absorbed into the bloodstream.

> Drugs enter the bloodstream by a process called absorption.

Distribution

After a drug is absorbed into the bloodstream, it is distributed to tissues, other body fluids, and ultimately to organs throughout the body. Not all organs are affected equally by drugs that are administered, however. This is because some areas of the body do not allow the drugs to infiltrate as quickly as other areas.

The most important rate-limiting factor for distribution of a drug is blood flow. Protein binding is another important factor related to drug distribution. Most drugs, to some extent, bind to proteins in the blood. The activity of a drug is directly proportional to the concentration of free drug in the bloodstream. Drug molecules that bind to protein in the blood are bound and unable to reach the intended site of action. Unbound, or free, drug particles are available to reach the site of action.

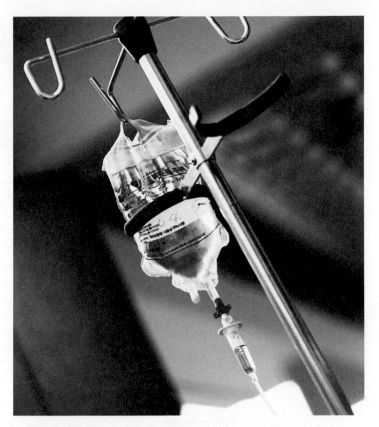

Drugs administered intravenously have 100% bioavailability—that is, total physical availability—because they are injected directly into the bloodstream.

Disease states can affect protein binding. Drugs can also bind to proteins other than those in the blood, such as proteins in tissues. Drug particles that bind to proteins in tissues would also be unable to reach the desired site of action.

The blood-brain barrier is a natural system that functions to keep harmful chemicals from entering the cerebrospinal fluid (CSF) from the blood. Many drugs are not able to get to the central nervous system (CNS) because they are water soluble, while other medications may penetrate the blood-brain barrier and cause unwanted side effects.

> The activity of a drug depends on the amount of free drug in the bloodstream.

> The most important rate-limiting factor for distribution of a drug is blood flow.

Metabolism

Drug **metabolism** is the process of biochemical modification or degradation of a drug in the body. As the drug is distributed throughout the body, some of it is transferred to the liver, where it is metabolized. Metabolism changes the chemical structure of the drug to a more water-soluble form so that it can eventually be excreted by the kidneys. The byproduct or the substance into which the drug is converted when it is metabolized is called a **metabolite**. In some cases, the metabolite is the one responsible for the pharmacological effect. In other cases, the drug is metabolized to an inactive substance or a less-toxic substance. The sequence by which a drug is converted to its metabolite is referred to as a **metabolic pathway**.

Some drugs can pass directly from the gastrointestinal tract to the liver. In these cases, the amount of active ingredient is reduced before it even enters the bloodstream. Other drugs are not metabolized in the liver at all and are excreted in the urine unchanged.

Different influences can affect the metabolism of a drug, including age, gender, diet, genetics, other diseases, and other drugs. Sometimes, when two or more drugs are administered together, one drug can decrease the metabolism of another drug by competitive or complete inhibition of the enzyme responsible for the metabolism of that drug. This results in an increased pharmacologic response to the other drug or toxicity. This process is referred to as **inhibition**. Other times, one drug can enhance the metabolism of another drug by inducing the enzyme responsible for the metabolism of the other drug, resulting in a decreased pharmacologic response to the other drug. This process is referred to as **induction**.

> Metabolism changes the chemical structure of the drug so that it can eventually be excreted by the kidneys.

> Age, gender, diet, concurrent diseases, and other drugs can affect the metabolism of a drug.

Elimination/Excretion

Elimination is the removal of the drug from the body. Excretion is usually associated with urination, but a drug can be also be excreted in feces, sweat, breast milk, semen, or exhalation. Drugs that are not eliminated from the body properly can lead to toxicity.

> Not all drugs are tested by the manufacturer for excretion into breast milk. A doctor must use his or her judgment when prescribing these drugs for patients who are breastfeeding.

Pharmacokinetic Properties

Understanding the pharmacokinetics of a particular drug enables researchers to determine how a drug should be administered to achieve an intended response while minimizing toxicity. For a drug to be effective, it must get to the site of action in concentrations large enough to allow the drug to exert its effect, but not so large that it produces toxicity. A basic understanding of pharmacokinetic principles is also necessary for the development and testing of drugs.

Bioavailability

Bioavailability is the degree to which or the proportion of the drug that is available to the site of action or target tissue to produce the desired effect. All drugs are metabolized in different ways and at different times. How much of the drug is actually available to produce the intended effect is an important consideration when deciding which drug to use and how often.

Drugs that are administered intravenously (IV) have a bioavailability of 100%. The bioavailability of drugs administered by other routes such as oral, topical, subcutaneous, or intramuscular injection varies. Some drugs pass directly from the gastrointestinal tract to the liver (**first-pass effect**), where they are metabolized before the active ingredient even enters the bloodstream, thereby reducing its bioavailability.

If a drug given orally undergoes considerable first-pass metabolism, its bioavailability will be decreased. In this case, drugs are often given in higher doses or by intravenous administration to counter this effect. Drugs administered intravenously bypass the first-pass effect because they are injected directly into the bloodstream.

> The proportion of drug that is available to the site of action is referred to as its bioavailability.

Half-Life

Half-life ($t_{1/2}$) is the amount of time it takes the plasma concentration of the drug to decrease by 50%, or reach half of the original concentration. An easier way to think about half-life is that it is the amount of time it takes the body to metabolize and excrete one-half of the drug. For example, if a person takes a medication that has a half-life of five hours, that means in five hours, one-half of the drug will be eliminated from the blood stream. Note that it takes about three to five half-lives to reach steady state with continuous dosing. A longer half-life means that the drug has a longer duration of action. The half-life of a drug is important because it enables you to calculate when the drug will be eliminated from the body, which helps determine the drug's dosing interval. By knowing the half-life of a drug, you can avoid accumulation of the drug and toxicity.

> Half-life is the amount of time it takes for the plasma concentration of the drug to decrease by 50%.

> Different drugs have different half-lives.

Therapeutic Window

Some drugs have a **therapeutic window**—that is, a range of serum concentrations at which the drug is most effective with minimal toxicity. When the amount of drug in the bloodstream elicits the desired response, the drug is said to be at the therapeutic level. If a drug is underdosed, it has little therapeutic benefit. If it is overdosed, it can lead to toxicity and death.

> The therapeutic window of a drug tells you the range of serum concentrations at which the drug is most effective.

The length of time a drug is within the therapeutic window is referred to as its **duration of action** FIGURE 2.2 . To maintain serum concentrations within the therapeutic window, the patient should receive **maintenance doses** of the drug. In some cases, a **loading dose** is required to bring serum concentrations of the drug to a therapeutic level quickly. To determine the loading dose, it is important to know the volume of distribution of a drug. The **volume of distribution** tells you the relationship between the amount of drug in the bloodstream and the dose of the drug given.

Some drugs such as digoxin (Lanoxin) or carbamazepine (Tegretol) have a narrow therapeutic window. A narrow therapeutic window describes a situation in which there is very little difference between a drug's therapeutic level and toxic level. These drugs require monitoring of serum concentrations to ensure that levels do not rise above (toxicity) or fall below (sub-therapeutic) the therapeutic window.

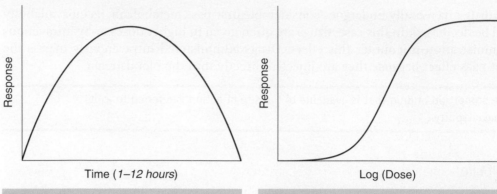

FIGURE 2.2 Duration of action. Serum drug concentrations must reach a minimum therapeutic level for therapeutic effect.

FIGURE 2.3 Dose-response curve. The larger the dose, the greater the response, until the response no longer improves with increased dosing. This is called a ceiling effect.

The duration of action of a drug tells you how long the serum concentrations remain within the therapeutic window.

A loading dose can bring serum concentrations of a drug to a therapeutic level quickly. Maintenance doses are needed to keep serum concentrations within the therapeutic window.

A **dose-response curve** defines the relationship between the dose of the drug and the response or effect of the drug at that dose **FIGURE 2.3**. As the dose of the drug increases, the response to the drug also increases, until increases in the dose of some drugs have no further effect above a particular dosage level. When this happens, it is called a **ceiling effect**. Acetaminophen (Tylenol) is an example of a drug with a ceiling effect.

Uses of Drugs

Drugs can be classified according to their use or pharmacologic effect. Some medications may belong in more than one category.

A **therapeutic agent** is any drug that relieves symptoms of a disease, stops or delays disease, or maintains health. Examples of therapeutic agents include vitamins, analgesics, antibiotics, and antidepressants. A **pharmacodynamic agent** is any drug that alters bodily functions. Examples include drugs used to increase or decrease blood pressure, general anesthetics to cause loss of consciousness, and caffeine to keep us awake. A **diagnostic agent** is any drug used in the diagnosis or identification of a disease.

A *pharmacodynamic agent* alters body functions to elicit a desired response.

A *diagnostic agent* is any drug that is used for diagnostic purposes.

A *therapeutic agent* maintains health, relieves symptoms, combats illness, or reverses the disease process.

Most diagnostic agents are chemicals that contain radioactive isotopes. An **isotope** is a form of a chemical element that contains the same number of protons as the regular element, but a different number of neutrons. Radioactive isotopes give off energy in the form of radiation, which can be used for diagnosis and treatment. One example of a radioactive isotope is iodine-131 (^{131}I).

A **prophylactic agent** is any drug that prevents a disease or illness from occurring. Examples of prophylactic agents include vaccines or antibiotics given for the prevention of disease. A **destructive agent** is a drug that destroys or kills abnormal and sometimes normal cells. Destructive agents can also kill bacteria, fungi, or viruses. Examples include penicillin, **antineoplastic drugs**, which are used to treat cancer, and radioactive iodine.

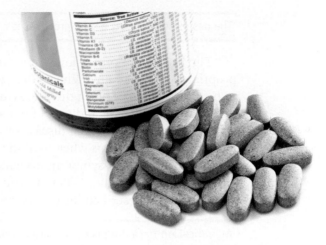

Vitamins are therapeutic agents that maintain health.

A prophylactic agent is used to prevent an illness from occurring.

A destructive agent destroys or kills abnormal or normal cells.

Drug Effects

The pharmacokinetics of an individual drug provides insight into the possible effects, both therapeutic and adverse, of a drug. The reaction to a drug varies from person to person. Response to drug therapy must be monitored to ensure that the therapy produces the desired effect, while minimizing the chances of side effects.

Therapeutic Effect

A drug is given to produce a desired effect on the body, either to treat a disease or to relieve symptoms. This is referred to as a drug's **therapeutic effect**. Sometimes drugs are administered to prevent the occurrence of an infection or disease. When a drug is administered in this fashion, its effect is referred to as **prophylaxis**. Drugs can have a local or systemic effect. When a drug has a **local effect**, the effect is confined to one area or organ of the body. An example of this would be local anesthesia, when an anesthetic medication is administered directly into one part of the part of the body, such as procaine (Novocain) being administered into the gums during a dental procedure. When a drug has a **systemic effect**, the effect is on the entire body. An example of a systemic drug is a chemotherapy agent used to treat cancer. It affects all the cells in the body, not just the cancer cells.

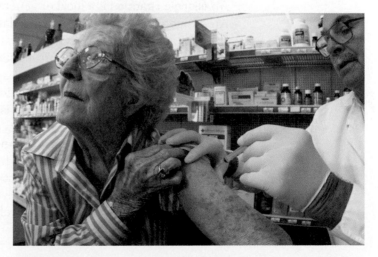

Prophylactic agents such as vaccines prevent an illness or disease from occurring.

The desired effect that a drug produces is called a therapeutic effect.

The healthcare professional must assess each individual patient to determine appropriateness of therapy. When a drug is given according to its labeling and is known to be of benefit for a given disease, symptom, or condition, it is an **indication** for that drug. Even if a drug is indicated for a specific patient, the physician must weigh the benefits of the drug for that disease or condition with the risks to the patient. Often, a drug can be dangerous when used in certain situations. When a patient has a certain condition, disease, or symptom for which the drug should not be used, it is a **contraindication** for that drug. When a drug is contraindicated for a particular patient, it should not be prescribed for that patient.

An indication for a drug is the disease, symptom, or condition that may be treated by using the drug (FDA-approved use). When a drug is used off-label, it means that it is being prescribed for a purpose other than that indicated on its label (non-FDA approved use).

A contraindication for a drug is a disease, condition, or symptom for which the drug is not indicated or will cause harm.

Side Effects

A **side effect** is an unintended response to a drug. Examples of common side effects include nausea, diarrhea, vomiting, constipation, lethargy, and drowsiness. Side effects can vary in severity, ranging from mild to serious. Often, drugs are prescribed because of their side effects. Some drugs have been marketed for use in one disease because of the side effects noted while using the same drug for treatment of another disease. One example of this is sildenafil. Although it was originally developed to treat heart disease, it was noticed in trials to enhance penile erections. This resulted in the approval of the drug Viagra to treat erectile dysfunction.

A side effect is any unintended response to the drug. Common side effects include nausea, diarrhea, vomiting, lethargy, and drowsiness.

Allergic Reactions

An **allergic reaction** is a local or general response of the immune system to an antigen. An **antigen** is a molecule that stimulates an immune response. Allergic reactions can manifest in a variety of ways. The first response the body has to an allergen is usually little or no reaction. Upon subsequent exposure, the body remembers the antigen and responds with a more severe response. These responses can vary from mild to severe to life threatening. The reactions themselves could be immediate or delayed responses to the antigen. **Histamine** is the chemical your body releases when you are having an allergic reaction. Examples of ways that an allergic reaction could manifest include rash, hives (urticaria), itching (pruritis), wheals (red, blistery areas), fluid accumulation in tissues, sneezing, wheezing, and swelling. A severe allergic response to an allergen is called an **anaphylactic reaction**. It is an immediate, life-threatening reaction that involves respiratory distress (difficulty breathing) followed by shock. Often, the response to a drug is unrelated to the dose of that drug. This is called an **idiosyncratic reaction**.

Drug Dependence

Drug dependence means the body needs the drug to function normally, and that abruptly stopping the drug will lead to withdrawal symptoms. **Addiction** is the perceived need to use the drug to attain physical and psychological effects, despite it being dangerous. A common sign of drug addiction is lack of control. One can be dependent on a drug without being addicted to the drug.

Physical dependence to a drug occurs when physical symptoms of withdrawal, such as sweating, racing heart, and difficulty breathing, present when the use of the drug is stopped. **Psychological dependence** to a drug is when psychological symptoms, such as irritability, inability to sleep, or depression, occur when the use of the drug is stopped. Patients with drug dependence can experience physical dependence, psychological dependence, or both.

Drug abuse is any use of a drug for purposes other than that for which it was prescribed or in amounts other than that prescribed. Often, drug abuse can lead to drug addiction.

Tolerance

Tolerance is a decrease in the pharmacological response to a drug that occurs with continued administration. To overcome tolerance, the dosage or interval at which the drug is administered may need to be increased.

Drug Interaction

One drug can exert an effect on another drug. Food, alcohol, herbal preparations, vitamins, and nicotine can also interact with prescription and over-the-counter drugs. Drugs can interact with other drugs by inhibiting (decreasing the activity) or inducing (increasing the activity) the enzymes responsible for the metabolism of the other drug. Drugs can also have an additive effect on each other. That means the combined effect of both drugs is additive.

A common way in which foods or drugs interact is by a system of enzymes called cytochrome P450 (CYP450). Grapefruit juice is one example of a food that inhibits a CYP450 isoenzyme found primarily in the intestines. Inhibition of CYP450 isoenzymes by grapefruit juice results in less of a drug undergoing first-pass metabolism, resulting in increased serum concentrations of the drug. For this reason, consumption of grapefruit and its juice are not recommended when taking certain drugs.

Following are some common drug interactions:

- Additive: The combined effect of both drugs is equivalent to the sum of the effects of each drug taken alone.
- Antagonism: One drug blocks the action of another drug.
- Synergism: The combined effect of both drugs is greater than the sum of the effects of each drug taken alone.
- Potentiation: One drug increases the potency of the other drug. The combined effect is greater than the sum of the effects of each drug taken alone.

Drug Names

The manufacturer of each drug assigns a chemical name, a generic name, and a brand name (also called a trade name) to each drug TABLE 2.1. The chemical name describes the chemical structure of the drug. The generic name is often a shortened version of the chemical name. It describes the drug without any indication to the name of the

Table 2.1　Drug Names		
Chemical Name	**Generic Name**	**Brand Name**
N-acetyl-p-aminophenol	Acetaminophen	Tylenol
[R-(R*, R*)]-2-(4-fluorophenyl)-β, δ-dihydroxy-5-(1-methylethyl)-3-phenyl-4-[(phenylamino) carbonyl]-1H-pyrrole-1-heptanoic Acid, calcium salt (2:1) trihydrate	Atorvastatin calcium	Lipitor
Acetylsalicylic acid	Aspirin	Bayer Aspirin
($\pm$)-N-methyl-3-phenyl-3-[(α,α,α-trifluoro-p-tolyl)oxy]propylamine hydrochloride	Fluoxetine	Prozac

manufacturer. The brand name is the name under which the manufacturer markets the drug and is the name that is found on the product's official label. The brand name is protected by a patent; only the company that holds the patent has the right to market that product under that name. Different manufacturers are allowed to market the same generic drug under different brand names, or by simply using the generic name.

Regulation of Drugs

The manufacturing, distributing, and dispensing of drugs is highly regulated. Federal and state laws and regulatory bodies ensure that drugs that are dispensed are safe and effective, and that they are dispensed in a regulated and controlled manner.

Federal Laws

Federal laws and subsequent amendments were established to set the standards of practice for pharmacy and to protect the public from the unregulated manufacturing, distribution, and dispensing of unsafe drugs. Regulatory bodies assist in the administration and enforcement of these laws to ensure the safe use of drugs. These agencies follow written rules or established guidelines to carry out federal or state laws. (Refer to Chapter 1 for more on regulatory bodies.)

The Pure Food and Drug Act of 1906, the first federal law regulating drugs, prevented the manufacture, sale, or distribution of inaccurately labeled food and drugs across state lines. It also required that labels not contain false information of a drug's strength and purity.

The Pure Food and Drug Act required labels to have accurate information regarding a drug's strength and purity.

The Federal Food, Drug, and Cosmetic Act (FD&C), which created the Food and Drug Administration (FDA), was passed in 1938 because the Pure Food and Drug Act was not worded strictly enough. The FDA is the oldest consumer-protection agency in the country. This act required all drug manufacturers to file a New Drug Application (NDA) to provide evidence of a drug's safety when used as directed on the label before the drug could be approved for marketing. It also gave the FDA the authority to approve or deny NDAs and to conduct inspections of manufacturing facilities to ensure compliance with regulations. The manufacturer also had to ensure the purity, packaging, and strength of the medication. Pharmaceutical manufacturers were also required to conduct animal studies and human clinical trials and to submit the results of these studies before approval of a new drug would be granted. Pharmaceutical manufacturers were also required to include patient package inserts (PPIs) and directions to the consumer.

All manufacturers of new drugs must file a New Drug Application (NDA) with the FDA to be approved for marketing.

This act also clarified and extended the definitions of adulterated drugs (**adulteration** deals with the preparation and storage of a medication) and misbranded drugs (**misbranding** is making false or exaggerated claims that can mislead a consumer). The act also defined the *United States Pharmacopeia* and the *National Formulary* as official compendia.

Misbranding is making false or exaggerated claims that can mislead a consumer.

Adulteration deals with the preparation and storage of a medication.

In 1951, the Durham-Humphrey Amendment added more instructions for pharmaceutical manufacturers and established clear criteria for the classification of prescription and nonprescription over-the-counter medications. It prohibited the dispensing of legend prescription drugs without a prescription and required each prescription medication to bear the following legend: "Caution: Federal Law prohibits dispensing without a prescription."

The Drug-Approval Process

To receive approval for marketing, the FDA has regulations for the way a manufacturer researches and develops a new drug. It requires that all manufacturers or drug sponsors submit a New Drug Application (NDA) to provide evidence of a drug's safety and efficacy, gathered through an intensive testing process in animals and humans. (Before any new drug can be tested in humans, the manufacturer must receive approval from the FDA.) The NDA will contain the results of these tests, the proposed labeling for the new drug, a description of the chemical composition of the drug, pharmacokinetic studies, and details of the manufacturing and packaging process. If the FDA determines that the new drug is indeed safe and effective when used according to the package labeling, it will be approved for marketing.

First, the drug is tested in the laboratory to assess its activity, potency, selectivity, and toxicity in animals. It is also tested for safety. If it meets all necessary criteria, the manufacturer or sponsor will develop a plan for testing the drug in humans. This plan is submitted to the FDA in the form of an **Investigational New Drug (IND) application**. The FDA reviews the IND application for assurance that the trials do not place humans at risk of harm. If the IND application, sometimes called an INDA, is approved by the FDA, clinical studies in humans can begin.

The FDA also plays an important role in guiding the design and conduct of clinical

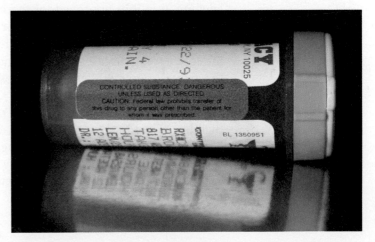

A prescription showing the legend required by the Durham-Humphrey Amendment.

trials required for approval. Clinical trials involve testing new drugs or therapies in humans to determine whether they are safe and effective. During a clinical trial, patients are usually separated into a placebo or control group and an experimental group. The placebo or **control group** receives an inactive substance (called a **placebo**) or a standard treatment for the disease or illness in question. The experimental group receives the new drug or therapy in question. In most cases, neither the trial participants nor those running the study know who is receiving placebo and who is receiving the experimental treatment. This type of study is referred to as a **double-blind trial**.

Healthcare practitioners should know the pregnancy categories of the most commonly prescribed drugs.

A placebo is an inactive substance that has no pharmacological effect. It is sometimes referred to as a "sugar pill."

Clinical trials of new drugs can be divided into four phases:

- Phase I trials are generally conducted by the manufacturer or sponsor to evaluate safety in small numbers of healthy volunteers (between 20 and 80 people). These studies also determine a safe dosage range and identify side effects. The data obtained in phase I trials are used to design future clinical studies.

- Phase II trials are often conducted by academicians on larger groups of patients (up to 300 people) who have the illness or disease the drug is intended to treat. These studies assess drug activity, dosing requirements, and efficacy, as well as safety. If the results of these trials are promising, phase III trials are conducted.

- Phase III trials are often conducted in hundreds or thousands of patients to provide a broader assessment of safety and efficacy of the drug at various doses. During this phase, the new drug is often compared to drugs that are already available on the market for the same disease or illness. If the new drug being investigated is promising after phase III trials, a manufacturer can submit an NDA to the FDA.

- Phase IV studies, also referred to as post-marketing studies, continue to test and monitor the safety of the drug after it has been approved for marketing by the FDA. These studies also identify safety issues associated with widespread and long-term use.

The NDA will contain the results of phase I–III clinical trials. If the FDA determines that the new drug is indeed safe and effective when used according to the package labeling, it will be approved for marketing.

On average, it takes 12 years for a drug to be approved. However, the FDA has instituted reforms that shorten the review process for drugs used to treat serious or life-threatening diseases. Applications are reviewed based on priority. Drugs that have the greatest potential benefit and those that offer a significant medical advantage over existing therapies are given priority.

The approval of a drug by the FDA is based on the information that is available at that time. The FDA determines that a drug is safe for approval by weighing the potential benefits of the new drug or therapy against its potential risks. Sometimes, safety issues can only be uncovered when the drug is being used by millions of people over a period of time. Although the FDA has an extensive drug-review process, some drugs make it to the market only to be removed or relabeled due to safety concerns **FIGURE 2.4**.

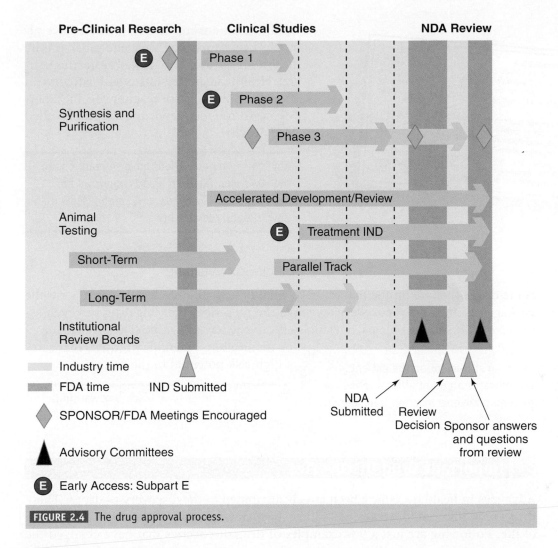

FIGURE 2.4 The drug approval process.

Pregnancy

Drugs are not actively tested on pregnant women, but clinical data is gathered from pregnant women taking medications. The FDA classifies all drugs by placing them into one of five pregnancy categories. These categories determine the level of risk to the fetus. The pregnancy categories are as follows:

- A: No risk to the fetus
- B: No evidence of risk to human fetuses
- C: Risk to the fetus cannot be ruled out
- D: Definite risk to the fetus
- X: Contraindicated—do not use

> Some healthcare professionals may not feel comfortable asking a woman if she is pregnant. Even so, pregnancy categories should be considered whenever medication is dispensed to a woman of childbearing age. Pharmacists often need to ask women if they are pregnant or plan to become pregnant.

Post-marketing Surveillance

Post-marketing surveillance (phase IV studies) is important because it ensures the continual safety and quality of drugs that are already available on the market. These

WARNING: TARDIVE DYSKINESIA
Chronic treatment with metoclopramide can cause tardive dyskinesia, a serious movement disorder that is often irreversible. The risk of developing tardive dyskinesia increases with the duration of treatment and the total cumulative dose. The elderly, especially elderly women, are most likely to develop this condition.

Metoclopramide therapy should routinely be discontinued in patients who develop signs or symptoms of tardive dyskinesia. There is no known treatment for tardive dyskinesia; however, in some patients symptoms may lessen or resolve after metoclopramide treatment is stopped.

Prolonged treatment (greater than twelve weeks) with metoclopramide should be avoided in all but rare cases where therapeutic benefit is thought to outweigh the risks to the patient of developing tardive dyskinesia.

A black-box warning label.

studies also ensure that drugs that have already been approved that endanger public health are promptly removed from the market. Healthcare professionals and patients can report serious adverse reactions to the FDA's Medical Products Reporting Program, called MedWatch.

> Anyone can report serious adverse reactions to the FDA's MedWatch Program, which can be found at http://www.fda.gov/Safety/MedWatch/HowToReport/default.htm.

Black-Box Warning

Some drugs that are on the market have what is termed a black-box warning on the package insert. A **black-box warning** warns the prescriber that this drug has been associated with some problems, but still is effective when used as directed. It is required on medications and other products that carry a high risk potential to the patient.

A black-box warning statement on the patient package insert indicates a potential for a serious or even life-threatening adverse reaction from a drug.

> Thousands of drugs have black-box warnings.

Important Drug Discoveries

Advances in health care have been largely attributed to the discovery of drugs. These drugs have allowed for increases in life expectancy and improvements in the quality of life. Following are just a few examples of drug discoveries that have changed the way we maintain our health.

The Smallpox Vaccine

In 1796, Dr. Edward Jenner observed that milkmaids who caught the cowpox virus did not get smallpox. He realized that inoculation with one disease (cowpox) resulted in immunity to another disease (smallpox). Exposure to cowpox produced antibodies that had cross-immunity with smallpox. An **antibody** is a complex molecule that is made in response to the presence of an antigen or foreign substance. This theory—that inoculation with a specific pathogen prior to infection may prevent occurrence of a disease—formed the basis of the discovery of subsequent vaccines. A **vaccine**, such as for hepatitis B, influenza, or polio, is a substance that is given to stimulate the immune system to produce antibodies to build immunity against a particular disease. Because of the smallpox vaccine, smallpox has been eradicated worldwide.

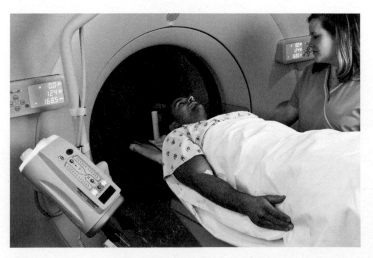
Patient receiving an MRI.

Radioactive Drugs

In the early 1900s, Madame Marie Curie developed methods for the separation of radium from radioactive residues in enough quantities to allow for the careful study of its therapeutic properties. She promoted the use of radium to alleviate the suffering of soldiers during World War I. The discovery of radioactivity formed the basis of nuclear imaging for the diagnosis and treatment of disease. Without this discovery, there would be no CAT scans or magnetic resonance imagings (MRIs). There would also be no radiation therapy for diseases such as cancer.

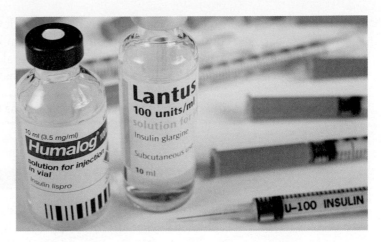

Examples of insulin.

Insulin

In the 1920s, Sir Frederick Banting and his assistant, Charles Best, discovered insulin. Building upon previous research that showed a link between the pancreas and diabetes, they isolated and purified a substance they termed insulin. Prior to the discovery of insulin, diabetics had high rates of complications and death. This discovery has improved the quality of life and life expectancy for diabetic patients.

Penicillin

In 1928, Dr. Alexander Fleming and his colleagues discovered penicillin, the first antibiotic. Fleming noticed that some of his bacterial Petri dishes were contaminated with a fungus and that there was a zone around an invading fungus where the bacteria did not seem to grow. He isolated this substance from the invading fungus, identified it as an organism from the *Penicillium* genus, and named it penicillin. The discovery of this antibiotic saved many lives during World War II. Penicillin was mass-produced in 1945 and brought to the commercial market.

The discovery of penicillin has changed the world of modern medicine by introducing useful antibiotics for the prevention and treatment of bacterial infections. Although there are many antibiotics available, continued research is needed to overcome bacterial resistance.

Penicillin causes the most drug allergies. Update the patient's allergy history profile when receiving a prescription for an antibiotic. Patients with a penicillin allergy may also have cross-sensitivity to other antibiotics.

The Polio Vaccine

Polio is a disease that attacks the central nervous system. Once a patient is infected, there is no cure for polio. Treatment of symptoms involved the use of an iron lung, which artificially maintained respiration until the patient could breathe by himself. In 1953, Jonas Salk created a vaccine containing inactivated viruses from three kinds of polio strains from animal cultures. Using the chemical formalin, he killed the whole virus.

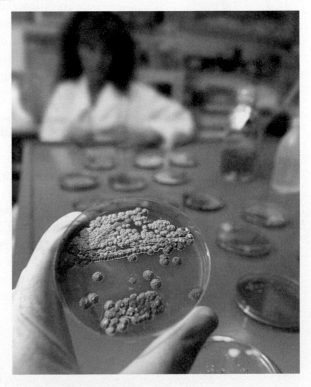

Fungus growing in a petri dish.

A few years later, Albert Sabin developed an oral form of the polio vaccine that contained a live but attenuated form of the virus (that is, the infectious part of the virus was inactive). In 1963, the oral vaccine became available for widespread use. Because of the polio vaccine, polio has been eradicated worldwide.

It is important to reassure patients of the benefits of routine vaccinations.

National Drug Code

The Drug Listing Act of 1972 mandated the assignment of a unique drug code to each medication after it is approved by the FDA. This code is known as the National Drug Code (NDC). It consists of 10 or 11 characters, divided into three segments that identify the manufacturer, medication and dosage form, and size and type of packaging **FIGURE 2.5**. The first four or five digits (labeler code) identify the manufacturer or distributor of the drug. (Note that a manufacturer can have multiple manufacturer codes.) The next three or four digits (product code) identify the product, strength, and dosage form of the medication. The last two digits (package code) identify the packaging size and type. The NDC can be used to verify that a medication is correct when it is dispensed. When processing medications through insurance, the NDC must match what is being billed.

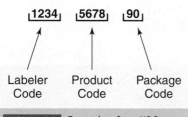

Although the manufacturer may label a product with 10 digits, the National Council for Prescription Drug Programs (NCPDP) requires an 11-digit NDC, with the following format: 55555-4444-22. If you are using a computer system to enter information about a drug that has an NDC with only 10 digits, you must add a leading zero to whichever section—5, 4, or 2—that does not have the appropriate number of digits.

1234   5678   90

Labeler   Product   Package
Code   Code   Code

FIGURE 2.5 Example of an NDC.

When a manufacturer discontinues a drug product, its product code may be reassigned to another drug product five years after the expiration date of the discontinued product or, if there is no expiration date, five years after the last shipment of the discontinued product into commercial distribution. Reuse of product codes may occur, under the specified conditions, regardless of the NDC, product code, and package code configuration used.

References Used in Pharmacy

Drug information reference texts are important tools available to pharmacists and pharmacy technicians. Various healthcare professionals constantly ask pharmacists questions about the use of medications. Knowing which reference book to choose and how to access this information is necessary to provide reliable and accurate information, save time, and avoid frustration.

Most drug references have a section on how to use the text. Being familiar with using these references will enable the technician to find the correct information. This section discusses only the most common references found in a pharmacy setting. Most references available to pharmacists and technicians also come in a variety of formats: text and online.

The FDA Orange Book is used to determine whether a generic drug is bioequivalent to a brand-name product.

With the Internet, you can have instant access to an enormous amount of information. But because information posted on the Internet is not regulated, you should be wary of its accuracy. Always ascertain the sponsor of the site. Determine the source of information and whether its credentials are reliable. Websites of pharmacy organizations, of pharmacy associations, and at universities are good places to look for information.

Approved Drug Products with Therapeutic Equivalence Evaluations: The FDA *Orange Book*

The FDA *Orange Book* contains a list of all drugs approved for use by the FDA. It can be used to determine whether a generic drug or a drug with a different brand name and the same chemical composition is **bioequivalent**, meaning it can be safely substituted for the brand-name product. It lists the drug products that the FDA considers to be therapeutically equivalent to other pharmaceutical products. It also contains information on discontinued drugs and orphan drugs. It is published annually, but the online version is updated more frequently.

> A patient brings in a prescription for Tegretol with the instructions "Brand Medically Necessary." Given the situation, the technician should prepare to dispense Tegretol rather than carbamazepine, which is the generic form of Tegretol. If the "dispense as written" or "brand medically necessary" comments are not on this prescription, the pharmacy technician may prepare to dispense carbamazepine, which is determined to be bioequivalent to Tegretol, the brand-name product, per the FDA *Orange Book*.

Drug Facts and Comparisons

Drug Facts and Comparisons provides quick and easy access and comparative tables for drug comparison. It contains information on product availability, formulations, dosages, indications, mechanisms of action, adverse effects, drug interactions, and patient information. It is available as a loose-leaf binder with monthly updates, a hardcover, a pocket guide, and online.

United States Pharmacopeia–National Formulary (USP-NF)

This reference is a combined edition of the *United States Pharmacopeia* and the *National Formulary*. It establishes the criteria and standards for pharmaceutical manufacturing when submitting a new drug application to the FDA and quality control and legal standards for drugs in the United States. It contains standards for medicines, dosage forms,

Drug Facts and Comparisons provides comparative tables and information on drug formulations, dosages, indications, mechanisms of action, adverse effects, drug interactions, and patient information.

drug substances, medical devices, and dietary supplements. The standards originate from sponsors who provide draft standards and supporting data to either create new or revise existing monographs and general chapters. USP's scientific staff and volunteer experts review this input, conduct laboratory tests (if necessary), and forward the new or revised monograph or general chapter to Pharmacopeial Forum (PF) for public review and comment. The public process helps to refine and finalize USP standards for publication as official text in the USP–NF. USP's expert committees, composed of volunteer scientists elected on the basis of their knowledge and expertise, approve USP–NF standards. It is available in hardcover, online with a subscription, or on CD-ROM.

The USP-NF establishes standards for pharmaceutical manufacturing and quality control and legal standards for drugs.

The PDR contains pictures that can be helpful in identifying unknown drugs by color, shape, or markings. It also contains contact information for manufacturers that have paid a fee to be included in this book.

Physician's Desk Reference (PDR)

This book is a compilation of the patient package inserts (PPIs) from pharmaceutical manufacturers that have paid a fee to be included into the reference. It contains pictures of these drugs and can be helpful in identifying unknown drugs by color, shape, or markings. The PDR also contains contact information for these manufacturers. This book is used primarily by physicians and is updated annually. It is available in hardcover, on CD-ROM, and online.

Drug Topics Red Book

The Drug Topics Red Book *contains average and wholesale pricing for drugs.*

This book contains information on the average and wholesale prices of drugs. It also has charts for easy and quick referencing that provide information such as which drugs should not be crushed. It includes tables with dosing instructions converted into Spanish. This book is available in paperback and CD-ROM.

American Hospital Formulary Service Drug Information (AHFS DI)

AHFS DI is useful in a hospital setting because it contains information on parenteral drugs.

This reference is used primarily in hospitals. It contains drug monographs (mainly for parenteral administration, which means any route other than into the gastrointestinal tract). **Monographs** provide drug information, including approved and off-label uses, dosages, indications, adverse effects, drug interactions, mechanisms of action, pharmacology, pharmacokinetics, and stability. It is available in hardcover, CD-ROM, and online.

Handbook of Nonprescription Drugs

This reference is published by the American Pharmacists Association. It provides information and dosing information on nonprescription medications (OTCs), nutritional supplements, medical foods, and homeopathic medications. It is available in hardcover or as a textbook that can be downloaded.

Remington's Pharmaceutical Sciences: The Science and Practice of Pharmacy

Remington's contains information on drug stability and compatibility.

This reference contains particularly useful information on drug stability and compatibility. It also contains information on medication safety, immunology, disease-state management, specialization in pharmacy practice, and professional communication. It is available in hardcover with a companion CD-ROM.

Trissel's Handbook on Injectable Drugs

This reference is used in the hospital setting for information on parenteral agents, including administration, stability, and compatibility with other parenteral solutions and drugs. It is available in hardcover, CD-ROM, and via PDA.

Goodman & Gilman's The Pharmacological Basis of Therapeutics

This reference contains information on pharmacokinetics and pharmacodynamics, membrane transporters and drug response, pharmacogenetics, and principles of therapeutics in all systems of the body.

The Lawrence Review of Natural Products

This reference is published by Facts and Comparisons, a division of Wolters Kluwer, and contains scientific information on herbal medications.

Martindale's The Complete Drug Reference

This reference provides information on drugs in clinical use, investigational and herbal drugs, diagnostic agents, pesticides, coloring agents, preservatives, and noxious substances used worldwide. It is available in hardcover or CD-ROM.

WRAP UP

Chapter Summary

- Drugs have allowed for increases in life expectancy and improvements in the quality of life.
- Pharmacology is the study of drugs and their actions on the body.
- Drugs are derived from sources such as animals, plants, minerals, chemicals, and recombinant DNA technology.
- The FDA sets regulations that require manufacturers to provide evidence of a drug's safety and efficacy before it can be approved for marketing.
- Laws were established to set the standards of practice for pharmacy and to protect the public from the unregulated manufacturing, distribution, and dispensing of unsafe drugs.
- Regulatory bodies follow written rules or established guidelines to carry out federal or state laws
- A drug's active ingredient is responsible for the drug's therapeutic effect. An inert ingredient, also called an inactive ingredient, has little or no therapeutic value.
- Drugs that are derived from chemicals can be further categorized as synthetic, synthesized, or semi-synthetic.
- Drugs can be categorized as therapeutic, pharmacodynamic, diagnostic, prophylactic, or diagnostic, depending on their use.
- Pharmacokinetics is the study of the effects the body has on a drug. The processes can be divided into absorption, distribution, metabolism, and elimination.
- Some drugs exert their action by binding to receptors on or within the body to mimic or block the action of chemical messengers, while others compete with another drug for its receptor.
- One drug can exert an effect on another drug. Food, alcohol, and nicotine can also interact with prescription and over-the-counter drugs.
- Drugs have therapeutic effects, adverse reactions, and side effects.
- Drug information reference texts are important tools available to pharmacists and pharmacy technicians.

Learning Assessment Questions

1. Which of the following books is created from patient package inserts (PPIs) from the manufacturers?
   A. *Drug Topics Red Book*
   B. USP-NF
   C. PDR
   D. *Drug Facts and Comparisons*

2. Which reference book is the best source for quickly comparing several medications?
   A. *Drug Facts and Comparisons*
   B. *Handbook of Nonprescription Drugs*
   C. USP DI
   D. *PDR*

3. Which reference book is the best source for finding information on the average and wholesale price of a drug?
   A. *Drug Topics Red Book*
   B. *Handbook of Nonprescription Drugs*
   C. USP DI
   D. *Drug Facts and Comparisons*

4. An active ingredient exerts which of the following?
   A. The therapeutic effect
   B. The placebo effect
   C. The inert effect
   D. No physiologic effect

5. Which of the following is a substance that is introduced into the body to produce immunity to disease?
   A. An inert ingredient
   B. A vaccine
   C. An antibody
   D. A radioactive isotope

6. A therapeutic agent does which of the following?
   A. Maintains health
   B. Relieves symptoms
   C. Stops or delays the disease
   D. All of the above

7. Iodine-131 (^{131}I) is an example of which of the following?

   A. Prophylactic agent

   B. Destructive agent

   C. Pharmacodynamic agent

   D. Diagnostic agent

8. Clinical trials can be divided into how many phases?

   A. Two phases

   B. Five phases

   C. Four phases

   D. Six phases

9. What are warning statements on the patient package insert that indicate a serious or even-life threatening adverse reaction from a drug called?

   A. Black-box warnings

   B. Indications for use

   C. Side effects

   D. Patient medication guides

10. Which of the following references would be helpful in determining if a generic drug is bioequivalent to a brand name drug?

    A. The FDA *Orange Book*

    B. PDR

    C. USP-NF

    D. Patient medication guides

11. Banting and Best are known for their discovery of what?

    A. Radiopharmaceuticals

    B. Insulin

    C. Polio vaccine

    D. Digoxin

12. The National Drug Code (NDC) does not identify which of the following?

    A. Product manufacturer

    B. Package size

    C. Package type

    D. Pregnancy category

13. A drug that has a pregnancy category X rating means it is which of the following?

    A. Safe for use only in the first-trimester

    B. Safe for use only in the second-trimester

    C. Safe for use only in the third-trimester

    D. Contraindicated for use in pregnancy

14. What is the study of how the body affects a drug over time?

    A. Pharmacology

    B. Pharmacokinetics

    C. Biology

    D. Pharmacotherapeutics

15. What is the most important rate-limiting factor for distribution of a drug?

    A. Blood flow

    B. Solubility

    C. Half-life

    D. Bioavailability

16. Pharmacokinetics is the study of which parameters of a drug?

    A. Absorption

    B. Distribution

    C. Elimination

    D. All of the above

17. Half-life is the time required for which of the following?

    A. 50% of the drug to be eliminated from the body

    B. 25% of the drug to be eliminated from the body

    C. 100% of the drug to be eliminated from the body

    D. 75% of the drug to be eliminated from the body

18. A severe allergic reaction is called an

    _____.

    A. Antigen

    B. Allergen

    C. Anaphylactic reaction

    D. Addiction

19. Healthcare professionals and patients can report serious adverse reactions to the FDA's Medical Products Reporting Program, also called which of the following?
    A. MedReporting
    B. MedWatch
    C. FDA hotline
    D. TIPs

20. The NDA will contain the results of which of the following?
    A. Phase I–III clinical trials
    B. Phase IV trials
    C. Phase 0 trials
    D. Phase 6 trials

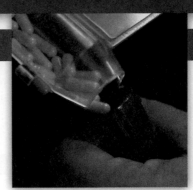

Basic Math Review

OBJECTIVES

After reading this chapter, you will be able to:

- Identify whole numbers.
- Perform basic calculations using addition and subtraction.
- Perform basic calculations using multiplication and division.
- Set up and use fractions.
- Compare fractions, express them as decimals, and find common denominators.
- Perform basic mathematical calculations using fractions and decimals.
- Understand and use percentages.
- Perform basic mathematical calculations using percentages.

KEY TERMS

Addition	Factor	Percentages
Common denominator	Fractions	Product
Cross-multiplication	Improper fraction	Proper fraction
Decimal number	Mixed number	Quotient
Denominator	Multiplication	Subtraction
Difference	Number	Sum
Division	Numerator	Whole numbers

Chapter Overview

This chapter will review basic mathematical skills that are necessary to perform more complex calculations. Calculations in the pharmacy setting require a basic understanding of addition, subtraction, division, multiplication, fractions, percentages, and decimals.

Numbers

A **number** is a quantity or amount that is made up of one or more numerals. There are several kinds of numbers: whole numbers, fractions, and decimal numbers. Examples of whole numbers include 2, 10, 100, 2,000, and 5,000,000. Examples of fractions include ¼, ³/₁₀, and ⁷/₈. Examples of decimals include 0.2, 0.75, and 2.6.

A number is represented by one or more numerals.

Whole Numbers

Our number system is a base-10 number system. That is, it is based on the number 10. We use 10 digits, also called **whole numbers** (0, 1, 2, 3, 4, 5, 6, 7, 8, 9). Whole numbers are counting numbers.

We use whole numbers to count.

Addition and Subtraction

Many dosage calculations involve addition and subtraction. With **addition**, you add something to a given number **FIGURE 3.1**. The **sum** is the amount obtained when adding numbers (see **TABLE 3.1**). With **subtraction**, you take something away from a given number **FIGURE 3.2**. The **difference** is the amount obtained when subtracting numbers (see **TABLE 3.2**). There is an inverse relationship between addition and subtraction.

Addition means that you are adding or increasing the quantity by a given number.

Adding a zero to a number does not change the value of the original number. The value of zero is nothing. Examples: 0 + 5 = 5; 10 + 0 = 10; 210 + 0 = 210.

Subtraction means that you are taking away or reducing the quantity by a given number.

Subtracting a zero from a number does not change the value of the original number. The value of zero is nothing. Examples: 7 − 0 = 7; 128 − 0 = 128; 21 − 0 = 21.

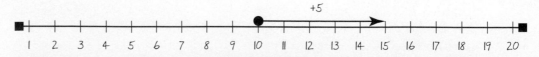

FIGURE 3.1 Addition example using a number line.

Table 3.1 Addition Strategy

Fact Strategy	Example	Answer (Sum)
Plus 0	8 + 0	8
Plus 1	8 + 1	9
Plus 2	8 + 2	10
Plus 3	8 + 3	11
Plus 4	8 + 4	12
Plus 5	8 + 5	13
Plus 6	8 + 6	14
Plus 7	8 + 7	15
Plus 8	8 + 8	16
Plus 9	8 + 9	17
Plus 10	8 + 10	18

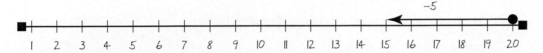

FIGURE 3.2 Subtraction example using a number line.

Table 3.2 Subtraction Strategy

Fact Strategy	Example	Answer (Difference)
Minus 0	10 – 0	10
Minus 1	10 – 1	9
Minus 2	10 – 2	8
Minus 3	10 – 3	7
Minus 4	10 – 4	6
Minus 5	10 – 5	5
Minus 6	10 – 6	4
Minus 7	10 – 7	3
Minus 8	10 – 8	2
Minus 9	10 – 9	1
Minus 10	10 – 10	0

Multiplication and Division

Multiplication and **division** are used constantly in performing pharmacy calculations. Sometimes, you must enlarge or reduce the quantity or determine a part or portion of a quantity needed. Multiplication and division are the mathematical processes used to do this. The **product** is the amount obtained by multiplying numbers. The **quotient** is the amount obtained by dividing one number by another number. TABLE 3.3 shows a multiplication chart.

Table 3.3		Multiplication Chart									
1	**2**	**3**	**4**	**5**	**6**	**7**	**8**	**9**	**10**	**11**	**12**
2	4	6	8	10	12	14	16	18	20	22	24
3	6	9	12	15	18	21	24	27	30	33	36
4	8	12	16	20	24	28	32	36	40	44	48
5	10	15	20	25	30	35	40	45	50	55	60
6	12	18	24	30	36	42	48	54	60	66	72
7	14	21	28	35	42	49	56	63	70	77	84
8	16	24	32	40	48	56	64	72	80	88	96
9	18	27	36	45	54	63	72	81	90	99	108
10	20	30	40	50	60	70	80	90	100	110	120
11	22	33	44	55	66	77	88	99	110	121	132
12	24	36	48	60	72	84	96	108	120	132	144

Division is the inverse relationship of multiplication.

Example: $9 \times 5 = 45$
$45 \div 9 = 5$
$45 \div 5 = 9$

Example: $7 \times 6 = 42$
$42 \div 7 = 6$
$42 \div 6 = 7$

When multiplying numbers, any number multiplied by zero always equals zero.

Example: $126 \times 0 = 0$
Example: $546 \times 0 = 0$
Example: $4 \times 0 = 0$

When dividing numbers, any number divided by one always equals the number.

Example: $978 \div 1 = 978$
Example: $69 \div 1 = 69$
Example: $78 \div 1 = 78$

Fractions

Many dosage calculations use amounts other than whole numbers—for example, fractions. Pharmacy technicians work with these amounts to fill orders and complete pharmaceutical calculations. Pharmacy technicians must be able to recognize fractions and understand what amounts they represent.

Fractions express a quantity or portion that is a part of a whole number **FIGURE 3.3**. It is a ratio of a part to the whole. The number above the fraction line is called the **numerator**. The number below the fraction line is called the **denominator**. The denominator tells how many equal parts are in the whole or set. The numerator tells you the number of those parts you are expressing.

Fractions express a quantity that is a part of a whole number.

The numerator is the number above the fraction line.

The denominator is the number below the fraction line.

Another way to think about fractions is by dividing a pie into parts. For example, imagine a pie that has been divided into eight pieces or parts. Each piece is a fraction, or ⅛ of the whole pie **FIGURE 3.4**.

A number line can be a useful tool when thinking about fractions **FIGURE 3.5**.

A **proper fraction** has a numerator that is smaller than the denominator. The value of this type of fraction is always less than 1. Examples of a proper fraction include ⅕, ⅔, and ⅜.

The value of a proper fraction is always less than 1.

An **improper fraction** has a numerator that is equal to or larger than the denominator. The value of this type of fraction is always equal to or greater than 1. When the numerator and denominator are the same, the value of the fraction is always 1, because any number divided by itself always equals 1. Examples of an improper fraction include 2/2, 4/3, and 9/7.

The value of an improper fraction is always equal to or greater than 1.

A **mixed number** contains both whole numbers and fractions. Examples of mixed numbers include 1⅔ and 2⁴/₇.

A mixed number has whole numbers and fractions.

You can convert a mixed number to an improper fraction by multiplying the denominator by the whole number and adding the numerator **FIGURE 3.6**.

You can rewrite a fraction greater than 1 as a mixed number or as a whole number **FIGURE 3.7**. For example, to write ⁷/₄ as a mixed number, follow these steps:

1. Divide the numerator by the denominator.
2. Use the remainder to write the fraction part of the quotient.

A fraction is in its simplest form when its numerator and denominator have no common factor other than 1 **FIGURE 3.8**. A **factor** is a number that you multiply by another number, which is also a factor, to make yet another number. For example, the simplest form of ⁶/₁₈ is ⅓.

When a fraction is in its simplest form, the numerator and denominator have no common factor other than 1.

You can divide the numerator and denominator by common factors until the only common factor is 1.

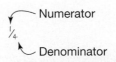

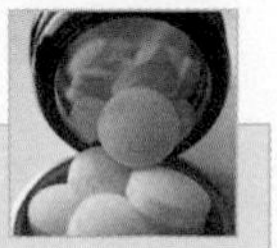

Numerator

¼

Denominator

FIGURE 3.3 Defining a fraction.

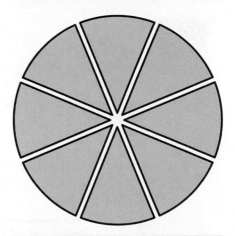

FIGURE 3.4 Fraction example using a pie.

$$0 \quad \tfrac{1}{4} \quad \tfrac{1}{2} \quad \tfrac{3}{4} \quad 1$$

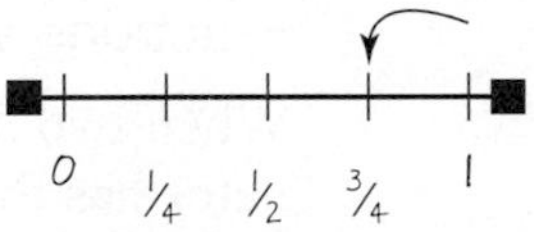

FIGURE 3.5 Fraction example using a number line.

$$1\tfrac{2}{3} = \frac{\left((3\times1)+2\right)}{3} = \tfrac{5}{3}$$

FIGURE 3.6 Converting a mixed fraction to an improper fraction.

$$7 \div 4 = 1\tfrac{3}{4}$$

FIGURE 3.7 Division example using fractions.

$$\frac{6}{18} = \frac{6\div6}{18\div6} = \frac{1}{3}$$

FIGURE 3.8 Simplifying a fraction.

To convert a mixed number to an improper fraction, multiply the denominator by the whole number. Then add the numerator to this calculated amount and place it over the same denominato

Reduce every mixed number and improper fraction.

To simplify a fraction, divide the numerator and denominator by a common factor until the only common factor is 1.

Comparing Fractions

Comparing fractions helps to ensure that correct calculations are used in the practice of pharmacy and in the normal work tasks of pharmacy technicians. Fractions can most easily be compared by using denominators that are the same. Fractions can also be compared when the denominators are different, as well as when the numerators are the same or different. Using fractions in pharmacy work is a simple and helpful mathematical concept to be mastered by the pharmacy technician.

Fractions with Like Denominators

Comparing fractions with the same denominators is similar to comparing whole numbers **FIGURE 3.9**. When comparing fractions that have the same denominator, the fraction with the larger numerator will have the larger value. For example, ³⁄₅ is greater than ²⁄₅.

> When two fractions have the same denominator, the fraction with the larger numerator has a larger value.

Fractions with Like Numerators

When two fractions have the same numerator, the fraction with the smaller denominator has the larger value **FIGURE 3.10**.

> When two fractions have the same numerator, the fraction with the smaller denominator has a larger the value.

If the numerator is the same, the smaller the denominator, the larger the value **FIGURE 3.11**.

If the denominator is the same, the smaller the numerator, the smaller the value **FIGURE 3.12**.

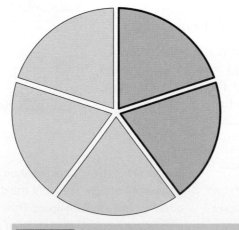
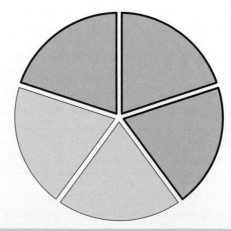

FIGURE 3.9 Same denominator fraction graph.

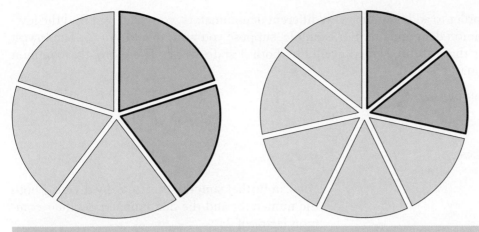

FIGURE 3.10 Different denominator fraction pie graph.

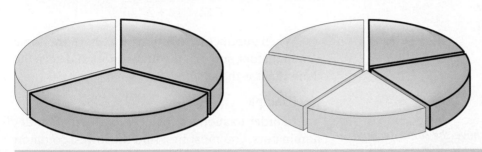

FIGURE 3.11 Which tablet is bigger?

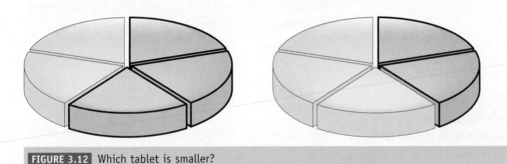

FIGURE 3.12 Which tablet is smaller?

Adding and Subtracting Fractions

When you add and subtract fractions, you need to find the lowest common denominator. A **common denominator** is a number into which both denominators can divide evenly.

If both fractions have the same denominators, add the numerators and keep the denominator the same.

When adding fractions that have the same denominators, add the numerators and keep the denominator the same.

Example: $\frac{1}{7} + \frac{2}{7} = \frac{3}{7}$

Rules for Adding Fractions

When adding fractions, first convert the fractions to the lowest common denominator (if necessary). Then, add the numerators, placing the sum over the denominator. Finally, reduce the resulting fraction.

In order to add fractions with different denominators, you must first find the lowest common denominator. For example, suppose you want to add $\frac{1}{3} + \frac{2}{4}$. The lowest number that can be divided evenly by both 3 and 4 is 12. Therefore, the common denominator is 12.

Example: $\frac{1}{3} + \frac{2}{4}$
$\frac{1}{3} \times \frac{4}{4} = \frac{4}{12}$
$\frac{2}{4} \times \frac{3}{3} = \frac{6}{12}$

Answer: $\frac{4}{12} + \frac{6}{12} = \frac{10}{12}$

When adding fractions with different denominators, first find the lowest common denominator.

If both fractions have the same denominator, subtract the numerators and keep the denominator the same.

When subtracting fractions with different denominators, first find the lowest common denominator.

You can further simplify this to $\frac{5}{6}$ by dividing both the numerator and the denominator by their common factor of 2:

$$\frac{10}{12} = \frac{10 \div 2}{12 \div 2} = \frac{5}{6}$$

When subtracting fractions that have the same denominators, subtract the numerators and keep the denominator the same.

Example: $\frac{5}{7} - \frac{2}{7} = \frac{3}{7}$

In order to subtract fractions with different denominators, you must first find the lowest common denominator. For example, suppose you want to subtract $\frac{8}{10} - \frac{2}{5}$. The lowest number that can be divided evenly by both 10 and 5 is 10. Therefore, the common denominator is 10.

Example: $\frac{8}{10} - \frac{2}{5}$
$\frac{8}{10} \times \frac{1}{1} = \frac{8}{10}$
$\frac{2}{5} \times \frac{2}{2} = \frac{4}{10}$

Answer: $\frac{8}{10} - \frac{4}{10} = \frac{4}{10}$

You can further simplify this answer to $\frac{2}{5}$ by dividing both the numerator and the denominator by the least common factor, which is 2:

$$\frac{4}{10} = \frac{4 \div 2}{10 \div 2} = \frac{2}{5}$$

Rules for Subtracting Fractions

When subtracting fractions, first convert the fractions to the lowest common denominator (if necessary). Next, subtract the numerators, placing the difference over the denominator. Finally, reduce the resulting fraction.

Multiplying and Dividing Fractions

It is important to understand the mathematical concepts used in multiplying and dividing fractions. Many dosage calculations will require the pharmacy technician to calculate the amount of drug required using multiplication and division with fractions prior to a final check by the pharmacist.

Multiplying Fractions

To multiply fractions, multiply the numerators of each fraction and the denominators of each fraction.

Example: $\frac{2}{3} \times \frac{4}{5}$

$2 \times 4 = 8$

$3 \times 5 = 15$

Answer: $\frac{8}{15}$

Rules for Multiplying Fractions

When multiplying fractions, first convert any mixed numbers into improper fractions (if necessary). Next, multiply the numerators to obtain a new numerator. Then multiply the denominators to obtain a new denominator. Finally, reduce the resulting fraction.

Dividing Fractions

To divide fractions, invert or reverse the numbers of the second fraction in the equation. Then multiply the numerators of each fraction and the denominators of each fraction, as you do when multiplying fractions. This is known as "invert and multiply."

Example: $\frac{1}{3} \div \frac{1}{8}$

$\frac{1}{3} \times \frac{8}{1}$

$\frac{1}{3} \times 8$

Answer: $\frac{8}{3}$, which simplifies to $2\frac{2}{3}$

Rules for Dividing Fractions

When dividing fractions, first convert any mixed numbers into improper fractions (if necessary). Next, find the reciprocal of the divisor (the second fraction). Then multiply the first number by the reciprocal. Finally, reduce the resulting fraction.

Decimals

Not every number is a whole number. **Decimal numbers** are numbers that are written using place value. The decimal system includes 10 digits (0, 1, 2, 3, 4, 5, 6, 7, 8, 9). Using these digits, you can express numbers of all sizes using a decimal point. The decimal point, which looks like a period, is the central character in the decimal system. Any value can be expressed using a combination of these numerals. Digits to the left of the decimal point indicate whole numbers, and digits to the right indicate fractions of a whole. The value of a digit increases by a multiple of 10 each time it moves one space to the left. Equally, the value of a digit decreases by a multiple of 10 each time it moves one space to the right.

The scheme of the decimal system is depicted in **TABLE 3.4**. In this case, the number 63,207.5184 is used to illustrate decimal-system notation.

The total value of a number expressed by the decimal system is the sum of all its digits according to their place to the right or left of the decimal point. Therefore, in the sample number, 63,207.5184 is equal to the following:

- 60,000.0000 (6 ten-thousands)
- + 03000.0000 (3 thousands)
- + 00200.0000 (2 hundreds)

Table 3.4   Decimal System Notation

Value	Ten-thousands	Thousands	Hundreds	Tens	Ones	Decimal point	Tenths	Hundredths	Thousandths	Ten-thousandths
Sample Number	6	3	2	0	7	.	5	1	8	4

- + 00000.0000 (0 tens)
- + 00007.0000 (7 ones)
- + 00000.5000 (5 tenths)
- + 00000.0100 (1 hundredth)
- + 00000.0080 (8 thousandths)
- + 00000.0004 (4 ten-thousandths)

Any fraction can be written in decimal form. The position of a number in relation to the decimal point indicates the value of that number. Digits to the left of the decimal point indicate whole numbers, and digits to the right of the decimal point indicate fractions of a whole. Each place value is multiplied by 10 as you move left from the decimal point. Each place value is divided by 10 as you move right from the decimal point.

Think of money to help understand decimals and their place values. One dollar can be thought of as having 100 parts, with each part being equal to one penny. A dollar can also be thought of as having 10 parts, with each part then being equal to one dime.

In pharmacy practice, when using the decimal system to express a number less than 1, a leading zero (0) is placed to the left of the decimal point. Trailing zeros, or zeros that are placed to the right of the final digit, are not used in pharmacy. These techniques help eliminate errors when reading decimals. If a leading zero is not included or a trailing zero is included, and the decimal point may not be read. That means a dose may be misinterpreted by a factor of 10, 100, or even 1,000.

For example, consider the following: $\frac{2}{5} = 2 \div 5 = 0.4$. This would not be written as .4, .40, or 0.40. In this case, if 0.4 represented a dose, and if a leading zero were not included, the value could be misinterpreted as 4 or 40, resulting in respective overdoses of 10 or 100 times the intended dose. Or, if a dose of 10mg was written as 10.0, the value could easily be interpreted as 100mg.

Always include a leading zero when expressing doses that are less than 1.

A leading zero is placed to the left of the decimal point when expressing a number less than 1.

Do not include a trailing zero in pharmacy calculations, except when it is critical to the accuracy of the measurement. Never use a trailing zero when a dose is expressed as a whole number.

The exception to the rule of no trailing zeros is when the zero is considered significant to the dose or calculation, or when rounding results in a trailing zero—for example, 0.799 rounded to the nearest hundredth is 0.80 (written with a trailing zero). Another example is the use of a trailing zero in calculations involving currency **FIGURE 3.13**. For

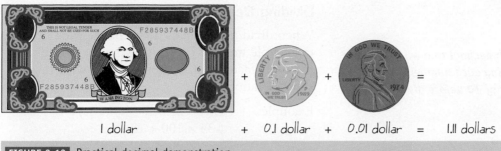

I dollar + 0.1 dollar + 0.01 dollar = 1.11 dollars

FIGURE 3.13 Practical decimal demonstration.

Table 3.5 Different Ways to Express a Decimal

Form	Example
Standard	45.38
Word	forty-five and thirty-eight hundredths
Expanded	$(4 \times 10) + (5 \times 1) + (3 \times 0.1) + (8 \times 0.01)$

example, 10 dollars and 70 cents is written mathematically as $10.70, not as $10.7, without the trailing zero.

There are many ways to write the same decimal, as shown in **TABLE 3.5**.

Adding and Subtracting Decimals

When adding and subtracting decimals, the numbers should be placed in columns so that the decimal points are all aligned. For example:

Align the decimal points before adding and subtracting decimal numbers.

$$
\begin{array}{r}
4.3 \\
2.16 \\
+\ 3.289 \\
\hline
9.749
\end{array}
$$

Multiplying Decimals

When multiplying decimals, you multiply them as whole numbers, and then move the decimal the total number of places that were in the two numbers being multiplied **FIGURE 3.14**. There is an implied decimal point for all whole numbers, which is placed at the end of the smallest or last digit in the number. For

Multiply the decimals as whole numbers first and then move the decimal over the total number of places.

example, the whole number 76 is also the same as 76.0, with the decimal point and zero being the implied decimal. Thus, when multiplying decimals, the starting point for moving the decimal begins with the implied decimal point at the end of the whole number. For example, to multiply 23.6×45.29, you first multiply $236 \times 4529 = 1,068,844$. The implied decimal point is 1,068,844.0 and the movement of the decimal places begins after the number four in the ones digit place. Next, count from right to left three decimal places (because there are three total decimals in 23.6 and 45.29) and place the decimal point there: 1,068.844.

1068.844.

FIGURE 3.14 Moving decimals.

> *Change each decimal to a whole number by multiplying each number by the same factor of 10 before dividing decimals.*

Dividing Decimals

When dividing decimals, first change each decimal to a whole number by multiplying each number by the same factor of 10. Then proceed with the division operation.

Example: 1.34 ÷ 2.1
              1.34 × 100 = 134
              2.1 × 100 = 210

Answer: 134 ÷ 210 = 0.638

Example: 2.5 ÷ 1.25
              2.5 × 100 = 250
              1.25 × 100 = 125

Answer: 250 ÷ 125 = 2

Percentages

Pharmacy calculations often require the use of **percentages**. A percentage is represented by the % symbol and is used to express the number of parts of one hundred. It represents the same number as a fraction whose denominator is 100. Examples include the following:

- $0.9\% = {}^{0.9}/_{100}$.
- $2\% = {}^{2}/_{100}$
- ${}^{5}/_{100} = 5\%$

Tech Math Practice

Question: **What is the sum of 143 + 211?**

Answer: 354

Question: **What is the sum of 29 + 33?**

Answer: 62

Question: **What is the difference of 187 – 96?**

Answer: 91

Question: **What is the difference of 435 – 78?**

Answer: 357

Question: **What is 8 × 6?**

Answer: 48

Question: **What is 12 × 11?**

Answer: 132

Question: **What is 99 ÷ 9?**

Answer: 11

Question: **What is 108 ÷ 9?**

Answer: 12

Question: **What type of fraction is $^4/_3$?**

Answer: Improper fraction

Question: **What type of fraction is $^2/_7$?**

Answer: Proper fraction

Question: **What type of fraction is $1^7/_8$?**

Answer: Mixed number

Question: **What is the simplest form of the fraction $^{20}/_{40}$?**

Answer: $^{20}/_{40} \div ^2/_2 = ^{10}/_{20} \div ^2/_2 = ^1/_2$

Question: **What is the simplest form of the fraction $^8/_{24}$?**

Answer: $^8/_{24} \div ^4/_4 = ^2/_6 \div ^2/_2 = ^1/_3$

Question: **What is the simplest form of the fraction $^{12}/_{16}$?**

Answer: $^{12}/_{16} \div ^4/_4 = ^3/_4$

Question: **Which of the following doses of drug is the smallest dose? $^3/_{10}$ mg tablet, $^7/_{10}$ mg tablet, or $^2/_{10}$ mg tablet?**

Answer: The $^2/_{10}$ mg tablet is the smallest dose because when fractions have the same denominator, the fraction with the smaller numerator has the smallest value.

Question: **Which of the following doses of drug is the largest dose? $^1/_{15}$ mg tablet, $^3/_{15}$ mg tablet, or $^7/_{15}$ mg tablet?**

Answer: The $^7/_{15}$ mg tablet is the largest dose because when fractions have the same denominator, the fraction with the larger numerator has the largest value.

Question: **Which of the following tablets is the smallest dose?** $^3/_{10}$ **mg tablet,** $^3/_{12}$ **mg tablet, or** $^3/_{20}$ **mg tablet?**

Answer: The $^3/_{20}$ mg tablet is the smallest dose because when fractions have the same numerator, the fraction with the larger denominator has the smallest value.

Question: **Which of the following tablets is the largest dose?** $^4/_7$ **mg tablet,** $^4/_{12}$ **mg tablet, or** $^4/_{15}$ **mg tablet?**

Answer: The $^4/_7$ mg tablet is the largest dose because when fractions have the same numerator, the fraction with the smallest denominator has the largest value.

Question: **What is the sum of** $^1/_6$ + $^4/_6$**?**

Answer: $^5/_6$

Question: **What is the sum of** $^3/_8$ + $^2/_8$**?**

Answer: $^5/_8$

Question: **What is the sum of** $^1/_5$ + $^2/_{10}$**?**

Answer: To obtain the sum, first determine the lowest common denominator: $^1/_5 \times ^2/_2 = ^2/_{10}$. Then complete the addition operation: $^2/_{10} + ^2/_{10} = ^4/_{10}$, which simplifies to $^2/_5$.

Question: **What is the sum of** $^2/_3$ + $^3/_7$**?**

Answer: To obtain the sum, first determine the lowest common denominator: $^2/_3 \times ^7/_7 = ^{14}/_{21}$ and $^3/_7 \times ^3/_3 = ^9/_{21}$. Then complete the addition operation: $^{14}/_{21} + ^9/_{21} = ^{23}/_{21}$. Note that $^{23}/_{21}$ is an improper fraction, and can be simplified to $1^2/_{21}$.

Question: **What is the difference of** $^8/_9$ − $^3/_9$**?**

Answer: $^5/_9$

Question: **What is the difference of** $^3/_5$ − $^1/_5$**?**

Answer: $^2/_5$

Question: **What is the sum of** $^3/_8$ + $^3/_{12}$**?**

Answer: To obtain the sum, first determine the lowest common denominator: $^3/_8 \times ^3/_3 = ^9/_{24}$ and $^3/_{12} \times ^2/_2 = ^6/_{24}$. Then complete the addition operation: $^9/_{24} + ^6/_{24} = ^{15}/_{24}$, which can be simplified to $^5/_8$.

Question: **What is the difference of** $^4/_{12}$ − $^2/_6$**?**

Answer: To obtain the difference, first determine the lowest common denominator: $^4/_{12} \times ^1/_1 = ^4/_{12}$ and $^2/_6 \times ^2/_2 = ^4/_{12}$. Then complete the subtraction operation: $^4/_{12} − ^4/_{12} = 0$.

Question: **What is the product of $\frac{2}{5} \times \frac{3}{4}$?**

Answer: $\frac{6}{20}$, which simplifies to $\frac{3}{10}$.

Question: **What is the product of $\frac{3}{5} \times \frac{4}{7}$?**

Answer: $\frac{12}{35}$

Question: **What is the product of $\frac{4}{12} \times \frac{3}{8}$?**

Answer: $\frac{12}{96}$, which simplifies to $\frac{1}{8}$.

Question: **What is the quotient of $\frac{4}{7} \div \frac{3}{7}$?**

Answer: $\frac{28}{21}$, which simplifies to $1\frac{1}{3}$.

Question: **What is the quotient of $\frac{2}{11} \div \frac{1}{2}$?**

Answer: $\frac{4}{11}$

Question: **What is the quotient of $\frac{4}{9} \div \frac{5}{8}$?**

Answer: $\frac{32}{45}$

Question: **What is the value of the digit 4 in 369.045?**

Answer: The digit 4 is in the hundredths place. It has a value of 0.04, or 4 hundredths.

Question: **What is the value of the digit 2 in 364.0782?**

Answer: The digit 2 is in the ten-thousandths place. It has a value of 0.0002, or 2 ten-thousandths.

Question: **What is the sum of 3.42 + 2.76 + 3.2?**

Answer: 9.38

```
  3.42
  2.76
+ 3.2
------
  9.38
```

Question: **What is the sum of 2.3 + 1.4 + 1.22?**

Answer: 4.92

```
  2.3
  1.4
+ 1.22
------
  4.92
```

Question: **What is the difference of 3.5 − 1.1?**

Answer: 2.4

$$
\begin{array}{r}
3.5 \\
-\ 1.1 \\
\hline
2.4
\end{array}
$$

Question: **What is the quotient of 6.6 ÷ 2.2?**

Answer: To determine the quotient, first multiply the dividend (the first number) by 10: $6.6 \times 10 = 66$. Next, multiply the divisor (the second number) by 10: $2.2 \times 10 = 22$. Finally, solve the problem: $66 \div 22 = 3$.

Question: **What is the quotient of 4.8 ÷ 1.2?**

Answer: To determine the quotient, first multiply the dividend by 10: $4.8 \times 10 = 48$. Next, multiply the divisor by 10: $1.2 \times 10 = 12$. Finally, solve the problem: $48 \div 12 = 4$.

Question: **What is the quotient of 4.9 ÷ 0.7?**

Answer: To determine the quotient, first multiply the dividend by 10: $4.9 \times 10 = 49$. Next, multiply the divisor by 10: $0.7 \times 10 = 7$. Finally, solve the problem: $49 \div 7 = 7$.

Question: **How do you write ¼ as a percent?**

Answer: To write ¼ as a percent, first find the equivalent fraction with a denominator of 100: $\frac{1}{4} \times \frac{25}{25} = \frac{25}{100}$. $\frac{25}{100} = 25\%$. Another method is to divide the top of the fraction (the numerator) by the bottom of the fraction (the denominator) and multiply the result by 100: $1 \div 4 = 0.25 \times 100 = 25\%$.

Question: **How do you write $^2/_{20}$ as a percent?**

Answer: To write $^2/_{20}$ as a percent, first find the equivalent fraction with a denominator of 100: $\frac{2}{20} \times \frac{5}{5} = \frac{10}{100}$. $\frac{10}{100} = 10\%$.

WRAP UP

Chapter Summary

- Numbers can be represented as whole numbers, fractions, and decimals.
- Each type of number can be used in addition, subtraction, multiplication, and division.
- Addition and subtraction involve adding numbers to each other or taking numbers away from each other, respectively.
- Multiplication involves changing the quantity of a number by multiplying a number by another number.
- Division involves changing the quantity of a number to determine a part or portion of a quantity needed.
- Cross-multiplication is a mathematical concept that is very useful to the pharmacy technician when performing calculations.
- Fractions are used to express a quantity or portion that is a part of a whole number. It is a ratio of a part to the whole. The numerator is the number above the fraction line, while the denominator is the number below the fraction line. The denominator tells you how many equal parts are in the whole or set. The numerator tells you the number of those parts you are expressing.
- Decimals are numbers that are written using place value. Any fraction can be expressed as a decimal.
- Percentages are used to express the number of parts of 100. A percentage represents the same number as a fraction whose denominator is 100, and is denoted by the % symbol.
- Fractions, decimals, and percentages can be converted to each other and used in addition, subtraction, multiplication, and division operations.
- When adding fractions, first convert the fractions to the lowest common denominator (if necessary). Then, add the numerators, placing the sum over denominator. Finally, reduce the resulting fraction.
- When subtracting fractions, first convert the fractions to the lowest common denominator (if necessary). Next, subtract the numerators, placing the difference over the denominator. Finally, reduce the resulting fraction.
- When multiplying fractions, first convert any mixed numbers into improper fractions (if necessary). Next, multiply the numerators to obtain a new numerator. Then multiply the denominators to obtain a new denominator. Finally, reduce the resulting fraction.
- When dividing fractions, first convert any mixed numbers into improper fractions (if necessary). Next, find the reciprocal of the divisor (the second fraction). Then multiply the first number by the reciprocal. Finally, reduce the resulting fraction.
- Pharmacy technicians need to be comfortable performing basic mathematical equations with all the concepts in this chapter.

Learning Assessment Questions

1. Which of the following fractions has the highest value?
   A. $1\frac{1}{3}$
   B. $\frac{2}{3}$
   C. $\frac{4}{9}$
   D. $\frac{5}{9}$

2. What is a fraction with a value of less than 1 called?
   A. Mixed number
   B. Proper fraction
   C. Improper fraction
   D. Whole number

3. What is a fraction with a value greater than 1 called?
   A. Mixed number
   B. Proper fraction
   C. Improper fraction
   D. Whole number

4. What is $\frac{12}{16}$, reduced to its simplest form?
   A. $\frac{12}{16}$
   B. $\frac{6}{8}$
   C. $\frac{3}{4}$
   D. $\frac{4}{7}$

5. Which dose is larger?
   A. ¼ of a 300mg tablet
   B. ½ of a 300mg tablet
   C. ⅓ of a 300mg tablet
   D. ¹/₁₀ of a 300mg tablet

6. What is the value of the digit 3 in 2,476.9432?
   A. 0.3
   B. 0.003
   C. 0.03
   D. 0.0003

7. A percentage represents the same number as a fraction whose denominator is?
   A. 50
   B. 25
   C. 100
   D. 0

8. What is the product of 9 × 7?
   A. 54
   B. 63
   C. 72
   D. 45

9. What is the sum of 10.3 + 2.7 + 3.65?
   A. 16.65
   B. 16.62
   C. 12.67
   D. 16.66

10. What is the value of the digit 7 in 3,045.2783?
    A. 0.7
    B. 0.07
    C. 0.007
    D. 70

11. What is the value of the digit 4 in the number 567.431?
    A. 4 tenths
    B. 4 hundredths
    C. 4 thousandths
    D. 40

12. What is the product of 0.25 × 0.2?
    A. 0.005
    B. 50
    C. 0.5
    D. 0.05

13. ¹²/₂₀ is the same as what percent?
    A. 50%
    B. 60%
    C. 30%
    D. 20%

14. ¾ is the same as what percent?
    A. 25%
    B. 55%
    C. 75%
    D. 33%

15. Convert 0.40 to a fraction.
    A. ⁸/₁₀
    B. ⅕
    C. ⁴/₁₀
    D. ⁴⁰/₁₀

16. Convert ⁴/₈ to a decimal.
    A. 0.5
    B. 0.2
    C. 0.4
    D. 0.8

WRAP UP

17. What is the difference in 12.8 – 3.4?
    A. 9.4
    B. 9.3
    C. 6.6
    D. 4.9

18. What is the product of 3.62 × 3.3?
    A. 11.469
    B. 11.649
    C. 11.946
    D. 19.4

19. What is the sum of 987 + 0?
    A. 0
    B. 978
    C. 980
    D. 987

20. What is the quotient of 978,657 ÷ 0?
    A. 978,657
    B. 987,756
    C. 0
    D. 978,665

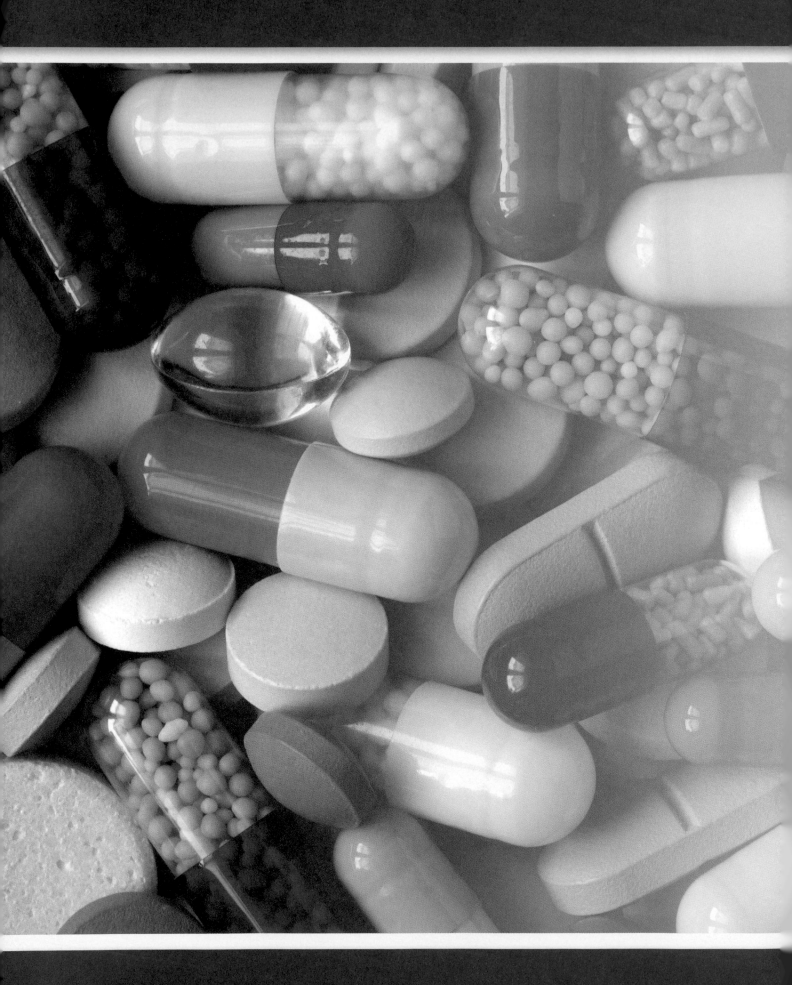

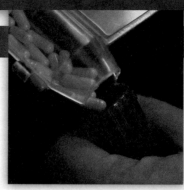

Dosage Forms, Routes of Administration, and Dispensing Medications

OBJECTIVES

After reading this chapter, you will be able to:

- Outline the components of a prescription, including commonly used abbreviations.
- Understand the "rights" of correct drug administration.
- Describe common dosage forms.
- Explain the most common routes of administration.
- Summarize the factors that influence the effects of drugs, particularly in elderly and pediatric populations.
- Explain the difference between dosage form and route of administration.
- Describe the properties of solid, semisolid, liquid, inhalation, and transdermal dosage forms.
- Describe inactive ingredients, various tablet coatings, and their functions.
- Describe various delayed-release dosage formulations.
- Compare and contrast different types of emulsions such as ointments, creams, and gels.
- Discuss the advantages of a transdermal dosage form.
- Explain the major routes of administration and the advantages and disadvantages associated with each route of administration.
- Explain the correct techniques for administration of eye drops, metered-dose inhalers, vaginal medications, and injections.

KEY TERMS

Additives	Immediate-release	Rectal
Aerosol	Incontinence	Ring
Alcoholic solution	Infection	Route of administration
Aqueous suspension	Infusion	Signa
Aromatic water	Inhalation	Solute
Binders	Inscription	Solution
Bolus dose	Intradermal	Solvent
Buccal	Intramuscular	Sprinkles
Caplet	Intravenous	Subcutaneous
Capsule	Irrigating solution	Sublingual
Chewable tablet	Lotion	Sugar-coated
Controlled-release	Lozenges	Suspension
Cream	Nasal	Spansule
Delayed-release	Noncompliance	Spirit
Depot	Oil-in-water (O/W)	Spray
Diluents	emulsion	Sprinkles
Dispersion	Ointment	Suppository
Dosage form	Ophthalmic	Sustained-release
Elixir	Oral disintegrating	Syringe
Emulsion	tablet (ODT)	Syrup
Emulsifying agent	Order	Tablet
Enteric-coated	Otic	Tincture
Excipients	Parenteral solution	Topical
Extended-release	Paste	Transdermal patch
Extract	Peroral (PO)	Urethral
Film-coated	Polypharmacy	Vaginal
Gel	Powder	Water-in-oil (W/O)
Granules	Prescription	emulsion
Homogenous	Preservatives	
Hydroalcoholic solution	Reconstitution	

Chapter Overview

The legal form that a prescriber utilizes to order a medication, medical device, or piece of medical equipment to be dispensed to a patient by a licensed pharmacist is called a prescription. A valid prescription must contain all the information necessary for a pharmacist to complete the prescriber's order. A pharmacy technician plays a key role in the preparation and dispensing of prescription products. This chapter covers the legally required elements of a prescription, as well as many of the common abbreviations used by prescribers to create prescription orders. To effectively read prescriptions and prepare prescription orders, it is essential for a pharmacy technician to possess a thorough understanding of common prescription abbreviations.

The Prescription

A **prescription** is a legal order for a specific product, to be dispensed to a patient by a licensed pharmacist. A prescription order can be made by any healthcare professional with prescribing authority. Although the most common issuer of prescription orders is a physician, prescription orders can also be issued by dentists, podiatrists, optometrists, physician assistants, nurse practitioners, and veterinarians in all 50 states.

Additionally, some states have granted limited prescribing authority to clinical psychologists and pharmacists. Physicians have broad prescribing authority, which means there are no limitations to what prescription products they may prescribe. Other healthcare professionals may have limited prescribing authority, which means there are specific restrictions in place for these prescribers. These restrictions are related to each professional's individual scope of practice and vary from state to state. For example, a dentist cannot order a medication for a patient's back pain and a veterinarian cannot order medications for a human patient.

Prescription orders are sometimes given to patients by their prescriber. A patient might then mail or hand-deliver a prescription to a pharmacy. Other times, prescriptions are transmitted by the prescriber or an agent of the prescriber (for example, a nurse in the prescriber's practice) directly to the pharmacy. A prescriber has several options for transmitting prescription orders to a pharmacy. Prescribers may mail prescriptions to the pharmacy, relay them via telephone, transmit them via fax, or use an e-prescribing service, which is a secure system that utilizes an Internet connection to deliver prescriptions directly to the pharmacy computer. Written prescription orders, whether given to the patient, faxed, or mailed to the pharmacy, must be signed by the prescriber. Telephone orders and e-prescribing orders are valid as long as they are relayed to the pharmacy by the prescriber or by an authorized agent of the prescriber. There are many special laws that relate to prescription orders for controlled substances, but these vary from state to state. For more information on these regulations visit your state board of pharmacy's Web site.

In an institutional setting, the term prescription is not used. Instead, the prescriber's request is referred to as an **order** or a **medication order**.

Patient Name   **Perscription Number**

> **PHARMACY**
> WEGMANS FOOD MARKETS, INC.
> 1 MAIN STREET
> ROCHESTER, NY 14624   AW-6116861
>
> **REFILLS: (123) 456-7890**
> **Pharmacy # 123**
> **Rx# 6000561**
> (123) 456-7890
>
> **SMARTFILL, MARY JANE**   01/18/10
> 123 MAIN STREET, ROCHESTER, NY 14620
> **TAKE ONE TABLET BY MOUTH EVERY 8 HOURS AS NEEDED FOR PAIN.**
>
> **IBUPROFEN 800 MG TABLET**
>   **QTY: 90**
>
> ANDREW SMITH
> **2 REFILLS BY 01/18/11**

Number of Refills Remaining

FIGURE 4.1 The essential components of a prescription.

The Components of a Hard-Copy Prescription

Prescription components may vary from state to state, but typically should contain the following information **FIGURE 4.1**:

- The prescriber's name, address, and phone number
- The name of the patient
- The date the prescription was written
- The name, strength, dosage form, and quantity of medication or product ordered (also called the **inscription**)
- Directions for use (also called the **signa**, often referred to as "sig")
- The number of refills allowed
- If the prescriber requests "no generic substitution," it must be clearly noted

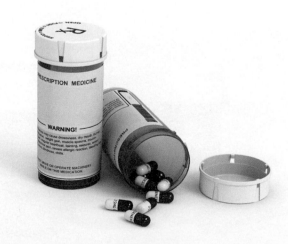

A medication bottle that has the Rx symbol can only be dispensed with a legal prescription.

- If it is a prescription for a controlled substance, the prescriber's Drug Enforcement Administration (DEA) number
- The prescriber's hand-written signature

When accepting a prescription order from a customer, the role of a pharmacy technician begins with double-checking the prescription for accuracy and ensuring that all legal requirements have been met.

The Components of a Patient Prescription Label

Components of prescription labels may vary from state to state, but typically should contain the following information:

- The name of the patient
- The name of the prescriber
- The date the prescription was filled
- The number of refills remaining
- The date the prescription expires
- The date the product expires
- The name, strength, dosage form, and quantity of product dispensed (also called the inscription)
- Directions for use (also called the **signa**, often referred to as the "sig")
- The name, address, and phone number of the pharmacy
- The Rx number
- If it is a prescription for a controlled substance, the statement "Caution: Federal law prohibits the transfer of this drug to any person other than the patient for whom it was prescribed" must be printed on the label
- Any necessary auxiliary labels

If a medication has the symbol Rx on the bottle, it can only be dispensed pursuant to a prescription.

Commonly Used Abbreviations

In most cases, the directions (signa) are written in shorthand, or an abbreviated form that allows for the easy writing of directions. Directions generally include how and when to take the medication ordered.

To fill the prescription safely, the pharmacy technician must have knowledge of commonly used abbreviations found in prescription orders. These abbreviations are standard usage for prescribers, pharmacists, and pharmacy technicians, but must be spelled out as simply as possible for the patient to ensure that the patient uses the medication properly. Never assume that directions are easily understood by a patient.

TABLE 4.1 contains a list of abbreviations used in writing prescriptions.

Here are several examples of the use of commonly used abbreviations, and their translations:

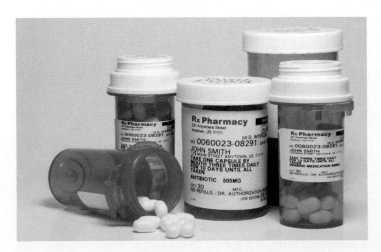

The label on a prescription bottle.

Table 4.1   Commonly Used Abbreviations

Abbreviation	Translation
ac	Before meals
am	Morning
AD	Right ear
AS	Left ear
AU	Both ears
bid	Twice a day
c̄	With
cap	Capsule
DAW	Dispense as written
D/C	Discontinue
g or gm	Gram
gr	Grain
gtt	Drop
h or hr or °	Hour
IM	Intramuscular
INH	Inhalation
IV	Intravenous
L	Liter
mcg	Microgram
mEq	Milliequivalent
mL	Milliliter
NKA	No known allergies
NKDA	No known drug allergies
npo	Nothing by mouth
OD	Right eye
OS	Left eye
OU	Both eyes
pc	After meals
PO	By mouth
PR	Per rectum
prn	As needed
q	Every
qid	Four times a day
qs	A sufficient quantity
SL	Sublingual
stat	Immediately
tab	Tablet
tid	Three times a day
top	Topically
ud	As directed
wk	Week

Example: iii gtts OS qid ud
Translation: Instill three drops into the left eye, four times a day as directed.

Example: 1 tab po tid×5 days
Translation: Take one tablet by mouth three times a day for five days.

Example: 1 supp pr bid prn
Translation: Insert one suppository rectally twice a day as needed.

Example: 0.5 mL SQ tid prn
Translation: Inject 0.5mL subcutaneously three times a day as needed.

Example: ii gtts OU qid
Translation: Instill two drops into both eyes, four times a day.

Example: 1 tab SL bid prn
Translation: Place one tablet under the tongue twice a day as needed.

Because of the concern over drug errors that have occurred from misinterpretation of prescription orders, the Institute for Safe Medication Practices (ISMP) has compiled a list of the most common misread abbreviations ▐TABLE 4.2▌.

> The ISMP has a list of error-prone abbreviations, symbols, and dose designations, which can be found at http://www.ismp.org/tools/errorproneabbreviations.pdf.

Table 4.2   Problematic Abbreviations Found on Prescription Orders

Abbreviations	Intended Meaning	Misinterpretation	Correction
µg	Microgram	Mistaken as "mg"	Use "mcg"
AD, AS, AU	Right ear, left ear, each ear	Mistaken as OD, OS, OU (right eye, left eye, each eye)	Use "right ear," "left ear," or "each ear"
OD, OS, OU	Right eye, left eye, each eye	Mistaken as AD, AS, AU (right ear, left ear, each ear)	Use "right eye," "left eye," or "each eye"
BT	Bedtime	Mistaken as "BID" (twice daily)	Use "bedtime"
cc	Cubic centimeters	Mistaken as "u" (units)	Use "mL"
D/C	Discharge or discontinue	Premature discontinuation of medications if D/C (intended to mean "discharge") has been misinterpreted as "discontinued" when followed by a list of discharge medications	Use "discharge" and "discontinue"
IJ	Injection	Mistaken as "IV" or "intrajugular"	Use "injection"
IN	Intranasal	Mistaken as "IM" or "IV"	Use "intranasal" or "NAS"
HS Hs	Half-strength, At bedtime, hours of sleep	Mistaken as bedtime Mistaken as half-strength	Use "half-strength" or "bedtime"
IU**	International unit	Mistaken as IV (intravenous) or 10 (ten)	Use "units"

Table 4.2   Problematic Abbreviations Found on Prescription Orders *(Continued)*

Abbreviations	Intended Meaning	Misinterpretation	Correction
o.d. or OD	Once daily	Mistaken as "right eye" (OD-oculus dexter), leading to oral liquid medications administered in the eye	Use "daily"
OJ	Orange juice	Mistaken as OD or OS (right or left eye); drugs meant to be diluted in orange juice may be given in the eye	Use "orange juice"
Per os	By mouth, orally	The "os" can be mistaken as "left eye" (OS-oculus sinister)	Use "PO," "by mouth," or "orally"
q.d. or QD**	Every day	Mistaken as q.i.d., especially if the period after the "q" or the tail of the "q" is misunderstood as an "i"	Use "daily"
qhs	Nightly at bedtime	Mistaken as "qhr" or every hour	Use "nightly"
qn	Nightly or at bedtime	Mistaken as "qh" (every hour)	Use "nightly" or "at bedtime"
q.o.d. or QOD**	Every other day	Mistaken as "q.d." (daily) or "q.i.d." (four times daily) if the "o" is poorly written	Use "every other day"
q1d	Daily	Mistaken as q.i.d. (four times daily)	Use "daily"
q6PM, etc.	Every evening at 6 PM	Mistaken as every 6 hours	Use "daily at 6 PM" or "6 PM daily"
SC, SQ, sub q	Subcutaneous	SC mistaken as SL (sublingual); SQ Mistaken as "5 every"; the "q" in "sub q" has been mistaken as "every" (e.g., a heparin dose ordered "sub q 2 hours before surgery" misunderstood as every 2 hours before surgery)	Use "subcut" or "subcutaneously"
ss	Sliding scale (insulin) or ½ (apothecary)	Mistaken as "55"	Spell out "sliding scale;" use "one-half" or "1/2"
SSRI	Sliding scale regular insulin	Mistaken as selective-serotonin reuptake inhibitor	Spell out "sliding scale (insulin)"
SSI	Sliding scale insulin	Mistaken as Strong Solution of Iodine (Lugol's)	
i/d	One daily	Mistaken as "tid"	Use "1 daily"
TIW or tiw (also BIW or biw)	TIW: 3 times a week	T/W mistaken as "3 times a day" or "twice in a week"	Use "3 times weekly"
	BIW: 2 times a week	B/W mistaken as "2 times a day"	Use "2 times weekly"

Table 4.2   Problematic Abbreviations Found on Prescription Orders *(Continued)*

Abbreviations	Intended Meaning	Misinterpretation	Correction
U or u**	Unit	Mistaken as the number 0 or 4, causing a 10-fold overdose or greater (e.g., 4U seen as "40" or 4u seen as "44"); mistaken as "cc" so dose given in volume instead of units (e.g., 4u seen as 4cc)	Use "unit"
UD	As directed ("ut dictum")	Mistaken as unit dose (e.g., diltiazem 125 mg IV infusion "UD" misinterpreted as meaning to give the entire infusion as a unit [bolus] dose)	Use "as directed"

Dose Designations and Other Information	Intended Meaning	Misinterpretation	Correction
Trailing zero after decimal point (e.g., 1.0 mg)**	1 mg	Mistaken as 10 mg if the decimal point is not seen	Do not use trailing zeros for doses expressed in whole numbers
No leading zero before a decimal point (e.g., .5 mg)**	0.5 mg	Mistaken as 5 mg if the decimal point is not seen	Use zero before a decimal point when the dose is less than a whole unit
Drug name and dose run together (especially problematic for drug names that end in "l" such as Inderal40 mg; Tegretol300 mg)	Inderal 40 mg Tegretol 300 mg	Mistaken as Inderal 140 mg Mistaken as Tegretol 1300 mg	Place adequate space between the drug name, dose, and unit of measure
Numerical dose and unit of measure run together (e.g., 10mg, 100mL)	10 mg 100 mL	The "m" is sometimes mistaken as a zero or two zeros, risking a 10- to 100-fold overdose	Place adequate space between the dose and unit of measure
Abbreviations such as mg. or mL. with a period following the abbreviation	mg, mL	The period is unnecessary and could be mistaken as the number 1 if written poorly	Use mg, mL, etc. without a terminal period
Large doses without properly placed commas (e.g., 100000 units; 1000000 units)	100,000 units 1,000,000 units	100000 has been mistaken as 10,000 or 1,000,000; 1000000 has been mistaken as 100,000	Use commas for dosing units at or above 1,000, or use words such as 100 "thousand" or 1 "million" to improve readability

Drug Name Abbreviations	Intended Meaning	Misinterpretation	Correction
ARA A	vidarabine	Mistaken as cytarabine (ARA C)	Use complete drug name
AZT	zidovudine (Retrovir)	Mistaken as azathioprine or aztreonam	Use complete drug name
CPZ	Compazine (prochlorperazine)	Mistaken as chlorpromazine	Use complete drug name
DPT	Demerol-Phenergan-Thorazine	Mistaken as diphtheria-pertussis-tetanus (vaccine)	Use complete drug name
DTO	Diluted tincture of opium, or deodorized tincture of opium (Paregoric)	Mistaken as tincture of opium	Use complete drug name

Table 4.2   Problematic Abbreviations Found on Prescription Orders *(Continued)*

Abbreviations	Intended Meaning	Misinterpretation	Correction
HCl	hydrochloric acid or hydrochloride	Mistaken as potassium chloride (The "H" is misinterpreted as "K")	Use complete drug name unless expressed as a salt of a drug
HCT	hydrocortisone	Mistaken as hydrochlorothiazide	Use complete drug name
HCTZ	hydrochlorothiazide	Mistaken as hydrocortisone (seen as HCT250 mg)	Use complete drug name
MgSO4**	magnesium sulfate	Mistaken as morphine sulfate	Use complete drug name
MS, MSO4**	morphine sulfate	Mistaken as magnesium sulfate	Use complete drug name
MTX	methotrexate	Mistaken as mitoxantrone	Use complete drug name
PCA	procainamide	Mistaken as patient controlled analgesia	Use complete drug name
PTU	propylthiouracil	Mistaken as mercaptopurine	Use complete drug name
T3	Tylenol with codeine (No. 3)	Mistaken as liothyronine	Use complete drug name
TAC	triamcinolone	Mistaken as tetracaine Adrenalin, cocaine	Use complete drug name
TNK	TNKase	Mistaken as "TPA"	Use complete drug name
ZnSO4	zinc sulfate	Mistaken as morphine sulfate	Use complete drug name
Stemmed Drug Names	**Intended Meaning**	**Misinterpretation**	**Correction**
"Nitro" drip	nitroglycerin infusion	Mistaken as sodium nitroprusside infusion	Use complete drug name
"Norflox"	norfloxacin	Mistaken as Norflex	Use complete drug name
"IV Vanc"	intravenous vancomycin	Mistaken as Invanz	Use complete drug name
Symbols	**Intended Meaning**	**Misinterpretation**	**Correction**
ʒ	Dram	Symbol for dram mistaken as "3"	Use the metric system
♏	Minim	Symbol for minim mistaken as "mL"	Use the metric system
x3d	For three days	Mistaken as "3 doses"	Use "for three days"
> and <	Greater than and less than	Mistaken as opposite of intended; Mistakenly use incorrect symbol; "< 10" Mistaken as "40"	Use "greater than" or "less than"
/ (slash mark)	Separates two doses or indicates "per"	Mistaken as the number 1 (e.g., "25 units/10 units" misread as "25 units and 110 units")	Use "per" rather than a slash mark to separate doses
@	At	Mistaken as "2"	Use "at"
&	And	Mistaken as "2"	Use "and"
+	Plus or and	Mistaken as "4"	Use "and"
°	Hour	Mistaken as a zero (e.g., q2° seen as q 20)	Use "hr," "h," or "hour"
Ø	zero, null sign	Mistaken as the numerals 4, 6, or 9	Use the number "0" or the word "zero"

**These abbreviations are included on The Joint Commission's "minimum list" of dangerous abbreviations, acronyms, and symbols that must be included on an organization's "Do Not Use" list, effective January 1, 2004. Visit www.jcaho.org for more information about this Joint Commission requirement.

Most pharmacies will also give the patient an information sheet with more details regarding the proper administration of the medication, possible side effects, and adverse drug interactions.

In some cases, the prescription directions may be difficult to interpret. If there is a question regarding the information on the prescription, the pharmacist should be notified. In most cases, the pharmacist will be able to clarify the information or if necessary; call the physician for clarification.

The "Rights" of Correct Drug Administration

When a pharmacy technician fills a patient's prescription, it is important to remember the basic "rights" of a patient with regard to medication safety. These rights offer useful guidelines when filling prescriptions. The rights of a patient to medication safety are as follows:

- The right patient—Always verify that the medication prescribed is for the correct patient. Use at least two patient identifiers.
- The right drug—Always check the medication bottle and medication against the original prescription, making sure to take into account the patient's disease state.
- The right dose—Always check the original prescription to verify the strength of the medication, paying particular attention to the age of the patient.
- The right route—Always check the prescriber's prescription order to make sure it agrees with the drug's specified route of administration.
- The right time—Always check the prescription to determine the correct frequency and duration for the medication to be administered.

Dosage Forms

Drugs are seldom administered in pure form. They are formulated into various dosage forms to facilitate ease of administration and ensure safety and efficacy. A **dosage form** is a system or device by which the drug is delivered to the body. In a dosage form, the active ingredient is combined with the inert ingredients that facilitate administration of the drug.

The most common dosage forms are those that are administered orally. Taking an oral medication is the most convenient method to deliver medication, which in turn makes it the most in demand, which leads to mass production and ultimately lower manufacturing costs. Some medications are not available in oral form because they cannot be properly absorbed in the GI tract. For instance, heparin is only available as an injectable formulation because it is ineffective when administered orally. The route of administration and dosage form are also determined by other factors, including the age of the patient, the disease being treated, the area of the body that the drug needs to reach, the ease of administration, and the characteristics of the drug.

The active ingredient is responsible for a drug's therapeutic effect.

An inert ingredient has little or no therapeutic value.

Dosage forms may also contain the following:

- Additives—**Additives** are inert ingredients that may be needed for a successful preparation of the dosage form.
- Binders—**Binders** promote adhesion of active and inactive ingredients in the tablets.
- Diluents—**Diluents** are additives used to increase the bulk weight or volume of a dosage form.
- Excipients—**Excipients** are inactive substances used as a carrier for the active ingredient.
- Preservatives—**Preservatives** are substances that prevent or minimize the growth of bacteria or other microorganisms in the dosage form, typically used in multi-dose vials. Single-dose vials are discarded immediately after use, while multi-dose vials, once opened, may be stored for a period. After a vial has been opened, however, the risk of bacterial overgrowth increases. To prevent or minimize the risk of bacterial overgrowth, preservatives are added to the medication.

Many top-selling drugs are available in several different dosage forms. It is important to know what dosage form is being requested because the strength of the medication may depend on the dosage form. It also ensures that the patient does not use a dosage form incorrectly, such as swallowing a suppository. Knowing the dosage form can serve as a double-check when a prescription calls for a certain strength of medication that is available in more than one dosage form.

The strength of the same medication can vary from one dosage form to another.

Solid Dosage Forms

Solid dosage forms include tablets, capsules, caplets, lozenges/troches, pastilles, powders, and granules. Solid dosage forms offer several advantages:

- Increased stability
- Ease of packaging, storage, and dispensing
- Convenience
- Little or no taste or smell

Solid dosage forms also allow for accurate dosing. The entire dose is contained within the contents of the solid dosage form, which minimizes measuring errors. Solid dosage forms may, however, be difficult to swallow, have a slow onset of action, and may be degraded by the acidic contents in the stomach.

Tablets/Caplets

Tablets are available in variety of sizes, shapes, colors, and thicknesses. They are formed in molds or produced by compression, and are composed of one or more active ingredients and one or more inert substances.

Some pharmaceutical manufacturers manufacture a hybrid of the capsule and tablet, called a caplet. A **caplet** is a tablet that is shaped like a capsule, but smooth-sided like a tablet. It is often easier to swallow than large tablets, and is more stable than capsules (discussed in a moment).

Most tablets and caplets are designed to be swallowed whole and dissolve in the gastrointestinal tract, but some are also made to be administered sublingually (under the tongue), buccally, or vaginally. Some tablets are available in a scored form so they may be easily broken in halves or quarters. Tablets can be formulated with delayed-release characteristics to allow for less-frequent dosing and/or side effects.

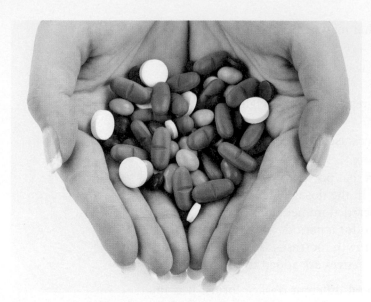

Tablets are manufactured in a variety of sizes and colors.

A **chewable tablet** is designed to be chewed. Chewable tablets contain a base that is flavored or colored. They are convenient for patients who have difficulty swallowing tablets or for children who are unable to swallow large tablets. An **oral disintegrating tablet (ODT)** is designed to dissolve in the mouth without water. These tablets are useful for pediatric and geriatric patients who have difficulty swallowing medication and in patients who are experiencing nausea and vomiting. Another benefit of ODTs is that they cannot be "cheeked" by patients who may attempt to be non-compliant with medication therapy that is administered by a caregiver, as with a nursing home patient.

Enteric-Coated Tablets

Tablets may have a coating applied to the outside to mask unpleasant flavor or odor, or to protect the drug from stomach contents. **Enteric-coated** tablets are coated with a substance that prevents dissolution of the drug in the stomach. They are meant to dissolve in the intestine to protect the drug from being broken down in the stomach or to protect the stomach lining from the drug. Enteric-coated dosage forms should not be chewed, broken, or crushed. Examples of drugs that are available in enteric-coated formulations include aspirin and potassium chloride.

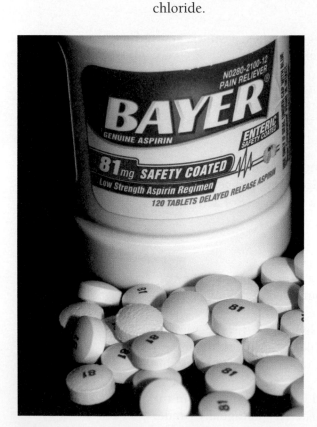

Enteric coated tablets prevent dissolution of the drug in the stomach.

Film-Coated Tablets

Film-coated tablets are coated with a thin outer layer of water-soluble material that dissolves rapidly in the stomach. The coating is designed to cover the unpleasant taste or smell of the medication or protect sensitive drugs from deterioration due to air and light. Erythromycin is an example of a medication available as a film-coated tablet.

Sugar-Coated Tablets

Sugar-coated tablets are coated with an outside layer of sugar that protects the medication and improves the taste and the appearance of the medication.

Capsules

Capsules are a solid dosage form in which the drug is enclosed within a hard or soft gelatin shell. The gelatin shell dissolves in the stomach, releasing the drug. The gelatin shell may be transparent, semitransparent, or opaque. A capsule may contain powders, granules, crushed tablets, or liquids with one or more active ingredients and one or more inert ingredients. Capsules can be formulated with delayed-release characteristics to allow for less-frequent dosing and/or side effects.

Spansules are capsules that are filled with granules that dissolve at different rates, in effect causing a sustained release of the active ingredients. **Sprinkles** or sprinkle capsules are similar to spansules but unique in that they are designed to be pulled apart and the contents sprinkled onto food, making it easier to administer the medication. The medication inside a sprinkle capsule is specially coated to allow the medication to be delivered after the contents have been ingested. They are convenient for patients who have difficulty swallowing large capsules or for children who are unable to swallow capsules.

Sizes of capsules range from 000 (largest) to 5 (smallest). The volume of powder that can be placed in a given capsule varies depending on the density of the powder being placed in the empty capsule.

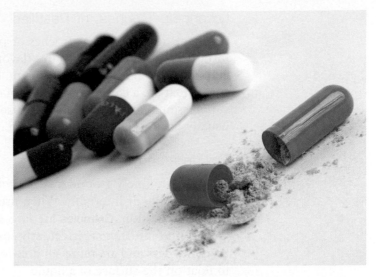

Capsules come in a variety of sizes.

Dosage Formulations Designed to Alter the Rate of Release

Tablets and capsules can be designed in **immediate-release** formulations, in which the medication is released within a short period of time after the drug is taken. They can also be designed in **delayed-release** formulations, which administer the drug over an extended period of time. A delayed-release formulation may be enteric coated, thus delaying the release of the medication until the formulation has passed through the stomach. Dosage forms designed to vary the rate or extent of release include the following:

- Controlled release—**Controlled-release** dosage forms regulate the rate of release of the active ingredient. They are designed to vary the dissolution rate or release of the active drug. These dosage forms are also referred to as long-acting and timed-release formulations.
- Sustained release—**Sustained-release** dosage forms allow the frequency of dosing of a medication to be reduced compared to that of immediate-release dosage forms.
- Extended release—**Extended-release** dosage forms are formulated so that the active ingredient is released at a constant rate for a prolonged period so that the frequency of dosing is less than that of immediate-release dosage forms. They usually allow for once-daily dosing, as the contained medication is available over an extended period of time following ingestion of the formulation.

Compared to immediate-release preparations, advantages of extended-release dosage forms include the following:

- Constant drug levels following long-term administration
- Reduction in adverse side effects
- Reduction in the frequency of administration
- Increased patient compliance

Immediate-release formulations are designed to release the medication within a short period of time.

Lozenges, Troches, or Pastilles

Lozenges, also known as troches or pastilles, are hard, oval, or discoid solid dosage forms with a drug contained in a flavored sugar base. They are dissolved in the mouth and generally have local therapeutic effects. Over-the-counter lozenges for relief of sore throat are a common example of this dosage form. Antibiotics, analgesics, cough suppressants, and antiseptics are also available as lozenges. Troche sizes vary; they usually have a chalky consistency in order to dissolve in the mouth.

Powders and Granules

Powders are finely ground mixtures of dry drugs and inactive ingredients that can be used topically or internally. When used internally, they should be dissolved in water prior to ingestion. **Granules** are larger than powders and are wetted, allowed to dry, and ground into coarse, irregularly shaped pieces. Granules are generally more stable than powders and are more suitable for use in solutions because they are not as likely to float on the surface of a liquid.

Semisolid Dosage Forms

Semisolid agents are different in their composition from liquids or solids. They are usually intended for topical application. They may be applied to the skin, placed on mucous membranes, or used in the nasal, rectal, or vaginal cavity. These dosage forms are too thick to be considered a liquid dosage form and not solid enough to be considered a solid dosage form. Examples include ointments, creams, lotions, gels, pastes, and suppositories.

An **emulsion** is a type of semi-solid dosage form. It is a mixture of two substances that are unblendable. One substance is dispersed in the other. An **oil-in-water (O/W) emulsion** contains a small amount of oil dispersed in water. A **water-in-oil (W/O) emulsion** contains a small amount of water dispersed in oil. An emulsion, which has a different composition than the two individual liquids that are mixed together, is dispensed in containers that hold liquids.

An emulsion is a mixture of two liquids that do not blend.

Ointments

An **ointment** is applied externally to the skin or mucous membranes. An ointment is an example of a W/O emulsion because it contains a small amount of water dispersed throughout oil. Ointments can also be formulated and sterilized for use in the eye. Ointments contain medication in a glycol or oil base and can effectively cover the surface of the skin. Examples of ointments include erythromycin ophthalmic ointment and Neosporin. Ointments are generally greasier than creams or gels, and can leave an oily residue at the site of application.

An ointment is an example of a water-in-oil (W/O) emulsion.

Creams

A **cream** contains suspensions or solutions of drugs intended for external use. A cream is an example of an O/W emulsion because it contains a small amount of oil dispersed in water. Creams can be easily massaged into the skin, without leaving an oily residue. They usually have medications in a base that is part oil and part water.

Creams can also be formulated for vaginal or rectal use. Examples of creams include hydrocortisone cream, benzoyl peroxide cream, and betamethasone valerate cream.

> A cream is an example of an oil-in-water (O/W) emulsion.

Lotions

A **lotion** is an O/W emulsion that is thinner than a cream because its base contains more water. Lotions penetrate into the skin and can cover large areas without leaving an oily residue. Examples of lotions include calamine lotion and hydrocortisone lotion.

> A lotion is an example of an oil-in-water (O/W) emulsion that is thinner than a cream.

Gels

A **gel** contains solid medication particles, like a suspension, in a thick liquid. It can be used internally and externally. The particles in a gel are ultrafine and are linked to form a semisolid. Gels penetrate the skin without leaving a residue. Examples of gels include aluminum hydroxide gel and benzocaine gel.

Pastes

A **paste** contains more solid material and less liquid base than a solid. Pastes are like ointments, but are stiffer, less greasy, and applied more thickly. One example of a paste is zinc oxide.

Suppositories

A **suppository** is designed to be inserted rectally, vaginally, or urethrally. The suppository base is an inactive ingredient, which melts or dissolves in the body cavity, releasing the medication. Some suppositories are designed for local action, while others are used as vehicles for systemic drugs. A hydrocortisone rectal suppository is used for local relief. Suppositories are often used in children and in adults who are unable to take oral medications. Rectal suppositories bypass the stomach, which is helpful if the patient has nausea or vomiting. They are also used to treat inflammatory bowel disease or pain. Vaginal suppositories are used to treat yeast infections and vaginal atrophy. Examples of suppositories include miconazole vaginal suppositories and bisacodyl rectal suppositories.

Liquid Dosage Forms

Liquid dosage forms contain one or more active ingredients in a liquid vehicle such as a solution, suspension, or emulsion. The drug may be dissolved in the vehicle or suspended as very fine particles. They can be administered by many routes, but are often less stable than medications in solid dosage forms.

Liquid dosage forms offer several advantages:

- They allow for easier dosage adjustments, particularly for pediatric patients.
- They are easier to swallow, particularly for pediatric and geriatric patients.
- The onset of action is faster than that of solid dosage forms.
- They are easier to place down a feeding tube.

Liquid dosage forms have several disadvantages:

- Loss of potency occurs faster than with solid dosage forms.

- There is difficulty in masking bitter taste or odor.
- There is a need for preservatives because liquid doses provide an excellent medium for the growth of microorganisms.
- There is a potential for dosing inaccuracy.
- They are inconvenient.

Solutions

A **solution** is an evenly distributed (**homogenous**) mixture of one or more dissolved medications (**solutes**) in a liquid vehicle (**solvent**). Solutions can be classified by vehicle as an **aqueous solution** (water-based), an **alcoholic solution** (alcohol-based), or a **hydroalcoholic solution** (water- and alcohol-based). Solutions can be for internal and external use.

Solutions can also be classified by their contents:

- Aromatic water—**Aromatic water** is a solution of water that contains oil or other substances that are volatile. They usually have a pleasant smell.
- Elixir—An **elixir** is a clear, sweet solution that contains dissolved medication in a base of water and ethanol (hydroalcoholic).
- Syrup—**Syrup** is a sugar-based solution that may be medicated or non-medicated. Syrups mask the taste of the drug.
- Extract—An **extract** is a powder or liquid derived from animal or plant sources in which all or most of the solvent has been evaporated.
- Tincture—A **tincture** is an alcoholic or hydroalcoholic solution that contains plant extracts.

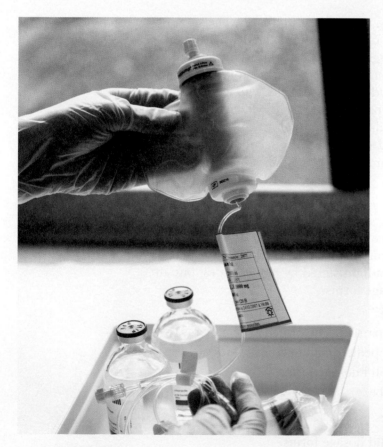

Various injectable dosage forms.

- Spirit—A **spirit** is an alcoholic or hydroalcoholic solution that contains volatile, aromatic ingredients.
- Irrigating solution—An **irrigating solution** is a solution that is used for cleansing an area of the body.

Solutions can also be classified by their method of administration as topical, systemic, epicutaneous, percutaneous, oral, otic, ophthalmic, parenteral, vaginal, or urethral.

A **parenteral solution** is a sterile solution that is administered by a needle or catheter via injection or infusion. It can be administered in an **intravenous (IV)**, **intramuscular (IM)**, **subcutaneous (SC)**, or **intradermal (ID)** manner.

Injectable dosage forms are marketed in ampules, vials, pre-filled syringes, and pre-filled infusion bags. Most vials contain solutions up to 50mL. A vial will contain either a single dose, which is meant for withdrawal of one dose before the vial is discarded, or multidose, which means the vial can be pierced multiple times to retrieve multiple doses. Some vials come in powder form and will need to have diluents added before administration. The addition of a diluent to a powder vial is called

reconstitution. The vial will give information as to how much and which diluent is needed to obtain a specific concentration. Pre-filled syringes or infusion bags have the medication in ready-to-administer form.

Dispersions

Some drugs do not dissolve in the solvents that are used to prepare liquid dosage forms. In a **dispersion**, the medication is not dissolved, but distributed throughout the vehicle. A **suspension** is a mixture of undissolved, very fine, solid particles distributed through a gas, liquid, or solid. Most suspensions contain medications distributed in water; this type of suspension is called an **aqueous suspension**. Suspensions are used for drugs that are not able to dissolve readily into a solution. Suspensions need to be shaken prior to use and should contain a "shake well" auxiliary label. The pharmacy tech must shake a suspension prior to pouring an amount from a stock bottle into a bottle for dispensing.

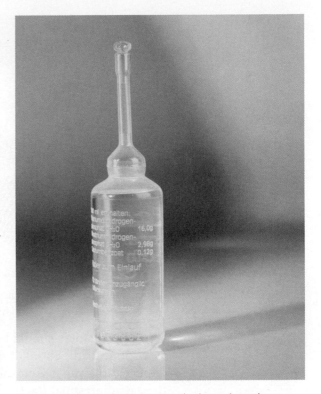

Injectable suspensions allow for insoluble drugs to be administered intramuscularly or subcutaneously. They are often used for **depot** therapy, where the drug is released over a long period of time.

Enemas can be used to evacuate the lower intestine.

Suspensions have the following characteristics:

- The suspended material should be evenly distributed when the container is shaken.
- It should pour freely from the bottle or pass easily through a syringe or needle.
- When used externally, it should dry quickly and spread easily over the affected area.

As mentioned, an emulsion is a mixture of two liquids that are immiscible (do not blend). It is a dispersion, with one liquid being dispersed in the other. They vary in their viscosity from liquids such as lotions to semisolid dosage forms such as ointments and creams. In an emulsion, one liquid is broken into small particles and evenly scattered throughout the other liquid. The liquid that is in small particles is called the internal phase, and the other liquid is called the external phase. The two liquids will separate into two phases unless an **emulsifying agent**, an ingredient used to bind together substances that normally do not mix, is used. An emulsifying agent is a chemical that has water-loving and lipid-loving properties that can keep oil and water together.

Enemas

Enemas are used to deliver medication, rectally, a way that bypasses the stomach. Enemas are manufactured in a water base and can also be used to evacuate the lower intestine to prepare for surgeries or examinations involving the intestine.

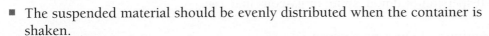

An enema can be used to deliver medication to bypass the stomach.

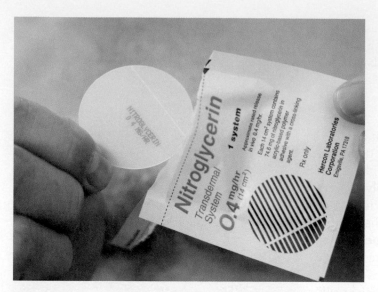

Nitroglycerin is available in a transdermal patch formulation.

Inhalation Dosage Forms

Some patient populations, such as asthmatic patients, need to have their medications delivered to a specific site in the body, such as the bronchial tree. Gases, vapors, aerosols, powders, sprays, solutions, and suspensions intended to be inhaled via the nose or mouth are known as inhalations, after the term **inhalation**, or the acts of inhaling or breathing in. The medication particles must be extremely fine to reach these areas effectively. Devices that enable the medication to reach the lungs easily include vaporizers, humidifiers, and nebulizers.

An **aerosol** is a spray that contains very fine liquid or solid drug particles in a gas propellant that is packaged under pressure. An aerosol dosage form consists of the medication, the container, and the propellant. Pressurized aerosol containers should be stored away from heat. The medication may be released as a spray, foam, or solid, depending on the formulation of the product and on the design of the valve. Aerosols have a rapid onset of action because the drug bypasses the gastrointestinal tract.

A **spray** consists of a container that has a valve assembly unit that contains various bases, such as alcohol or water, in a pump-type dispenser. When activated, it emits a fine dispersion of liquid, solid, or gaseous material.

Transdermal Dosage Forms

A **transdermal patch** dosage form is designed to hold a specific amount of medication to be released into the skin and absorbed into the bloodstream over time via a patch or disk. The patch consists of a backing, drug reservoir, control membrane, and adhesive layer. The backing is removed and the adhesive layer is applied to the skin. The drug is slowly absorbed across the membranes of the skin and into the skin where optimal absorption into the bloodstream will occur. Patches are convenient because they can be applied easily and minimize stomach upset. They can also improve compliance because they eliminate the need for more frequent dosing that is often associated with oral dosage forms. Drugs such as nitroglycerin, fentanyl, scopolamine, and nicotine are administered in this manner for their systemic effects.

Not all medications designed to be administered transdermally are in the form of patches. Some gels are also formulated to be administered transdermally. These gels are also designed to hold a specific amount of medication to be absorbed into the skin and bloodstream over time. The drug is slowly absorbed across the membranes of the skin and into the skin, where optimal absorption in the bloodstream will occur.

Routes of Administration

Medications can be administered by many different routes. A **route of administration** is the way to get a drug into or onto the body. Sometimes, combinations of routes are used at the same time. The age and condition of the patient often determines the route of administration. The oral route is the most common route of administration. Following is a list of routes of administration:

- Buccal—Administered inside the mouth on the mucosa of the cheek
- Dental—Application to teeth or gums
- Epidural—Injection on or outside the dura meter of the spinal cord
- External—Applied externally to the skin or hair
- Implant—Placing a drug form, drug-delivery device, or other device at the desired administration site by insertion in a body tissue or body cavity by surgical or other appropriate insertion procedures
- In vitro—Occurs within the laboratory or controlled experimental environment rather than in the body
- Inhalation—Drug administration into the lungs (either during a drawn or forced breath)
- Injection—A set of one or more injectable routes or the route of injection is not specified
- Intra-arterial—Injection into an artery or intra-arterial port
- Intra-articular—Injection into a joint
- Intracavernosal—Injection into the corpora cavernosa
- Intradermal—Injection within the epidermis (skin)
- Intramuscular—Injection into a muscle group
- Intraocular—Injection, implantation, or surgical irrigation within the eyeball
- Intraperitoneal—Administration into the intraperitoneal cavity, commonly by injection or instillation into an intraperitoneal catheter port
- Intrapleural—Injection into the pleura or pleural cavity
- Intrathecal—Injection into a subarachnoid or subdural space
- Intrauterine—Administered into the uterus
- Intravenous—Injection directly into a vein or into a venous line port
- Intravesical—Administered into the bladder
- Irrigation—To flush a body cavity or site with a stream of liquid
- Mouth/Throat—Applied to a mucus membrane of the oral cavity or throat
- Nasal—Administered via the nose
- Ophthalmic—Administered onto the surface of the eyeball or into the conjuctival sac
- Oral—Taken by mouth
- Otic—Commonly administered into the external ear canal
- Perfusion—Administration (pumping) of a fluid through an organ or tissue
- Rectal—Administered into the rectum (in the anal canal beyond the anal sphincter)
- Subcutaneous—Injection through the skin into the loose subcutaneous tissue under the skin
- Sublingual—Administered under the tongue
- Transdermal—Applied topically (e.g., a patch or ointment), with absorption through the skin for local or systemic effect
- Translingual—Drug absorption through the tongue into systemic circulation after application on the tongue
- Urethral—Administered via insertion or instillation into the urethra
- Vaginal—Administered into the vagina

Peroral

The **peroral (PO)** route is commonly referred to as the oral route. It means that the drug is administered orally through the mouth and swallowed to reach the stomach. It must then undergo dissolution in the stomach, absorption in either the stomach or small intestine, activation in the liver, and distribution to the tissue before it exerts its therapeutic effect.

Advantages of the oral route are that it is safe and convenient and easy to tolerate. In addition, the medications are usually less expensive, and are available in extended-release forms. A patient can take one or more tablets or, if the tablet is scored, a portion of the tablet. Sustained-release and extended-release tablets provide a longer duration of action and, in some cases, fewer side effects. Liquid solutions and suspensions are useful in those patients who have difficulty swallowing. They also work more quickly than tablets and capsules because they are already in liquid form and ready to be absorbed.

Disadvantages include a time delay between administration of the drug and the onset of action, the possible interference of food and other drugs with absorption of the drug, and the possible degradation of the drug by gastrointestinal fluids. Side effects that occur with sustained-release medications also take longer to subside. Liquid formulations sometimes have an unpleasant taste, which may make compliance more difficult. Patients who are experiencing nausea or vomiting or who are sedated or otherwise unable to swallow should not take medications via the oral route.

Sublingual (under the tongue) and **buccal** (between the check and gum) routes of administration are used when a rapid onset of action is needed. The medication is absorbed directly by the blood vessels under the tongue or in the lining of the mouth. When taking the medication sublingually, the patient should hold the tablet under the tongue until the medication dissolves **FIGURE 4.2**. Nitroglycerin is the most commonly used sublingual tablet. Drugs administered sublingually have a rapid onset of action because they enter the bloodstream directly. When taking the medication buccally, the patient should place the tablet between the gums and cheek and hold the tablet there until it dissolves.

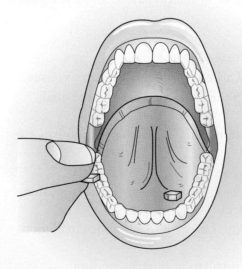

FIGURE 4.2 The correct way to take a medication that is administered sublingually.

Following Directions with Oral Medications

Patients should receive verbal and written instructions from the pharmacist about what foods and behaviors to avoid while taking their medication. Auxiliary labels added to the medication container can help ensure that the drug is taken correctly.

Dispensing Oral Medications

Dispensing measuring spoons, oral syringes, droppers, and cups with the liquid medication can help ensure that the patient or caregiver measures the dose correctly. Many directions, both on prescription and over-the-counter products, include use of teaspoonful or tablespoonful, but most household utensils are often inaccurate. Many over-the-counter liquid preparations come with a measuring cup for ease of administration. Most pharmacies will provide measuring spoons or cups, syringes, or droppers with the medication.

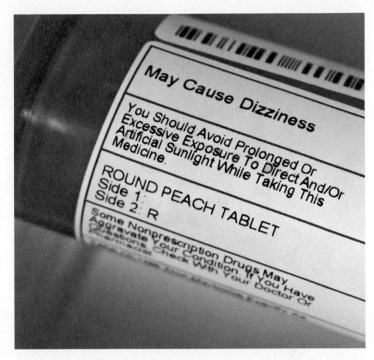

Auxiliary labels provide important information to help the patient take the drug correctly.

An oral syringe is often used to deliver a precise amount of liquid medication to children. It is a calibrated syringe that has a plunger and barrel, which is used to slowly administer liquid medication to infants and small children or to patients who have difficulty opening their mouth.

Droppers can be used to deliver a small amount of medication to an infant. It consists of a small squeezable bulb and a hollow tube with a narrow point. The size of the drop can vary from one medication to another, depending on the thickness or viscosity of the medication.

Some solutions and suspensions have specific storage requirements and limited dates of expiration. Some antibiotics must be refrigerated after reconstitution and are only good for 7 to 14 days. Suspensions must be shaken before administration to ensure that the medication is uniformly distributed into solution.

> Suspensions must have an auxiliary label, "Shake Well," to ensure that the medication is shaken before administration.

Parenteral

The parenteral route of administration bypasses the gastrointestinal tract. Drugs that are administered by this route can be given over a short (seconds to minutes) or extended (days) period of time. This route of administration distributes the drug systemically throughout the body to exert a systemic effect. Parenteral administration may be necessary when drugs are inactivated in the stomach or undergo significant first-pass metabolism, so swallowing them

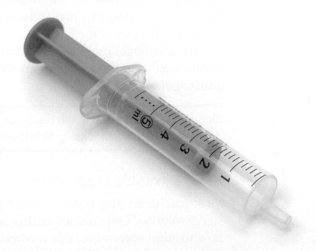

Use of dosing aids can promote more accurate dosing for infants and young children who need to take liquid medications.

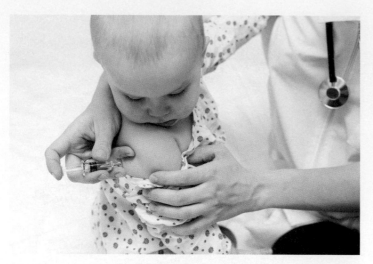

Some drugs can be administered intramuscularly.

would be ineffective. The majority of drugs for parenteral administration are formulated as solutions, but they may also be emulsions or suspensions. Drugs that are administered by this route are given via injection and must be sterile and free from particles. Drugs that are administered by this route are administered into the vein (IV), subcutaneously (SC), intradermally (ID) or intramuscularly (IM). When a drug is given all at once or over a short period of time, it is called a **bolus dose** and is administered by IV push via a syringe or needle. If it is infused into a vein over hours or days, it is called a constant infusion.

Advantages of this route include that it can be used in patients who cannot take medications orally, it has a faster onset of action, and it can be used for drugs that are unstable in the acidic environment of the stomach. The IV route is the fastest route of drug administration.

Disadvantages of this route include pain at the injection site, risk of infection, and the drugs are usually more expensive. Another disadvantage is that, because injectable drugs exert their action quickly, there is little or no time to alter its availability if the wrong dose is given or an adverse reaction occurs. IV injections must be free from air bubbles and particulate matter to prevent an embolism or blockage. Absorption of the drug by the IM or SC route is not as predictable as the IV route, but drugs administered via this route may have a longer duration of action because they can be given as depot formulations, and thus are not metabolized quickly.

When a drug is administered by injection into a muscle, it is called intramuscular (IM). The most common sites for intramuscular injection are the upper arm, the thigh, or the buttock. The advantages of IM injection include a more rapid onset of action than oral dosage forms. The disadvantages of this route of administration include that it is difficult to reverse, it may cause pain or bruising, absorption may be incomplete, and only a small volume of drug can be injected. It should also be used cautiously in patients with decreased muscle mass.

When a drug is administered below the skin, it is called subcutaneous (SC, SQ, or subQ). Drugs that are administered by this route are absorbed more slowly than by IV or IM routes. The main advantage of this route is that patients can be taught to self-administer their medication.

Disadvantages include only a limited volume of drug can be injected and it should also be used cautiously in patients with bleeding disorders or those who are receiving anticoagulants.

Drugs that are available in injectable formulations and given parenterally can be administered intravenously, subcutaneously, or intramuscularly.

Using Injectable Medications

Most parenteral preparations are prepared in a sterile-water, normal saline, or other sterile solution. Only trained healthcare professionals or patients who have been taught how to administer injectable medications should give injections.

A **syringe** is a calibrated medical instrument that is used to accurately draw up, measure, or deliver medication to a patient. The two types of syringes that are commonly used for injections are glass syringes and plastic syringes. Glass syringes are expensive and must be sterilized prior to use. Plastic syringes are easier to use because they are disposable and do not need to be sterilized prior to use. Syringe barrels can vary in size, depending upon the volume of medication needed. A needle is attached to the syringe to facilitate delivery of medication to the patient or to pierce the core of a vial to draw up the medication.

All drugs administered IV, SC, or IM must be sterile.

Intravenous Injections or Infusions

A medication can be given via an intravenous injection or as an **infusion**. It can be used to deliver antibiotics, IV fluids, pain medications, or nutritional supplements. These medications are usually administered into the vein of the arm.

Intramuscular Injections

Intramuscular injections (IM) can be used to deliver a small volume of medication (2 to 3mL). It can be used to deliver antibiotics, pain medications, vitamins, iron, and some vaccines. IM injections are usually injected into the upper, outer portion of the buttock. In children, it can also be given in the deltoid muscles of the shoulder. IM injections are administered at a 90-degree angle with a 22 to 25 gauge, $1/2$- to 1-inch needle FIGURE 4.3 .

Subcutaneous Injections

Subcutaneous injections (SC) can be used to deliver a small volume of medication (less than 1mL) into the subcutaneous tissue. SC injections are usually injected on the outside of the upper arm, the top of the thigh, or the

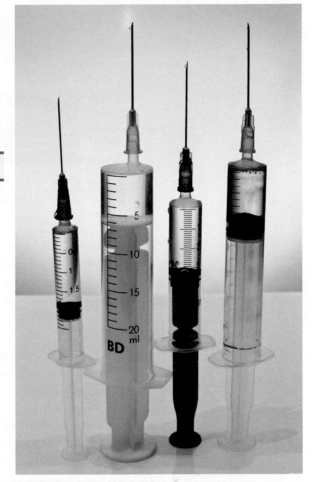

Syringes come in a variety of sizes. The syringe that should be used will depend on the volume of medication needed.

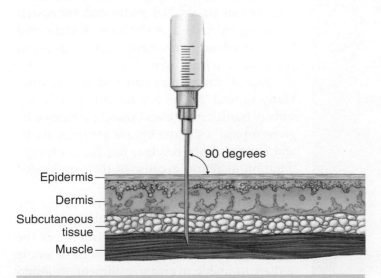

FIGURE 4.3 The correct way to administer an IM injection.

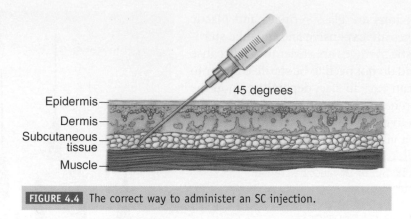

FIGURE 4.4 The correct way to administer an SC injection.

lower part of the abdomen. SC injections are administered at a 45 degree angle with a 25 to 26 gauge needle (with diabetic needle gauges now available up to 31 gauge) and a $^3/_8$- to $^5/_8$-inch needle **FIGURE 4.4**. In lean or obese patients, the injections should be administered closer to a 90-degree angle.

Topical

Topical route of administration refers to the application of a drug to the surface of the skin or mucous membranes. Drug forms administered this way include creams, ointments, gels, lotions, sprays, powders, aerosols, and transdermal formulations. The effects of topical preparations range from systemic (affecting the entire body) to localized (affecting a small area). The skin has many openings, including sweat glands, hair follicles, and pores through which drugs can pass through the skin. Topical agents can be used to fight skin infections, reduce inflammation, and protect the skin.

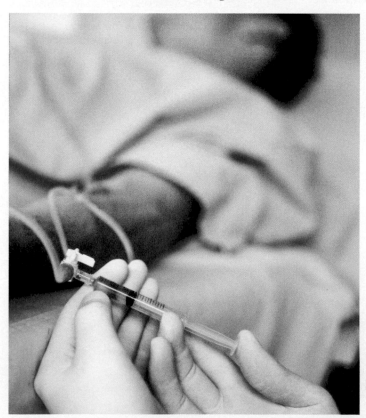

A patient receives medication intravenously.

Advantages of topical agents include ease of application, fewer adverse effects than the same drug administered orally, and rapidity of action at the site of application. Most drugs that are applied topically are not well absorbed systemically, thereby reducing the incidence of side effects. Creams and gels are more cosmetically appealing and less greasy than ointments. Lotions can be applied easily and are easiest to use on hairy parts of the body. Transdermal formulations are convenient to use, and patient compliance is improved.

Topical drugs may cause skin irritation. Many topical agents are not adequately absorbed transdermally and therefore cannot be given topically. Ointments are generally sticky and leave an oily residue, but have a longer duration of action because of their prolonged contact time with the skin.

Medications can be administered via the **ophthalmic** route by instilling one drop or drops of medication into the conjunctival sac of the eye. All ophthalmic preparations must be sterile and are available in cream, ointment, or liquid formulations. Most ophthalmic medications are used to treat eye infections, inflammation, or conditions such as glaucoma. Drugs can also be administered via the **otic** route by instilling one drop or drops of medication into the ear. Medications used to treat ear conditions do not need to be sterile because they do not typically penetrate a sterile environment. They can be used to treat an ear infection, remove earwax buildup or reduce pain. If the patient has a tube in the ear, a suspension should be used instead of a solution. Most medications administered via this route are solutions and suspensions. Ophthalmic medications can be used to treat ear conditions, but otic medications cannot be used in the eye.

Medications can also be administered via the **nasal** route by instilling one or more drops of medication or one or more sprays into the nasal passages. Most nasal sprays are used to treat symptoms of colds and allergies.

Medications administered by the **rectal** route, through the anus and into the rectum, are commonly in the form of a suppository or an enema. They can be used if a person is vomiting and cannot take the medication orally or if the person is unconscious and needs medication. Rectal administration is preferred for drugs that are destroyed by stomach contents or that are metabolized too quickly by the liver. Ointments and creams are available for use rectally to treat inflammation. Drugs administered by this route may provide a local or systemic effect. The disadvantage of this route is that most people don't feel comfortable using this route of administration. The amount of drug absorbed rectally is also unpredictable and varies from one person to another depending on the retention time of the suppository.

Medications administered by the **vaginal** or **urethral** route come in suppositories, creams, ointments, foams, gels, and **rings**, which are vaginal dosage forms used to administer hormones for birth control or hormone-replacement therapy. An etonogestrel/ethinyl estradiol vaginal ring (Nuvaring) is considered birth control, while the estradiol acetate vaginal ring (Femring) is considered hormone-replacement therapy. Drugs must be inserted into the vagina or urethra to exert either a local or systemic effect. When used for a local effect, the drug provides a higher concentration of medication at the site and minimizes side effects seen when the drug is absorbed systemically. They can be used to treat infection, to treat inflammation, or for local or systemic birth control. These medications are sometimes difficult to use and can be uncomfortable.

Proper application or use of topical medications can ensure that the desired therapeutic effect is achieved. Improper technique or use can increase the risk of systemic absorption and side effects.

Ointments, Creams, Lotions, Gels

Some topical preparations have special instructions for use. In order to use them safely, patients should receive proper instructions on how to use them. For example, capsaicin cream, available over the counter, should be applied with gloves because the active ingredient can cause burning and irritation if accidentally rubbed near the eyes. Some drugs such as topical corticosteroids should be applied sparingly because using a thick layer can increase systemic absorption and increase the incidence of adverse effects.

Transdermal Patches

Patches can be applied to the arm, chest, back and behind the ear, usually in a hair-free area. The site of application should be rotated to minimize skin reactions. The duration of action for each transdermal formulation varies from one drug to another. Some patches should be changed daily, while others are changed every three to seven days. Some patches, such as nitroglycerin patches, exert their effect for 24 hours when worn for only 12 hours. Doctors recommend removing the patch at bedtime to minimize the development of tolerance. Localized heat from sun exposure, heating pads, electric blankets, hot tubs, and hot lamps should be avoided when using some transdermal formulations because it can increase absorption of the active drug into the bloodstream, resulting in an increase in adverse effects or toxicity.

The duration of therapeutic effect of a transdermal formulation varies from one drug to another.

Ophthalmic Medications

Proper installation of an ophthalmic preparation is necessary to avoid contamination of the eye. Ophthalmic medications must be at room or body temperature before instillation into the eye. Follow the manufacturer's recommendations for storage of ophthalmic preparations to ensure drug stability and minimize bacterial overgrowth.

Proper hand-washing techniques should be followed to prevent contamination of the application site or the medication container. The tip of the medication container should not touch the eye; this will help minimize contamination of the medication.

To instill a drop into the eye, the patient's head should be tilted back **FIGURE 4.5A**. A finger should be placed in the corner of the eye to prevent loss of the medication through the tear duct. Only one drop of medication should be administered at a time, and the eye should be kept closed for one to two minutes after application. If instilling more than one medication, wait at least five to 10 minutes between administrations of different drugs. If a solution or suspension and ointment are to be administered at the same time, administer the solution or suspension first and then wait five to 10 minutes before applying the ointment. To apply an ointment into the eye, the lower eyelid should be pulled down with one or two fingers to create a pouch **FIGURE 4.5B**. Only one thin layer of medication should be applied in the pouch at a time, and the

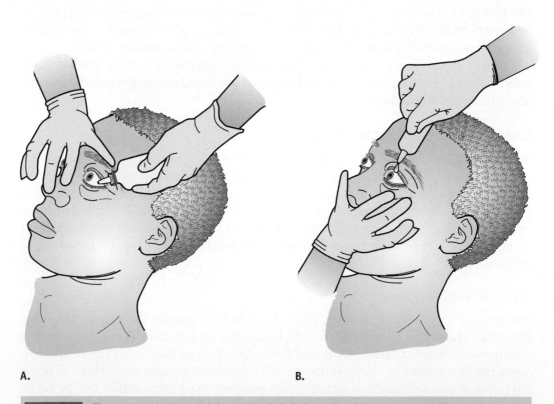

A.   **B.**

FIGURE 4.5   The correct way to administer an ophthalmic medication. A. Drops. B. Ointment.

eye should be kept closed for 30 seconds after application to let the ointment absorb.

An otic preparation should never be used in the eye, but an ophthalmic preparation can be used in the ear.

Otic Medications

Otic preparations must be at room or body temperature before instillation into the ear. Otics that are too hot could rupture the eardrum; those that are too cold can cause discomfort or pain.

To instill a drop into the ear, the patient's head should be tilted to the side so that the ear faces up. Patients who are under three years old should have their earlobes pulled back and down and those older than three should have their earlobes pulled back and up. After instillation, the patient should remain in this position for five minutes.

Inhaled Medications

Medications can also be administered via inhalation. This route delivers the medication from the mouth to the respiratory system. There are two types of inhalers: those that use a propellant to push the drug into the lungs (metered-dose inhaler) and those that use a dry powder to release the medication as the patient takes a deep, quick breath. The type of inhaler needed depends on the medication and the level of convenience required. Advantages of inhalants include convenience and portability. The onset of action is usually quick, but when used incorrectly, the medication will not be able to reach the lungs.

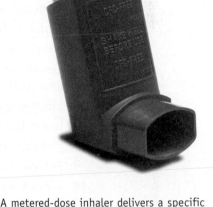

Proper administration of inhaled medications is necessary to ensure that the medication reaches the lungs. Some medications require that patients rinse their mouths thoroughly after each dose, not only to remove the aftertaste, but more importantly, to avoid developing an oral fungal infection. Spacer devices can ensure that a higher concentration of medication is inhaled and help improve drug delivery to the lungs.

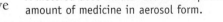

A metered-dose inhaler delivers a specific amount of medicine in aerosol form.

Here is the proper technique for using a metered-dose inhaler:

1. Take off the cap and shake the container.
2. Breathe out all the way.
3. Hold the inhaler 1 to 2 inches in front of mouth.
4. Breathe in slowly through your mouth and press down on the inhaler. Breathe in as deeply as you can.
5. Hold your breath and count to 10.
6. Repeat if more than one puff is required.

Vaginal Medications

The vaginal route is used to treat bacterial or fungal infections or to provide hormone-replacement therapy. Some vaginal creams or ointments require the use of an applicator tube. This route is also used for some forms of contraception.

Here is the proper technique for the administration of vaginal medications:

1. Empty the bladder.
2. Wash the vaginal area and dry thoroughly.
3. Wash hands thoroughly.

4. Attach the applicator to the opening of the tube and squeeze the medication into the applicator until it reaches the recommended dose.
5. Lie down, spread your legs, and open the labia with your free hand. (You can also stand with your feet apart and knees bent.)
6. Gently insert the applicator about 2 inches into the vagina and release the labia.
7. Push the plunger of the applicator until it stops.
8. Remove the applicator from the vagina and wash hands.
9. If the applicator is reusable, wash and dry the applicator.

Rectal Medications

Rectal medications are administered for a localized effect on the rectum or for a systemic effect when a patient is vomiting, unable to swallow, or unconscious. Rectal medicine is most commonly used as a localized treatment for constipation or as a topical treatment for rectal inflammation or **infection**.

Here is the proper technique for the administration of rectal suppositories:

1. Wash hands thoroughly.
2. If the suppository is soft, place in cold water to harden it before removing it from the wrapper.
3. Remove the suppository from the foil wrapper.
4. Lubricate the suppository with Vaseline or K-Y Jelly.
5. Lie on your side with the lower leg straightened out and the upper leg bent in toward the stomach.
6. Lift the upper buttock to expose the rectum.
7. Insert the pointed end of the suppository into the rectum.
8. Hold the buttocks together for a few seconds.
9. Remain lying down for 15 minutes.
10. Wash hands thoroughly.

Factors That Influence Drug Action

Many factors can influence the effect that a drug has on the body. For example, age, gender, and the presence of disease can affect the metabolism and elimination of a drug in the body. Children and the elderly often require a reduced dose because of their reduced weight or because of the inability of the liver to metabolize the medication adequately.

Patients with concomitant diseases are often unable to absorb, metabolize, or eliminate certain medications. Diseases that alter the normal gastrointestinal flora or change the environment of the stomach may also adversely affect the metabolism of drugs. In addition, impaired liver or kidney function may affect the metabolism and elimination of some drugs. Finally, nutritional status can affect the metabolism of some drugs. Before a medication is prescribed, the patient should have a medical evaluation.

Psychological and genetic factors can also influence the way a drug is metabolized in the body or eliminated from the body. Genes can control the release of chemicals and enhance or decrease the metabolism of certain drugs. Psychological factors can influence the body's ability to release certain chemicals necessary for the metabolism of certain drugs, or may interfere with the body's ability to absorb a drug.

Elderly Patients

Aging affects both the physiological processes in the body as well as the pharmacokinetic and pharmacodynamic processes that drugs undergo in the body. Elderly patients also tend to take more medications because they tend to have multiple chronic diseases. This can also increase the risk of drug-drug interactions and adverse side effects.

Changes in Physiology

Physiological changes that occur in the body do not occur at the same rate for each individual. The normal changes that occur in physiologic function with age are not related to disease. It is often difficult to predict when these changes will occur. Changes that occur as a result of aging can affect the metabolism and elimination of some drugs. Following is a list of some of the changes that can occur with age:

- Optic changes—Visual changes can occur and acuity can be compromised as the lenses of the eye become less elastic and more dense. Macular degeneration and cataracts can also occur in the elderly.
- Auditory changes—Hearing loss, especially in higher frequencies, can occur. Impairment of perception is common, which also results in a delay in the processing of auditory stimulation.
- Gastrointestinal changes—Decreases in esophageal motility, rate of gastric emptying, and saliva production are common complaints in the elderly.
- Pulmonary changes—Reduced oxygen in the blood, increased carbon dioxide in the blood, and a decrease in maximum intake and exhalation can occur as a result of increased rigidity of the chest wall. Complicating matters is the fact that many elderly patients have diseases such as chronic obstructive pulmonary disease (COPD) and cardiac disease.
- Cardiovascular changes—Elderly patients with cardiovascular disease have limited ability to meet the demand for increased oxygen to maintain cardiac output.
- Urinary changes—Instability of the bladder muscle, overflow, and sphincter weakness can result in **incontinence** (inability to hold urine in the bladder) or leakage. Elderly patients also have a higher incidence of renal insufficiency.
- Hormonal changes—Changes in hormone levels are a normal part of the aging process.
- Body changes—The amount of lean body mass and total body mass decreases with age, while the proportion of fat increases. The production of albumin, a blood plasma protein, also decreases with age. This can affect the amount of drug that is bound to plasma protein and the amount of free drug available to exert a therapeutic effect.

Response to Medication

Changes in the body can alter the response to medication. These physiological changes that occur as a result of aging can also affect the absorption, distribution, metabolism and elimination of some drugs.

- Absorption—Decreases in GI fluid secretion and motility can delay the absorption of some drugs. Absorption of some drugs can also be delayed by a reduction in the rate of gastric emptying. Changes in the gastrointestinal flora and environment of the stomach can also affect the dissolution and degradation of certain drugs.

- Distribution—The amount of free drug that is available can be altered by changes in body composition. In the elderly, a drug that is highly protein-bound can be toxic even when administered at normal doses because the amount of albumin decreases with age.
- Metabolism—Blood flow decreases by about 1% a year, beginning at age 35. This decline results in a decrease in clearance of the drug, allowing the drugs to accumulate to potentially toxic levels.
- Elimination—Most elderly patients have some degree of renal or hepatic dysfunction. The reduced filtration rate and reduction in blood flow and tubular secretions that result with aging can also affect the amount of drug that can be eliminated by the kidney.

Elderly patients tend to have multiple, chronic diseases that require long-term treatment with multiple medications. As a result, they are more likely to experience multiple adverse drug reactions. The term used to describe concurrent use of multiple medications is **polypharmacy**. When many drugs are prescribed for a patient, the potential for drug interactions is also high. The majority of adverse drug reactions in the elderly are the result of three drugs: warfarin, insulin, and digoxin.

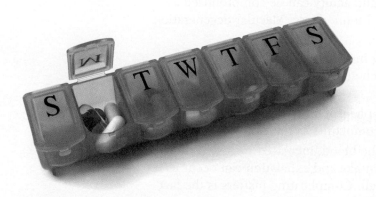

Tools such as a pillbox can help patients who take multiple medications remember when to take them.

The Beers list was initially created to help clinicians determine which medications should be avoided in nursing-home patients because seniors in nursing homes are particularly at risk for suffering medication-related problems. It was written by Dr. Mark Beers, a physician specializing in medical issues pertaining to the elderly. It is now useful for elderly patients in other settings. This list is periodically updated.

The Beers list is a list of medications that should be avoided or used cautiously in the elderly.

Aging can also affect the memory. The inability to adequately understand or remember directions for medication administration can lead to unintentional underdosing or overdosing, failure to take the drug, or taking a drug prescribed for another person. **Noncompliance** or failure to adhere to the prescribed drug regimen is especially common in the elderly. The pharmacy technician can play an important role in ensuring that elderly patients get written information and dosing aids that can help them remember to take their medication.

Noncompliance is the failure to adhere to the prescribed drug regimen.

Children

As children grow, their bodies undergo physiologic changes that can affect the absorption, distribution, metabolism, and elimination of a drug. Understanding these changes can help eliminate underdosing or overdosing that can occur in this patient population.

Body-surface area is the best measure to use to determine a dose because it correlates with all body parameters. Age is often used to determine the dose of a medication, but it does not take into account the weight of a child or the variation in the relationship between age and the degree of physiologic development. Body weight is most often used because it is easy to obtain. Children who are small for their age should receive doses at the lower end of the recommended dosage range, and those who are large for their age should receive doses at the higher end of the recommended dosage range. Larger children may also need a dose that is recommended for the next-higher age bracket.

> Always double-check all calculations, make sure the dose is appropriate for the child's age, and reevaluate all dosages.

Tech Math Practice

Question: **Calculate the quantity to dispense for the following:**
Sig: one tablet tid for 30 days.

Answer: The abbreviation tid means three times a day.
3 tablets/day × 30 days = 90 tablets.

Question: **Calculate the quantity to dispense for the following:**
Dispense a 10-day supply.
Sig: 3 cap bid.

Answer: The abbreviation bid means twice a day.
3 capsules/dose × 2 doses/day = 6 capsules/day.
6 capsules/day × 10 days = 60 capsules.

Question: **Calculate the quantity to dispense for the following:**
Dispense a 30-day supply.
Sig: 1$\frac{1}{2}$ tab bid.

Answer: The abbreviation bid means twice a day.
1$\frac{1}{2}$ tablets/dose × 2 doses/day = 3 tablets/day.
3 tablets/day × 30 days = 90 tablets.

Question: **Calculate the quantity to dispense for the following:**
Dispense a 15-day supply.
Sig: $\frac{1}{2}$ tab bid po.

Answer: The abbreviation bid means twice a day.
$\frac{1}{2}$ tab/dose × 2 doses/day = 1 tab/day.
1 tab/day × 15 days = 15 tablets.

Question: **Calculate the quantity to dispense for the following:**
Dispense a 30-day supply.
Sig: 1$\frac{1}{2}$ tab qid po.

Answer: The abbreviation qid means four times a day.
1$\frac{1}{2}$ tablets/dose × 4 doses/day = 6 tablets/day.
6 tablets/day × 30 days = 180 tablets.

Question: **A prescription for an ophthalmic solution reads "Instill one drop in affected eye twice a day" and instructs the pharmacy to dispense a 10-day supply. The medication is available as 20gtts/mL in a 1mL and 5mL bottle. Which bottle size should be dispensed?**

Answer: 1 drop/dose × 2 doses/day = 2 drops/day.
2 drops/day × 10 days = 20 drops.
20 drops ÷ 20gtts/mL = 1mL.
The 1mL size bottle should be dispensed.

WRAP UP

Chapter Summary

- A prescription is a written or verbal request for a medication.
- The "rights" for correct drug administration offer useful guidelines when filling prescriptions.
- Drugs can be administered in a variety of dosage forms. The choice of dosage form will depend on the patient, the desired effect, the dose required, the duration of desired effect, and the properties of the medication.
- Solid dosage forms include tablets, capsules, and caplets. They can be coated to mask the taste, prolong the duration of action, or to protect the medication from degradation in the stomach.
- Liquid dosage forms include suspensions, solutions, and emulsions. They have a faster onset of action than solid dosage forms.
- Topical dosage forms include creams, gels, ointments, and transdermal patches.
- Routes of administration include oral, topical and parenteral. The decision of which route to use will depend on the site, medication, desired effect, and duration of action.
- Topical administration includes the ophthalmic, inhalation, nasal, vaginal, urethral, and rectal routes of administration.
- Parenteral administration includes IV, IM, and SC routes of administration.
- Elderly and pediatric patients have special needs that can affect the way their medication should be administered and the way their bodies react to drugs.

Learning Assessment Questions

1. Parenteral medications are often used for which of the following reasons?
   - A. They have a faster onset of action.
   - B. They bypass the acidic secretions of the stomach.
   - C. The patient cannot take medication by mouth.
   - D. All of the above.

2. Administration of a medication between the cheek and gum is called which of the following?
   - A. Buccal
   - B. Sublingual
   - C. Topical
   - D. Intramuscular

3. An ointment is an example of which of the following?
   - A. W/O emulsion
   - B. O/W emulsion
   - C. Dispersion
   - D. Elixir

4. Which of the following routes of administration has the fastest onset of action?
   - A. Oral
   - B. Intravenous
   - C. Transdermal
   - D. Sublingual

5. To what does the abbreviation PO refer?
   - A. By mouth or orally
   - B. Rectally
   - C. Intradermally
   - D. Subcutaneously

6. The parenteral route of administration bypasses which of the following?
   - A. Veins
   - B. Gastrointestinal tract
   - C. Heart
   - D. All of the above

7. Lozenges are also known as which of the following?
   - A. Capsules
   - B. Pastilles
   - C. Suppositories
   - D. All of the above

8. Drugs administered into the eye are given by what route?

   A. Otic

   B. Rectal

   C. Ophthalmic

   D. Oral

9. Which of the following is not a solid dosage form?

   A. Emulsion

   B. Tablet

   C. Capsule

   D. Powder

10. Medication dosage forms include which of the following?

    A. Liquids

    B. Solids

    C. Semisolids

    D. All of the above

11. The rectal route of administration is useful if the patient is which of the following?

    A. Unconscious

    B. Vomiting

    C. Nauseated

    D. All of the above

12. Where are intramuscular injections given?

    A. Under the skin

    B. In the muscle

    C. In the vein

    D. In the artery

13. Extended-release tablets should not be which of the following?

    A. Crushed

    B. Cut without specific directions from the manufacturer for cutting along a scored tablet

    C. Chewed

    D. All of the above

14. Injection of a drug into the subcutaneous layer of fat is known as what route of administration?

    A. IM

B. SC

C. IV

D. ID

15. A prescription label must have which of the following?

    A. The patient's name

    B. The name of the drug

    C. The name and address of the pharmacy

    D. All of the above

16. Which of the following drugs causes the most ADRs in the elderly?

    A. Warfarin

    B. Heparin

    C. Nitroglycerin

    D. Aspirin

17. If the prescriber directs usage, a drug prepared for the ophthalmic route may also be used where ?

    A. In the ear

    B. In the nose

    C. In the rectum

    D. In the vagina

18. Drugs administered into the ear are given by what route?

    A. Rectally

    B. Ophthalmic

    C. Otic

    D. Buccal

19. Advantages of transdermal patches include which of the following?

    A. Convenience

    B. Improved patient compliance

    C. Ease of administration

    D. All of the above

20. The abbreviation TID means which of the following?

    A. Three times daily

    B. Twice a day

    C. Four times a day

    D. Immediately

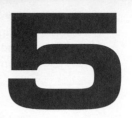

Pharmaceutical Measurements and Calculations

OBJECTIVES

After reading this chapter, you will be able to:

* Implement systems of measurement commonly used in pharmacy practice.
* Practice operations involving ratios and proportions.
* Calculate drug doses.
* Describe four systems of measurement commonly used in pharmacy, and convert units from one system to another.
* Explain the meanings of the prefixes most commonly used in metric measurement.
* Convert from one metric unit to another (e.g., grams to milligrams).
* Convert Roman to Arabic numerals
* Convert standard time to 24-hour military time.
* Convert temperatures to and from the Fahrenheit and Celsius scales.
* Round decimals up and down.
* Perform basic operations with proportions, including identifying equivalent ratios and finding an unknown quantity in a proportion using cross-multiplication.
* Convert percentages to and from fractions, ratios, and decimals.
* Perform fundamental dosage calculations and conversions.
* Solve problems involving powder solutions and dilutions.
* Use the alligation method to prepare solutions.
* Identify the basic units and prefixes of the metric system.
* Convert units within the metric system by moving the decimal place, using the ratio-proportion method, and using the dimensional-analysis method.
* Calculate drug doses using the ratio-proportion and dimensional-analysis methods.
* Calculate doses based on weight and body surface area (BSA).
* Calculate a pediatric dose using the patient's weight or age and the appropriate adult dose.

KEY TERMS

Accuracy	Concentration	Proportion
Admixture	Dilution	Ratio
Alligation	Dose	Ratio strength
Body-surface area (BSA)	Dosage	Specific gravity
Compounding	Precision	

Chapter Overview

Mathematics is important in pharmacy practice. A mistake in a calculation or measurement could lead to serious consequences, such as underdosing or overdosing. This, in turn, may lead to inadequate treatment or drug toxicity.

Virtually all tasks within pharmacy practice relate to mathematics and calculations: dispensing the correct volume of a solution, compounding a medication or determining a dose. These tasks involve basic arithmetic as well as an understanding of fractions, rounding numbers, ratios and proportions, and percentages. This chapter covers important topics relating to pharmaceutical measurements and calculations.

Numbers and Numerals

Number refers to a total quantity or amount, while a *numeral* is a word or symbol that represents a number. The Arabic, or decimal, system and Roman numerals are the most commonly recognized and used systems of notation in pharmacy practice.

Roman Numerals

The Roman system of notation uses combinations of eight letters whose position indicates addition or subtraction from a succession of base numbers **TABLE 5.1**. Bases include ½, 1, 5, 10, 50, 100, 500, and 1,000. Roman numerals are used for expression only and are not used for calculations. The values of each letter are shown here.

By combining letters, quantities other than the base values can be expressed. The letters indicate a sum of their values when they are represented in equal or successively smaller values. For example:

II = 2

III = 3

VI = 6

Table 5.1   Roman Numeral Base

Letter	Value
SS or ss	½
I or i	1
V or v	5
X or x	10
L or l	50
C or c	100
D or d	500
M or m	1,000

VII = 7
VIII = 8
XI = 11
LI = 51
LV = 55
CX = 110

> *In Roman-numeral notation, letters are not repeated more than three times in a row. For example, XXX = 30, but XL = 40.*

If a smaller value precedes a larger value, then the smaller value is subtracted from the larger value before the quantities are added together. For example:

IV = 4
IX = 9
XIV = 14
XIX = 19
XL = 40
XCIX = 99
CM = 900

Usually, capital letters are used to express years, while lowercase letters are used to express numerical values. Traditionally, capital Roman numerals have been used in pharmacy practice on prescriptions to designate the number of units prescribed or the quantity of medication to be administered. However, Roman numerals are increasingly being replaced by the decimal system in pharmacy practice.

Roman numerals are sometimes preferred on prescriptions because they cannot be easily altered.

Systems of Measurement Used in Pharmacy Practice

Several systems of measurement are employed in pharmacy: the common household system, the avoirdupois system, the apothecary system, and the metric system. Other notations of quantity and measurement include international units and milliequivalents. Pharmacy technicians should be familiar with all these systems, and be able to use them interchangeably. However, the metric system is the most common, and safest, system used in pharmacy practice.

Advise

Help patients understand how to convert between the metric system and the household measuring system. Many will be more familiar with teaspoonfuls than milliliters.

Household and Avoirdupois Systems of Measurement

The household and avoirdupois systems are the common measurements used in the United States for selling goods and food products, although they have been replaced in most other countries throughout the world by the metric system.

The household system of measurement is the one with which patients in the United States will be the most familiar. This system includes teaspoons, tablespoons, pints, quarts, and gallons for measuring liquid. The household system and the avoirdupois system are synonymous for measuring weight, and include ounces and pounds. In both systems, a pound is 16 ounces.

Communicate

Household measuring devices vary in actual capacity. Remind patients to use the calibrated administration devices that come with medications.

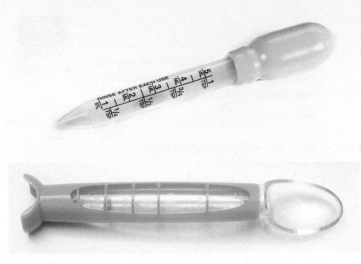

Calibrated spoons and droppers for medications administered by mouth often display household and metric units.

Instructions to patients are often provided in the household measuring system. In these cases, pharmacy representatives should caution patients, because household measuring instruments vary considerably in their actual capacity.

The Apothecary System of Measurement

The apothecary system is an outdated system of measurement previously used in medicine and science. Unlike the household and avoirdupois systems, the pound in the apothecary system is based on 12 ounces. The only equivalent unit of measure between the apothecary system and the avoirdupois system is the grain, used for measuring dry weight. Interestingly 1 grain is equal to 64.79891 milligrams, but this can be expressed as 64.8, 65, and in some cases 60. Remnants of this unit of measure can be seen in older drugs like aspirin 325mg (equal to 5gr), ferrous sulfate 325mg, Tylenol with codeine #2 ($\frac{1}{4}$gr codeine), Tylenol with codeine #3 ($\frac{1}{2}$gr codeine), and Tylenol with codeine #4 (1gr codeine). In general, the use of the apothecary system is discouraged in pharmacy practice today because of safety concerns and inaccuracies. Two common exceptions are thyroid medications and phenobarbital dosing.

Metric System of Measurement

The metric system is by far the most commonly used system of measurement throughout the world, as well as throughout science and medicine. The metric system is the legal standard of measurement for pharmacy and medicine in the United States. The metric system is based on the decimal system, and all units are described as multiples of 10. The correlations among units of measure are more distinct than in other systems of measurement, simplifying calculations and aiding in the **accuracy** (that is, how well a measurement represents the true value) and **precision** (that is, how well a series of measurements can be reproduced or how close the measurements are to each other) of measurements.

One cubic centimeter (cm³) of water is equivalent to one milliliter. One gram is equivalent to the weight of 1cm³ of water at 4°C.

The basic units of measurement in the metric system are the meter (m), for measuring length or distance; the liter (L), for measuring liquid volume; and the gram (g), for measuring dry weight. The gram is based on an actual cylinder of metal that is considered *the* kilogram. A cylinder locked away in Paris serves as the basis for all metric weight measurements. It was determined to be exactly 1kg in 1889. Copies were made to match it; then, it was locked up and has only been weighed two other times.

Prefixes Used in the Metric System

In the metric system, prefixes are added to the base units to specify a particular measurement. Common prefixes and conversions used in pharmacy practice are provided in TABLE 5.2 .

The use of the abbreviation m for micro is discouraged because it can be easily misinterpreted. Instead, mc is the preferred abbreviation for micro.

Table 5.2	Common Prefixes and Conversions in the Metric System

Prefix	Symbol	Meaning	Conversion
Kilo	K	one thousand times	Base unit $\times 10^3$
Hecto	H	one hundred times	Base unit $\times 10^2$
Deci	D	one tenth	Base unit $\times 10^{-1}$
Centi	C	one hundredth	Base unit $\times 10^{-2}$
Milli	M	one thousandth	Base unit $\times 10^{-3}$
Micro	mc or μ	one millionth	Base unit $\times 10^{-6}$

Table 5.3	Common Systems of Measurement and Equivalents Used in Pharmacy Practice

	System	Unit (Symbol)	Equivalent
Volume	Apothecary	Minim (♏)	0.06mL
		Fluidram (f℥)	60♏ = 5mL
		Fluidounce (f℥)	6 f℥ = 30mL
		Pint (pt)	16f℥ = 480mL
		Quart (qt)	2pt = 32f℥ = 960mL
		Gallon (gal)	4qt = 8pt = 3,840mL
	Household	Teaspoon (tsp or t)	5mL
		Tablespoon (tbsp or T)	3tsp = 15mL
		Fluid ounce (fl oz)	2tbsp = 30mL
		Cup (c)	8fl oz
		Pint (pt)	2c = 480mL
		Quart (qt)	2pt = 4c = 960mL
		Gallon (gal)	4qt = 16c = 3,840mL
Weight	Avoirdupois	Grain (gr)	65mg
		Ounce (oz)	437.5gr = 30g
		Pound (lb)	16oz = 7,000gr = 454g
	Apothecary	Grain (gr)	65mg
		Scruple (℈)	20gr = 1.3g
		Dram (℥)	3℈ = 60gr = 3.9g
		Ounce (℥)	8℥ = 480gr = 30g
		Pound (#)	12℥ = 5760gr = 373.2g
	Household	Ounce (oz)	30g
		Pound (lb)	16oz = 454g

Converting Between Systems of Measurement

The base units and equivalents of the primary systems of measurement used in pharmacy for measuring weight and volumes are provided in **TABLE 5.3**.

Some discrepancies exist when converting from one system to another. For example, 1f ℥ in the apothecary system actually contains 3.75mL, but the value is often rounded to 5mL, or one household

In the apothecary system, fluidram and fluidounce are written as one word, but in the household system, fluid ounce is separated into two words.

Abbreviations for the apothecary system are discouraged, because they can be easily misinterpreted—for example, ℳ could be read as mL, and ℥ or ℈ read as 3. If the apothecary system must be used, write out the entire word indicating the units.

Table 5.4 Common Equivalents Used in Pharmacy Practice	
1mL = 16.23ℳ	1mg = 1,000mcg
1pt = 473mL	1g = 1,000mg
1g = 15.432gr	1kg = 1,000g
1gr = 64.8mg	1in = 2.54cm
1oz = 28.35g	1m = 39.37in
1kg = 2.2lb	1cm = 0.394in

Do not abbreviate cup. The common abbreviation, c, can be easily misinterpreted as a 0 or a c with a horizontal line over it, indicating "with."

Get the Pharmacist

When in doubt, ask the pharmacist to double-check abbreviations, conversions, and calculations.

teaspoonful. Similarly, if ℥ in the apothecary system and 1 fl oz in the household system contain 29.57mL, but this is often rounded to 30mL. This difference is negligible at small volumes, but accounts for more significant differences at larger quantities such as the gallon. For the purposes of practice exercises in this chapter, the rounded volumes will be used. However, the actual values of common equivalents are presented in **TABLE 5.4**, and should be committed to memory for future pharmacy practice.

International Units

The international unit (IU) expresses drug amounts. Examples of drugs measured in international units include insulin and vitamin D. They are most frequently used in hospital pharmacy practice. The IU per milligram varies with each drug, so standard conversion factors are not possible. If necessary, the conversion factor will be provided by the drug manufacturer.

The use of the abbreviations t and tsp for teaspoon and T and tbsp for tablespoon are discouraged in pharmacy because they can be easily misinterpreted. Instead, write out "teaspoonfuls" or "tablespoonfuls."

Milliequivalents

The milliequivalent expresses electrolyte concentration. A milliequivalent is the number of positively charged ions per liter of salt solution and indicates the composition of intravenous fluids. Examples of electrolytes measured in milliequivalents per a volume of solution include potassium acetate 2mEq/mL or sodium chloride 38.5 mEq/L. One equivalent (Eq) equals 1,000mEq, and is determined by dividing the molecular weight of a substance by its valence, both of which are found in the periodic table of the elements.

Measuring Time

In hospital and institutional settings, time is expressed in 24-hour military style, also called international time. This reduces errors and ambiguity in medication administration. Military time is based on a 24-hour clock rather than the commonly used 12-hour clock. One day is divided into 24 one-hour segments, noted from 0000 through 2300. The first two digits indicate the hours passed since midnight, and the last two digits, the minutes.

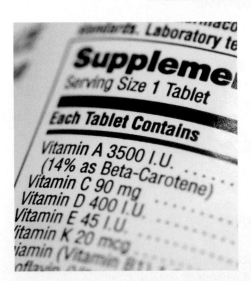

International units (IUs) are often used to denote the quantity of vitamins present in a multivitamin tablet.

Example: 0000 means midnight

Example: 0630 means 6:30 in the
            morning, or 6:30 a.m.

Example: 1200 means noon

Example: 1845 means 6:45 in the
            evening, or 6:45 p.m.

In military time, no "a.m." or "p.m." is used, reducing confusion and eliminating potential errors.

Measuring Temperature

As with systems of weight and liquid measurement, the most commonly used system for measuring temperature in the United States, the Fahrenheit scale, is not the preferred system within medicine or pharmacy. The Fahrenheit scale, used daily in many households to evaluate temperature, identifies 32°F as the temperature when water freezes and 212°F as the temperature when water boils.

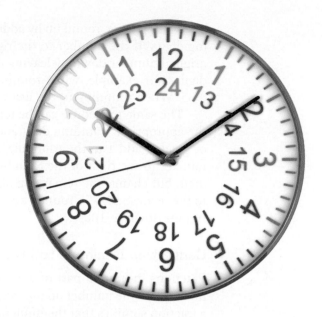

In institutional settings, time is indicated by 24-hour notation, based on a 24-hour clock, rather than 12-hour notation.

An alternative is the Celsius scale, which uses 0°C as the temperature when water freezes and 100°C as the temperature when water boils. The Celsius scale is used commonly throughout the world, and in science and health care.

Because proper storage of drugs and medical devices often relies on accurate temperatures, pharmacy technicians must be able to correctly convert from one temperature scale to the other. In most pharmacy settings, it is the pharmacy technician's responsibility to maintain daily records of refrigerator and freezer temperatures. Additionally, technicians may be asked to help interpret temperatures for patients.

Every 5° change in the Celsius scale is equivalent to a 9° change in the Fahrenheit scale. Therefore, several equations exist to convert between the two scales:

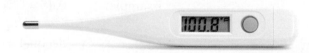

To convert from Fahrenheit to Celsius:
°F = (1.8 × °C) + 32°

To convert from Celsius to Fahrenheit:
°C = (°F − 32°) ÷ 1.8 or 5 × °F = 9 × °C + 160

At one temperature, the values on the Celsius and Fahrenheit scales are equal. That is −40°F = −40°C.

Rounding Decimals

In pharmacy, calculations are commonly rounded to the nearest one-tenth, but carrying the calculation out to the nearest hundredth or thousandth to ensure accuracy may be appropriate for certain medications or certain patients.

To round decimals, choose the place that is appropriate for rounding (the rounding digit). Then, look at the number directly to the right. If this num-

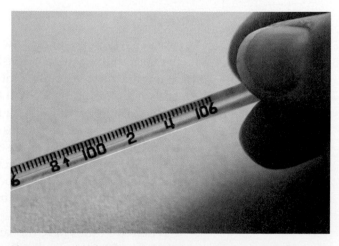

Pharmacy technicians may be asked to interpret or convert temperatures taken by digital or alcohol- or mercury-filled glass thermometers.

ber is 5 or greater, round up by adding 1 to the rounding digit and omitting the remaining digits. If the number to the right of the rounding digit is less than 5, round the original number down by leaving the rounding digit as is and omitting the remaining digits. For example, when rounding to the nearest hundredth, 0.847 rounds up to 0.85. When rounding to the nearest thousandth, 0.5134 rounds down to 0.513.

The same procedure can be followed for rounding whole numbers. Simply locate the appropriate rounding digit and look at the digit to the right. If this number is 5 or greater, add 1 to the rounding digit and change the digits to the right to 0. If the number to the right of the rounding digit is less than 5, do not change the rounding digit, but change the remaining digits to the right to 0. For example, when rounding to the nearest 10, 756 rounds up to 760. When rounding to the nearest hundred, 135 rounds down to 100.

Converting Decimals to Fractions

Fractions indicate a part of a whole. A fraction is represented by two numbers: the numerator (the number on top) and the denominator (the number on bottom). Simply, a fraction signifies that the numerator is to be divided by the denominator. Therefore, fractions can be noted as a numerator and a denominator, or as a decimal value. For example, $\frac{3}{4} = 3 \div 4 = 0.75$. The value of a fraction, or the result of the division, is called the quotient.

Any decimal can be converted to a fraction using a denominator that is a multiple of 10. To convert a decimal to a fraction, first use the decimal value as the numerator and place it over a denominator of 1. Next, multiply both the numerator and the denominator by 10 for each digit to the right of the decimal point. The numerator will become a whole number. For example, if there are two numbers to the right of the decimal point, multiply the numerator and the denominator by 10 two times, or 100. Once the decimal is expressed as a fraction, the fraction can be reduced, or simplified, by multiplying by a factor of one.

Example: $0.3 = \frac{0.3}{1}$

$\frac{0.3}{1} \times \frac{10}{10} = \frac{3}{10}$

Example: $0.45 = \frac{0.45}{1}$

$\frac{0.45}{1} \times \frac{10}{10} \times \frac{10}{10}$ (because two numbers are to the right of the decimal $= \frac{45}{100}$ which can be further reduced to $\frac{9}{20}$)

Ratios

A **ratio** is a representation of how two similar quantities are related to each other. A ratio may express either the relationship between two parts of one whole or between one part and the whole. Simply, a ratio is a comparison. Traditionally, ratios are expressed in odds notation, using a colon to separate the numbers, such as 1:2. Alternatively, a ratio can also be expressed as a fraction, such as $\frac{1}{2}$.

In pharmacy practice, ratios are often used to express the concentration of a drug in solution or the weight or dose of a drug in a delivery unit or volume. For example, a tablet that contains 25mg of active ingredient can be expressed as 25mg:1 tablet or 1 tablet:25mg. Similarly, this value can be expressed as a fraction: $\frac{25mg}{1\ tablet}$ or $\frac{1\ tablet}{25mg}$. Similarly, a solution that contains 1g of drug per 100mL can be expressed as a ratio (1g:100mL) or a fraction ($\frac{1g}{100mL}$).

When two ratios have the same value, they are equivalent. You can find equivalent ratios by multiplying or dividing both sides of the ratio by the same number. This is the same process as finding equivalent fractions.

Example: 1:2

Multiply both sides by 2 to get 2:4 (1 × 2):(2 × 2) = 2:4

Multiply both sides by 4 to get 4:8 (1 × 4):(2 × 4) = 4:8

Multiply both sides by 100 to get 100:200 (1 × 100):(2 × 100) = 100:200

Example: 50:100

Divide both sides by 25 to get 2:4 (50 ÷ 25):(100 ÷ 25) = 2:4

Divide both sides by 50 to get 1:2 (50 ÷ 50):(100 ÷ 50) = 1:2

When two ratios are equivalent and expressed as fractions, the product of the first numerator multiplied by the opposite denominator is equivalent to the product of the first denominator multiplied by the opposite numerator. That is, 3:5 = 6:10. Therefore, $\frac{3}{5} = \frac{6}{10}$. Note: 3 × 10 = 5 × 6.

Proportions

A **proportion** is an equation that states two ratios are equal. When the terms of a proportion are multiplied, the cross products are equal.

Example: $\frac{2}{8} = \frac{5}{20}$

                2 × 20 = 8 × 5

Answer: 40 = 40

A practical application of ratios comes in the form of a proportion. A proportion is the expression of equality between two equivalent ratios. A proportion is designated by a double colon (::) between two ratios or as a fraction—for example, 3:5::6:10 or $\frac{3}{5} = \frac{6}{10}$. In a proportion, the inside numbers are termed the "means" and the outside numbers are termed the "extremes." As with equivalent ratios expressed as fractions, the product of the means always equals the product of the extremes in a proportion.

Calculating the Value of a Missing Term in a Proportion

The ratio-proportion method is based on comparing a known ratio with an unknown ratio.

Because this relationship is always true in a proportion, it can be used to calculate the value of a missing term in a proportion. For example, if a:b::c:d, then $\frac{a}{b}$ = $\frac{c}{d}$ and a × d = b × c. Therefore, if any one of the variables is unknown, you can use the three known variables and solve for the unknown using basic algebra.

Ratio-Proportion Method for Pharmacy Calculations

A stock solution is a solution of known concentration. It may be supplied from a manufacturer or made in advance of dispensing by a pharmacist.

The ratio-proportion method is commonly used to calculate drug doses in pharmacy practice. For example, the concentration of a stock solution and the dose needed for administration are often known. The volume of the dose is the unknown. A ratio or proportion can be established to solve for the missing value.

Cross-Multiplication

Cross-multiplication is the multiplication of the numerator of the first fraction by the denominator of the second fraction, and the multiplication of the denominator of the first fraction by the numerator of the second fraction (see **FIGURE 5.1**). Cross-multiplication is used frequently within pharmacy practice to determine correct doses

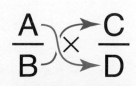

FIGURE 5.1 Cross-multiplication.

and amounts of drugs needed to mix medications or to make specific doses for a prescription.

To cross multiply is to go from $^a/_b \times {^c/_d}$ to ad = bc. This is used when the value of a is proportional to the value of c and the value of b is proportional to the value of d.

If one term of the proportion is unknown—meaning that three of the four values are known, cross-multiplication can be used to find the value of the unknown term.

Example: $x \div 8 = 5/20$

$20x = 8 \times 5$

$20x = 40$

$20x/20 = 40/20$

Answer: $x = 2$

Percents

Like fractions and ratios, percentages are parts of a whole. More specifically, percentages and their symbol (%) refer to parts per a total of 100 parts. Therefore, a percentage can be expressed as a percent, a fraction, a decimal, or a ratio. For example, 1% = $^1/_{100}$ = 0.01 = 1:100.

Converting Between Ratios and Percents

To convert a ratio to a percent, first convert the ratio to a fraction, selecting the first number as the numerator and the second number as the denominator. Next, multiply the fraction by 100. Express the final value followed by a percent sign.

Reverse the process to convert a percent to a ratio. First, express the percent as a fraction, with a denominator of 100. Then reduce the fraction to its most simplified form, if possible. Finally, express the final value as a ratio, designating the numerator as the first number and the denominator as the second number.

Converting Between Percents and Decimals

To convert a percent to a decimal, remove the percent symbol and divide the number by 100. This is equivalent to moving the decimal point two places to the left.

Conversely, to convert a decimal to a percent, multiply by 100, moving the decimal point two spaces to the right, and add a percent sign.

Calculating Drug Doses, Dosages, and Quantities

One of the critical functions of pharmacy practice is ensuring that patients get the correct drug for the most appropriate length of time. There are many methods for accurately calculating drug quantity, as well as expressing and communicating the treatment regimen. Regardless of the drug or how the quantity is determined, accuracy and appropriateness must be verified by the pharmacist.

Dose and Dosage

A **dose** of a drug is the quantity that is intended to be administered, usually taken at one time or during one specified period such as per day. **Dosage** refers to the determination and regulation of the size, frequency, and number of doses. The dosage is the entire regimen or schedule of doses. Although often used interchangeably, the terms "dose" and "dosage" do have slightly different connotations. The dose refers to a quantity of drug. The dosage implies treatment duration and a cumulative effect.

Doses can be expressed as a single dose, a daily dose, or a total dose. A daily dose, in turn, may be expressed as divided doses.

Example:	A dose of 50 mg is prescribed once daily for 10 days.
Solution:	In this case, the single dose, as well as the daily dose, is 50mg.
Total dose:	50mg/day × 10 days = 500mg

Example:	A dose of 500mg, three times daily, is prescribed for seven days.
Solution:	The single dose = 500mg.
Daily dose:	500mg × 3 = 1,500mg
Total dose:	1,500mg/day × 7 days = 10,500mg

Doses and dosage regimens are highly variable among substances. Each is determined by a drug's biochemical and physical properties, the route of administration, and individual patient factors. A dose may be based on age, body weight, body-surface area (BSA), overall health, liver or kidney function, or the specific illness or condition being treated. Additionally, prescription recommendations may be based on clinical trials, studies, or manufacturers' guidelines.

Determining the Number of Doses in a Quantity of Drug

To determine the number of doses in a given quantity of drug, simply divide the total amount of drug available by the size of the dose. Note that the total amount of drug and the dose must be expressed in the same units.

Example:	The total amount of drug available is 1,000mg and each dose is 100mg. Determine the number of doses available in 1,000mg.
Solution:	1,000mg ÷ 100mg/dose = 10 doses (Note that the total amount of drug and the amount of dose are both expressed in milligrams.)

Determining the Size of a Dose

To determine the size of a dose, given the total number of doses in a quantity of drug, divide the total amount of drug available by the number of doses. As always, check the units to ensure accuracy in calculations.

Example:	A 10g vial of vancomycin is used to make eight doses. Determine the number of milligrams in each dose.
Solution:	First convert the grams to milligrams: 10g × 1,000mg/g = 10,000mg. Then divide the total amount of the drug by the number of doses: 10,000mg ÷ 8 doses = 1,250mg/dose.

Determining the Total Amount of a Drug to Be Administered

To determine the total amount of drug to be administered given the total number of doses and the quantity of drug in each dose, multiply the number of doses by the quantity of each dose.

> *It is most efficient to convert the units to the denomination in which the final answer should be expressed.*

Example:	A nurse practitioner writes an order for 2 grams of Rocephin IV to be given once daily for six weeks for home IV therapy. Determine the total amount of drug to be administered over that period of time.

Solution: Use the following calculation: 2 g/day × 7 days/week × 6 weeks = 84 g.

The pharmacy technician often places the drug order. This type of calculation is used when determining how much drug to order. In this case, the pharmacy would need to have in the inventory 14 grams of Rocephin each week for making the patient's IV medication.

Determining Doses Based on Weight

The usual adult dose for most drugs is based on an average body weight of 70kg (154lb). However, some drugs act differently in the body depending on body size and composition and the concentration of drug desired at the site of action. Therefore, some doses need to be increased or decreased for particularly lean or overweight individuals. Also, body weight is often used to determine pediatric doses because age may not be a reliable indicator of body composition or function in children.

When drugs are intended to be dosed based on body weight, the dose will usually be expressed as a quantity of drug (usually in milligrams) per kilogram body weight. Therefore, to determine the dose, multiply the patient's body weight by the dose required.

Example: An antibiotic is dosed 15mg/kg/day. Determine how many milligrams the patient will receive in his daily dose if he weighs 85kg.

Solution: Use the following equation to solve for the dosage in milligrams: 15mg/kg × 85kg = 1,275mg.

As with all calculations, note the units. If a patient's weight is given in pounds, but the dose is prescribed in mg/kg, the weight must first be converted to kilograms before proceeding with the calculation.

Determining Doses Based on Body-Surface Area

Body-surface area (BSA) is a representation of a patient's weight and height relative to each other. Some patient populations or certain drugs require dosing based on BSA, such as cancer patients receiving chemotherapy and pediatric patients who require special assessment for drug response or adverse reactions.

BSA is calculated using the following equation:

$$BSA\ (m^2) = [Height\ (cm) \times Weight\ (kg)/3600]^{1/2}$$

Usual adult doses are based on a weight of 70kg and a BSA of 1.73m².

If inches and pounds are used to measure height and weight, respectively, the following equation can be used:

$$BSA\ (m^2) = [Height\ (in) \times Weight\ (lb)/3131]^{1/2}$$

The average adult has a BSA of 1.73m². Using this value, a pediatric dose can be calculated by using the ratio-proportion method, defining the pediatric dose as a relative portion of the adult dose.

Alternatively, to determine a pediatric dose based on an adult dose and BSA, convert the child's BSA to a percent or fraction of usual adult BSA and multiply the result by the adult dose.

Considerations for Pediatric Patients

Patient age is often considered in calculating doses, particularly for very young or very old patients. For example, both newborns and the elderly are especially sensitive to the actions of certain drugs because of immature or abnormal liver or kidney function, which are required for healthy drug metabolism.

Several rules have been established to estimate the pediatric dose based on age or weight of the patient relative to the usual adult dose of a drug. However, these calculations are generally no longer used because age and weight are not always considered single reliable criteria for determining pediatric doses. Also, these calculations relate a pediatric dose to an adult dose, assuming that a child is simply a small adult. This is not always the case, however, because of different body composition and organ function between children and adults. Therefore, doses based directly on a child's BSA or body weight are the safest and most common choices to establish pediatric doses. Also, manufacturers often provide pediatric dosing tables with the drug information to aid in determining doses.

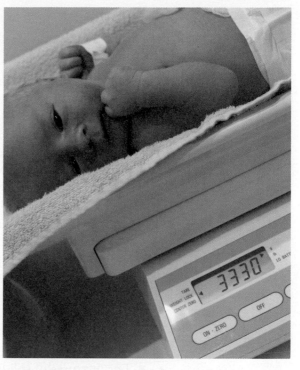

Doses based on body weight are often most accurate for pediatric patients.

Young's Rule

Young's rule for determining pediatric doses is based on age:

Pediatric dose = [age of child (years) ÷ (age of child [years] + 12)] × adult dose

Clark's Rule

Clark's rule for determining pediatric doses is based on weight:

Pediatric dose = (weight of child [pounds] × adult dose) ÷ 150lb, where 150lb is the average weight of an adult

Preparing Solutions and Compounded Products

Solutions are liquids containing one or more drugs dispersed in a solvent. Pharmaceutical solutions are used for oral administration, topical application, nasal, otic or ophthalmic instillation, parenteral administration, or irrigation of body cavities or wounds. Solutions are a flexible dosage form because they can be used in any route of administration and the doses can be easily adjusted.

When converting between pounds and kilograms, 1lb = 2.2kg. This conversion can be used to solve dosing problems based on patient weight.

However, not every drug is suitable for preparation in a solution. Some drugs are not stable as liquids, and some drugs are not soluble in liquid. Also, solutions are more difficult to store and transport than dry, solid dosage forms.

Compounding is the preparation of a drug product pursuant to a prescription or medication order. Solutions may need to be compounded to achieve a specific concentration of drug that is not commercially available or to accommodate an individual's medical or dietary restrictions. Solid and semi-solid dosage forms may also need to be compounded for the same reason. In any case, compounding and preparing drug products require accurate calculations to ensure proper doses and safety and consistency in the dosage form.

%w/v = grams of substance/100mL of liquid vehicle

%v/v = milliliters of a liquid/100mL of liquid vehicle

%w/w = grams of a substance/100g of solid vehicle

Concentration

Concentration indicates the amount of active ingredient per total volume or weight of a substance.

- For solutions or suspensions of solids in liquids, the concentration is expressed as weight-in-volume; the percent weight-in-volume (%w/v) is presented as the number of grams of a substance per 100mL of liquid vehicle.

  Example: A 5%(w/v) solution of dextrose in water contains 5g of dextrose in every 100mL of total vehicle, or 5g dextrose/100mL total vehicle. Note: The volume of water needed to make 100mL of total solution will be less than 100mL.

- For solutions of liquids in liquids, the concentration is expressed as volume-in-volume; the percent volume-in-volume (%v/v) is presented as the number of milliliters of a liquid per 100mL of liquid vehicle.

  Example: A 70% (v/v) isopropyl alcohol contains 70mL of isopropyl alcohol in every 100mL of total solution, or 70mL isopropyl alcohol/100mL total solution Note: Less than 30mL of water must be added to 70mL of isopropyl alcohol to obtain 100mL of 70% solution.

- For mixtures of solids, the concentration is expressed as weight-in-weight; the percent weight-in-weight (%w/w) is presented as the number of grams of a substance in 100grams of a solid vehicle.

  Example: A 10% (w/w) hydrocortisone cream contains 10g of hydrocortisone in every 100g of cream, or 10g hydrocortisone/100g cream.

Ratio Strength

The **ratio strength** is used to express the concentration of weak solutions. Ratio strengths and percent concentrations may be converted to ratios or proportions for ease of calculations.

Example: Epinephrine is available in very dilute concentrations, such as 1:200,000. For every 200,000 total parts of epinephrine solution, only one part is epinephrine. What is the percent concentration of a 1:200,000 concentration epinephrine ampule?

Solution: As a percent concentration, this is equivalent to 0.0005%, because 1/200,000 = 0.000005 × 100% = 0.0005%.

Reconstitutable Powder Preparations

Sometimes, a drug must be reconstituted before it is dispensed or administered to a patient. In such cases, the drug product is a dry powder to which a specified volume of diluent must be added. A diluent is an inactive liquid used to increase the volume and decrease the concentration of another substance. The powder volume is the amount of volume occupied by the dry substance.

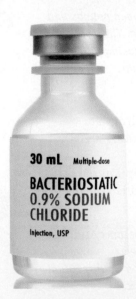

The percent concentration of sodium chloride solution indicates that there are 0.9 grams of sodium chloride in every 100mL of liquid.

The powder volume equals the final volume of the product minus the diluent volume after the powder has been mixed with the vehicle.

    Example: A vial of powder contains 1.5g of a drug. The manufacturer instructs adding 3.3mL of sterile water to obtain 4mL of solution with a final concentration of 375mg/mL. Why would you add 3.3mL of sterile water instead of 4mL of sterile to the vial?

    Solution: If 4mL of sterile water were added to the vial, the concentration would be less than the required 375mg/mL, because the powder displaces some volume of vehicle. The powder occupies 0.7mL in the final solution.

Dilutions

Dilution is the process of decreasing the concentration of a liquid. A dilution may be necessary to obtain the correct quantity for administration, to individualize a dose, or to accurately measure a final quantity. Pharmaceutical products are often diluted by adding a diluent to the original preparation. Additionally, an **admixture**—that is, a mixture of small volumes of drugs in a large volume of fluid of lower strength—can be added to a higher-strength product to achieve a dilution. Admixtures are often prepared to administer doses of concentrated medications that could cause toxicity or tissue damage when administered alone.

    Example: Promethazine cannot be administered in single doses of greater than 100mg. How does the pharmacy technician dilute the promethazine dose?

    Solution: Concentrated promethazine doses must be diluted in normal saline to a concentration of 25mg/mL.

Stock solutions are available in a pharmacy for ease of dispensing. These solutions contain a known concentration of drug and allow pharmacy staff to dispense small quantities of active drug in larger volumes of solution.

If a solution or product requires dilution, the amount of active drug in the final product will remain constant, but the volume will increase. The relationship between the concentration and the volume is inversely proportional. That is, as the percent of concentration or ratio strength decreases, the total quantity of product increases.

This fact is expressed in the following equation:

Quantity of the first solution × Concentration of the first solution = Quantity of the second solution × Concentration of the second solution

This equation can also be expressed as follows:

$$Q1 \times C1 = Q2 \times C2$$

That is, the quantity of the first product multiplied by its concentration is equivalent to the quantity of the final product multiplied by its concentration. In this equation, the first product is the stock solution or product that requires dilution, and the second product is the final product produced after dilution. Therefore, calculating the quantities or concentrations needed for a final product becomes simple algebra.

Further, if the concentration and quantity of a final product are known, the amount or concentration of the stock solution can be determined.

Alligation Method for Compounded Products

Alligation is a mathematical problem-solving method that involves mixing solutions or solids that have different strengths of the same active ingredient in order to obtain another strength of the ingredient. In pharmacy practice, alligation may be necessary if a physician prescribes a concentration of drug that is not available commercially. In this case, two different-strength solutions containing the same active ingredient can be combined to achieve the desired strength.

Simply, alligation is the weighted average of a mixture of two or more substances. The percentage strength of each component is expressed as a decimal fraction and multiplied by its quantity. The sum of all the products is divided by the total quantity and converted to a percent to present the final strength of the compounded product. The alligation method may be used for weight or volume.

The alligation method can be used to calculate the amounts of a high-strength product and a low-strength product that must be added together to make an intermediate-strength product.

Alternatively, a matrix arrangement may be used to visualize the known quantities and solve for the unknown value. Subtract on the diagonals and read the answers across the horizontals.

(highest concentration)		(highest concentration parts)
	(desired concentration)	
(lowest concentration)		(lowest concentration parts)

1. Draw a box or matrix. In the upper-left corner, place the highest concentration as a whole number. In the lower-left corner, place the lowest concentration. In the center of the box, place the desired concentration.

2. Write the difference between the upper-left number and the center number in the lower-right corner, subtracting the smaller number from the larger number. Next, write the difference between the lower-left number and the center number in the upper-right corner. The numbers on the right represent the parts of each solution that are required to make the new solution.

3. Read across the box to determine the strength and amount of each original solution. Add the numbers in the right column to determine the total parts needed for the new solution.

Finally, the results of the alligation calculation can be established as ratios. Then, you can proceed with calculations of weight or volume as previously described. In the previous example, the ratio of 70% solution to 20% solution is 10:40, or 1:4; the ratio of 70% solution to the final 30% solution is 10:50, or 1:5; and the ratio of 20% solution to the final 30% solution is 4:5. Therefore, for a total of five parts of 30% solution, one part will be 70% solution and four parts will be 20% solution.

If 20mL is desired, then determining the volume of each solution proceeds with simple ratio calculations:

| Example: | 5 parts 30% solution/1 part 70% solution = 20mL/xmL |
| Solution: | Solving for x, $x = 4$mL of 70% solution. |

| Example: | 5 parts 30% solution/4 parts 20% solution = 20mL/ymL |
| Solution: | Solving for y, $y = 16$mL of 20% solution. |

Knowledge of basic mathematics and calculations is essential to safe and effective pharmacy practice. Always check units to ensure consistency, and double-check calculations. These simple reminders will help minimize medication errors and maintain patient safety.

Specific Gravity

Specific gravity is the ratio of the weight of a substance to the weight of an equal volume of water at

Specific gravity has no units.

the same temperature. Or, specific gravity is a ratio of the density of a substance to the density of water. Specific gravity itself is a value that has no units, but when you calculate specific gravity, you use units of milliliters for volume and grams for weight. Specific gravity can be calculated using the following equation:

Specific gravity = weight of substance ÷ weight of an equal volume of water

Because the reference standard of 1mL of water weighs 1g, the specific gravity of water is 1. And because 1mL of water weighs 1g, the equation can be converted to the following:

Specific gravity = number of grams of a substance ÷
number of milliliters of a substance

Alternatively, if the specific gravity is known, the volume or weight of a desired quantity can be determined.

If different quantities of two or more liquids with known specific gravities must be combined, the alligation method can be used to determine the relative quantities of each component.

A specific gravity greater than 1 indicates a solution or substance that is thick and viscous. Substances with a specific gravity of greater than 1 are heavier than water. A specific gravity less than 1 indicates a solution or substance that contains volatile chemicals or is prone to evaporation. Substances with a specific gravity of less than 1 are lighter than water.

Similarly, a matrix can be used to solve for unknown quantities when compounding a product with a desired specific gravity.

The relative amounts can be established as ratios or proportions, as previously described, and calculations may proceed to determine the weights or volumes of each component required.

Tech Math Practice

Question: **How do you convert 0.513 to a fraction?**

Answer: To convert 0.513 to a fraction, first use the decimal value as the numerator and place it over a denominator of 1: $^{0.513}/_1$. Then note how many numbers are to the right of the decimal point—here, three. Next, multiply the value in the numerator by 10 three times: $0.513 \times 10 \times 10 \times 10 = 513$. Then multiply the value in the denominator by 10 three times: $1 \times 10 \times 10 \times 10 = 1,000$. The fraction, then, is $^{513}/_{1,000}$.

Question: **How do you convert 0.82 to a fraction?**

Answer: To convert 0.82 to a fraction, first use the decimal value as the numerator and place it over a denominator of 1: $^{0.82}/_1$. Then note how many numbers are to the right of the decimal point—here, two. Next, multiply the value in the numerator by 10 two times: $0.82 \times 10 \times 10 = 82$. Then multiply the value in the denominator by 10 two times: $1 \times 10 \times 10 = 100$. The fraction, then, is $^{82}/_{100}$. Divide that fraction by a factor of one to simplify it: $^{82}/_{100} \div ^2/_2 = ^{41}/_{50}$.

Question: **If a stock solution contains 25mg of drug per 5mL, and the patient needs a dose of 37.5mg, how many milliliters are in each dose?**

Answer: First, determine the equation using the ratio proportion method: $^{x\,mL}/_{37.5mg} = ^{5mL}/_{25mg}$. Next, solve for x: $x = (37.5mg \times 5mL) \div 25mg = 7.5mL$. Therefore, the dose needed is 7.5mL. To confirm the answer, establish a proportion and verify that the product of the means equals the product of the extremes:

  5mL:25mg::7.5mL:37.5mg = 5:25::7.5:37.5

  $(5 \times 37.5) = (25 \times 7.5)$

  $187.5 = 187.5$

Question: **What is the value of x in the following proportion: $^4/_5 = ^x/_{20}$?**

Answer: First, multiply the first numerator by the second denominator: $4 \times 20 = 80$. Next, multiply the first denominator by the second numerator: $5 \times x = 5x$. The result is the following equation: $80 = 5x$. To solve for x, divide both sides of the proportion by 5: $80 \div 5 = 16$ and $5x \div 5 = x$. So $x = 16$.

Question: **What is the value of x in the following proportion: $^3/_7 = ^x/_{21}$?**

Answer: First, multiply the first numerator by the second denominator: $3 \times 21 = 63$. Next, multiply the first denominator by the second numerator: $7 \times x = 7x$. The result is the following equation: $63 = 7x$. To solve for x, divide both sides of the proportion by 7: $63 \div 7 = 9$ and $7x \div 7 = x$. So $x = 9$.

Question: **What is the result of converting 1:4 to a percent?**

Answer: To convert 1:4 to a percent, first convert the ratio to a fraction: $1:4 = ^1/_4$. Next, multiply the fraction by 100: $^1/_4 \times 100 = 25\%$.

Question: **What is the result of converting 2:1 to a percent?**

Answer: To convert 2:1 to a percent, first convert the ratio to a fraction: 2:1 = $\frac{2}{1}$. Next, multiply the fraction by 100: $\frac{2}{1} \times 100 = 200\%$.

Question: **What is the result of converting 80% to a ratio?**

Answer: To convert 80% to a ratio, express the percent as a fraction: $\frac{80}{100}$, which simplifies to $\frac{4}{5}$. The ratio, then, is 4:5.

Question: **What is the result of converting 5% to a ratio?**

Answer: To covert 5% to a ratio, first express the percent as a fraction: $\frac{5}{100}$, which simplifies to $\frac{1}{20}$. The ratio, then, is 1:20.

Question: **What is the result of converting 3% to a decimal?**

Answer: To convert 3% to a decimal, use the following equation: $3 \div 100 = 0.03$.

Question: **What is the result of converting 25% to a decimal?**

Answer: To convert 25% to a decimal, use the following equation: $25 \div 100 = 0.25$.

Question: **What is the result of converting 150% to a decimal?**

Answer: To convert 150% to a decimal, use the following equation: $150 \div 100 = 1.5$.

Question: **What is the result of converting 0.18 to a percent?**

Answer: To convert 0.18 to a percent, use the following equation: $0.18 \times 100 = 18\%$

Question: **What is the result of converting 5.2 to a percent?**

Answer: To convert 5.2 to a percent, use the following equation: $5.2 \times 100 = 520\%$

Question: **What is the result of converting 0.004 to a percent?**

Answer: To convert 0.004 to a percent, use the following equation: $0.004 \times 100 = 0.4\%$

Question: **If each dose is 5mL, and the total amount of drug to be administered is 200mL, what is the total number of doses available?**

Answer: The total number of doses available is 200mL ÷ 5mL = 40 doses.

Question: **If the dose is 100mg, and the total amount to be administered is 4g, what is the total number of doses available?**

Answer: To calculate this, the quantities must first be converted to the same unit: 4g = 4×10^3mg = 4,000mg. Then, the total number of doses to be administered is 4,000mg ÷ 100mg = 40 doses.

Question: **How many milliliters will be in each dose if 1 fluid ounce of medicine contains 60 doses?**

Answer: First, convert 1 fluid ounce to the same units as the dose: 1 fluid ounce = 30mL. Then, divide the number of milliliters by the number of doses: 30mL ÷ 60 doses = 0.5mL/dose.

Question: **What is the total amount of drug to be administered if each dose is 25mg and the total number of doses is 40?**

Answer: Multiply the number of doses by the quantity of each dose: 25mg/dose × 40 doses = 1,000mg.

Question: **What is the total amount of drug to be administered at a dose of 1,200mg, three times daily, for seven days?**

Answer: Multiply the number of doses by the quantity of each dose: 1,200mg/dose × 3 doses/day × 7 days = 25,200mg.

Question: **What is the total dose for a man weighing 70kg and requiring a dose of 0.5mg/kg?**

Answer: The total dose is 70kg × 0.5mg/kg = 35mg.

Question: **What is the total dose for a woman weighing 110lb and requiring a dose of 2mg/kg?**

Answer: First, convert her weight to kg: 110lb × 1kg/2.2lb = 50kg. Then proceed with the dose calculation: 50kg×2mg/kg = 100mg.

Question: **If an average adult with a BSA of 1.73m^2 requires a dose of 20mg, what would be the dose for a pediatric patient with a BSA of 0.63m^2?**

Answer: First, establish a proportion: $\frac{\text{Child's dose}}{\text{child's BSA}} = \frac{\text{Adult dose}}{\text{adult BSA}}$, or $\frac{x\text{mg}}{0.63\text{m}^2} = \frac{20\text{mg}}{1.73\text{m}^2}$. Cross-multiplying and solving for the unknown variable yields $x\text{mg} = \frac{(20\text{mg} \times 0.63\text{m}^2)}{1.73\text{m}^2} =$ 7.28mg.

Question: **Referring to the previous question, if the average adult dose is 20mg and a child has a BSA of 0.63m^2, what is the child's dose?**

Answer: First, convert the child's BSA to a fraction of adult BSA: $\frac{0.63\text{m}^2}{1.73\text{m}^2} = 0.364$. The child's dose equals the fraction of the adult BSA multiplied by the adult dose: 0.364 × 20mg = 7.28mg.

Question: **The adult dose of a medication is 325mg. What is the dose for an 8-year-old child who weighs 55 pounds, based on Young's rule?**

Answer: Dose = (8y ÷ (8y + 12y)) × 325mg = 130mg.

Question: The adult dose of a medication is 325mg. What is the dose for an 8-year-old child who weighs 55 pounds, based on Clark's rule?

Answer: Dose = (55lb × 325mg) ÷ 150lb = 119.2mg.

Question: How do you calculate the ratio strength of a 0.05% solution?

Answer: The ratio strength of a 0.05% solution can be calculated as follows: $\frac{0.05\%}{100\%} = \frac{1\ part}{x\ parts}$. Solving for x, $x = 2,000$. Therefore, the ratio strength is 1:2000.

Question: How do you express the ratio strength of 1:4,000 as a percent concentration?

Answer: To express the ratio strength of 1:4,000 as a percent concentration, convert the values to fractions: $\frac{1\ part}{4,000\ parts} = \frac{x\%}{100\%}$. Solving for x, $x = 0.025\%$.

Question: Suppose the manufacturer directs adding 15mL of distilled water to the powder to reconstitute 1g of an antibiotic. If the final concentration is 250mg/5mL, what is the powder volume of the dry antibiotic?

Answer: First, determine the amount of active drug ingredient in 1g of powder: 1g = 1,000mg.

The total number of milliliters that will contain the active drug is represented by fractions: $\frac{250mg}{5mL} = \frac{1,000mg}{x\,mL}$. Solving for x, $x = 20mL$. Subtracting the diluent volume from the final volume yields the powder volume: 20mL – 15mL = 5mL.

Question: If 250mL of a 10% solution is diluted with 750mL of diluent, what is the concentration of the final product?

Answer: Using Q1 × C1 = Q2 × C2, calculate the concentration of the final product, where Q1 and C1 are the respective volume and concentration of the first solution, and Q2 and C2 are the respective volume and concentration of the final product: 250mL × 10% = (250+750)mL × C2. Solving for C2, $C2 = \dfrac{250mL \times 10\%}{(250+750)mL} = \dfrac{2,500}{1,000} = 2.5\%$. .

Question: If 25mL of a 1:20 solution is needed, and the stock solution is a 1:5 solution, what is the quantity needed to make the final product?

Answer: Using Q1 × C1 = Q2 × C2, calculate the quantity of the final product, where C1 is the initial concentration, Q2 is the second or final quotient, and C2 is the second or final concentration: $Q1 \times \frac{1}{5} = 25mL \times \frac{1}{20}$. Solving for Q1, Q1 = 6.25mL. In this example, 6.25mL of the stock solution will contain the required amount of active drug. This volume will be increased with an inactive diluent to the total volume of 25mL required for the final product.

Question: What is the final strength of a product that was compounded by combining 200g of 5% ointment and 100g of 1% ointment?

Answer: To calculate the final strength of the product, express the strengths as decimal fractions and multiply by the known quantities: 0.05 × 200g = 10g active ingredient, and 0.01 × 100g = 1g active ingredient. Adding the total grams and dividing by the total quantity yields the following: (10g + 1g active ingredient) ÷ (200g + 100g ointment) = 0.0367. Finally, converting the decimal fraction to a percent yields the final concentration of the compounded product: 0.0367 × 100 = 3.67%.

Question: **How do you mix a 30% solution from a 70% solution and a 20% solution?**

Answer: First, place the known quantities in a matrix:

70 (highest concentration)		
	30 (desired concentration)	
20 (lowest concentration)		

Next, subtract 30 from 70 and write the difference in the lower-right corner. Then subtract 20 from 30 and write the difference in the upper-right corner.

70 (highest concentration)		10 parts
	30 (desired concentration)	
20 (lowest concentration)		40 parts

Reading across the matrix, 10 parts of 70% solution and 40 parts of 20% solution are needed to make 50 parts (10 parts + 40 parts) of a 30% solution.

Question: **What is the specific gravity of a liquid if 100mL of it weighs 85g?**

Answer: To calculate the specific gravity of the liquid, divide the weight by the volume: 85g ÷ 100mL = 0.85.

Question: **If the specific gravity of a solution is 1.2, and 20g of the liquid is needed, what is the total volume required?**

Answer: The total volume required is determined by basic algebra: Specific gravity = number of grams of a substance ÷ number of milliliters of a substance, or 1.2 = 20g ÷ *x*mL. Solving for *x*, *x* = 16.67mL.

Question: **If the specific gravity of a solution is 0.5, and 35mL is available, what is the total weight of the solution?**

Answer: Specific gravity = number of grams of a substance ÷ number of milliliters of a substance, or 0.5 = *x*g ÷ 35mL. Solving for *x*, *x* = 17.5g.

Question: **How do you calculate the specific gravity of a compounded product made from the following ingredients:**

- 500mL of a solution with a specific gravity of 1.2
- 300mL of a solution with a specific gravity of 0.75
- 600mL of a solution with a specific gravity of 0.9

Answer: First, multiply the specific gravity of each component by its volume. Then add the products and divide by the total volume:

- $1.2 \times 500 = 600$
- $0.75 \times 300 = 225$
- $0.9 \times 600 = 540$
- $(600 + 225 + 540) \div (500 + 300 + 600) = 0.975$

The specific gravity of the final product is 0.975.

Question: **If a final product with a specific gravity of 0.8 is desired, and the available products possess specific gravities of 1.25 and 0.6, what are the relative quantities needed of each component?**

Answer: You can use a matrix to calculate the relative quantities needed of each component:

1.25 (highest specific gravity)		
	0.8 (desired specific gravity)	
0.6 (lowest specific gravity)		

Subtracting on the diagonals yields the following:

1.25 (highest specific gravity)		0.2 parts
	0.8 (desired specific gravity)	
0.6 (lowest specific gravity)		0.45 parts

Reading across the matrix, 0.2 parts of the solution with a specific gravity of 1.25 and 0.45 parts of the solution with the specific gravity of 0.6 are needed to compound a final product with a specific gravity of 0.8.

WRAP UP

Chapter Summary

- An understanding of basic mathematics and calculations is essential to pharmacy practice to ensure safe, accurate, and effective drug administration.

- The decimal system is the primary system used for calculations in pharmacy. The scheme of the decimal system is based on powers of 10.

- Roman numerals are used to express quantity, but are not used much in pharmacy today.

- The household system of measurement is familiar to patients.

- The metric system is the most accurate, and preferred, system of measurement in pharmacy. Prefixes are added to base units of measurement in the metric system to denote larger or smaller quantities.

- The apothecary system is an antiquated system of measurement whose use is discouraged because of inaccuracies and safety concerns. However, thyroid medications and phenobarbital are often dosed in grains, the base unit of the apothecary system of dry weight.

- In hospitals, time is expressed using 24-hour or military time. In this case, time is based on a 24-hour clock rather than a 12-hour clock. This reduces ambiguities and errors in medication administration.

- The preferred system for measuring temperature in pharmacy and medicine is the Celsius scale. In this scale, water freezes at a temperature of 0°C and boils at 100°C.

- In the Fahrenheit scale, water freezes at a temperature of 32°F and boils at 212°F.

- Fractions represent part of a whole. Fractions contain a numerator and a denominator.

- A ratio represents how two quantities are related to each other. A ratio may also be expressed as a fraction, and vice versa.

- Proportions are equivalent ratios, often used to calculate unknown quantities or concentrations in pharmacy.

- Percents are the number of parts per 100 total parts. A percent can also be expressed as a fraction or a ratio.

- Concentrations, quantities, specific gravities, doses, and dosage regimens can be determined using basic algebra or the ratio-proportion method, when some of the values are known.

- Doses of drugs are highly variable and can be based on the drug's chemical composition or physical properties, the route of administration, or the condition being treated. Alternatively, patient factors such as age, body weight, body-surface area, or organ function may be used to calculate the correct dose.

- Pediatric patients require special consideration when determining doses, because children have immature organ function and a different body composition from adults.

Learning Assessment Questions

1. 68°F is equivalent to how many degrees Celsius?
   A. 20°C
   B. 154.4°C
   C. 64.8°C
   D. 37.8°C

2. Aminophylline contains 80% theophylline. The concentration of an aminophylline injection is 25mg/mL. How many milliliters of aminophylline are needed to provide a dose of 640mg theophylline?
   A. 25.6mL
   B. 512mL
   C. 20.5mL
   D. 32mL

3. The ratio 4:25 is equivalent to what percent?
   A. 4%
   B. 25%
   C. 16%
   D. 40%

4. If 8g of powder are needed to make 50mL of a product, how many grams of powder are needed to make 725mL of product?

   A. 35g

   B. 116g

   C. 55g

   D. 290g

5. If a patient is prescribed 2 teaspoonfuls of medicine four times daily for 10 days, what is the total dose of medicine the patient will receive?

   A. 100mL

   B. 8mL

   C. 80mL

   D. 400mL

6. How many ounces are in 6 avoirdupois pounds?

   A. 96oz

   B. 72oz

   C. 454oz

   D. 30oz

7. How is 37 expressed in Roman numerals?

   A. XLVII

   B. XXLIIIX

   C. XXXVII

   D. VIIXX

8. How is the following Roman numeral expressed in the Arabic system: MCMLIX?

   A. 1959

   B. 2199

   C. 2011

   D. 1987

9. How many grains of aspirin are in one 325mg tablet?

   A. 65gr

   B. 21gr

   C. 5gr

   D. 15gr

10. If the concentration of an antibiotic solution is 200mg/5mL, how many milligrams of drug will be in 1 ounce of solution?

    A. 40mg

    B. 1,200mg

    C. 200mg

    D. 13.3mg

11. A physician orders a drug at a dose of 2mg/kg. The patient weighs 187lb. What is the correct dose?

    A. 42.5mg

    B. 374mg

    C. 170mg

    D. 823mg

12. If the dose of a drug is 75mcg, how many doses are contained in 0.35g?

    A. 4666.67 doses

    B. 4.67 doses

    C. 26.25 doses

    D. 466,667 doses

13. A physician prescribes 2 teaspoonfuls of a medication three times daily for seven days. What is the total volume that should be dispensed to the patient?

    A. 630mL

    B. 42mL

    C. 210mL

    D. 35mL

14. If the adult dose of a drug is $0.8mg/m^2$, what dose should be administered to a child with a body-surface area of $1.32m^2$? (Remember, the average adult BSA is $1.73m^2$.)

    A. $10.5mg/m^2$

    B. $1.38mg/m^2$

    C. $1.06mg/m^2$

    D. $0.61mg/m^2$

15. What is the body-surface area of an adult woman who is 5'4" tall and weighs 115lb?

    A. $1.42m^2$

    B. $1.53m^2$

    C. $1.02m^2$

    D. $1.17m^2$

16. What times should a medication be given, expressed in 24-hour time, if it is ordered to be given every eight hours beginning at midnight?

    A. 0000M, 08 a.m., and 16 p.m.

    B. 8:00 a.m. and 4:00 p.m.

    C. 0000, 0800, 1600

    D. 0, 8, 16

17. What time is 2130, expressed in 12-hour time?

    A. 9:30 p.m.

    B. 2:13 a.m.

    C. 1:30 p.m.

    D. 3:21 a.m.

18. A syrup contains 0.1% (%w/v) active ingredient. If a physician prescribes 8 ounces to be dispensed, how many milligrams will be contained in the total prescription?

    A. 80mg

    B. 240mg

    C. 800mg

    D. 378mg

19. A lotion contains 15mg drug in 750mg base. What is the percentage concentration (%w/w) of the lotion?

    A. 200%

    B. 0.2%

    C. 2%

    D. 50%

20. If 250mL of a 1:750 (v/v) solution is diluted to 1,000mL, what is the ratio strength (v/v) of the final product?

    A. 1:187.5

    B. 1:333

    C. 1:425

    D. 1:625

21. How many milliliters of water should be added to 1 pint of 70% solution to prepare a 30% solution?

    A. 1,120mL

    B. 640mL

    C. 205mL

    D. 2.4mL

22. Round the following number to the nearest hundredth: 345.648.

    A. 345.6

    B. 300

    C. 345.65

    D. 345.680

23. A physician prescribes three tablets to be taken four times daily. If 100 tablets are dispensed, how many days supply will the patient receive?

    A. 8.3 days

    B. 33.3 days

    C. 12.6 days

    D. 25 days

24. How many milligrams are equivalent to 6g?

    A. 600mg

    B. ⅙mg

    C. 6,000mg

    D. 60,000mg

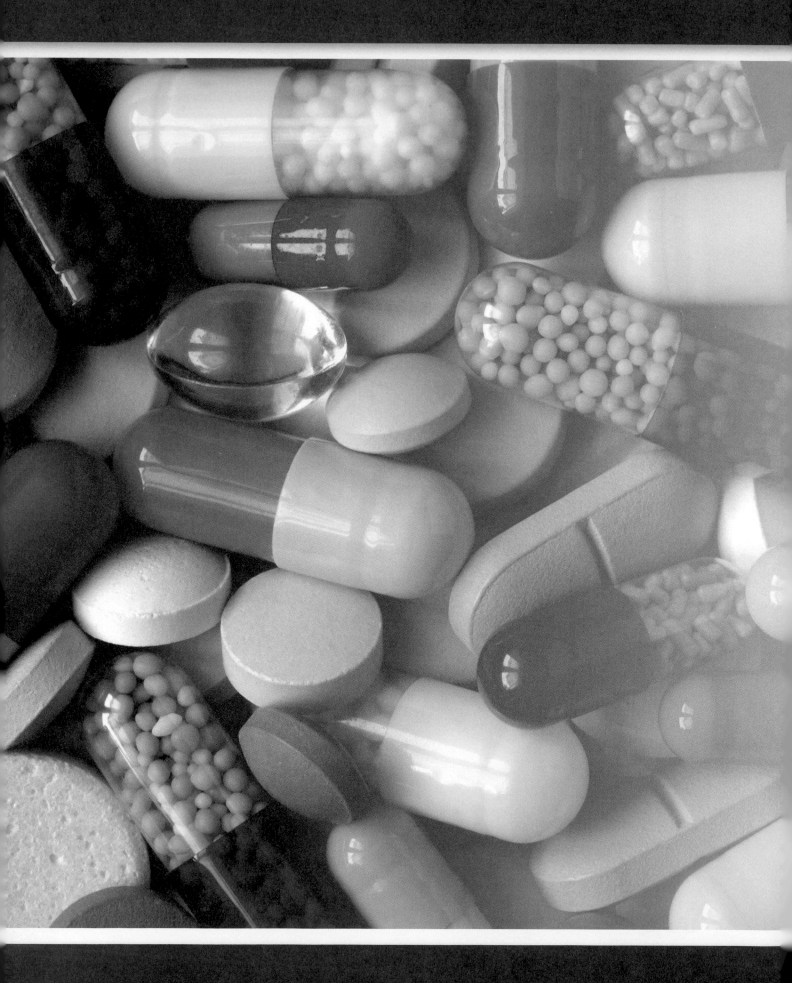

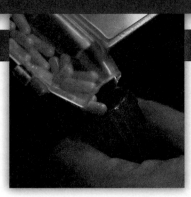

Medication Safety

OBJECTIVES

After reading this chapter, you will be able to:

- Identify problems patients would experience with over-the-counter purchases and take appropriate action to intervene.
- Identify commonly prescribed drugs.
- Identify look-alike and sound-alike medications.
- Discuss strategies in preventing medication errors.
- Understand the extent of medical and medication errors and their effects on patient health and safety.
- Review specific categories and medication errors.
- List examples of medication errors commonly seen in pharmacy practice settings.
- Apply a systematic evaluation to search for medication error potential to a pharmacy practice model.
- Define strategies, including use of automation, for preventing medication errors.
- Identify the common systems available for reporting medication errors.
- Compare common over-the-counter and prescription medications.
- Evaluate the effects of medication errors on patient health and safety.
- Participate in strategies for preventing and reporting medication errors.
- Explain categories and common uses of antibiotic classes.

KEY TERMS

Aerobic
Anaerobic
Anaphylaxis
Bactericidal antibiotic
Bacteriostatic antibiotic
Chelation
Electronic medication
    administration
    record (eMAR)
Empirical treatment
Extra-dose error
Human-failure error
Immunocompromised

Institute for Safe
    Medication Practices
    (ISMP)
Look-alike sound-alike
Medical error
Medication error
Medication Error
    Reporting Program
    (MERP)
MEDMARX
MedWatch
Nephrotoxicity
Omission error

Organizational-failure
    error
Ototoxicity
Perioperative
Prescribing error
Ribonucleic acid (RNA)
Sentinel event
Substrate
Technical-failure error
Wrong–dosage form
    error
Wrong-dose error
Wrong-time error

Chapter Overview

Medication use is abundant in the United States, with an estimated 82% of adults taking at least one medication on a regular basis, and 29% taking five or more. Medications can be used to treat an acute disease, manage the symptoms of a chronic condition, or prevent the onset of new symptoms. Medications are rigorously tested and proved to be safe and effective when used in accordance with directions provided by a prescriber or the manufacturer. However, medications are not without risk. With the increased use of medications to prevent disease, an aging population that requires more medical intervention, and the discovery of new medications, safety is of the utmost concern in health care today. Every member of the healthcare team plays an important role in ensuring that all patients receive the most effective medication with the fewest possible risks and side effects. Knowledge and awareness of medication safety will empower patients, strengthen morale of healthcare providers, and improve quality of health care provision.

Over-the-Counter (OTC) Medications

An over-the-counter (OTC) medication is classified as any medication product that can be purchased without a prescription. There are more than 80 therapeutic classes of OTC medications recognized by the FDA. OTCs can treat conditions like cough and cold symptoms, pain, acne, topical fungal infections, motion sickness, sleeplessness, and many other conditions. OTC drugs also include products like mouthwash, toothpaste, antiperspirants, medicated shampoos, sun block, and smoking-cessation aids, just to name a few.

The safety and efficacy requirements for OTC products are identical to the requirements for prescription drugs. The difference between a prescription and an OTC drug is that the FDA states that OTC drugs generally have the following characteristics:

- Their benefits outweigh their risks.
- The potential for misuse and abuse is low.
- Consumers can use them for self-diagnosed conditions.
- They can be adequately labeled.
- Health practitioners are not needed for the safe and effective use of the product.

Many drugs are introduced to the market as OTCs, while others are first introduced as prescriptions and later gain OTC status. In order for a drug to switch from prescription to OTC, the medication must meet the aforementioned criteria. Some drugs that have made this switch in recent years include Prevacid, Prilosec, Zyrtec, Miralax, and Claritin. All of these drugs are available over the counter in the same strength that was formerly available as prescription only. Other drugs may become available over the counter, but at lower strengths than what may be available as prescription. For example, ibuprofen is available OTC as a 200mg tablet, but is available by prescription only in strengths of 400mg, 600mg, and 800mg per tablet. Some OTC medications are not recommended for long-term use without instructions from a physician, but many can be taken routinely with no concern, as long as the patient follows the printed directions.

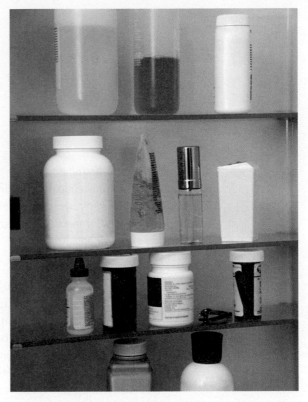

The use of OTC medications is increasing because of rising healthcare costs, inadequate health-insurance coverage, convenience, and a desire for patient autonomy. In about one-third of health-related problems, consumers do nothing at all, choosing to ignore symptoms or to do nothing to treat them. Of the remaining two-thirds of cases, one-quarter will enter the healthcare system at some level. The remaining consumers self-diagnose and self-treat illnesses and conditions. Most of these people will choose an OTC product. Consumers generally view OTC products as safer and easier to use than prescription products. But, this ready access to a plethora of drug products does not mean that the use of OTC products is of no concern.

Nearly all Americans take at least one medication every day.

Safety of OTC Medications

Some OTC medications specifically indicate on their labels that they should not be used for more than a specified number of days without the advice of a healthcare professional. This is common with products that may alleviate symptoms of a more serious underlying condition that may require medical attention. Drugs like antihistamines, antiperspirants, and mouthwash may be taken continually without consulting a healthcare professional.

All medications, even those available without a prescription, pose a risk of side effects and drug interactions. Not all drugs are appropriate for all patients. Therefore, pharmacy technicians and pharmacists in a community practice are routinely approached for advice concerning the proper choice and use of OTC products. A pharmacy technician may help patients by reading medication labels and warnings or comparing drug products, but questions regarding proper drug selection, indications, dose, administration, therapeutic effects, side effects, contraindications, and interactions should be referred to a pharmacist.

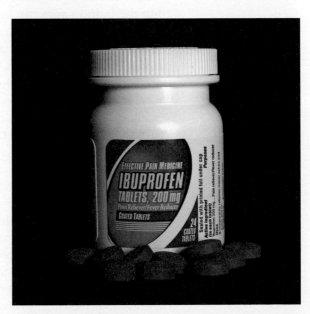

Ibuprofen is available as a prescription and an OTC product.

OTC products should be used for the short-term treatment of self-limiting conditions.

Clear and concise labeling enables consumers to choose the most appropriate medication for their symptoms and to avoid taking similar medications or drug classes simultaneously.

Labeling Requirements for OTC Medications

Because consumers purchase and use most OTC medications without the direction of a physician or pharmacist, it is important that all OTC medications contain ample and adequate directions, written in easy-to-understand language for the every-day consumer. The FDA requires that prominent labeling on OTC products includes the product's active and inactive ingredients, purpose for use, directions for use, warnings, and age-appropriate dosing information. An expiration date is also required.

Potential Problems with OTC Medications

Due to the abundance of advertising for OTC drugs, patients are likely to become confused about the most appropriate choice of product. In addition, it is often difficult to recognize and identify the source of symptoms, resulting in an inaccurate self-diagnosis.

Some patients may not know the names of the other medications they are taking, causing them to misinterpret clearly presented safety information. For example, the labeling of cimetidine (Tagamet) contains a warning that it interacts with warfarin. If a patient knows he is taking brand-name Coumadin, but does not know that it is the same drug as warfarin, he may unknowingly put himself at risk of a potentially serious drug interaction.

It is important that pharmacy technicians and pharmacists be aware of brand and generic names of OTC products. Of the more than 300,000 OTC medications sold in most community retail establishments, there are only 700 distinct active ingredients. Therefore, pharmacy technicians and pharmacists must educate the public on OTC products with different names but the same ingredients. There are also products with the same name that contain different ingredients, as in the case of Mylanta preparations and Afrin products. Additionally, Tylenol is the brand name for acetaminophen, but the brand name can be used on products that do not contain acetaminophen. It is extremely important to read the labels and become familiar with the ingredients in over the counter medications. This enables the pharmacy technician to assist customers when purchasing OTC medications. When patients are better informed, they are better advocates for their own health. In turn, safety is maintained and patients receive appropriate treatment.

OTC Cough and Cold Products   OTC products intended to treat cough, cold, and allergy symptoms are a significant source of confusion and medication errors. These products are intended to treat coughing, chest or nasal congestion, itchy eyes, or sneezing. These products will not cure a cough, cold, or allergies; they are only intended to make the patient more comfortable. These products often contain decongestants, antihistamines, and analgesics, either alone or in combination.

Serious adverse events have been reported when children take OTC cough and cold products. In 2008, the FDA released a public health advisory warning parents that giving any OTC cough and cold product to a child under two years of age could be dangerous or even fatal, and is not recommended. The American Academy of Pediatrics supports these recommendations. The FDA-approved age for specific dosing and use is listed by the manufacturer on the label and packaging. Several studies report that these products are not effective in children younger than six years old.

One of the most significant sources of errors among adult and pediatric products is the availability of combination products. Consumers may unknowingly give themselves or their children an overdose of medication, not realizing that a combination product contains several active ingredients. Surveys of parents routinely demonstrate that consumers do not understand that brand-name and generic-name drugs are the same ingredient. In addition, most do not know how to accurately measure and administer OTC medications.

Cough, cold, and allergy symptoms are usually self-limiting and will resolve on their own. Consumers should not continue to self-medicate with OTC products that may not be providing relief of symptoms. Continued treatment of chronic symptoms may be ineffective and potentially unsafe. In this situation, patients should be advised to seek the advice of a healthcare provider.

Homeopathic Medications

The use of homeopathic medications is controversial in the practice of pharmacy. Homeopathy is based on the principle of "like cures like," and uses very small quantities of natural products diluted often in a large percentage of water. Homeopathy is rooted in the idea that these natural products stimulate the body's own immune system. There is little scientific data to support this idea, however. Homeopathy was first practiced over 200 years ago and has changed little since its inception. The FDA recognizes some products as being homeopathic. Most homeopathic products are available OTC, but there are a few prescription-only homeopathic remedies.

FDA-approved OTC homeopathic products are usually intended for short-term use for conditions that do not require a medical diagnosis or monitoring. However, many homeopathic medications that are not FDA approved are available over the counter, or specially prepared by homeopathic doctors or practitioners, who may claim to treat severe and chronic conditions. Patients should be aware that homeopathic products may pose a risk for drug interactions with certain foods, prescription medications, and OTC medications. Patients should be advised to tell their physician and pharmacist about all homeopathic remedies they are taking.

Dietary and Nutritional Supplements

Dietary and herbal supplements include vitamins, minerals, and herbs. These supplements are loosely regulated in the United States, with most of the control governed by the Dietary Supplement Health and Education Act (DSHEA) amendments of 1994. Other than when patient safety is a concern, the FDA has no jurisdiction over diet supplements. Therefore, the quality, safety, and origin of many of these products is questionable. Supplements must contain a disclaimer stating, "This statement has not been evaluated by the FDA. This product is not intended to diagnose, treat, cure, or prevent any disease."

Patients should be advised to follow the dosing recommendations provided by the manufacturer, and not to exceed these doses without the advice of a trained healthcare provider. As with homeopathic remedies, it is important for pharmacy and healthcare providers to be aware of all drugs and supplements that a patient is taking in order to make drug interactions milder.

Technicians should not counsel patients on OTC products.

Common Prescription Drugs

Prescription drug sales exceeded $307 billion in 2010, growing at a rate of more than 2.3% from the previous year. Oncologics achieved the most sales in terms of dollar amount, followed by respiratory agents. Lipid regulators and anti-diabetes agents were the third and fourth top-selling drugs by therapeutic class, respectively. Atorvastatin (Lipitor), manufactured by Pfizer, was the single highest grossing drug in 2010, with a revenue of $7.2 billion.

In terms of number of prescriptions dispensed, analgesics rank first. Other classes of frequently prescribed drugs include antidepressants, cholesterol-lowering drugs, antihypertensives (blood pressure–lowering drugs), antibiotics, thyroid medications, diabetes drugs, and asthma-controlling drugs. The top-selling drugs in the United States do not vary much from year to year. Some of the most commonly prescribed drugs sold in the United States, and their generic equivalents, are provided in TABLE 6.1 .

Table 6.1   Top Prescription Drugs in the United States

Drug Class/Action	Generic Ingredient	Brand Name (If Applicable)
Antidepressants	Duloxetine	Cymbalta
	Escitalopram	Lexapro
	Fluoxetine	Prozac
	Sertraline	Zoloft
	Trazodone	Desyrel
	Venlafaxine	Effexor XR
Antibiotics	Amoxicillin	Amoxil
	Amoxicillin/clavulanate	Augmentin
	Azithromycin	Zithromax
	Cephalexin	Keflex
	Levofloxacin	Levaquin
	Sulfamethoxazole/trimethoprim	Bactrim
Analgesics	Celecoxib	Celebrex
	Hydrocodone/acetaminophen	Lortab, Vicodin, and others
	Oxycodone/acetaminophen	Percocet
	Pregabalin*	Lyrica
	Tramadol	Ultram
Antihypertensives	Amlodipine	Norvasc
	Atenolol	Tenormin
	Lisinopril	Prinivil, Zestril
	Metoprolol	Lopressor, Toprol XL
	Valsartan	Diovan
Cholesterol-lowering agents	Atorvastatin	Lipitor
	Ezetimibe/simvastatin	Vytorin
	Fenofibrate	Tricor
	Rosuvastatin	Crestor
	Simvastatin	Zocor

Table 6.1 Top Prescription Drugs in the United States (Continued)

Drug Class/Action	Generic Ingredient	Brand Name (If Applicable)
Asthma- and chronic obstructive pulmonary disease–controlling medications	Fluticasone/salmeterol	Advair Diskus
	Mometasone	Nasonex
	Montelukast	Singulair
	Prednisone	Many
Anti-diabetic agents	Insulin	Many
	Metformin	Glucophage
	Pioglitazone	Actos
Proton-pump inhibitors	Esomeprazole	Nexium
	Lansoprazole	Prevacid
	Omeprazole	Prilosec
Anti-anxiety agents	Alprazolam	Xanax
	Clonazepam	Klonopin
Thyroid hormone	Levothyroxine	Synthroid
Erectile dysfunction	Sildenafil	Viagra
Sleep aid	Zolpidem	Ambien
Anticoagulant	Warfarin	Coumadin
Antiplatelet agent	Clopidogrel	Plavix
Antipsychotic	Quetiapine	Seroquel
Osteoporosis prevention and treatment	Alendronate	Fosamax

*Pregabalin is also used as an anticonvulsant.

Medical Errors

A **medical error** is any action, inaction, or decision that contributes to an unintended consequence in health care. A medical error may be an inaccurate or incomplete diagnosis, an inappropriate or ineffective treatment of a disease or condition, or an injury, syndrome, or behavior that results from a medical treatment. Ultimately, a medical error is an adverse event that could have been prevented given the current state of medical knowledge. Medical errors may be seemingly small, resulting in no actual harm. For example, if a laboratory sample is drawn at the wrong time, the results may not accurately reflect the level of drug in a patient's body. Another example is a medication that is administered late, perhaps preventing a patient from achieving optimal drug levels as quickly as possible and delaying overall treatment. A third example is a patient who receives a regular diet in the hospital instead of the low-salt diet ordered by his physician. While these errors may not cause a direct or substantial injury, they contribute to less-than-optimal care and convenience for the patient. Moreover, a delay in overall therapeutic effect may lead to lost productivity or increased healthcare costs.

More-serious medical errors may result in significant disability or death. For example, filling a prescription incorrectly with a higher dose of the drug than prescribed can cause an overdose of medication, which could be fatal depending on the drug. Or dispensing the wrong anesthetic could very likely result in patient death. The pharmacy technician as part of the pharmacy team must integrate the prevention of medical errors into the filling of every prescription. A double-check process to ensure the correct medication is dispensed according to the prescription must always be in place to ensure patient safety.

Cost of Medical Errors

Regardless of which stage of the healthcare process in which they occur, medical errors are costly. It is estimated that in hospitals alone, as many as 98,000 people die each year in the United States from medical errors. This far exceeds the number of people who die as a result of motor-vehicle accidents, breast cancer, or complications related to the acquired immune deficiency syndrome (AIDS). The total costs related to medical errors that result in injury may reach nearly $30 billion annually. (Healthcare costs represent half of this total.) Opportunity costs are also high for medical errors, resulting in increased financial, personnel, and time resources directed toward repeated tests, additional therapy, or prolonged hospital stays.

No less significant are the indirect costs associated with a loss of trust in the healthcare system. Both patients and healthcare providers are increasingly dissatisfied with the outcomes of the healthcare system. A loss of morale and frustration in the healthcare system result in lost productivity, reduced school attendance by children, and lower levels of overall population health.

Many circumstances contribute to medical errors, but every individual on the healthcare team must take responsibility for his or her own actions and be vigilant about preserving the safety, well-being, and trust of patients. Most medical errors can be prevented, and attention to safety details is paramount in improving the quality of care provided in today's healthcare system.

Medication Errors

According to the National Coordinating Council for Medication Error Reporting and Prevention, a **medication error** is defined as follows:

> Any preventable event that may cause or lead to inappropriate medication use or patient harm while the medication is under control of the healthcare professional, patient, or consumer. Such events may be related to professional practice, healthcare products, procedures, and systems, including prescribing; order communication; product labeling, packaging, and nomenclature; compounding; dispensing; distribution; administration; education; monitoring; and use.

A **prescribing error** has been further defined as any action in the prescribing decision or prescription-writing process that leads to an unintentional significant reduction in the probability of treatment being timely and effective or an increase in the risk of harm when compared with generally accepted practice. Many medication errors do originate with the prescriber—the person who made the decision about choice of therapy and dosage. Determining why the error occurred and preventing future errors is far more important than pointing blame at one group of healthcare providers.

Significance of Medication Errors

In pharmacy, a medication error may occur at any point in the process of selecting, prescribing, transcribing, dispensing, administering, or monitoring drug therapy. Medication errors are among the most common medical errors, and are considered almost entirely preventable. Of the 98,000 people who die as a result of a medical error, 7,000 of the deaths are attributed to a medication error.

Each year, nearly 1.5 million preventable medication errors result in harm, including 380,000 to 450,000 among hospitalized patients. Each year in the United States, medication errors and problems

A 2006 report by the Institute of Medicine (IOM) indicates that medication errors occur at a rate of one per patient per day in hospitals.

account for 116 million additional physician visits, 76 million additional prescriptions, 17 million
emergency room visits, and 3 million admissions to
long-term–care facilities. While most information
regarding medication errors is collected from hospital
data, it is estimated that nearly 2% of all prescriptions
dispensed in a community pharmacy contain some
type of medication error.

*Medication errors are a significant
source of healthcare costs, death, and
disability in the United States.*

Causes of Medication Errors

Pharmacy technicians can be especially vigilant to monitor, prevent, and report
medication errors that occur in pharmacies daily. There are several primary types of
medication errors, and the causes of each are multifaceted. Although one healthcare
provider cannot prevent all medication errors, one provider can establish safe practices
to do his or her part to reduce medication errors as much as possible.

Individual Causes

Some medication errors occur because of patient response. Individuals have unique
physiological and social characteristics that influence the effect of medications. In
this way, it is impossible to predict exactly who will have an adverse reaction to a
medication or when it will occur.

Physiological causes of medication errors include age-related organ dysfunction or
a genetically determined high or low level of enzymes necessary for drug metabolism.
For example, many drugs rely on kidney or liver function for proper metabolism,
and chronic kidney or liver disease affects a patient's ability to properly metabolize or
eliminate drugs in the body. When patients have a compromised kidney or liver, many
medications must be dosed differently to accommodate these conditions. If the patient's
medication dosing is assessed and properly based on these conditions, this would be
a preventable medication error. A medication error occurs when organ function is not
measured and the dose of a medication is not adjusted appropriately.

Social causes of medication errors most often occur in the outpatient setting and
are not entirely preventable by a healthcare provider, although steps can be taken to
reduce the likelihood of errors occurring. Usually, patients incorrectly administer their
medications, both prescription and OTC products, resulting in ineffective treatment
or adverse effects. Some patients are simply noncompliant with medication therapy
instructions because of conditions such as costs or language barriers. Additionally,
patients may not understand the instructions, or may fail to get a prescription filled
at all. Some patients simply stop taking a drug or start taking a new one without
seeking the advice of a physician or pharmacist. Any of these situations could lead to
inappropriate medication-therapy management, ranging from an ineffective underdose
to a toxic overdose.

Technicians can help assess individual causes of medication errors by thoroughly
reviewing a patient's medication history and refill history to establish compliance. Once
brought to the pharmacist's attention, such examples of social causes of medication
errors can be addressed when the pharmacist counsels the patient.

Classification of Medication Errors

The cause of most medication errors is difficult to determine, often attributable to
multiple systemic or organizational weaknesses. The errors themselves, however, are
divided into five main categories.

- An **omission error** occurs when a prescribed dose is not administered as ordered.
- A **wrong-dose error** occurs when a dose is either above or below the correct dose.
- An **extra-dose error** occurs when a patient receives more doses than were actually prescribed by the prescriber.
- A **wrong–dosage form error** occurs when the dose is not administered to the patient by the route intended by the prescriber.
- A **wrong-time error** occurs when the drug is not given at the correct time.

Alternatively, the reasons for the errors can be grouped into three categories.

- A **human-failure error** occurs at an individual level and is performance-related. Human failures may include a lack of proper training or education, or a failure to follow organizational protocols or policies and procedures. Often, human failures are cited in combination with other factors that contributed to a medication error.
- A **technical-failure error** results from environmental or location factors or equipment malfunctions. Technical failures may include such issues as lighting, noise, staffing levels, distractions in the pharmacy workspace, or a failure of machinery or equipment to operate correctly.
- An **organizational-failure error** occurs when rules or policies direct the inappropriate selection, preparation, or administration of a medication.

According to a large-scale evaluation of medication-error reports, the three most-frequently reported medication errors are omission errors, wrong-dose errors, and prescribing errors. These three types of errors account for 68% of reported errors. The types of errors that most frequently resulted in harm were wrong–route of administration or wrong dosage–form errors and wrong-dose errors. The leading causes of failures included performance deficits, failure to follow a procedure or protocol, and inaccurate order communication

Preventing Medication Errors

The American Hospital Association provides five categories to help determine why and how medication errors occur:

- Incomplete patient information, including patient allergies, other medications patients are taking, previous diagnoses, or lab results
- Unavailable drug information, including the most up-to-date warnings
- Miscommunication of drug orders, including poor handwriting, confusion between two similar drug names, misuse of zeros and decimal points, confusion of units, and inappropriate abbreviations
- Lack of appropriate labeling as the drug is prepared and/or repackaged
- Environmental factors, including interruptions and distractions for healthcare professionals

Focusing on why and how medication errors happen allows for the development of techniques and reporting systems to identify and prevent future errors. In 1992, the FDA began monitoring medication-error reports that were received by the **Institute for Safe Medication Practices (ISMP)**, which is an organization that monitors medication errors and makes recommendations on how to prevent them, and the United States Pharmacopeia (USP). Today, the **MedWatch** program, the FDA's adverse drug event–reporting system for healthcare providers, patients, and consumers, also monitors potential medication errors. As a result, the ISMP and the FDA have launched programs to educate healthcare providers on strategies to reduce common medication errors. Overall, the ISMP has developed 10 key elements that have the greatest impact on safe medication use:

1. Patient information
2. Drug information
3. Medication-related communication
4. Drug labeling, packaging, and naming system
5. Drug standardization, storage, and distribution
6. Medication-delivery selection
7. Environmental factors
8. Staff competency and education
9. Patient education
10. Quality-improvement processes and risk management

ISMP promotes the following:

- Having up-to-date information available for prescribers and healthcare providers
- Collaboration between all healthcare team members and the patient
- Restricting access to drugs commonly reported in medication errors
- Systems for identifying, reporting, analyzing and reducing the risk of medication errors

ISMP also advocates for a nonpunitive culture of safety within the healthcare system. Often, the pharmacy is very busy, and medication errors are either overlooked or not reported. These unreported errors contribute to safety issues with medications. When medication errors go unreported, the safety data on specific medications is not complete and it may take longer to identify adverse events that are occurring due to a specific drug. There is also an ethical component involved with reporting medication errors. Not only does it protect the patient by providing additional drug-safety information to the FDA and the drug manufacturer, it also assists in providing the best of care to the patient. Pharmacy staff may not want to report a medication error if it involves a co-worker. Turning someone in for making a medication error is just plain tough. However, the only way to change policies or procedures and to learn from the error is to identify and report it accordingly. Only then can changes to improve patient safety and provide better care to the patient occur. The Institute for Safe Medication Practices provides extensive information to assist with medical-error reporting and the personal responsibility of reporting medication errors.

Unapproved Abbreviations

One of the well-publicized campaigns promoted by the FDA and the ISMP is the publication of the "List of Error-Prone Abbreviations, Symbols, and Dose Designations." This list emphasizes the need for safety first in the written communication of medication orders. TABLE 6.2 displays some of the common abbreviations and symbols involved in medication errors that are included on the ISMP's full list.

Table 6.2 Commonly Misinterpreted Abbreviations and Symbols	
Unapproved Abbreviation	**Correct Form, to Be Written Out Completely**
>	"greater than"
<	"less than"
cc	"mL" or "milliliter"
μ	"micro" or "mc"
hs	"half-strength" or "at bedtime"
IU	"International Unit"
qd	"daily" or "every day"
U	"units"
$MgSO_4$	"Magnesium sulfate"
MSO_4	"Morphine sulfate"

Look-Alike Sound-Alike Medications

So-called **look-alike sound-alike** medication names are a source of confusion for medical and pharmacy personnel. With tens of thousands of brand and generic medication names available, the chance for confusion is likely. In addition to looking or sounding like other drug names, poor handwriting, similar packaging, or similar therapeutic uses contribute to frequent mistakes in interpreting drug names.

The ISMP's "List of Confused Drug Names" includes pairs of medications whose names have been involved in medication errors. The Joint Commission, the organization that provides accreditation to hospitals and healthcare programs and organizations, requires that all accredited programs have a look-alike sound-alike list within the organization. An abbreviated version of the ISMP list is presented in **TABLE 6.3**.

To reduce the incidence of medication errors involving look-alike sound-alike medications, several strategies may be implemented:

- Minimize the use of verbal or telephone orders as much as possible.
- Carefully read the label each time a medication is obtained from the stock shelves or cabinets. Do not merely rely on visual recognition or location to verify a drug product.
- Legibly print all drug names and doses to prevent confusion.
- Use "tall-man" lettering if necessary to emphasize differences in drug names, as in the preceding list.
- Implement storage strategies such as color-coding or boldface labeling for commonly confused medications.

Tall-man lettering is the capitalization of portions of names that differ among look-alike sound-alike drug names.

Clinical Recommendations

In addition to the ISMP, several other organizations have published clinical pharmacy service recommendations to reduce medication errors. These include the Agency for Healthcare Research and Quality (AHRQ), the Institute for Healthcare Improvement (IHI), the Institute of Medicine (IOM), the National Quality Forum, and Pathways for Medication Safety.

The AHRQ is a division of the United States Department of Health and Human Services. It has identified two distinct pharmacy services that have a high potential to reduce medication errors: pharmacist consultation services and information transfer

Table 6.3   Common Look-Alike Sound-Alike Drug Names

Accupril/Aciphex	Doxil/Paxil	Panlor DC/Pamelor
AcetaZOLAMIDE/acetoHEXAMIDE	Enjuvia/Januvia	Patanol/Platinol
Aciphex/Aricept	Evista/AVINza	Paxil/Taxol
Actonel/Actos	Fioicet/Fiorinal	Paxil/Plavix
Adacel (Tdap)/Daptacel (DTaP)	Flovent/Flonase	Percocet/Procet
Adderall/Inderal	Folic acid/folinic acid	PENTObarbital/PHENObarbital
Advair/Advicor	Foradil/Fortical	Pilocar/Dilacor XR
Aggrastat/argatroban	Foradil/Toradol	Plendil/Isordil
Alora/Aldara	GuanFACINE/guaiFENesin	Polycitra/Bicitra
ALPRAZolam/LORazepam	Heparin/Hespan	Precare/Precose
Amantadine/amiodarone	Statins/nystatin	PrednisoLONE/prednisone
Amaryl/Reminyl	HydrALAZINE/hydrOXYzine	QuiNIDine/quiNINE
Antacid/Atacand	Inderall/Adderall	Qwell/Kwell
Antivert/Axert	InFLIXimab/riTUXimab	Rabeprazole/aripiprazole
Aricept/Azilect	Iodine/Lodine	Retrovir/ritonavir
AVINZza/INVanz	LaMICtal/LamISIL	Rifampin/rifaximin
Benazepril/Benadryl	Lanoxin/naloxone	Tiazac/Ziac
CeleBREX/Cerebyx	Lunesta/Neulasta	TiZANidine/tiaGABine
CeleXA/CeleBREX	MS Contin/Oxycontin	Tricor/Tracleer
CeleXA/Cerebyx	Neulasta/Neumega	VinBLASTine/vinCRISTine
Clindets/Clindesses	Neumega/Neupogen	Xanax/Zantac
Cymbalta/Symbyax	Neurontin/Motrin	Zebeta/Diabeta
DACTINomycin/DAPTOmycin	Oracea/Orencia	Zocor/Cozaar
DAUNorubicin/DOXOrubicin	Os-Cal/Asacol	Zyvox/Zovirax
Denavir/indinavir	Pamelor/Tambocor	

between inpatient and outpatient pharmacies. Overall, the AHRQ notes several opportunities for the implementation or expansion of pharmacy services to reduce the likelihood of medication errors:

- Implementing computerized order-entry systems with decision-making support
- Implementing automated medication-dispensing devices
- Limiting antibiotic use
- Improving **perioperative** management (that is, management of the period of time during and around a surgical procedure)
- Providing geriatric and pain-consulting services

The IHI recommends three key practices to reduce medication errors:

- Pharmacy-based dosing for certain high-risk medications
- Pharmacy-based dosing for patients with impaired kidney function
- Assigning pharmacists to patient-care units

Similarly, the IOM and the National Quality Forum recommend increasing pharmacist involvement in direct patient care, such as making pharmacists available for consultation during preparation of medication orders, having pharmacists participate

Strategies and clinical recommendations are available from several organizations to help reduce medication errors.

in hospital rounds, and having pharmacists counsel hospital patients. The Pathways for Medication Safety furthers such recommendations by emphasizing that pharmacists should routinely adjust doses for patients with kidney or liver dysfunction and provide in-service education to medical staff.

The Role of the Pharmacy Technician in Preventing Medication Errors

Although most of these clinical recommendations are more applicable to pharmacists than to pharmacy technicians, the technician is responsible for supporting the pharmacist's activities so that the pharmacist may be available to provide clinical support or recommendations to physicians, nurses, or other healthcare providers. However, the technician is the primary member of the pharmacy staff responsible for filling

Observe and report information affecting drug safety or effectiveness to the pharmacist.

prescriptions, in both community and hospital settings. As such, the pharmacy technician has ample opportunities at each stage in the process to recognize, correct, report, and prevent medication errors. By diligently maintaining safe working conditions and monitoring for sources of errors, technicians make significant contributions to patient safety. Transversely, if the pharmacy technician makes an error, a pharmacy may be more likely to make an error. All pharmacy workers must be sure to verify their own and each other's work.

Receiving the Prescription

First, the pharmacy technician will likely be the first to receive and review the prescription and the last staff member to review the final filled prescription before it leaves the pharmacy. The pharmacist performs the final check, but the pharmacy technician usually dispenses it directly to the patient or delivers it to the healthcare practitioner who administers it. The technician is responsible for verifying that the information provided is complete and legible. In some states, pharmacy technicians may take verbal or telephone orders, and spelling or repeating names is often useful for transcribing accurate information. Reading back a verbal or telephone order is sensible practice, and it is wise to note on the prescription "VORB" (verbal order read back) or "TORB" (telephone order read back) along with your name.

Verify all unclear or incomplete information before proceeding with filling the prescription. The patient information must be complete, including date of birth, address, phone number, and medication allergies, as well as the prescriber's name, address, phone number, signature, and DEA number, in the case of controlled substances. The drug, dose, route of administration, refills, directions for use, and dosing schedule must

Always verify patient information, prescriber information, and medication information contained on a written prescription.

be complete, as well as the date the prescription was written. Use any available resources, including the patient or her family members, the patient profile, the pharmacist, or a nurse or physician in a hospital setting to complete and verify any information that is unclear.

Data Entry for the Prescription

If all information required on the prescription is complete, the technician may proceed with entering the prescription into the computerized system. Accurate data entry is essential to avoiding medication errors. This will require the technician to verify brand and generic names of drugs, match prescribed dose and available strengths and routes of administration, and read the prescription for leading or trailing zeros. Once entry into the computerized system is complete, the technician should once again verify the information entered against the original prescription to ensure accuracy. Once a prescription label is generated, the label should also be verified against the original prescription.

Filling the Prescription

Next, the technician will retrieve the medication from the stock shelves or cabinets. Many products have similar packaging or labeling, and extra care should always be taken to double-check the product against the prescription. Use National Drug Code (NDC) numbers, drug names and doses, and any other information available to verify that the correct medication was retrieved and used to fill the prescription.

When filling the prescription, make sure all equipment is clean and calibrated, and the workspace is free of distractions or interruptions. If dispensing solid dosage forms, always count the quantity twice. If compounding a product, double-check your calculations. If measuring a liquid, use the appropriate size container to measure. Place auxiliary labels on the prescription bottle in a clean, legible manner.

Always read drug labels carefully. Do not rely on visual cues or location to choose the correct product.

Finally, review the prescription and prepare for the pharmacist's review by asking yourself several key questions:

- Does the pharmacist have complete information regarding the patient's medical history?
- Can the pharmacist verify the original prescription against the label provided?
- Can the pharmacist verify the calculations and measurements?
- Has the pharmacist been informed of any potential barriers to safe medication administration or sources of errors?

Final Check

After review by the pharmacist, store the medication appropriately until the patient is ready to receive the medication. Avoid errors in storage temperature, light, or humidity that may affect the integrity of the final product.

Deliver the Prescription

Deliver the medication to the patient, or the nurse in a hospital setting. Once again, verify the patient name and other unique patient identifiers to confirm his or her identity before delivering the final medication.

Communicate. Use more than one unique identifier to verify patient identity when delivering medications.

Although technicians cannot legally counsel patients, technicians can encourage patients to become proactive and educate themselves regarding their health and medications, as well

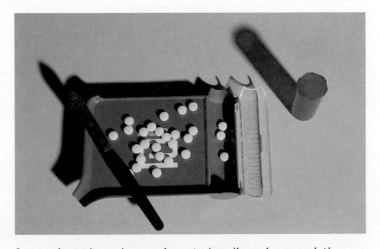

Count twice and use clean equipment when dispensing prescriptions.

Encourage patients to ask questions about their prescriptions

as ensure that the patients are comfortable asking the pharmacist for advice or counsel. Patients should always know some basic information about their medications. This includes the following:

- The brand and generic names
- What the medication looks like
- Why they are taking it

- How long they will take it
- How much to take and how often
- What to do if they miss a dose
- Common side effects or precautions of which they should be aware
- How to store the medication

AHRQ Recommendations for Patients to Prevent Medication Errors

- Be an active member of your healthcare team.
- Make sure your doctors know every prescription, OTC, or dietary supplement you are taking.
- Make sure your doctor knows about any allergies or adverse reactions you have had to medicines.
- Make sure you can read your doctor's prescription.
- Ask for information about your prescription medications when they are prescribed and when you receive them.
- When you pick up your medication from the pharmacy, ask, "Is this the medicine my doctor prescribed?"
- If you have any questions about the directions on the medication label, ask.
- Ask your pharmacist for the best device to measure a liquid medication, and know how to use it.
- Ask for written information about the side effects of your medicines.

The most common medication error is incorrect drug identification, although many occur during prescribing and administration. Ideally, every patient will achieve the "five R's" of patient drug administration:

- Right patient
- Right drug
- Right strength
- Right route
- Right time

All members of the healthcare team must work together to ensure these five rights are preserved to achieve the best outcome possible.

Strategies to Prevent Medication Errors

A patient's five rights: right patient, right drug, right strength, right route, right time

As mentioned, medication errors are costly to patients, the healthcare system, and society. A comprehensive approach is needed to prevent medication errors. Such an approach requires input and changes in practice from medical, nursing, and pharmacy staffs; government and regulatory agencies; hospitals and other healthcare institutions; and patients themselves. Specific strategies that focus on small pieces of the healthcare puzzle are producing significant results toward the big-picture goal of preventing medication errors.

Innovations that Reduce Errors

Although plenty of human steps can be taken to reduce medication errors, technology is innovating the way pharmacy is practiced and reducing the potential for medication errors at the same time. Automation in pharmacy is becoming widespread in both hospitals and community pharmacy practice settings. In some cases, a computerized system recognizes and compares National Drug Codes selected by pharmacy staff against the original prescription information entered in the order-entry system, minimizing the risk of choosing the wrong stock bottle off the shelf. Other systems offer computerized verification of the prescription, in which the computer displays images of the correct tablet that the pharmacist can view compared to what has actually been dispensed.

Robotic systems have reduced medication errors substantially. Also, automated dispensing cabinets and bar-coded patient validation are reducing medication errors in hospitals. Automated processes are significantly reducing errors involving look-alike sound-alike medications.

Additionally, in hospitals, the use of an **electronic medication administration record (eMAR)** reduces medication errors because all medication-related actions, from prescribing to dispensing to administering, are documented electronically, often with a hand-held computer.

Personal Strategies

A pharmacy can be a stressful work environment. For all pharmacy staff, taking better care of oneself results in improved patient care. Get plenty of sleep, exercise regularly, and eat a balanced diet to maintain workplace focus and stamina. And, never be afraid to ask for help. It is imperative that the pharmacy technician take breaks. Pharmacies get very busy and sometimes staff will skip or work through their scheduled breaks and breaks required by law. An overworked pharmacy employee who is not rested can contribute to medical errors.

Finally, all steps in the provision of health care should be carried out by qualified, well-trained personnel. Pharmacy technicians are essential in the provision of pharmacy services, and remaining up to date on training and education is paramount to the provision of quality health care.

Patient-Related Strategies

Reducing the risk of patient-related medication errors involves providing patients and their caregivers with written medication information—in their primary language, if necessary—and promoting education and awareness. Developing strategies to accommodate patients with other barriers or limited healthcare knowledge is essential to promote the safe and effective use of medications.

Reporting Medication Errors

Many anonymous reporting systems have been established to collect information about medication errors. Data obtained from these systems is used to identify sources for improvement in medication safety and to implement policies or procedures that improve overall quality of care.

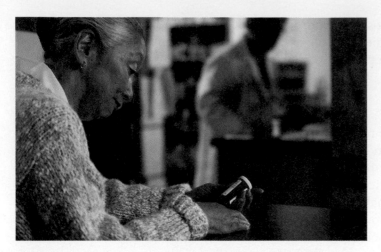

Patients should understand their prescriptions to prevent medication errors.

The Joint Commission released the Sentinel Event Policy in 1996 to promote reporting of medication errors. A **sentinel event** is an unanticipated event in health care that results in death or serious physical or psychological injury to a patient, or has the potential to do so. When an organization reports a sentinel event, it is expected to analyze the cause of the event, correct the cause, monitor the changes made as a result, and determine whether the risk was eliminated. The Joint Commission requires medication error–reporting systems for healthcare organizations to receive its accreditation.

MEDMARX is a reporting system supported by the USP. It is an Internet-based system that enables hospitals and healthcare providers to anonymously document and track adverse events for a specific institution. Additionally, the **Medication Error Reporting Program (MERP)** is supported by the USP and ISMP. It is a voluntary and confidential program that enables healthcare professionals to report errors directly. The information obtained through MEDMARX and MERP is used to publish lists of drugs commonly involved in errors, as well as to make recommendations for avoiding common mistakes.

The MedWatch program is another voluntary system for reporting serious adverse drug events to the FDA. Healthcare providers, patients, and consumers can report events to MedWatch involving not only prescription and OTC drug products, but also vitamins, nutritional supplements, infant formulas, and cosmetics.

Drug Insights: Antibiotics

Antibiotics are among the most frequently prescribed anti-infective drugs in the United States. Antibiotics are used in the treatment of bacterial infections. Antibiotics kill or stop the growth of infection-causing bacteria. **Bactericidal antibiotics** kill bacteria, while **bacteriostatic antibiotics** stop the growth or reproduction of bacteria. Antibiotics do not treat infections caused by viruses, such as the cold or flu. Medications to treat fungal and viral infections are discussed in Chapter 7.

There are many classes of antibiotics available for the treatment of bacterial infections. The following classes will be reviewed in this section:

- Sulfonamides
- Penicillins
- Cephalosporins
- Carbapenems
- Carbacephems
- Monbactams
- Tetracyclines
- Macrolides
- Ketolides
- Quinolones
- Aminoglycosides
- Miscellaneous antibiotics

There are many kinds of bacterial organisms that cause various types of infections and are thus treated with different antibiotics.

Bacteria primarily exist as spheres (cocci), rods (bacilli), and spirals (spirilla).

When choosing an antibiotic to treat an infection, an antibiotic will ideally be targeted to the specific infection-causing organism. There is a common misconception that some antibiotics are "stronger" or "weaker" than others. However, it is important to understand antibiotics are neither strong nor weak but are simply prescribed to treat a specifically targeted organism. But, when the cause of an infection is unknown or immediate treatment is required, a broad-spectrum antibiotic is used that is effective in fighting multiple types of bacteria. This type of treatment is known as **empirical treatment**. Empirical antibiotic therapy should be based on factors including likely bacteria at the site of the infection, patient history and recent exposure risks, and local susceptibility data. Of course, individual characteristics, such as allergies or other chronic diseases or medications, should be considered when selecting an antibiotic regimen.

Antibiotics need to treat the infection without causing harm to the patient.

Once therapy is initiated, all patients receiving antibiotics should be monitored for resolution of the signs and symptoms of infection, as well as adverse effects. If patients do not respond to antibiotic treatment in two or three days, the diagnosis should be reevaluated, or the drug therapy monitored to achieve optimal concentrations of drug at the site of infection. Sometimes, selection of a new antibiotic or addition of a second drug is necessary to overcome confounding factors contributing to the infection.

Patients should always be advised to consume the entire antibiotic prescribed. Patients must not stop taking the antibiotic when their symptoms improve. Nor should they share antibiotics with a friend or family member, even if they believe they have the same infection. Such actions are inappropriate and illegal, and contribute to the evolution of antibiotic-resistant bacteria.

Gram-Negative Versus Gram-Positive Bacteria

Bacteria are divided into two classes, based on a staining technique developed by Danish scientist Hans Christian Gram. The gram-staining technique uses a crystal violet dye. Due to structural differences, gram-positive bacteria will retain the dye and appear blue to purple after staining. Gram-negative bacteria will not retain the stain and appear pink to red.

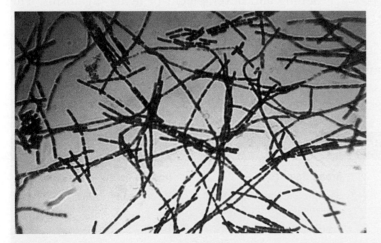

Gram-positive *Bacillus anthracis* appear dark purple after gram-staining.

Examples of gram-positive bacteria include the following:

- *Streptococcus spp.*
- *Staphylococcus spp.*

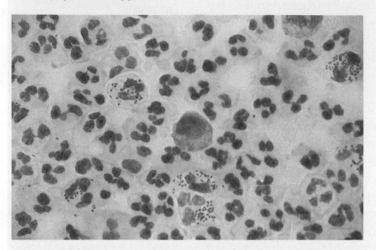

Gram-negative *Neisseria spp.* appear pink after gram-staining.

Examples of gram-negative bacteria include the following:

- *Spirochetes spp.*
- *Neisseria spp.*
- *Pseudomonas aeruginosa*

In biology, a species is the most descriptive classification of biological organisms in the taxonomic system. The word "species" is sometimes abbreviated "sp." The abbreviation "spp." indicates plural, or more than one, species. The conventional designation spp. refers to several species of the same genus.

Sulfonamides

Sulfonamides, or sulfa drugs, were the first antibiotics and are still in use today. They are bacteriostatic, exerting their effect by preventing the synthesis of folic acid in bacteria, which is needed to make deoxyribonucleic acid (DNA), the hereditary material that provides the genetic information for the functioning and development of living organisms. The sulfonamides are available as generic products, so pharmacy technicians should be familiar with both the brand and generic names within this class of drugs. **TABLE 6.4** lists commonly prescribed sulfonamide drugs, as well as their brand names and available dosage forms.

Table 6.4   Common Sulfonamides

Generic Name	Brand Name(s)	Dosage Forms Available
Sulfamethoxazole-trimethoprim	Bactrim, Bactrim DS, Cotrim, Cotrim DS, Septra, Septra DS	IV, oral liquid, tablet
Sulfasalazine	Azulfidine	Tablet
Sulfisoxazole	Gantrisin	Oral liquid, tablet

Sulfonamides are primarily used to treat urinary tract infections (UTIs), middle-ear infections in children, ulcerative colitis, and lower respiratory tract infections, and as prophylaxis against *Pneumocystis carinii* pneumonia in patients with compromised immune systems.

Allergies to sulfonamides are common, although they occur less frequently with today's sulfonamides than with older drugs in this class. The most common side effect is a rash. Other side effects of sulfonamides include nausea, drug fever, vomiting, jaundice, blood disorders, and kidney dysfunction.

Sulfonamides require auxiliary labels: Avoid sun exposure and drink plenty of water.

Sulfa drugs should always contain a label to avoid prolonged exposure to the sun while taking the medications, because this can lead to severe skin rashes. Also, patients taking sulfa drugs need to stay well-hydrated to avoid the formation of crystals in the urine. Therefore, sulfa drugs should be dispensed with an auxiliary label to take with fluids.

Nitrofurantoin

Nitrofurantoin is not a sulfonamide, but is related to this class. It is available under the brand names Macrobid and Macrodantin and is primarily used to treat urinary tract infections (UTIs), particularly when patients are allergic to or unable to take sulfonamides. It is a broad-spectrum antibiotic, but its exact mechanism of action is unknown. Patients should take nitrofurantoin with food to avoid nausea, as well as drink plenty of water to prevent the discoloration of urine and false-positive glucose urine tests. Also, alcohol should be avoided while taking nitrofurantoin. Nitrofurantoin requires auxiliary labels: Take with food, drink plenty of water, and avoid alcohol when patients undergo surgery or dental procedures.

Penicillins

The penicillins are antibacterial agents with a beta-lactam ring that are bactericidal or they kill susceptible bacteria. Their mechanism of action involves blocking cell-wall formation and thus killing bacteria. Many of the beta-lactam antibiotics work this way to kill bacteria. The most common side effect of the penicillins is diarrhea. Patients should take oral-dosage forms of penicillins on an empty stomach, and drink plenty of water. Technicians should place such auxiliary labels on a penicillin product before dispensing to the patient. The most prominent concern when taking penicillins, however, is the potential for an allergic reaction. Ten percent of people have an allergy to penicillins, which may vary from an itchy, red rash to breathing difficulties and **anaphylaxis**. If a patient has experienced an anaphylactic or allergic reaction to one of the penicillins, the prescriber should be notified and potentially another class of antibiotics prescribed.

Prophylactic regimens prior to dental procedures include 2g amoxicillin, 600mg clindamycin, or 500mg azithromycin.

Anaerobic bacteria do not need oxygen to survive.

Aerobic bacteria require oxygen to survive.

One of the primary limitations of penicillins is the ability of bacteria to become resistant to them. That is, with each exposure to an antibiotic, bacteria can develop ways to avoid the effects of the drug, thereby making the drug ineffective over time. Over-

Penicillins require auxiliary labels: Take on an empty stomach and drink plenty of water.

Table 6.5   Penicillin-Beta-Lactamase Combinations

Generic Name	Brand Name	Dosage Forms Available
Amoxicillin-clavulanate	Augmentin	Oral suspension, tablet
Ticarcillin-clavulante	Timentin	IV
Ampicillin-sulbactam	Unasyn	Injection, IV
Piperacillin-tazobactam	Zosyn	IV

use and inappropriate use of antibiotics has created a public health crisis in terms of antibiotic-resistant bacteria. To combat this resistance, some penicillins are combined with other agents to improve the effectiveness of the drug. One example is the beta-lactamase inhibitors combined with certain penicillins, which inhibit the bacteria's ability to work against the penicillin. Common examples of penicillins combined with beta-lactamase inhibitors are presented in TABLE 6.5 .

Antibiotic Resistance

The prevalence of antibiotic-resistant bacteria is increasing, primarily because of the misuse and overuse of current antibiotics. It is estimated that half of the 100 million antibiotics prescribed annually in the United States may be inappropriate. Inaccurate or uncertain diagnoses, patient demand for treatment, and time constraints are significant barriers to appropriate antibiotic use.

When antibiotics are used when they are not necessary, as in the case of infections caused by viruses, or used for too-short or too-long periods of time, bacteria can evolve and develop resistance mechanisms to antibiotics. Antibiotic-resistant bacteria are dangerous because, once they cause an infection, there may be no treatment option available. Resistant infections increase morbidity and mortality, as well as healthcare costs. They are particularly concerning to **immunocompromised** individuals (that is, individuals having a compromised or impaired immune system, often from illness or treatment).

All members of the healthcare team should promote education and awareness of antibiotic-resistant bacteria and advocate for the safe and judicious use of antibiotics.

What Would You Do?

Question: A mother calls the pharmacy to ask about a prescription she recently obtained for her child. The patient is a six-year-old girl who was diagnosed with a middle-ear infection three days ago. She was prescribed amoxicillin 800mg by mouth every 12 hours for 10 days. Her fever has subsided and she has had no adverse effects to the medication. Now, the patient's younger brother, who is three years old, has the same symptoms of an ear infection that his sister had. The mother wants to know if she can stop giving her daughter the amoxicillin, because she is feeling better, and give it to her son instead, because she believes it is the same infection. What should the pharmacy technician do?

Answer: After discussing with the pharmacist, advise the mother that her daughter should finish the entire course of antibiotics that was prescribed. Not completing the entire regimen will put the daughter at risk for a recurrent infection. This also contributes to the development of antibiotic resistance. Also, giving a prescription drug to any person for whom it was not prescribed is illegal and should not be advised. Antibiotics require a prescription so that healthcare providers can ensure accurate and safe use of the drugs. Tell the mother than her son should been seen by a pediatrician. He will receive his own prescription, if appropriate.

Cephalosporins

Cephalosporins work by a mechanism similar to penicillins, inhibiting cell-wall formation in bacteria. However, they are effective against different bacteria from penicillins. Because they are similar, though, cephalosporins possess a risk of allergic reaction in

A person with an allergy to penicillins has a 1% chance of having an allergy to cephalosporins.

patients allergic to penicillins. This is called a cross-reaction or cross-sensitivity. Often, if a patient is allergic to one class of drugs, both drug classes will be avoided.

The cephalosporins are divided into four generations, each with a different antibacterial spectrum.

- First-generation cephalosporins are used to treat mild-to-moderate community-acquired infections.

- Second-generation cephalosporins have broader antibacterial coverage than the first generation, especially against *Haemophilus influenza*. This generation is used to treat ear infections in children, as well as respiratory-tract infections and UTIs.

- Third-generation cephalosporins are used to treat severe infections such as UTIs and meningitis. Most third-generation agents have a long half-life, requiring infrequent dosing compared to earlier generations.

- Currently, only one fourth-generation cephalosporin is available. It possesses a broad antibacterial spectrum and is used to treat pneumonia, UTIs, and sepsis.

Commonly prescribed cephalosporins are presented in **TABLE 6.6** .

Oral first- and second-generation agents are used for prophylaxis during dental procedures and oral infections. Cefazolin is the drug of choice for surgical prophylaxis in heart and pacemaker procedures, neurosurgery, obstetrical and gynecological surgery, and orthopedic surgery. Cefepime (the fourth-generation cephalosporin) and ceftazidime (a third-generation cephalosporin) are effective in treating infections of *Pseudomonas aeruginosa*, which causes significant hospital-acquired infections.

The names of many cephalosporins look and sound similar. Double-check and clarify any ambiguous spelling or handwriting.

Table 6.6   Common Cephalosporins

Generation	Generic Name	Brand Name	Dosage Forms Available
First generation	Cefadroxil	Duricef	Capsule, oral liquid
	Cefazolin	Ancef	Injection, IV
	Cephalexin	Keflex	Capsule, oral liquid, tablet
Second generation	Cefaclor	Ceclor	Capsule, oral liquid
	Cefprozil	Cefzil	Oral liquid, tablet
	Cefuroxime	Ceftin, Zinacef	Injection, IV, oral liquid, tablet
Third generation	Cefdinir	Omnicef	Capsule, oral liquid
	Ceftazidime	Fortaz	Injection, IV
	Ceftriaxone	Rocephin	Injection, IV
	Cefpodoxime	Vantin	Oral liquid
Fourth generation	Cefepime	Maxipime	Injection, IV

Table 6.7	Common Carbapenems, Carbacephems, and Monobactams		
Class	**Generic Name**	**Brand Name**	**Dosage Forms Available**
Carbapenems	Ertapenem	Invanz	Injection, IV
	Imipenem-cilastatin	Primaxin	Injection, IV
	Meropenem	Merrem IV	IV
Cabacephems	Doripenem	Doribax	IV
	Loracarbef	Lorabid	Capsule, oral liquid
Monobacatams	Aztreonam	Azactam	IV

Oral suspensions of cephalosporins require auxiliary labels: Refrigerate and shake well prior to administration.

Because of their similarity in structure and function, cephalosporins share the same side effects as penicillins. In general, however, cephalosporins are well tolerated by most patients.

Other than cefdinir and cefixime, oral suspensions of cephalosporins must be refrigerated after reconstitution. (A suspension is a mixture that contains small particles of a substance dispersed throughout the liquid.) They should also contain an auxiliary label, advising patients to shake well immediately prior to administration.

Carbapenems, Carbacephems, and Monobactams

Several new drugs and drug classes that are structurally and functionally similar to penicillins and cephalosporins have been developed recently. They are broadly termed "beta-lactams" because of their biochemical structure. Individually, the classes are called carbapenems, carbacephems, and monobactams. Examples of each class are presented here in TABLE 6.7.

Imipenem-cilastatin has broad coverage against gram-negative and gram-positive bacteria. Seizures occur more frequently with imipenem-cilastatin than with related drugs. Meropenem is effective against the same types of bacteria as imipenem-cilastatin, but is less likely to cause seizures. Meropenem is most often used for bacterial meningitis and intra-abdominal infections. Ertapenem is a once-daily injection used for severe community-acquired infections.

Loracarbef requires an auxiliary label: Take on an empty stomach.

Doripenem is used for UTIs, and also presents a risk of seizures. Loracarbef is routinely given to children. Patients should be advised that Loracarbef should be taken on an empty stomach.

Tetracyclines

Tetracyclines are broad-spectrum antibiotics that block protein formation in bacteria by binding to ribosomes. Common tetracyclines are listed in TABLE 6.8.

Table 6.8	Common Tetracyclines	
Generic Name	**Brand Name**	**Dosage Forms Available**
Demeclocycline	Declomycin	Tablet
Doxycycline	Vibramycin, Oracea	Capsule, IV, oral liquid, tablet
Minocycline	Minocin, Soladyne	Capsule, IV
Tetracycline	Sumycin	Capsule, oral liquid, tablet

Drugs from the tetracycline class are used to treat acne, *Bacillus anthracis* infections (anthrax), chronic bronchitis, Lyme disease, *Mycoplasma pneumonia* infections (walking pneumonia), *Rickettsia* infections (Rocky Mountain spotted fever), and *Chlamydia* infections.

Nausea and vomiting are the most common side effects of tetracyclines. Antacids should not be consumed several hours before or after tetracyclines because of the risk of **chelation**, which will render the drug ineffective. Patients taking tetracyclines should avoid sun exposure due to photosensitization, as well as avoid eating dairy products. Also, tetracyclines should never be given to pregnant women or children under eight years old, as they can cause permanent tooth discoloration and affect bone growth.

Chelation involves the interaction of an organic molecule, such as a drug, and a heavy metal to form a ring structure.

Tetracyclines require auxiliary labels: Avoid sun exposure and avoid dairy products.

Tetracyclines that have reached their expiration date pose a risk of toxicity and fatal renal syndrome. Technicians should be diligent about checking the expiration dates of all drugs, but tetracyclines, in particular.

Tigecycline

Tigecycline (Tygacil) is a relatively new drug that is related to the tetracycline class. It is classified as a glycylcycline, but is currently the only drug in that class. Tigecycline is available only in IV form, and is used to treat skin and intra-abdominal infections.

Macrolides

Macrolides are bacteriostatic antibiotics. They primarily treat respiratory infections caused by *Legionella* and other gram-positive bacteria. Like tetracyclines, macrolides inhibit protein synthesis in bacteria by binding to ribosomes. Common macrolides are listed in TABLE 6.9.

As stated earlier, macrolides treat respiratory infections, including Legionnaires disease, and infections caused by *Streptococcus pneumoniae*, *M. pneumonia*, and *H. influenzae*.

When taken on an empty stomach, macrolides achieve faster absorption into the body. But, this may cause severe gastrointestinal upset, which is often decreased when these drugs are taken with a snack. Therefore, these products may be dispensed with labels directing patients to take with food.

Table 6.9 Common Macrolides

Generic Name	Brand Name	Dosage Forms Available
Azithromycin	Zithromax, Z-Pak, Zmax	Oral liquid, tablet
Clarithromycin	Biaxin	Oral liquid, tablet
Erythromycin base	Eryc, Ery-Tab	Capsule, tablet, topical
Erythromycin ethylsuccinate	EES, EryPed	Oral liquid, tablet
Erythromycin lactobionate	Erythrocin	Injection
Erythromycin stearate	Erythrocin	Tablet
Erythromycin-sulfisoxazole	Pediazole	Oral liquid

Erythromycin preparations require an auxiliary label: Take with food.

Telithromycin requires an auxiliary label: May cause blurred vision.

Ketolides

Ketolides also bind to bacterial ribosomes, inhibiting protein synthesis. Additionally, they inhibit the growth of newly forming ribosomes. Ketolides are used to treat infections in the lungs and sinuses. The currently available ketolide is telithromycin (Ketek), although others are in development. It is available in a tablet formulation and is used to treat community-acquired pneumonia, bacterial sinusitis, and acute exacerbations of chronic bronchitis. This drug may cause blurred vision, so patients should not drive or participate in tasks that require intense focus while taking this drug. Ketek poses a more serious, but rare, risk of irregular heartbeat. Ketolides are metabolized by cytochrome P450 3A4 enzymes, and, as such, are prone to a host of drug interactions with other medications and foods.

Cytochrome P450 Enzymes

The cytochrome P450 (CYP) family of enzymes is responsible for the metabolism of many drugs in the body. A majority of CYP enzymes are located in the liver.

A drug can act as an inducer (increasing the activity), an inhibitor (decreasing the activity), or a **substrate** or substance of which an enzyme acts. In this case, the CYP enzymes. Some drugs fall into more than one of these categories. Therefore, several drug interactions can occur related to the CYP enzymes, resulting in drug toxicity, reduced therapeutic effect, or adverse reactions.

CYP3A4 is one of the most active members of the CYP family, and caution should be advised when multiple drugs acting on or with CYP3A4 are administered simultaneously. While multiple-drug regimens may not always be avoidable, dose adjustments may be necessary to optimize therapy.

Common substrates of CYP3A4 include the following:

- Alprazolam
- Calcium channel blockers
- Erythromycin
- HIV protease inhibitors
- Tacrolimus

Common inhibitors of CYP3A4 include the following:

- Amiodarone
- Cimetidine
- Clarithromycin
- Diltiazem
- Grapefruit juice (which may be taken to swallow medications)
- Ketoconazole
- Macrolides (not azithromycin)
- Omeprazole
- Propofol
- Ritonavir
- Verapamil

Common inducers of CYP3A4 include the following:

- Carbamazepine
- Dexamethasone
- Phenobarbital
- Phenytoin
- Rifampin
- Ritonavir

Quinolones

Quinolones are rapid-acting bactericidal antibiotics that are effective against most gram-negative bacteria and many gram-positive bacteria. They cause DNA breakage and cell death in replicating bacteria. Common quinolones are listed in TABLE 6.10.

Quinolones are used to treat bone and joint infections, skin infections, UTIs, bronchitis, pneumonia, and tuberculosis. Ciprofloxacin gained notoriety as for a treatment for anthrax infections as a result of possible bioterrorism attacks. Nausea and vomiting are the most common side effects of quinolones. Antacids interfere with quinolone absorption, so patients should avoid taking antacids several hours before or after a quinolone. Quinolones can increase the risk of theophylline toxicity, so these drugs are rarely administered together. Quinolones can also cause joint swelling and malformation, and may cause tendon injuries. The risk of tendon injuries is highest among patients also taking corticosteroids, organ-transplant recipients, and patients over 60 years of age. Quinolones are generally not recommended for children or pregnant women.

Aminoglycosides

Aminoglycosides are bactericidal antibiotics and exert their activity by binding to bacterial ribosomes and inhibiting protein synthesis. The use of aminoglycosides is limited to serious, mostly life-threatening infections, sepsis, or peritonitis. Dosing of aminoglycosides is based on monitoring blood levels of the drug in conjunction with patient response. The most common aminoglycosides are presented in TABLE 6.11.

Aminoglycosides present a substantial risk of **nephrotoxicity** (damage to the kidney) and **ototoxicity** (damage to the organs of hearing). Therefore, drug levels must be monitored routinely. Dose adjustment or less-frequent dosing may be necessary for patients at high risk for adverse effects.

One strategy to reduce the risk of aminoglycoside toxicity is once-daily dosing. In this case, peak drug levels do not need to be checked on a regular basis. Only one

Table 6.10   Common Quinolones

Generic Name	Brand Name	Dosage Forms Available
Ciprofloxacin	Cipro	IV, oral liquid, otic preparation, tablet, topical;ophthalmic
Gatifloxacin	Tequin	IV, tablet, ophthalmic
Levofloxacin	Levaquin	IV, oral liquid, tablet
Moxifloxacin	Avelox	Tablet, ophthalmic
Norfloxacin	Noroxin	Tablet
Ofloxacin	Floxin	IV, otic preparation, tablet

Table 6.11 Common Aminoglycosides		
Generic Name	Brand Name	Dosage Forms Available
Amikacin	Amikin	Injection, IV
Gentamicin	Garamycin	Injection, IV, ophthalmic preparation
Neomycin	Mycifradin, Neo-Fradin, Neo Rx	Oral liquid, topical preparation
Streptomycin	None	Injection, IV
Tobramycin	Nebcin	Injection, IV

level is usually required, prior to the second dose, to ensure adequate drug elimination from the patient's body.

Miscellaneous Antibiotics

Several antibiotics are the only, or the primary, agent in a given class of drugs. These agents are listed in TABLE 6.12 .

The streptogramins include quinupristin and dalfopristin and are always supplied together in one dosage form. Like several other classes of antibiotics, streptogramins inhibit protein synthesis in the bacterial ribosome. They treat *Enterococcus faecium* infections, as well as infections that are resistant to vancomycin and methicillin. Streptogramins are structurally related to quinolones and pose similar risks of adverse effects, with nausea and vomiting being the most prevalent. Joint swelling and dizziness may also occur. Synercid must be stored in the refrigerator. Quinupristin and dalfopristin inhibit CYP3A4 enzymes and, therefore, pose a significant risk of drug interactions with other medications and food.

Daptomycin is the only routinely used cyclic lipopeptide. It binds to the bacterial membrane, leading to depolarization of the membrane, inhibition of DNA and **ribonucleic acid (RNA)** synthesis, and cell death. (RNA is the genetic material that encodes the functioning and development of some viruses; it also aids in the reproduction and replication of DNA.) Daptomycin is used to treat complicated skin infections caused by aerobic gram-positive bacteria. It should not be taken with the group of cholesterol-

Table 6.12 Miscellaneous Antibiotics			
Class (If Applicable)	Generic Name	Brand Name	Dosage Forms Available
Streptogramins	Quinupristin-dalfopristin	Synercid	IV
Cyclic lipopeptides	Daptomycin	Cubicin	IV
	Vancomycin	Vancocin	IV, capsule
	Clindamycin	Cleocin	Capsule, injection, IV, oral liquid, topical preparation
	Metronidazole	Flagyl	Capsule, IV, tablet, topical preparations, vaginal preparations
	Pentamidine	NebuPent, Pentam	Injection, IV, inhalation
Oxazolidinones	Linezolid	Zyvox	IV, oral liquid, tablet

lowering medications known as the HMG-CoA-reductase inhibitors, more commonly known as statins. Side effects of daptomycin include low blood pressure, headache, insomnia, rash, gastrointestinal upset, and injection site pain and reactions.

Vancomycin is not included in a larger class of antibiotics because of its distinct structure, which is unlike any other available antibiotic. Vancomycin is a bactericidal antibiotic and inhibits bacterial cell-wall synthesis. Vancomycin is particularly useful in treating methicillin-resistant *Staphylococcus aureus* (MRSA) infections. MRSA is a significant public health threat, but vancomycin's usefulness against this disease is decreasing as bacterial resistance to vancomycin becomes evident. Vancomycin-resistant *enterocci* (VRE) is becoming more common. Consequently, most healthcare facilities and institutions, as well as the Centers for Disease Control and Prevention, have strict guidelines pertaining to the use of vancomycin to ensure prudent and judicious use of this novel antibiotic.

The oral formulation of vancomycin can be used to treat infections of the gastrointestinal tract caused by *Clostridium difficile*. Vancomycin can cause ototoxicity and nephrotoxicity. Dosing of vancomycin is based on a collection of individual characteristics, such as body weight and kidney function. Drug levels are monitored routinely to assess patient response and effectiveness.

Clindamycin is a broad-spectrum antibiotic that inhibits protein synthesis. It can be used to treat serious gram-positive infections, including bone infections, bowel infections, or gynecological infections, or as a prophylaxis against infections prior to abdominal surgery. However, it is most frequently used as a topical preparation to treat acne. The most serious side effect of clindamycin is pseudomembranous colitis, which causes bloody diarrhea. If this occurs, clindamycin must be discontinued.

Metronidazole effectively treats bacterial infections, as well as fungal infections. It is often used to treat gastrointestinal infections, such as those caused by *Clostridium difficile*, amoebic dysentery, and sexually transmitted diseases, particularly those caused by *Trichomonas*. Metronidazole may cause gastrointestinal upset, a metallic taste, rash, or intolerance to alcohol. A label warning patients not to drink alcohol while taking metronidazole must be attached to the prescription vial. Metronidazole causes a disulfiram-like reaction to alcohol, causing severe nausea and vomiting, flushing, and headache.

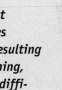

Disulfiram is a drug used to treat chronic alcohol abuse, and causes extreme sensitivity to alcohol, resulting in severe nausea, vomiting, flushing, headache, weakness, confusion, difficulty breathing, and anxiety when alcohol is consumed.

The mechanism of pentamidine is unknown. It is used as a second-line treatment option for *Pneumocystis carinii* infections. It is administered only once every four weeks. Sudden hypertension is a risk of pentamidine administration. Emergency drugs and equipment should be available when administering pentamidine.

Metronidazole is available in a variety of dosage forms, and technicians should verify the correct form when in doubt.

Linezolid is the first FDA-approved oxazolidinone. It inhibits bacterial-protein synthesis, and is used to treat infections caused by MRSA, vancomycin-resistant *E. faecium* (VRE), and other gram-positive infections. Linezolid should be administered alone in a separate IV line due to the presence of many chemical incompatibilities.

Metronidazole requires an auxiliary label: Avoid alcohol.

Tech Math Practice

Question: **A patient has been prescribed Lortab for pain control after surgery. Each tablet contains 7.5mg hydrocodone and 500mg acetaminophen. The patient has been instructed to take one tablet every four to six hours as needed. The patient has been taking the Lortab every four hours around the clock, and his pain is still not controlled, so he purchases an OTC pain reliever. He does not know what ingredients are in Lortab. If he purchases tablets containing 325mg acetaminophen in each tablet, and takes two tablets every six hours (according to the package directions), how much acetaminophen will he consume in one day?**

Answer: Lortab contains 500mg acetaminophen per tablet. If the patient takes one tablet every four hours, then he will consume 3,000mg acetaminophen per day with the Lortab. (500mg acetaminophen/tablet × 1 tablet ÷ 4 hours × 24 hours/day = 3,000mg acetaminophen.)

The OTC product contains 325mg acetaminophen per tablet. If the patient takes two tablets every six hours, then he will consume 2,600mg acetaminophen per day with the OTC product. (325mg acetaminophen/tablet × 2 tablets/6 hours × 24 hours/day = 2,600mg acetaminophen.)

Therefore, the total daily dose would be 5,600mg acetaminophen. The maximum recommended daily dose of acetaminophen is 4,000mg daily. Therefore, this patient would be at risk for side effects and toxicity related to an acetaminophen overdose.

Question: **A patient has been diagnosed with Lyme disease. He is prescribed amoxicillin 500mg every eight hours for 21 days. If your pharmacy has 500mg tablets available, what is the total quantity of tablets that needs to be dispensed?**

Answer: 500mg/1 tablet × 1 tablet/8 hours × 24 hours/day = 500mg, 3 times/day; 3 tablets/day × 21 days = 63 tablets.

Question: **A pediatric patient weighing 36 pounds receives a prescription for erythromycin ethylsuccinate 40mg/kg/day in three divided doses. If the oral suspension contains 200mg/5mL, how many milliliters will the patient receive at each dose?**

Answer: 36lb × 1kg/2.2lb = 16.4kg
16.4kg × 40mg/kg/day = 656mg/day
656mg/day ÷ 3 doses = 218.7mg/dose
218.7mg/dose × 5mL/200mg = 5.5mL/dose

Question: **A dose of vancomycin 15mg/kg every 12 hours is ordered for a 47-year-old male with normal renal function who weighs 150 pounds. How many milligrams of vancomycin will he receive with each dose?**

Answer: 150lb × 1kg/2.2lb = 68.2kg
15mg/kg × 68.2kg = 1,023mg

Question: **A patient arrives at the pharmacy with a prescription for Flagyl 250mg every eight hours for seven days. The pharmacy only has 15 250mg tablets left in stock. How many days' supply will the patient receive? How many tablets will the patient receive when she returns to obtain her remaining partial fill?**

Answer: Total dose: 1 tablet/8 hours × 24 hours/day = 3 tablets/day × 7 days = 21 tablets

Available dose: 15 tablets × 1 day/3 tablets = 5 days' supply

Remaining partial fill: 21 tablets − 15 tablets = 6 tablets

WRAP UP

Chapter Summary

- Most adults in the United States take at least one medication on a regular basis. Although tested for safety and efficacy, all medications expose patients to a risk of side effects and drug interactions. As members of the healthcare team, pharmacy technicians must be vigilant to maintain patient safety and ensure optimal drug therapy.

- Over-the-counter (OTC) medications can be purchased without a prescription, and without the advice of a physician or pharmacist. The use of OTC products is increasing due to costs, convenience, and patient autonomy. Most OTC medications should not be used for more than seven days without consulting a healthcare provider.

- OTC labeling requires the product's active ingredients, purpose for use, directions for use, warnings, age-appropriate dosing information, and an expiration date to be prominently displayed in easy-to-understand language.

- Due to the thousands of OTC products available, many with similar names or ingredients, consumers may need help in choosing an OTC product and determining what ingredients are actually in each product.

- Homeopathic medications are OTC drugs that are regulated by the FDA. They should be used only for short-term, self-limiting conditions, and patients should inform their physician and pharmacist about all the homeopathic products they are taking.

- Dietary supplements are not regulated by the FDA, and the safety, effectiveness, origin and quality of some products is questionable. As with all other medications or OTC products, patients should inform their physician and pharmacist about all the dietary supplements they are taking.

- Frequently prescribed drugs in the United States include antidepressants, cholesterol-lowering drugs, antihypertensives, antibiotics, thyroid medications, diabetes drugs, and asthma-controlling medications.

- Medical errors account for enormous costs, both direct and indirect, every year. An esti-

mated 98,000 hospitalized patients die each year due to a medical error. Many medical errors are preventable.

- Medication errors are medical errors that are directly related to the prescribing, dispensing, or administering of a medication. Medication errors account for 7,000 deaths each year in the United States. Medication errors may occur due to individual variability in drug response, or because of human, technical, or organizational failures.

- To prevent medication errors, healthcare team members must have up-to-date prescribing and drug information, collaborate among healthcare providers, and experience an atmosphere of safety—not one that will punish those who bring attention to medication errors.

- Unapproved abbreviations and look-alike sound-alike medication names are two potential sources of medication errors. Healthcare organizations are encouraged to have policies and practices in place to reduce confusion and mitigate these types of errors.

- Pharmacy technicians play a vital role in identifying, reporting, and preventing medication errors. There are many steps in the process of filling a prescription in which a technician may recognize a potential source for an error. Technicians should be encouraged to report these sources to the pharmacist.

- Technology and automated processes are reducing the incidence of medication errors. The use of computerized order-entry systems, computerized verification, robotic dispensing systems, bar-coded identification methods, and eMARs are effective measures to prevent medication errors.

- Patients should be educated on the safe and proper use of medications to prevent medication errors.

- Medication errors can be reported through MEDMARX, MERP, and MedWatch. The information is analyzed and clinical recommendations and guidelines are published to educate healthcare providers about possible sources of medication errors.

- Antibiotics kill or stop the growth of bacteria that cause infections. An antibiotic should be targeted to the specific infection-causing organism, but when this is not possible, a broad-spectrum antibiotic can be used to initiate empirical treatment.

- The misuse and overuse of antibiotics contributes to the development of antibiotic-resistant bacteria. Antibiotic resistance is a significant public health concern and leads to increased morbidity, mortality, and costs.

- The ideal antibiotic will target the specific infection-causing organism. When that is not known, empirical antibiotic therapy should be based on likely bacteria at the site of the infection, patient history and recent exposure risks, and local susceptibility data. Individual characteristics, such as allergies or other chronic diseases or medications, should be considered when selecting an antibiotic regimen.

Learning Assessment Questions

1. Which of the following drugs was originally available only by prescription, but is now available as an OTC product?
   A. Clindamycin (Cleocin)
   B. Metronidazole (Flagyl)
   C. Diphenhydramine (Benadryl)
   D. Amoxicillin (Amoxil)

2. Which of the following statements is *not* true for an OTC medication?
   A. An expiration date is required.
   B. Their benefits outweigh their risks.
   C. A prescription is required.
   D. They are available free of charge.
   E. They can be used for self-diagnosed conditions

3. Which of the following is a patient-related cause of a medication error?
   A. A nurse administers a drug to the wrong patient.
   B. A technician does not review the patient's history of compliance with medication therapy.
   C. A prescriber orders the wrong dose of a medication.
   D. A patient does not fill a prescription on time.

4. Which program should a patient use to report a medication error that occurred from an OTC product?
   A. MERP
   B. ISMP
   C. MedWatch
   D. MEDMARX

5. What information is *not* required to be on the label of an OTC product?
   A. Expiration date
   B. Date of manufacturing
   C. Possible side effects
   D. Indication for use

6. A medication error may occur at any of the steps in the healthcare process, *except* which of the following?
   A. When a patient picks up a prescription from a community pharmacy
   B. When a physician and a pharmacist consult about the best choice of antibiotic for a hospitalized patient
   C. When a technician is late for his shift in a community pharmacy
   D. When a nurse reports an adverse reaction she experienced due to a new cosmetic product

7. How many people are estimated to die each year in the United States due to medication errors?

   A. 7,000

   B. 1,998

   C. 98,000

   D. 1.5 million

8. Which of the following is *not* part of the pharmacy technician's role in preventing medication errors?

   A. Using multiple patient identifiers to confirm the identity of a patient

   B. Counseling the patient on what to do if he or she misses a dose of prescribed medication

   C. Double-checking all calculations when compounding a product

   D. Getting plenty of sleep prior to working a shift in the pharmacy

9. Which is an example of a wrong-time error?

   A. An intramuscular injection is scheduled to be given to a patient at 1600, but the nurse administers the same drug in a tablet form at 1600.

   B. A patient is going on vacation, so she refills all her prescriptions two weeks early.

   C. A patient is supposed to take one tablet at 0900, but he forgets and just takes his next scheduled dose at 1300.

   D. An oral suspension is prescribed to be given to a child at 1000, but the mother does not administer it until 1130.

10. Which of the following is an example of a human-failure error?

   A. A pharmacist not reading the most up-to-date drug information for a medication prior to dispensing

   B. A patient having chronic kidney disease

   C. A crowded workspace in a community pharmacy

   D. Inadequate staffing in a hospital pharmacy

11. Which of the following is *not* one of the five rights of patient drug administration?

   A. Right strength

   B. Right color

   C. Right time

   D. Right drug

12. Which strategy has significantly reduced medication errors in hospitals?

   A. Robotic systems

   B. Improved staffing requirements

   C. Color-coded storage systems

   D. Technician verification of missing prescription information

13. Which two classes of antibiotics exhibit a possibility of cross-reactivity when patients are allergic to one of the classes?

   A. Sulfonamides and nitrofurantoin

   B. Amoinoglycosides and vancomycin

   C. Macrolides and ketolides

   D. Pencillins and cephalosporins

14. Which of the following antibiotics *do not* need an auxiliary label relating to food?

   A. Telithromycin

   B. Pencillins

   C. Loracarbef

   D. Nitrofurantoin

15. Which antibiotic causes a disulfuram-like reaction when taken with alcohol?

   A. Nitrofurantoin

   B. Metronidazole

   C. Sulfamethoxazole

   D. Doxycycline

16. Why is antibiotic overuse a public health concern?

   A. Because drug interactions with antibiotics are dangerous

   B. Because people experience too many side effects

   C. Because inappropriate use of antibiotics is contributing to antibiotic-resistant bacteria

   D. Because antibiotics are expensive

17. Which of the following classes of drugs is *not* usually used to treat a urinary tract infection?

    A. Sulfonamides

    B. Penicillins

    C. Cephalosporins

    D. Quinolones

18. Antibiotics that are metabolized by cytochrome P450 enzymes are at risk of drug interactions with all *except* which of the following?

    A. Grapefruit juice

    B. Phenytoin

    C. Ritonavir

    D. Peanuts

19. Which of the following are essential to consider in choosing an antibiotic?

    A. The broadest spectrum of antibacterial activity available and which agent the patient's insurance will cover

    B. The location of the infection, likely pathogens, and local susceptibility patterns

    C. The amount of swelling at the infection site, the results of the gram stain, and patient preference

    D. Whether to wait three days before selecting an antibiotic to see if the infection resolves on its own

20. It is important for patients taking tetracyclines to do which of the following?

    A. Take the medication on an empty stomach.

    B. Avoid alcohol and avoid driving due to blurred vision.

    C. Avoid sun exposure and dairy products.

    D. Store the medication in the refrigerator and drink plenty of water.

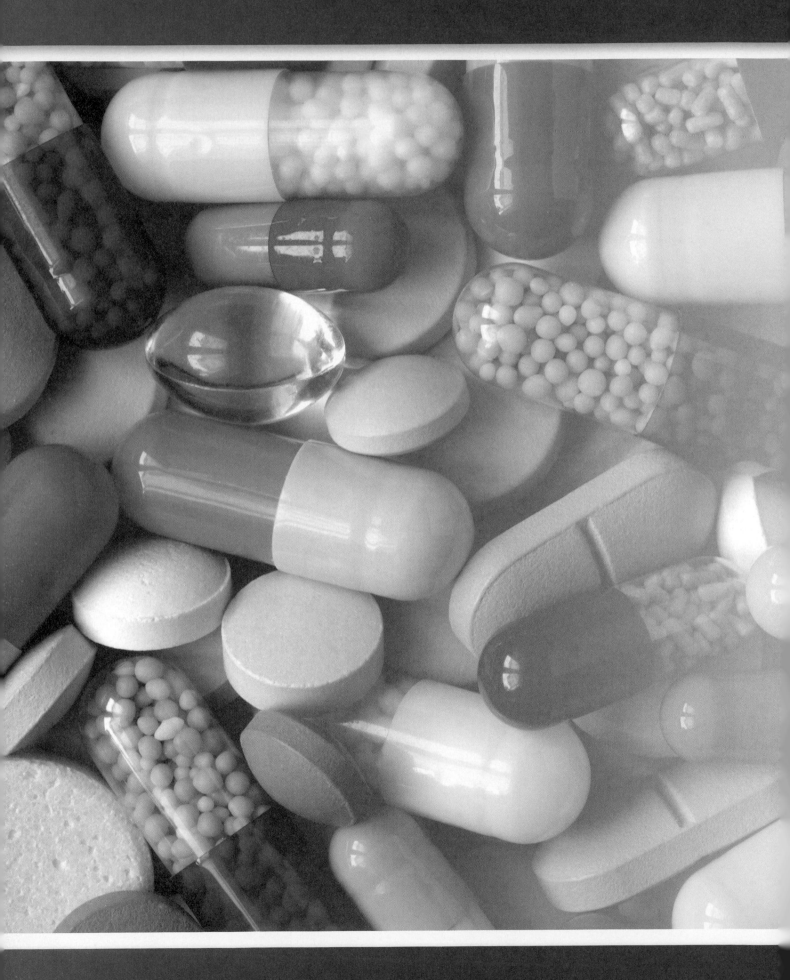

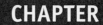
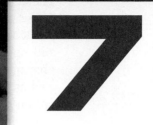
Labs for Drug References

OBJECTIVES

After reading this chapter, you will be able to:

- Use pharmaceutical reference texts and differentiate their functions.
- Understand the difference between fungi and viruses.
- Compare and contrast antifungal, antiviral, and antiretroviral drugs.
- Discuss the drugs used to treat fungal and viral infections
- Identify the drugs used for HIV and how the use of two or more drugs together leads to synergism in treatment.

KEY TERMS

Acquired immune
  deficiency syndrome
  (AIDS)
Adsorption stage
AIDS-defining illness
  (ADI)
Algae
Antifungal
Antiretroviral
Antiviral
Assembly stage
Average wholesale price
  (AWP)
Bacteria
Capsid
Chemokine coreceptor
  inhibitor
Direct price cost
DNA
Drug Facts and

Comparisons
Enteral feeding
Envelope
Eukaryotic organisms
Federal upper limit (FUL)
Fungus
Fusion inhibitors
Helminths
Human immunodeficiency
  virus (HIV)
Integrase inhibitor
Interferon
Investigational drug
Naked virus
National Drug Code
  (NDC)
Non-nucleoside reverse
  transcriptase
  inhibitors (NNRTIs)
Nucleoside reverse

transcriptase
  inhibitors (NRTIs)
Nucleotide reverse
  transcriptase
  inhibitors (NtRTIs)
Orange Book
Orphan drug
Penetration stage
Protease inhibitors (PIs)
Protozoa
Red Book
Release stage
Retrovirus
Synergism
Synthesis stage
Uncoating stage
Virion
Virus
Wholesale acquisition
  cost (WAC)

Chapter Overview

There are many pharmaceutical references available to the pharmacy technician. These pharmaceutical references are available in several different formats, including printed-book format, loose-leaf–binder format, pocket-sized booklets, foldout charts, and materials that can be posted in prominent places within the pharmacy. Many pharmaceutical references are available online, on electronic media such as CDs, as well as in printed form. The average pharmacy will have a combination of print and online pharmaceutical references available to the pharmacy technician. This chapter examines three of the most popular pharmaceutical references: *Drug Facts and Comparisons*, Micromedex, and *Red Book*.

This chapter also examines fungal and viral infections, as well as the drug-therapy options for treating these infections.

Drug References

Drug references are commonly used by the pharmacy technician. It is important to examine the contents and organization of each reference in addition to identifying how each specific reference can contribute to your successful pharmacy practice. The chapter starts with a look into *Drug Facts and Comparisons*.

Drug Facts and Comparisons

Facts & Comparisons, a product of Wolters Kluwer Health, publishes a bound version of **Drug Facts and Comparisons**, a pocket version of *Drug Facts and Comparisons*, and a loose-leaf *Drug Facts and Comparisons*. In addition, the group offers four online products: Facts & Comparisons eAnswers, Facts & Comparisons Clinical eAnswers, Facts & Comparisons Patient Facts Online, and The Formulary Monograph Service. Finally, a Facts & Comparisons eAnswers monthly and a Facts & Comparisons eAnswers single-user annual version are both available in CD-ROM format.

The bound and the loose-leaf versions of *Drug Facts and Comparisons* contain monographs for more than 20,000 prescriptions and over the counter (OTC) drugs, along with multiple charts and tables. Additionally, both these versions of *Drug Facts and Comparisons* contain commonly accepted treatment guidelines and a list of drug manufacturers and distributors. In both of these versions of *Drug Facts and Comparisons*, pharmacy personnel can find both the brand and generic name for each U.S. drug along with a list of Canadian drug brand names.

Subscribing to the Facts & Comparisons eAnswers online gives pharmacy personnel access to an entire range of routinely updated drug references. Included in this online package are the entire *Drug Facts and Comparisons*, as well as the following drug resources:

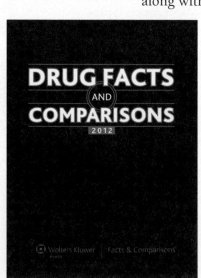

Drug Facts and Comparisons reference book.

- Drug Interaction Facts
- Drug Interaction Facts: Herbal Supplements and Food
- MedFacts patient information in English and Spanish
- Comparative Efficacy Content
- The Review of Natural Products
- A to Z Drug Facts
- Nonprescription Drug Therapy

- Off-Label Drug Facts
- Drug Identifier

In addition, subscribing to the Facts & Comparisons eAnswers online provides pharmacy personnel with a wide range of additional pharmacy related resources. The following items are included in the eAnswer online subscription:

- Clinical calculators
- Black-box warnings
- Pregnancy and lactation warnings
- Bioequivalence codes
- Investigational drugs
- Manufacturer index
- Orphan drugs
- Medication guides
- FDA MedWatch links
- Patient-assistance programs

Additional references that can be added to the online subscription include the following:

- Cancer Chemotherapy Manual
- 5-Minute Clinical Consult
- Trissel's IV-Chek
- ToxFacts Toxicology Treatment Guidelines
- Healthwise Patient Instructions
- The Formulary Monograph Service
- *Martindale—The Complete Drug Reference*

Advantages and Disadvantages of the Drug Facts and Comparisons Formats

Each of the different formats of *Drug Facts and Comparisons* has its own individual advantages and disadvantages. One of the primary advantages of all the formats is their ability to support pharmacy personnel by providing a source for rapidly locating drug information that is correct and reliable. All the formats allow for quick and reliable cross-referencing of drug information along with ways to locate related content. Each of the formats enhances pharmacy personnel's ability to make reliable therapeutic decisions, be that in relation to a generic substitution, dosing, or a drug-interaction question.

The hard-bound, complete version of *Drug Facts and Comparisons* contains almost 2,000 complete, detailed drug monographs, covering more than 20,000 drugs. This version provides extensive information for each drug monograph. The disadvantages of this version are the size of the book itself and the reader's inability to update the materials it contains except through the purchase of an entire new edition.

The loose-leaf *Drug Facts and Comparisons* provides all the advantages of the hard-bound complete version, with the additional advantage of being able to routinely update the information it contains. The loose-leaf version subscription includes an automatic updating system where new pages are sent to the pharmacy on a regular basis. This allows for the replacement of pages in the binder that needed updating. The disadvantage of this system is that these new pages can get lost, either in the mail or within the pharmacy itself, and thus the older pages may not be replaced. Two additional disadvantages are the need to assign specific personnel to routinely update the binder when new pages arrive and the cost to the pharmacy, which is much greater than with the bound version.

The bound pocket version of *Drug Facts and Comparisons* contains abridged monographs. The disadvantage of this version is the loss of information in comparison to the larger versions. The advantage is the ability to carry this version in your lab coat pocket.

You can obtain the most comprehensive amount of drug information by subscribing to the Facts & Comparisons eAnswers, the online product. The main advantage is the amount of information available, while one disadvantage is the learning curve required to utilize all the different references included in this service. Web access must be available to use these references, thus lack of Web availability is a disadvantage.

Using Drug Facts and Comparisons

Drug Facts and Comparisons can be an invaluable resource in the pharmacy, both for the pharmacist and the pharmacy technician. This reference contributes to a successful pharmacy operation specifically because of the large amount of drug information available within one reference. Having this information available in one place is a cost and time saver for the pharmacy. Pharmacy personnel can answer most drug-related questions quickly and correctly by simply accessing this reference. This cost and time savings can only be realized, however, if the pharmacy technician understands the layout of the reference and has practiced locating information.

Drug Facts and Comparisons begins with an introduction section that explains how to use the text itself. This reference ends with a Canadian drug index. Following the introduction are the drug-related chapters, which are organized by body system. Thus, to find a drug that would be used for kidney disease, one would look in the chapter entitled "Renal and Genitourinary Agents." The arrangement of these drug-related chapters is as follows:

- Chapter 1: "Nutrients and Nutritional Agents"
- Chapter 2: "Hematological Agents"
- Chapter 3: "Endocrine and Metabolic Agents"
- Chapter 4: "Cardiovascular Agents"
- Chapter 5: "Renal and Genitourinary Agents"
- Chapter 7: "Respiratory Agents"
- Chapter 8: "Central Nervous System Agents"
- Chapter 9: "Gastrointestinal Agents"
- Chapter 10: "Systemic Anti-Infectives"
- Chapter 11: "Biological and Immunologic Agents"
- Chapter 12: "Dermatological Agents"
- Chapter 13: "Ophthalmic and Otic Agents"
- Chapter 14: "Antineoplastic Agents"

Examining this list of drug-related chapters, you will quickly note the difficulty in finding a specific drug if you do not know what body system that drug is used for. A much easier method for locating a drug would be to search the index for the drug's name.

In addition to the introduction and the various drug-related chapters, this reference contains a "Keeping Up" section, which discusses investigational and orphan drugs. An **orphan drug** is a drug that is developed by a drug company specifically for a rare disease or condition. Drugs that have been designated orphan drugs follow a different approval process with the Food and Drug Administration (FDA). An **investigational**

drug is one that is currently in human testing, prior to being sent to the FDA for approval. Additionally, there is a chapter on diagnostic aids, which can prove helpful to the pharmacy technician when the pharmacy is filling a prescription for one of these medical aids or when the patient has a question if purchasing the product.

Another very important section in *Drug Facts and Comparisons* is the appendix. It contains useful information that relates to drug therapy, such as treatment guidelines, standard medical abbreviations, FDA pregnancy categories, guidelines for treatment of acute overdoses and hypersensitivity reactions, and even a reference on the international system of units. The appendix also contains a list of manufacturers and distributors.

Lab: Using Facts & Comparisons

Pharmacy technicians must be able to use the reference materials discussed in this chapter. This lab covers using Facts & Comparisons. To complete this lab, the pharmacy technician will need to access Facts & Comparisons. The most recent printed version of *Drug Facts and Comparisons* may be used, or the technician can access the online version of Facts & Comparisons, if available.

Using Facts & Comparisons, the pharmacy technician will complete the form in **Practice 7.1**, answering all the questions. More than one form may be assigned for completion by the technician based on instructor preference.

Facts & Comparisons Practice 7.1

Using the brand or generic name of the drug noted by the instructor on the form, the pharmacy technician will complete all questions.

Brand Name: _____   Generic Name: _____

Available Dosage Forms: _____

Drug Class: _____

Controlled Substance: _____ Yes   _____ No

If Yes, Control Schedule: _____

FDA-Approved Indications: _____

_____

Adult Dosage: _____

Pediatric Dosage: _____

Pregnancy Category: _____

Adverse Reactions: _____

_____

Drug Interactions: _____

_____

Warnings/Precautions: _____

_____

Contraindications: _____

_____

Micromedex

Micromedex, a product of Thomson Reuters Healthcare Inc., publishes Micromedex 2.0 and Micromedex 2.0 (Healthcare Series), CareNotes System, Formulary Advisor, and a PDR Electronic Library.

Micromedex is an online program that can be downloaded onto computers and PDAs and accessed through subscription portals. Access to Micromedex provides pharmacy personnel such user tools as the following:

- 360° View Dashboard
- Drug Interactions
- Trissel's 2 IV Compatibility
- Drug Identification
- Toxicology and Drug Product Lookup
- Drug Comparison
- Calculators
- CareNotes

360° View Dashboard

The 360° View Dashboard is just what it sounds like. From the dashboard, the user can access multiple search results for any drug. Micromedex information will include the following items in an easy-to-find DrugPoint Summary, organized in the following manner:

Micromedex information:
- Adult dosing
- Pediatric dosing
- FDA-labeled indications
- Non–FDA-labeled indications
- Contraindications/warnings
- Pregnancy category
- Drug interactions
- Adverse effects
- IV compatibility
- Mechanism of action/pharmacokinetics
- Administration/monitoring
- How supplied
- Toxicology
- Clinical teaching

Drug images:
- A photograph of all sides of oral solids

Drug consults:
- A list of pertinent information such as the American College of Gastroenterology (ACG) guidelines, information about **enteral feeding** (that is, feeding through a tube instead of normal swallowing), information about administering medication, and other miscellaneous information related to a specific drug

Comparative efficacy:

■ Information to enable the user to make a side-by-side comparison with other medications from the same class

Drug Interactions

The Drug Interactions tool enables the user to enter patient-specific allergies as well as the drugs the patient is taking. The program will then sort the interactions in the following manner:

■ Drug-drug
■ Ingredient duplication
■ Allergy
■ Food
■ Ethanol (alcohol)
■ Lab
■ Tobacco
■ Pregnancy
■ Lactation

The information reveals the drugs involved in the interaction, a level of severity (contraindicated, major, moderate, minor and unknown), documentation, and a summary of the interaction.

Trissel's 2 IV Compatibility

Trissel's 2 IV Compatibility database enables the user to select a parenteral drug and check its compatibility with other parenteral drugs or solutions when administered intravenously (by IV). The program identifies the compatibility for Y-site, admixture, and syringe combinations as one of the following:

■ Compatible
■ Incompatible
■ Caution
■ Variable
■ Uncertain
■ Not tested

Drug Identification

The Drug Identifications tool enables the user to search for the identity of a pill or capsule. The program uses several identifiers. The first is an imprint code. This is the easiest and safest identifier. If there is no imprint code, the program will call for the color of the dose, the shape of the dose, and any pattern that might assist in the identification. After identifying information has been entered, the program displays images with those characteristics with the corresponding drug name. Of course, if you enter the characteristics of a white, round, unmarked tablet, you will obtain more than 1,100 results.

Toxicity and Drug Product Lookup

The Toxicity and Drug Product Lookup tool enables the user to search for commercial or household products and chemicals by product name or other substance. The name is identified along with the strength or form, the manufacturer, the country of manufacture, the product ID, the American Association of Poison Control Centers (AAPCC) code, and a quick link to related documents, such as on POISINDEX.

Drug Comparison Results

The Drug Comparison Results program enables the user to select two drugs and compare the following items side by side:

- Dosing and indications
- Adult dosing
- Pediatric dosing
- FDA-labeled indications
- Non–FDA-labeled indications
- Contraindications/warnings
- "Do Not Confuse" warnings
- Contraindications
- Precautions
- Pregnancy category
- Breastfeeding
- Drug interactions (major, moderate)
- Adverse effects (common, serious)
- Name information (U.S. trade names, class, regulatory status, generic availability)
- Mechanism of action/pharmacokinetics
- Administration/monitoring
- How supplied
- Toxicology
- Clinical teaching
- References

Calculators

The Calculator section of Micromedex offers a variety of automatic formulas for the following:

- Antidote dosing and nomogram
- Laboratory values
- Dosing tools
- Clinical calculators
- Measurement calculators

These calculators are used primarily by clinical pharmacists when dosing medications for hospitalized patients.

CareNotes

The CareNotes section of Micromedex is a useful tool for educating patients about their medications. Pharmacy personnel can enter a drug into the program, and it will print patient-education information in any one of 15 languages for the patient to take home.

Micromedex would be the best reference to use when searching for drug interactions

Lab: Using Micromedex

Pharmacy technicians working in a pharmacy that prepares IV fluids should be familiar with the Trissel's section of Micromedex. Using Trissel's can help to prevent a drug incompatibility when mixing two different injectable drugs into one IV fluid for administration.

To complete this lab, the pharmacy technician should log on to the Micromedex Web site. Using Micromedex, the pharmacy technician will complete the **Practice 7.2** form by answering all the questions. More than one form may be assigned for completion by the technician based on instructor preference.

Micromedex Practice 7.2

Using the brand or generic name of the drug noted by the instructor on the form, the pharmacy technician will complete all questions. (Note: The instructor will need to choose a second drug for the IV-compatibility question.)

Brand Name: _____ Generic Name: _____

Available Dosage Forms: _____

Drug Identification Markings: _____

Drug Class: _____

Controlled Substance: _____ Yes _____ No

If Yes, Control Schedule: _____

FDA-Approved Indications: _____

_____

Adult Dosage: _____

Pediatric Dosage: _____

Pregnancy Category: _____

Adverse Reactions: _____

_____

Drug Interactions: _____

_____

Warnings/Precautions: _____

_____

Contraindications: _____

_____

*IV Drug Compatibility
When Mixed With: _____

Red Book

Red Book, published by Medical Economics Company, Inc. differs from *Drug Facts and Comparisons* in several ways, although certain sections of *Red Book* do contain the same information. One of the recent changes that separates *Red Book* from *Drug Facts and Comparisons* is the format in which *Red Book* is available. The familiar printed, hard-copy *Red Book*, always printed with a red cover as shown here, is no more. Beginning in 2011, the only *Red Book* format available will in fact not be a book at all, but a CD-ROM. This CD-ROM will be updated four times a year.

One of the most common reasons to use *Red Book* is the access it gives to thousands of healthcare prices, for both drug and non-drug healthcare items. The drug-price sections are especially useful for obtaining a manufacturer's **average wholesale price (AWP)**, suggested retail price for OTC drugs, and drug-reimbursement information. In addition to the AWP, *Red Book* is a resource for obtaining the **wholesale acquisition cost (WAC)** (that is, the cost of the drug from the wholesale drug distributor), the **direct price cost** (that is, the cost of a drug from the manufacturer), and the **federal upper limit (FUL)** price, which is the ceiling or highest price the federal government pays to pharmacies for the prescription drugs they dispense to Medicaid beneficiaries.

Red Book is especially useful for conducting a drug-pricing analysis or searching for a less-expensive generic substitution approved by the FDA. *Red Book* makes the question of generic substitution easier, as it provides the current *Orange Book* code for drug substitution. *Orange Book* is the official government list of drug safety, efficacy, and approved generic substitutions.

Red Book maintains a current list of **National Drug Codes (NDCs)** for every drug on the market in the U.S. When an NDC number changes, *Red Book* can be used to cross-reference to the new NDC. Another useful section of *Red Book* is the drug-picture section. If you are trying to identify a tablet or capsule, you can locate a picture of it in the picture section of *Red Book*.

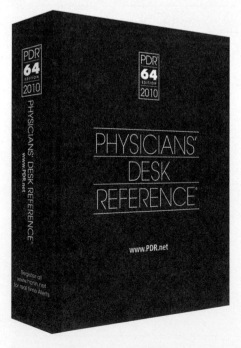

Red Book 2010, hard-copy edition.

Additional useful items found in *Red Book* include the following:

- Summaries of drug/food, drug/alcohol, and drug/tobacco interactions
- Sugar-free, alcohol-free, lactose- and galactose-free, and sulfite-containing product listings for customers with special needs
- A complete list of new molecular entities and generics approved by the FDA
- Comprehensive manufacturer, pharmaceutical wholesaler, and third-party administrator directories
- A vitamin-comparison table, with amounts of vitamins and minerals in more than 50 popular multivitamin products
- Common laboratory values, with answers to the most common patient questions about urine sugar level, cholesterol, blood pressure, and more
- A guide to leading alternative medicines
- A guide to pharmacy buying groups and group-purchasing organizations in the United States.
- National Council for Prescription Drug Programs (NCPDP) billing standards
- A controlled-substance inventory sheet

In today's busy pharmacy practice, two areas are of particular importance when searching a reference: clinical information about a drug, and drug pricing. The clinical information about a drug, including the drug indications, the correct dosage, common side effects, and interactions, can be located in several difference references. What *Red Book* brings to the pharmacy practice is a wide array of pricing information. Becoming adept at using *Red Book* is important for the pharmacy technician.

Red Book is the best reference text if one needs to locate the price of a drug.

What Would You Do?

Question: A customer comes to the prescription counter and asks you if severe abdominal cramps could be a side effect of the drug he picked up from the pharmacy yesterday. You know you could research this question in one of the available references in the pharmacy. Would you research the question and then advise the customer?

Answer: No. Because this question involves counseling the customer, you would relay the question to the pharmacist. A pharmacist should counsel the customer regarding all clinical questions.

What Would You Do?

Question: A customer comes to the window with a prescription for Diflucan. She asks if there is a generic drug available, and if so, what the price difference would be between the generic and the brand-name product. As the pharmacy technician, would you research this question and then advise the customer, or get the pharmacist?

Answer: The pharmacy technician can research the generic availability and pricing information to answer the customer's questions. These questions are not clinical in nature; the pharmacy technician is not counseling or giving medical advice to the customer.

Lab: Using *Red Book*

To complete this lab, the pharmacy technician will need to access *Red Book*. The most recent printed version of *Red Book* may be used, or the technician can access the online version if available.

Using *Red Book*, the pharmacy technician will complete **Practice 7.3** form by answering all the questions. More than one form may be assigned for completion by the technician based on instructor preference.

Red Book Practice 7.3

What is the Web site for reporting vaccine adverse events? _____

_____

What is the antidote for rattlesnake bite? _____

_____

What is the manufacturer ID number for Sandoz? _____

What is the NDC number for Depo Medrol 40mg/mL 5mL vials: _____

Note the address and phone number of your State Board of Pharmacy: _____

_____

_____

What is the Medicaid reimbursement formula for the State of Illinois? _____

_____

Is a generic form available for Ritalin?   _____ Yes _____ No

If yes, list the NDC_number: _____

_____

In how many dosage forms is Rocephin is available?   _____

In how many different-size vials is Rocephin available?   _____

What is the NDC number for Aveeno Skin Relief Bath Treatment? _____

Describe the appearance and ID markings of MS Contin 30mg: _____

_____

Describe the appearance and ID markings of Hyzaar 100mg/25mg: _____

_____

What is the average wholesale price (AWP) for Accupril 5mg?   _____

What is the suggested retail price for Tussin CF 115mL bottle? _____

Is Citrucel powder sugar free?   _____ Yes _____ No

Is Pediahist DM syrup alcohol free? _____ Yes _____ No

Drug Insights: Treatment of Viral and Fungal Infections

This section examines the drugs used to treat fungal and viral infections. The drugs used to treat these infections are very different from each other and from all the other drugs in the pharmacy.

Fungi that cause human infections have a very special lifestyle, reproductive cycle, and internal metabolism; thus, specific drugs are required to treat or kill them. These drugs are commonly called **antifungal** drugs. Viruses have a completely different reproductive mechanism from other organisms. They have no metabolism of their own. Thus, **antiviral** drugs are required to prevent their reproduction.

To understand the mechanism of action of antifungal and antiviral drugs, one must understand some of the basic differences between fungi, viruses, other infectious organisms, and our own human cells. This section begins its discussion of antifungal and antiviral agents by examining fungi and then the drugs that kill them. Following that, it moves on to examine viruses and the drugs that can stop them from reproducing—and, in some cases, actually kill them.

Microorganisms

Microorganisms have distinct characteristics that place them in one of two major classes: prokaryotic or eukaryotic. **Prokaryotic organisms** are simply organisms without any specific center structures, including no specific nucleus. Prokaryotic organisms are primarily bacteria, including those that cause human disease. **Eukaryotic organisms** have several internal structures that can be seen with an electron microscope, including a distinct nucleus. Animal cells, including human cells, are examples of eukaryotic cells.

In the study of microbiology, microorganisms are further divided into six different groups:

- Bacteria
- Fungus
- Virus
- Algae
- Protozoa
- Helminth

The first group of microorganisms are **bacteria**. Some bacteria cause disease in humans, while other bacteria are beneficial, such as the ones currently used to produce several different antibiotics. Bacteria do cause many of the human infectious diseases for which you will see drugs used. Most of these drugs are called antibiotics, which you studied in the previous chapter. The second and third groups of microorganisms are the **fungus** and **virus**. Both of these groups and their related drugs will be reviewed in this chapter. A fourth group of microorganisms is algae. **Algae** are a group of organisms that do not cause human diseases, but have some members that are beneficial to pharmacy. One example of this type of algae is seaweed, which is used as an ingredient to thicken some liquid drugs. The fifth and sixth groups of microorganisms, the **protozoa** and **helminth**, do cause disease in humans. These two groups include parasites and worms, which are discussed in Chapter 12, along with the drugs used to kill them.

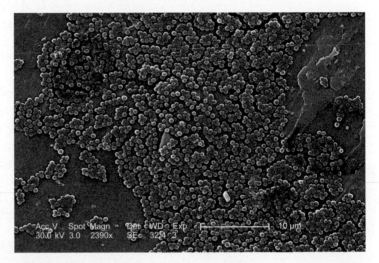

Bacteria.

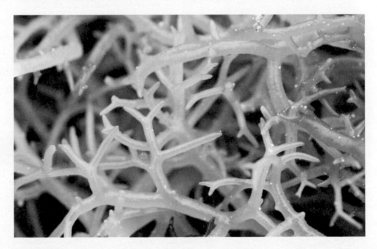

Common algae.

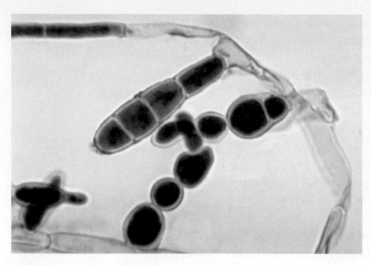

Common fungus.

Fungal Infections

Thousands of different types of fungi exist in the world. Some of these fungi are very large, like the toadstool mushroom, which can be seen with the naked eye. Other fungi, also called molds, can best be seen with a microscope. Some fungi are beneficial to humankind, while fungi can cause human diseases ranging from non-fatal nail fungus to fatal lung infections TABLE 7.1 .

One of these beneficial fungi, a mold, is penicillium, from which the drug penicillin was originally produced. Another beneficial fungus is yeast, without which we would not be able to produce most of the bread products that we eat. In contrast, *Aspergillus* is a harmful fungus that can grow on warm, wet walls in your house. It can cause a severe, sometimes fatal lung disease called aspergillosis. *Candida*, although a yeast, is a human pathogen and can cause candidiasis, which is a common vaginal infection. Some fungi, like *Candida*, can live in harmony with humans and cause no disease until our body's defense mechanism is lowered through disease or drug treatment for other medical conditions.

Unlike bacteria that cause human disease, fungi are eukaryotic organisms. As eukaryotic organisms, fungi are close to the human cell in structure, which makes treating them with drugs more difficult. The drugs used as antifungal agents (see TABLE 7.2) have a difficult time telling the difference between the fungus they are supposed to kill and our own cells; thus, antifungal drugs can be very toxic to the patient.

Fortunately, one major difference does exist between fungal cells and human cells. This difference is the way in which the outside cell wall is held together. In human cells, cholesterol is a primary ingredient. In fungal cells, ergosterol is the primary ingredient. Some fungal drugs work by inhibiting a special fungal enzyme, called fungal cytochrome P450, which is different from the cytochrome P450 found in the human liver. Antifungal drugs that utilize either of these two mechanisms of action are considerably less toxic to humans than agents that use different mechanisms.

Antifungal Drugs

Many antifungal drugs are very toxic. Extreme care must be taken when preparing these for dispensing. The IV antifungal agents are especially dangerous. When preparing one of these medications, every dispensing step is especially critical. That includes being

Table 7.1	Common Fungal Diseases	
Fungal Organism	**Common Name**	**Disease**
Pneumocystis jiroveci	PCP	Pneumonia in AIDS patients
Aspergillus spp.	Mold	Pneumonia, brain, skin, heart infections
Candida albicans	Yeast infection	Vaginal, lung, throat infections
Dermatophytes	Ringworm or tinea	Skin, nail infections
Coccidioides	Valley fever	Lung infections

Table 7.2 **Common Antifungal Drugs**				
Generic Name	**Brand Name**	**Availability**	**Mechanism of Action**	**Rx Y/N**
Amphotericin	Fungizone, Abelcet	IV, topical	Cell-wall interference	Y
Anidulafungin	Eraxis	IV	Ergosterol interference	Y
Caspofungin	Cancidas	IV	Ergosterol interference	Y
Clotrimazole	Lotrimin, Mycelex	Lozenge, vaginal cream, topical cream	Cell-wall interference	Y (lozenge); N (other forms)
Fluconazole	Diflucan	IV, liquid, tablet	P450 interference	Y
Itraconazole	Sporanox	IV, liquid, capsule	P450 interference	Y
Micafungin	Mycamine	IV	Ergosterol interference	Y
Miconazole	Monistat	Buccal tablet, vaginal cream/suppository, topical	Cell-wall interference	Y (tabs); N (other forms
Posaconazole	Noxafil	Liquid only	P450 interference	Y
Tolnaftate	Tinactin, Lamisil AT	Topical	Ergosterol interference	N
Voriconazole	Vfend	IV, liquid, tablet	P450 interference	Y

sure you choose the correct drug, calculating the correct dosage for the final IV mixture, and diluting the drug in the correct amount of IV fluid. When preparing to dispense the other dosage forms, especially the oral forms, double-checking yourself is very important. Dispensing the wrong drug or drug strength, or typing the directions incorrectly, could result in major side effects for the patient—in some cases, even death.

> You are preparing a nystatin oral liquid prescription for a customer. After calculating the dosage needed, you realize you will have to dispense two bottles of liquid for the ordered seven days of medication. If the patient refuses pharmacist counseling, you must communicate to the patient that he should use the medication for only seven days.

> Fungal cell structure is physically close to human cell structure. Thus, antifungal drugs can be very toxic to humans.

Viral Infections

Unlike bacteria or a fungus, a virus cannot live without a living host of some type. Because a virus cannot live by itself, there have been discussions for years as to whether a virus is really even alive. A virus must infect some other living organism, and then direct that organism's gene structure to produce more viruses. A virus does not even contain any mechanism for its own metabolism! The virus, once inside another

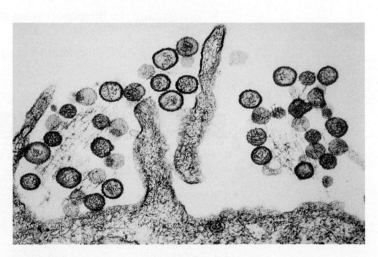

Hantavirus.

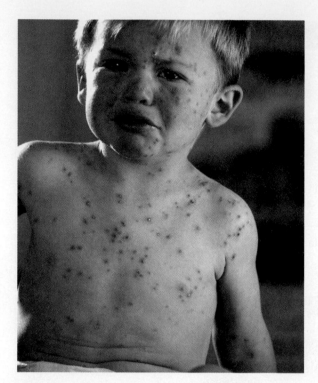

Chicken pox virus.

cell, uses that cell's metabolism to make new virus parts and assemble them. After the host cell makes the new virus, this virus is then released to infect another cell.

Because the virus must live inside the human cell, antiviral agents do not always kill a virus directly; this would also kill our human cells. Many antiviral drugs work by blocking the virus from replicating and moving to another human cell.

Whether you believe a virus is alive or not, viruses are one of the most common types of human infectious agents.

Thousands of different kinds of viruses exist, and can infect every type of living organism. Thus, they are not unique in just causing human disease. A virus is much smaller than a bacteria or a fungus, and some viruses even infect other viruses and bacteria. Some viruses infect plants and cause disease, while other viruses infect plants and cause the plant to display a beautiful array of colors. An example of this beneficial type of virus is the tulip mosaic virus, which gives many tulips their beautiful colors.

Viruses can be classified a couple of different ways. One way is by what type of internal core material the virus contains. Some viruses contain deoxyribonucleic acid (DNA), while other viruses contain ribonucleic acid (RNA). A virus never contains both DNA and RNA. This core material if protected by a protein shell called a **capsid**. Another way to differentiate viruses is by the presence or absence of another coating called an **envelope**. A virus without an envelope is called a **naked virus**. A fully formed virus is called a **virion**.

Viral Multiplication

Viruses can be spread through direct contact, eating contaminated food, drinking contaminated water, inhaling airborne particles, or being exposed to body fluids and/or contaminated equipment. **TABLE 7.3** comprises a list of common viral diseases. Once the body is infected, the virus follows six specific stages to reproduce **FIGURE 7.1**. These stages are as follows:

- Adsorption: In the **adsorption stage**, the virus attaches to a potential host cell.
- Penetration: In the **penetration stage**, the virus penetrates the host cell's outer wall.
- Uncoating: In the **uncoating stage**, the virus frees the core of either DNA or RNA.

Table 7.3   Common Viral Diseases

Virus Common Name	RNA or DNA Virus	Disease
Herpes simplex 1 virus	DNA	Fever blister, cold sores
Herpes simplex 2 virus	DNA	Genital herpes
Human papillomavirus	DNA	Several types of warts, cervical cancer
Hepatitis A virus	RNA	Short-term hepatitis
Influenza virus	RNA	Influenza or the flu

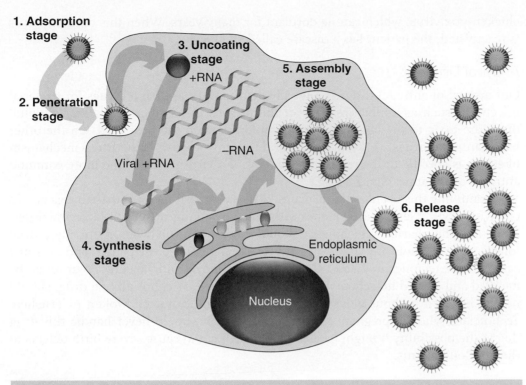

FIGURE 7.1 Viral replication process.

- Synthesis: In the **synthesis stage**, the virus controls the cell's mechanism, thus beginning the production of new virus components.
- Assembly: In the **assembly stage**, the viral parts are assembled.
- Release: In the **release stage**, a new virus is released.

Antiviral agents work by inhibiting one or more of these six stages.

All human cells contain DNA and RNA, while viral cells only contain *either* DNA or RNA.

Because the virus invades our own human cells and uses a cell's machinery to survive and duplicate, many antiviral drugs prevent the first infected cell from being able to make more. This process does not kill the first cell, because that is one of our own human cells. Our own immune system also aids the body in trying to rid itself of the virus. One way our body protects itself from a virus infection is by producing an agent called **interferon**. The infected cell sends out a messenger to surrounding cells, telling them it has been invaded by a virus and that they should protect themselves. This messenger is interferon, which additionally helps those cells protect themselves.

In the best-case scenario, the virus causes an acute infection, which quickly resolves on its own or with medications. This would include the common cold, the flu, and several other respiratory infections. Some viral infections become chronic. Their course of action usually starts with an acute phase. Then, the patient experiences periods of remission, followed by reoccurrences of the disease. Herpes virus infections are examples of viruses with this chronic course. Some viral diseases even lead to the death of the host due to cumulative damage within many cells and organs. AIDS would be an example of this type of viral infection.

Some viruses have the ability to become latent, which means they can lie dormant in the body and then, maybe years later, reappear. An example of this would be the chicken-pox virus, which can lie dormant for many years. When this dormant virus is reactivated, the patient has a disease called shingles.

Antiviral Drugs

Our arsenal of antiviral drugs is a lot smaller than our arsenal of drugs for bacterial infections, such as antibiotics. One of the reasons this is the case is that antiviral drugs are toxic to the host because they interfere with the host cells. On the other hand, antiviral drugs work only on viral infections because these drugs' mechanism of action is specific to the replication process of a virus. A list of the more common antiviral drugs appears in **TABLE 7.4** .

Examining this list of antiviral drugs, one can see that many of these drugs names end with a "vir." Generic drug names with this "vir" ending are usually antiviral drugs. That said, the pharmacy technician should not rely on this when preparing a drug for dispensing. Many antiviral drugs are very toxic, both to the patient and, in some cases, to the technician. Two of the drugs, gancyclovir and valgancyclovir, must be handled and treated like chemotherapy drugs. Valcyte, which is an oral drug, should not be handled without gloves, and the tablet should not be broken or crushed. Technicians who are pregnant or might be pregnant should never handle this drug due to the possibility it might be absorbed, which could cause severe birth defects to the developing fetus.

HIV-AIDS

Human immunodeficiency virus (HIV) is the virus, or viruses, that can progress in a patient to a point where that patient has **acquired immune deficiency syndrome (AIDS)**. AIDS is one of the few infectious diseases in which a specific causative agent is not isolated from the patient. AIDS is diagnosed when a patient has tested posi-

Table 7.4 Common Antiviral Drugs

Generic Name	Brand Name	Availability	Treatment Uses
Acyclovir	Zovirax	IV, oral suspension, topical	Chicken pox, herpes infections, shingles
Amantadine	Symmetrel	Capsule, tablet, oral solution	Influenza A
Cidofovir	Vistide	IV	Cytomegalovirus (CMV)
Famciclovir	Famvir	IV, tablet	Acute shingles, herpes infections
Foscarnet	Foscavir	IV	Cytomegalovirus
Ganciclovir	Cytovene	IV, oral, and ocular implant	Cytomegalovirus
Influenza vaccine live	Flumist	Intranasal	Seasonal influenza (flu)
Oseltamivir	Tamiflu	Oral	Influenza A and B
Ribavirin	Virazole, Rebetol	Aerosol, oral	Respiratory syncytial virus (RSV)
Rimantadine	Flumadine	Oral	Influenza A
Valacyclovir	Valtrex	Oral	Herpes infections
Valgancyclovir	Valcyte	Oral	Cytomegalovirus (CMV)
Zanamivir	Relenza	Inhalation	Influenza A and B

tive for the virus and has one or more clinical diseases, which only occurs in people with a suppressed immune system (hence the use of the word *immunodeficiency* in the syndrome's name). These diseases are called **AIDS-defining illnesses (ADIs)**. Some examples of these diseases include Kaposi's sarcoma, cytomegalovirus retinitis, and *Mycobacterium avium*.

HIV is a special kind of virus called a **retrovirus**. A retrovirus can copy its own genetic material, which is in the form of RNA, onto the host cell's DNA by using a special enzyme called reverse transcriptase. The mode of action of drugs that combat these types of viruses is to block this retroviral process; thus, they are called **antiretroviral** drugs `TABLE 7.5`. Like all antiviral agents, this class of drugs can have many side effects, from those that are rather mild to ones that are severe, including death. Currently, seven methods of this retroviral blocking action have been defined and then turned into drug therapies:

- The **nucleoside reverse transcriptase inhibitors (NRTIs)** method of action is to prevent the formation of the DNA copy from the viral RNA.
- The **non-nucleoside reverse transcriptase inhibitors (NNRTIs)** mode of action is to prevent this same step in replication, but through a method that obstructs the enzyme's mechanical action.

Table 7.5 Common Antiretroviral Drugs

Generic Name	Brand Name	Availability	Mechanism of Action
Albacavir	Ziagen	Oral	NRTIs
Amprenavir	Agenerase	Oral	PIs
Atazanavir	Reyataz	Oral	PIs
Darunavir	Prezista	Oral	PIs
Delavirdine	Rescriptor	Oral	NNRTIs
Didanosine	Videx	Oral	NRTIs
Efavirenz	Sustiva	Oral	NNRTIs
Emtricitabine	Emtriva	Oral	NRTIs
Enfuvirtide	Fuzeon	Injection	Fusion inhibitors
Fosamprenavir	Lexiva	Oral	PIs
Indinavir	Crixivan	Oral	PIs
Lamivudine	Epivir	Oral	NRTIs
Maraviroc	Selzentry	Oral	Chemokine coreceptor inhibitor
Nelfinavir	Viracept	Oral	PIs
Nevirapine	Viramune	Oral	NNRTIs
Raltegravir	Isentress	Oral	Integrase inhibitors
Ritonavir	Norvir	Oral	PIs
Saquinavir	Fortovase/Invirase	Oral	PIs
Stavudine	Zerit	Oral	NRTIs
Tenofovir	Viread	Oral	NtRTIs
Tipranavir	Aptivus	Oral	PIs
Zidovudine, AZT	Retrovir	IV, oral	NRTIs

Table 7.6   Antiretroviral Combination Drugs

Generic Names	Brand Name
Abacavir and lamivudine	Epzicom
Abacavir, lamivudine, and zidovudine	Trizivir
Efavirenz and tenofovir	Atripla
Emtricitabine and tenofovir	Truvada
Lamivudine and zidovudine	Combivir
Lopinavir and ritonavir	Kaletra

- The **nucleotide reverse transcriptase inhibitors (NtRTIs)** mode of action is very similar to the NRTI's, but with fewer side effects.
- The **protease inhibitors (PIs)** mode of action is to prevent the production of the protease enzyme, which is needed to make the new virions.
- The **fusion inhibitors** mode of action is to prevent the original HIV from entering the human immune cell, while the chemokine receptor blocker functions by not allowing the HIV virus to attach to the human immune cell.
- The **integrase inhibitors** mode of action is similar to the protease inhibitors, but this drug blocks a different enzyme called an integrase.
- The **chemokine coreceptor inhibitors** mode of action is to bind with the chemokine coreceptor cavities, thus inhibiting the HIV-1 entry into host cells and thereby assisting in the treatment of HIV infection.

HIV has become very good at adapting to some of these drugs, especially if the patient is only receiving one type. Thus, the patient with HIV and/or AIDS may take several of these drugs at the same time. As a result, patient compliance with treatment can become an issue, as the patient may forget to take some of the required doses, may forget to take one the different drugs, or may develop unpleasant side effects from taking so many different drugs at the same time.

One of the advances in drug therapy for HIV/AIDS is the advent of combination drugs **TABLE 7.6** . These combination drugs usually combine at least two drugs with two different mechanisms of action into one tablet or capsule. In addition to improving compliance, this combination of drugs leads to synergism in clinical results. **Synergism** means that both drugs together provide a more effective treatment than either drug by itself.

Antiretroviral Drugs

The pharmacy technician should use extra discretion and be aware of his or her surroundings and the presence of other patients when dispensing any of these medications. These medications are dispensed only to a patient who has been diagnosed as HIV positive or for HIV prophylaxis due to possible exposure to the virus as with a needle stick. This information should not be shared with anyone.

Antiviral drugs prevent the replication of additional viruses in our body. Antiviral drugs do not kill the cell that is already infected.

Tech Math Practice

Question: The pharmacy technician receives a prescription for Nystatin oral suspension. Directions: 200,000 units into each cheek, four times daily, for 10 days. How much Nystatin is required for the full therapy if the concentration of the Nystatin suspension is 100,000 units/mL?

Answer: 200,000 units/cheek × 2 cheeks/dose = 400,000 units/dose × 4 doses/day = 1,600,000 units/day × 10 days = 16,000,000 units required for full therapy. 16,000,000 units ÷ 100,000 units/mL = 160mL.

Question: The pharmacy technician receives a prescription for Mycostatin vaginal tablets, 100,000 units/tablet. Directions: Insert one tablet vaginally each day for 14 days. How many tablets will you dispense to complete the prescription if they come in boxes of 15 tablets per box?

Answer: 1 tablet/dose × 1 dose/day × 14 days = 14 tablets.

Question: The pharmacy technician is mixing a single 90mg dose of enfuvirtide (Fuzeon). The package insert says to reconstitute with 1.1mL of sterile water for injection, tap for 10 seconds, and then roll to mix. How many milligrams are in the reconstituted vial?

Answer: This is a single-dose vial containing 90mg. Despite the volume of diluents used to reconstitute the medication in the vial, the dose remains the same: 90mg.

Question: The technician is ready to fill a prescription in the IV room for fluconazole IV 200mg. The only stock you have is supplied in bags of fluconazole 2mg/mL in a 100mL size and a 200mL size. How many milliliters do you need to make a 200mg dose?

Answer: 2mg/mL × 100mL/bag = 200mg/bag, which is the dose prescribed. Thus, the 100mL bag of fluconazole would be dispensed.

Question: You are ready to fill a prescription in the IV room for fluconazole IV 200mg. The only stock you have is supplied in bags of fluconazole 2mg/mL in a 100mL size and a 200mL size. How many milliliters do you need to make a 200mg dose?

Answer: First, establish a proportion: $\frac{2mg}{1mL} = \frac{200mg}{x}$. Cross-multiplying and solving for the unknown variable yields $xmg = \frac{200mg \times 1mL}{2} = 100mL$.

Question: An 80kg patient is prescribed Zovirax 20mg/kg (max 800mg per dose), orally, five times daily for five days. The pharmacy carries 200mg capsules. How many capsules should be dispensed to complete the five-day therapy?

Answer: 20mg × 80kg = 1,600mg/dose. However, 800mg is the maximum approved dose, so each dose = 800mg. Your next step is to establish a ratio proportion: $\frac{200mg}{1capsule} = \frac{800mg}{x}$ $_{capsules}$. Then cross-multiply to solve for x: $x = 4$ capsules per dose. Finally, perform the following operations: 4 capsules/dose × 5 doses/day = 20 capsules/day × 5 days = 100 capsules total.

Question: A patient with HIV infection presents with a prescription for Retrovir 200mg orally, three times daily, for 30 days. The pharmacy only has 110 capsules of 100mg each (it only comes in 100mg or 300mg capsules) in stock. The patient is dispensed the 110 capsules that are in stock. How many more capsules does the patient need to complete the 30-day therapy?

Answer: 200mg/dose × 3 doses/day = 600 mg/day × 30 days = 1,800mg/day ÷ 100mg/capsule = 180 capsules/prescription. 180 capsules – 110 capsules = 70 capsules.

Question: Referring to the preceding question, how many days' supply will the 110 capsules of 100mg Retrovir provide to the patient at a dosage of 200mg, three times daily?

Answer: 600mg/day ÷ 100mg/capsule = 6 capsules/day. 110 capsules ÷ 6 capsules/day = 18.3 days.

Question: A patient presents to the pharmacy a written prescription for Famvir 750mg tid for seven days. There are 500mg and 750mg tablets in stock. What will the pharmacy technician prepare for dispensing?

Answer: When available, the pharmacy technician should always dispense the exact dose that is prescribed. The 750mg tablets should be selected to fill this prescription. Thus, 750mg tablets/dose × 3 doses/day = 3 tablets/day × 7 days = 21 tablets.

Question: A patient presents a written prescription for terbinafine (Lamisil). Directions: 250mg po qd for 12 weeks. The patient's insurance will pay for only 28 days of therapy at a time (per fill). How many times is this prescription going to be filled (including the original fill) to allow the patient 12 weeks of therapy paid for by the insurance?

Answer: 1 dose/day × 28 days = 28 doses of terbinafine. 250mg should be dispensed for the first prescription fill. 12 weeks × 7 days/week = 84 days ÷ 28 days/fill = 3 fills, including the first fill. This is an original fill plus two refills.

Question: You are making an IV solution for amphotericin. The final bag is 20mg of amphotericin in 500mL of dextrose, 5 percent in water. What is the concentration of the final solution?

Answer: 20mg amphotericin/500mL D_5W can be reduced to its final concentration by simple division: 20mg ÷ 500mL = 0.04mg/mL.

Question: When making the amphotericin solution in the preceding question the technician begins with a 50mg vial and uses 10mL of sterile water for dilution of the powder. This results in a concentration of 50mg/10mL of diluted drug. The order is for a 20mg dose. How much of the concentrated solution should be used to make the final bag of 20mg/500mL D_5W?

Answer: First, use a proportion ratio: $\frac{50mg}{10mL} = \frac{20mg}{xmL}$. Then cross-multiply: 50mg × xmL=20mg × 10mL. x = 200mg-mL ÷ 50mg = 4mL.

Question: **The pharmacy receives a prescription for Lotrisone cream, 45gm, with no refill. The pharmacy only stocks 15gm tubes and currently has only one tube in stock. The patient doesn't want to wait three days for a special order, so the pharmacy technician dispenses one 15gm tube and instructs the patient to return in three days for the remainder of the prescription. What is the remainder of the prescription?**

Answer: 45g prescribed – 15g dispensed = 30g owed to the patient. The pharmacy will need to dispense two 15g tubes to the patient upon return for the remainder of the prescription.

Question: **When making an amphotericin solution, you begin with a 50mg vial and use 10mL of sterile water to dilute the powder. You end up with a concentration of 50mg/10mL of diluted drug. Your order is for a 20mg dose. How much of the concentrated solution are you going to use to make the final bag of 20mg/500mL D$_5$W?**

Answer: First, establish a ratio proportion: $\frac{50mg}{10mL} = \frac{20mg}{x}$. Cross-multiplying and solving for the unknown variable yields $xmg = \frac{(20mg \times 10mL)}{50mg} = 4mL$.

Question: **You are making an IV solution for amphotericin. The final bag is 20mg of amphotericin in 500mL of dextrose 5% in water. What is the concentration of the final solution per milliliter?**

Answer: 20mg/500mL can be reduced to 0.04mg/mL, which is the concentration of the final solution.

WRAP UP

Chapter Summary

- Common pharmacy drug references used in pharmacies include *Drug Facts and Comparisons*, *Micromedex*, and *Red Book*.

- The pharmacy reference *Drug Facts and Comparisons* arranges the data primarily by body systems based on the drug's use.

- The drug references available include other information in addition to specific drug information. For example, a reference might contain potential drug interactions, pregnancy category, IV compatibility, and information regarding administration and monitoring parameters.

- The majority of pharmacies today access these references electronically yet generally have a hard copy on hand when available.

- One specific national drug code (NDC) is assigned to every drug that is manufactured in the U.S.

- Antifungal drugs are only effective against fungal diseases.

- Antifungal drugs can be very toxic because fungal cells resemble human cells.

- Antiviral drugs are only effective against diseases caused by a virus.

- Antibiotic drugs are only effective against diseases caused by a bacteria.

- A virus is not a living entity but requires a host for reproduction and metabolism.

- Antiviral drugs prevent the virus from replicating but do not kill the human cell that was originally infected by the virus.

- A virus contains either DNA or RNA required for replication, while human cells contain both DNA and RNA.

Learning Assessment Questions

1. The pharmacists gives you a list of four different generic drugs and asks you to perform a cost study to determine which manufacturer's generic would be the least expensive for the pharmacy to place in stock. Which reference would you use to perform this task?

A. *Drug Facts and Comparisons*

B. Micromedex

C. *Red Book*

D. A clinical reference book

2. A customer asks you if the pharmacy uses FDA-approved generics. To verify that all the generics the pharmacy stocks are listed as approved substitutions, which reference book would you use to determine the answer?

A. *Drug Facts and Comparisons*

B. Micromedex

C. The Formulary Monograph Service

D. *Orange Book*

3. When placing your drug order with a local wholesaler, you receive a notice that the NDC number you entered for a drug does not exist. You check the bottle of the same drug on the shelf, and note that the NDC you entered matches the NDC on the bottle. Realizing that the NDC may have changed, which reference could you check to find the updated NDC number (assuming the reference is the most recent version)?

A. *Drug Facts and Comparisons*

B. Micromedex

C. *Red Book*

D. A clinical reference book

4. You receive a prescription for valgancyclovir (Valcyte). As you are preparing the prescription for dispensing, you accidentally drop a tablet on the floor. What should you do?

A. Simply pick up the tablet from the floor and discard it.

B. Pick the tablet up using a paper towel or put on gloves first, and then discard it. This drug can be absorbed through the skin, and is toxic.

C. Pick up the tablet and return it to the bottle, because the tablet is very expensive.

D. None of the above

WRAP UP

5. You notice that a new drug has arrived from the manufacturer. Reading the drug information, you notice that the mechanism of action is that of a reverse transcriptase inhibitor. What is a disease for which this drug would be prescribed?

   A. HIV

   B. Fungal infections

   C. Bacterial infections

   D. High blood pressure

6. An antiviral drug will be effective against a bacterial disease.

   A. True

   B. False

7. Which of the following describes the direct price cost of a drug?

   A. The price if purchased from the manufacturer

   B. The price if purchased from the drug wholesale company

   C. The price if purchased from another retail pharmacy

   D. None of these

8. The NDC is the Federal ID number assigned to each pharmacy.

   A. True

   B. False

9. The FDA is a state regulation agency.

   A. True

   B. False

10. The *Orange Book* is the official government reference for drug doses.

    A. True

    B. False

11. All bacteria cause disease.

    A. True

    B. False

12. The mushroom in your salad is an example of what type of microorganism?

    A. Plant

    B. Algae

    C. Fungus

    D. Bacteria

13. Which of the following organisms can cause severe, sometimes fatal, lung disease?

    A. Candida

    B. Aspergillus

    C. Penicillinamine

    D. Tinea fungus

14. Fungus cells and human cells have many similar features.

    A. True

    B. False

15. Which of the following is a primary ingredient in fungal cell walls?

    A. Cholesterol

    B. Ergosterol

    C. Testosterone

    D. Cytoplasm

16. Which of the following drugs is *not* available in IV form?

    A. Amphotericin

    B. Posaconazole

    C. Voriconazole

    D. Micofungen

17. Many antifungal drugs have generic names that end in what?

    A. Amine

    B. Phyllin

    C. Cycline

    D. Zole

18. Which of the following drugs does not have a mechanism of action involving the cytochrome P450 interference?

    A. Voriconazole

    B. Clotrimazole

    C. Itraconazole

    D. Posaconazole

19. The cytochrome P450 mechanism can be found in which of the following human organs?

    A. Liver

    B. Brain

    C. Stomach

    D. Kidneys

20. One of the most common types of vaginal fungal infections is caused by which of the following?

    A. *Candida albicans*

    B. Dermatophytes

    C. Valley fever

    D. PCP

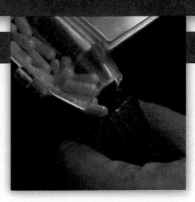

Communication

OBJECTIVES

After reading this chapter, you will be able to:

- Describe the role of the pharmacy technician as a member of the patient-care team.
- Discuss the primary employee rule for retail merchandising.
- Assess the importance of verbal and nonverbal communication skills.
- Convey which personal characteristics are desirable for the pharmacy technician.
- Communicate properly using the telephone in the pharmacy.
- Resolve linguistic and cultural differences when working with a patient.
- Identify and resolve problems related to a patient with a mental or physical disability.
- Define discrimination and harassment and understand how to properly deal with these issues.
- Demonstrate professionalism in the pharmacy.
- Advocate the importance of managing change.
- Realize the importance of being a team player in the pharmacy.
- Respond appropriately to rude behavior on the part of others in the workplace.
- Educate others on the role of pharmacy personnel in emergency situations in the community.
- Understand the importance of the Health Insurance Portability and Accountability Act (HIPAA) and when HIPAA regulations apply.
- Protect patient confidentiality.
- Compare and contrast the central nervous system (CNS) and the peripheral nervous system (PNS), their functions, and their relationship to drugs.
- Differentiate various drugs, dosage forms, and delivery systems for drugs that affect the PNS and CNS.
- Understand the concepts of general and local anesthesia.
- Identify the drugs used for anesthesia.
- Distinguish between controlled substances and non-controlled substances.
- Summarize the role of the technician in monitoring controlled substances.
- Discuss types of drugs used to treat migraine headaches.

KEY TERMS

Acute pain
Afferent system
Analgesics
Anesthetics
Autonomic nervous
    system (ANS)
Beta-blocker
Cerebrospinal fluid
Chronic pain
Chronic malignant pain
Controlled-substance
    schedules (CI, CII,
    CIII, CIV, CV)
Discrimination
Efferent system
Empathy
Equal Employment
    Opportunity
    Commission (EEOC)

Equal Employment
    Opportunity (EEO)
    laws
General anesthesia
Health Insurance
    Portability and
    Accountability Act
    (HIPAA)
Local anesthesia
Meninges
Monoamine oxidase
    inhibitor (MAOI) drug
Neuromuscular blocker
Neurotransmitters
Nonverbal
    communication
Open-ended question
Opiate
Opioid

Opium poppy
Parasympathetic
    nervous system
Patient identifier
Peripheral nervous
    system (PNS)
Selective serotonin
    reuptake inhibitor
    (SSRI) drug
Sense organs
Sensitivity
Sexual harassment
Somatic nervous system
Sympathetic nervous
    system
Triptans
Twilight sleep
Verbal communication
WHO

Chapter Overview

The role of effective, customer-oriented communication cannot be overemphasized in any form of business. But unlike many other types of businesses, where customers are purchasing something they desire, in the world of retail pharmacy, the patient is purchasing a prescription that was ordered by a healthcare provider. A customer's personal gratification is not usually part of the buying exchange between the retail-pharmacy patient and the pharmacy staff. In this exchange, patients are either buying something to make them well or buying a preventive medicine drug to keep them healthy. This somewhat forced type of purchase brings with it many different communication challenges, and a customer-centered approach is essential.

In a hospital pharmacy, effective communication is also essential, as the pharmacy technician will interact with many different healthcare providers. Effective, healthcare-provider–oriented communication will differ when communicating with different types of healthcare providers—for example, when communicating with a physician versus a nurse or a pharmacist versus another pharmacy technician.

In this chapter, you will learn the importance of both verbal and nonverbal communication in the pharmacy. The topic of communication involves a wide range of related issues, from the technician's personal-service characteristics, to proper telephone use, to how to deal with difficult people. Even dealing with change and being a team player in the pharmacy involve the use of effective communication. Communication relates to all aspects of your working life, so let us begin by examining the pharmacy-technician role as a member of the patient-care team.

The drug insights section of this chapter will address anesthetics and analgesics. The pharmacy technician will learn about the central nervous system (CNS) and drugs that are used in the CNS to treat various conditions such as those related to surgical procedures, pain, and migraine headaches.

The Patient-Care Team

Today, the pharmacy technician is a valued member of the patient-care team. The pharmacy technician's role has changed dramatically within the last few years. Originally, the technician's role revolved around simply counting and pouring drugs or preparing simple IV drugs. The role of the pharmacy technician has also expanded greatly due to the volume of prescriptions. Greater demand for prescription services and higher volumes of work in pharmacies have expanded the opportunities for pharmacy technicians. As the pharmacist's role has expanded from just the person who checks the prescription into more of a clinical specialist, so too, has the technician's role.

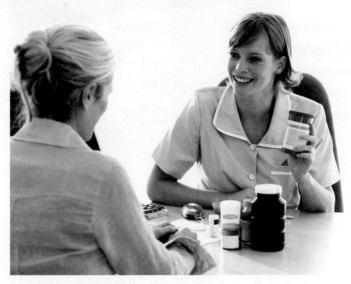

The patient-care team.

Retail Pharmacy

In the retail pharmacy, the pharmacy technician is a member of a team that also includes the pharmacy manager, pharmacists, pharmacy counter personnel, and other store employees. These other store employees could include cashiers, receiving and stocking employees, departmental employees such as the managers and employees of the photo or cosmetic departments, and even housekeeping and security employees.

As a member of this team, one of your primary responsibilities is customer service. When a patient comes to the pharmacy window to leave a prescription, the pharmacy technician or clerk is typically the first pharmacy employee this person sees and speaks with. Indeed, the pharmacy technician may be the first employee in the entire store who will interact with this patient. The attitude of the technician—from the courteous tone of his or her voice, to his or her focusing just on that patient—affects how that patient will view the entire store team. Pleasant, smiling pharmacy employees, functioning as a team, give patients the feeling that this is a good place to work, and thus a good place to bring their business. The patient in the retail pharmacy is also a customer; this customer-centered service will determine whether customers return to the pharmacy or go somewhere else with their next prescription.

In this retail setting, as a store team member, the pharmacy technician always represents the pharmacy and the store. This includes all of the merchandise available for purchase by the customer. Remember the primary employee rule for retail merchandising: No matter what task a pharmacy technician is performing in the store or the pharmacy, the pharmacy technician always represents the company to the patient. Especially in the pharmacy itself, the pharmacy technician is legally an agent of the employer. As an agent of the employer, a technician enters into a contract to provide care to the patient. The technician's employer, as well as the technician, is ultimately responsible for all the actions of the technician.

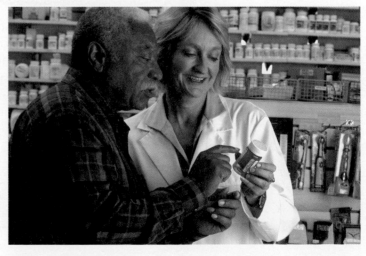

A retail pharmacy.

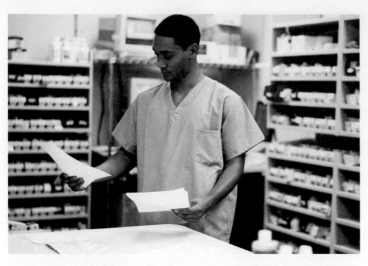
An institutional pharmacy.

Institutional Pharmacy

In an institutional pharmacy, the pharmacy technician is part of a team that includes the pharmacy manager, pharmacists, and other technicians. Outside the pharmacy, the pharmacy technician is part of a team that includes all other personnel working within the facility. These other personnel might include physicians, nurses, housekeepers, maintenance workers, and other departmental personnel. Many of the behaviors and the positive attitude described in the previous section are necessary in the institutional pharmacy; just the customers are different. Instead of having retail customers, the institutional pharmacy has other healthcare providers who require customer service.

Emergency Response

A rather new role for the pharmacy technician is that of emergency response. Pharmacy personnel can prepare themselves to be of service to the community in times of emergencies. To be of importance, pharmacy personnel should have an idea of what types of emergencies may occur in their area of practice. Understanding what type of disaster might occur in the area will help determine what type of preplanning the pharmacy should do. Preplanning for different types of emergencies such as flooding or earthquakes is considerably different, and should be considered in the pharmacy-planning process.

Pharmacists have a great opportunity to share their clinical knowledge during a disaster. Pharmacy technicians can be involved during a disaster by controlling inventory, restocking products, and obtaining necessary supplies from other centers. In addition, pharmacy technicians can become involved in inventory control and emergency preparedness prior to a disaster. Both pharmacists and pharmacy technicians should be involved in local and national disaster drills—both in the drills themselves and in the advance preparations.

Being the Best Pharmacy Technician

Being the best pharmacy technician one can be requires many different skills. As discussed previously, communication is one of these required skills. Even communication skills can be broken down further into effective verbal and nonverbal communication skills. The pharmacy technician must have a complete range of required clinical skills such as pharmacology knowledge, math competency, and problem-solving skills. The pharmacy technician has a wide range of behavioral and personal skills, a proper attitude, professional appearance and behavior, appropriate telephone skills, and a belief in providing service to others, be that customer service or service to a patient or other healthcare workers.

No matter what task is being performed within or outside the pharmacy, the pharmacy technician is representing the entire pharmacy.

Verbal and Nonverbal Communication

Verbal communication is a practiced skill. The need for this skill is particularly great when working in a healthcare setting. In the healthcare setting, the art of verbal communication often must include the trait of empathy. **Empathy**, or the ability to recognize and try to feel what other people feel, is a necessary communication component in the healthcare setting. Often, the pharmacy technician will interact with a sick patient, a parent with a sick child, or a person who may have just lost a family member to an accident or disease. Professional tone and appropriate pitch and pacing is highly encouraged when giving patients their medication use directions. Using slang or jargon, speaking loudly, interrupting, or exhibiting anything perceived to be rude behavior on the part of the pharmacy staff is discouraged. Patients need to feel comfortable with their verbal interaction and the information they have received regarding their prescription and any treatment or over-the-counter items they have purchased.

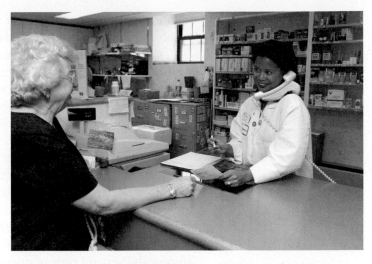

Talking on the telephone while helping a customer at the counter shows poor communication skills.

In the institutional setting, the pharmacy technician will need to have empathy when communicating with fellow healthcare workers who may be overworked, nurses who may be taking care of a sick or dying patient, direct patient-care staff who have been dealing with difficult family members, and workers facing many other issues of which you may not be aware.

The pharmacy technician's **nonverbal communication** skills must match their verbal skills for effective communication to occur. For example, typing a prescription into the computer terminal while talking to a different patient about his or her prescription is not an empathetic or effective communication method. Effective communication and empathy require that this technician devote his or her entire attention to the patient who is present at that moment. Acknowledging the patient by saying, "I will be right with you," lets the patient know you are going to finish what you are doing and then you will devote your full attention to him or her. Following this comment up by quickly completing your task and moving closer to the patient shows that patient that you care about him or her. This opens the door for effective, empathetic communication with that patient.

Maintaining a positive attitude is very important when working as a pharmacy technician. This can be as simple as smiling and making eye contact with the patient. In fact, smiling is one of the most important nonverbal communications available. However, the smile must be the outward sign of an actual positive attitude. Displaying an unreal or fake smile is a very negative nonverbal communication sign easily recognized by most patients and coworkers.

An important function of the pharmacy technician is that of gathering information, either from a patient or from another healthcare professional. In the retail-pharmacy setting, the pharmacy technician will be the first point of contact for the pharmacy patient. Thus, obtaining correct patient information is essential, as this will affect all future interactions with this patient. In the retail-pharmacy setting, this initial information will include such items as the patient's correct name, address, phone number, drug allergies, other medications the patient is currently taking, and any prescription insurance coverage the patient may have. In the retail setting, this information will be obtained from the patient, a caregiver, or a family member.

In the institutional setting, the initial information collected by the pharmacy technician will include such items as the patient's correct name, the patient's location (such as his or her room number), any allergies the patient has, a list of the patient's other medications, and the patient's height and weight. In the institutional setting, this information will be obtained either from patient admission records or from another healthcare professional such as a nursing unit clerk or a nurse.

Obtaining the correct information is essential in both settings. One way to do this is to ask the open-ended question. An **open-ended question** requires the patient to answer with a complete sentence, not just a yes or no answer. For example, asking the patient, "What is your current address?" will yield more correct information than asking the patient, "Is your current address 22937 West State Street?" A patient who is hard of hearing or who does not speak English as his or her first language could answer the second type of question with a "Yes," simply because he or she might not understand the question that was asked. If the pharmacy technician accepts that "Yes" answer and enters that information into the patient's records, major medical errors, or privacy violations could occur due to incorrect information and poor communication. For example, the patient could receive an incorrect medication or a medication that interacts with one the patient is currently taking. If the patient is to receive a delivery, it could go to the wrong address or potentially not reach the patient when he or she needs it for a specific dosing period. Privacy violations might occur if people receive someone else's information. Patients with language barriers very often do not fully understand the medication counseling provided by the pharmacist or specific directions from the pharmacy technician, and thus may not take their medications as directed. Using open-ended questions in this setting, pharmacy personnel may enable patients to better convey their understanding of the directions and appropriate use of the medication. It also alerts the pharmacy personnel as to whether or not the patient does understand.

What Would You Do?

Question: The cashier at the front of the store comes back to the pharmacy and asks the pharmacy technician what medication was just dispensed to her friend, who lives next door to her.

Answer: The technician should not tell the cashier the requested information. Additionally, the technician should remind the cashier that all patient information is confidential and protected by HIPAA regulations, including the name of the medication dispensed to a patient.

Lastly, the pharmacy technician must always remember that all patient information is confidential, and must not be shared with anyone other than the patient, designated caregiver, or healthcare provider. Extra care should be taken when obtaining patient information to ensure privacy for the patient. Patient information is even confidential when speaking to other healthcare workers. Unless that worker needs to know the information to perform a work-related task for that patient, confidential patient information should not be shared between healthcare workers.

Patient Sensitivity

In today's modern world, pharmacy technicians will have the opportunity to interact with patients and healthcare workers from different parts of the world. Additionally, pharmacy technicians will interact with patients who have a variety of physical or mental challenges. Dealing with patients or healthcare workers of different cultures or abilities presents extra challenges and opportunities to maintain or enhance customer service.

Being sensitive to the other person's views or abilities is the most important concept to learn and remember. **Sensitivity** to the other person's needs breaks down barriers, enabling the pharmacy to provide excellent customer service. Sensitivity starts with the realization that males and females may view each other differently in different cultures. However, in a patient-care setting, healthcare professionals must do their job to fill the prescriptions and counsel patients as is necessary. This should be done fairly and professionally with all patients regardless of beliefs, values, or culture. The healthcare worker may not agree with the patient's personal views or social or religious practices, but must respect them and be sensitive to their personal needs. All patients should be treated fairly and the same in pharmacy practice. It is imperative for the pharmacy technician to be sensitive and compassionate while also accurately and safely doing their job in the pharmacy.

Language differences can present a unique challenge for the pharmacy technician. Pharmacy technicians working in an area with a large population of people who speak a different language would benefit by having a good translation reference available. This will enable technicians to ask many of the required questions or to point

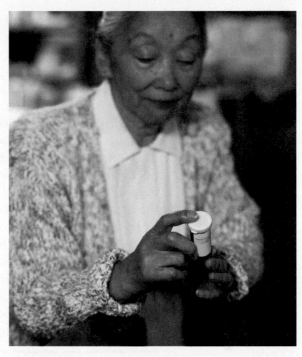

Awareness and sensitivity are critical when helping patients with hearing or vision impairment or who speak a different language.

to the question in the patient's language, with a choice of answers that are translated into the pharmacy technician's language. Identifying other employees who speak different languages is also beneficial to the pharmacy technician. When needed, this other employee can act as a translator. (The pharmacy technician must remind the other employee that all patient information is confidential, and should not be discussed elsewhere.) An important concept for the pharmacy technician to remember is that the person who speaks a different language does not understand what you are saying. Speaking louder or more slowly does not aid in comprehension, and can be offensive to the other person. The majority of pharmacy computer systems can print labels and patient information sheets in different languages. This information could be handed to the person who does not understand your language. Even if a pharmacy does have a computer system that prints labels in different languages, it is essential that someone in the pharmacy can read the printed label to assure that the translation was performed properly.

Another challenging communication area for pharmacy technicians is dealing with patients or other healthcare workers who have differing degrees of physical or mental challenges. Whether the pharmacy technician is dealing with a challenged patient in the retail setting or a coworker with disabilities in the institutional setting, enhanced communication strategies will need to be employed. The same basic strategies can be employed in either setting.

Depending on the location of the retail pharmacy, the pharmacy technician may routinely deal with a large percentage of elderly patients. Some of these elderly patients will have difficulty hearing, limited vision, or both. The pharmacy technician will need to take extra time and care when dealing with these types of patients. Speaking more slowly, speaking with great clarity, and increasing the volume of his or her voice may help the technician communicate with the hearing-impaired patient. If these techniques do not appear to improve the communication process, the technician may need to communicate through writing.

Communication with a patient who has limited vision can be enhanced through the use of handout materials printed with large print. If the patient is blind, the pharmacy technician will need to ensure that the patient understands all the verbal instructions that are being communicated. If the patient requires counseling or has questions regarding the information, the pharmacy technician needs to have the pharmacist communicate with the patient. Unless this patient has a sighted person living with him or her, that patient will not be able to refer to any printed materials, so comprehension of all verbal instructions is essential.

Communicating with a mentally challenged patient takes patience and understanding on the part of the pharmacy technician. The best method of communication will depend on the abilities of the patient, and thus will differ between patients. Giving the patient extra time to ask questions or repeat information back to you will give the technician an insight into comprehension. Whenever possible, the pharmacy technician should communicate with the mentally challenged on their level of understanding, thus enhancing the communication process.

A pharmacy technician will interact with many different people, including people with physical and mental disabilities. Patients with physical disabilities are protected from discrimination by special federal regulations. A combination of state and federal laws and regulations protect those people with mental disabilities.

Having a pleasant, caring attitude is the most important part of any type of communication.

The Americans with Disabilities Act (ADA) guarantees civil rights to every person with physical disabilities. These federal regulations are similar to those preventing discrimination based on race, color, sex, national origin, age, and religion. The ADA guarantees equal opportunity for individuals with disabilities in public accommodations, employment, transportation, state and local government services, and telecommunications (American with Disabilities Act 2011). State and federal laws protect the rights of people with mental disabilities while also establishing laws and regulations to protect the public from severely mentally ill people.

A patient with physical or mental disabilities may require a different style of interaction by the pharmacy technician. Examples of patients with physical disabilities would include patients in wheelchairs and those requiring a walker or a cane. Patients with physical disabilities might include a patient who has lost an arm or leg, a deaf patient, or a blind patient.

Being aware of the disability will enable the technician to be more customer friendly toward the patient. For example, when a new patient arrives at the pharmacy window, a patient history must be taken. If the patient is in a wheelchair, the pharmacy technician could take a chair and sit next to the patient while collecting the required information.

Being aware of a patient with a mental disability not only enables the technician to be more customer friendly, but also allows a better flow of information between both people. A person with a mental disability may have difficulty understanding complex sentences, and may be slower in assimilating new information and responding to questions. An example of a patient with a mental disability would be a Down syndrome patient. When interacting with a Down

Managing Change

In the pharmacy, managing change means keeping up with new drugs as they enter the market. Keeping up with new laws and their relationship to the pharmacy and your patients is another very important aspect of managing change. Lastly, managing change means working with new employees. Working with new employees, especially new pharmacy technicians, means assisting them in becoming good, empathetic communicators. Communication in all types of pharmacies involves using professional telephone etiquette and strong verbal communication skills.

syndrome patient, speaking slowly and using a very basic sentence structure will enable the technician to obtain more information.

Telephone Communication

One of the primary methods of communication with a pharmacy is by telephone. In both retail and institutional pharmacies, answering the telephone is usually a pharmacy technician's duty. Additionally, depending on the type of system in use, the pharmacy technician may be responsible for listening to and documenting information from the telephone voicemail system. Using common courtesies and maintaining a pleasant, upbeat tone of voice are very important when answering the phone. The following are some general rules to follow when answering the telephone:

- Always answer the phone with a pleasant, upbeat attitude, remembering the person calling you on the phone is a patient, a customer, or another healthcare professional.

- Always answer the phone with a pleasant statement that identifies yourself and pharmacy. Some pharmacies require a specific greeting when answering the phone. If yours does not, simply say something like, "Good morning, Hillcrest Pharmacy, this is Nick. How can I help you?" If working in an institutional pharmacy that is not open to the general public, simply say something like, "Good morning, pharmacy. This is Nick."

- Listen carefully to the first statement or question by the caller. This statement or question will determine whether you, as the technician, should continue with the conversation or transfer the call to a pharmacist. If the patient automatically requests the pharmacist, inform them that the pharmacist is busy with another customer and attempt to determine the nature of the call. The technician should decide if the pharmacist is needed, not the patient. If needed, refer the call to the pharmacist. Not taking this step may lead to the pharmacist being overloaded with calls that a technician may have fielded.

- In a retail setting, if the caller is calling in a refill prescription, the technician should document all the required information, such as the patient's name, the prescription refill number, and when the caller plans to pick up the refill. If the requested pickup time does not appear realistic based on the current workflow, the technician should politely explain this to the caller. This will prevent an unpleasant customer-service issue when the caller arrives and the prescription is not ready. For example, the technician should say to the caller, "We are very busy today and will try to have your refill ready by that time; however, you may have to wait a few minutes when you arrive." Document the pickup time requested. In most busy pharmacies, this refill request information is then placed in sequence with other refills waiting to be completed.

- If the caller asks whether his or her prescription is refillable or how many refills remain on the prescription, the pharmacy

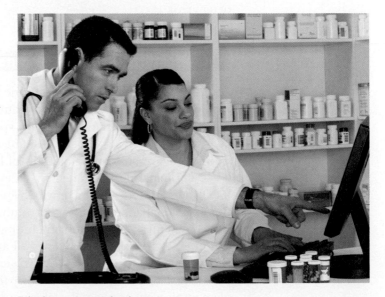

Telephone communication.

What Would You Do?

Question: A caller requests information about a medication, such as side effects, usual dosing, or interactions with other medications. What should the technician do?

Answer: This question is outside the scope of practice for a technician. Transfer the phone call to a pharmacist. This transfer should be preceded by the technician saying to the caller, "The pharmacist will have to answer that question for you. I am going to place you on hold and transfer you to the pharmacist. You will not be on hold for very long." As the technician who originally answered the call, it is your responsibility to monitor the amount of time your patient is on hold. If the pharmacist is very busy and is unable to answer the call in a timely manner, you should pick up the call again and explain this to the patient. As a part of good customer service, ask the caller if he or she would prefer to remain on hold or have the pharmacist return his or her phone call.

technician may provide this information in most states. Knowing the state law and your pharmacy policy will determine how you as the technician should handle this phone call.

- In an institutional setting, the caller is most commonly another healthcare provider. The pharmacy technician should know the state laws and policies of his or her institutional pharmacy with regard to what questions are within his or her scope of practice and what questions should be referred to a pharmacist. If the caller is requesting information about a medication, as noted in the next section, the technician should always transfer the call to a pharmacist.

- If the caller is a healthcare professional calling in a new prescription for a patient, in most states, the pharmacy technician would need to tell the caller that he or she is a technician and will transfer the call to a pharmacist. Knowing your state laws and pharmacy policy will dictate your response.

- If the caller has a medical emergency, the caller should be instructed to call 911.

- If the call is about a possible pharmacy error, the caller should politely be transferred to a pharmacist.

Telephone calls are an integral part of all pharmacies, as well as an integral part of the pharmacy technician's workday. Maintaining an upbeat, pleasant tone is essential when dealing with any phone caller. Making sure that all information you provide to the caller and that all information you record from the caller is accurate is very important. Incorrect information could result in a serious or even life-threatening drug error.

Discrimination, Harassment, and Rude Behavior

Discrimination, harassment, and rude behavior are all examples of improper forms of communication that should not occur nor be tolerated in the pharmacy. Workplace discrimination and harassment are specifically prohibited by both federal and state laws. Rude behavior, unless brought under proper control, can escalate into other forms of aggression and violations of both federal and state laws.

Discrimination is defined by federal laws called **Equal Employment Opportunity (EEO) laws** (EEOC, 2010(a)), which are enforced by the **Equal Employment Opportunity Commission**. Federal EEO laws prohibit preferential treatment or mistreatment of persons based on several factors, including age, religion, sexual orientation, race, national origin, and disability. These laws all apply in the workplace and cover such areas as the hiring and firing of employees, yearly evaluations, wages, and promotions.

Sexual harassment is defined by the United States Supreme Court as the creation of an unpleasant or uncomfortable work environment through sexual action, innuendo, or related means (EEOC, 2010(b)). Harassment can involve opposite-sex or same-sex coworkers. Harassment in the workplace could include such things as verbal, printed, or e-mailed jokes with a sexual connotation. Harassment would include any type of physical advances between employees, such as unwanted touching. Harassment laws are among the primary reasons that romantic or sexual involvement between coworkers is highly discouraged or even prohibited by most pharmacy policies. Either type of relationship becomes even more questionable when it involves a supervisory person with a subordinate.

Rude behavior can occur between coworkers, a supervisor and subordinate, different types of healthcare professionals or between a pharmacy worker and a patient. Many times rude behavior between workers occurs as part of a larger picture of conflict. The rude behavior should not be tolerated, however, and many times this behavior can be stopped through conflict resolution. If a coworker is displaying rude behavior toward you, one initial way to resolve this would be to talk one on one with this coworker in a non-confrontational manner to determine the root of the problem and thus resolve the behavior. Sometimes the rude behavior from another coworker stems from misinformation or gossip and can be stopped simply through communication. On the other hand, if the behavior continues, the problem should be taken to a supervisor.

Rude behavior toward another healthcare professional is unprofessional. If another healthcare professional expresses rude behavior toward you, calmly listen or walk away if possible. Do not escalate the behavior by responding with the same behavior. Immediately report the incident to a supervisor.

Rude behavior from patients many times is based on poor customer service or lack of understanding by the patient. Frustration on the part of a patient can be manifested as rude behavior. The majority of rude-behavior incidents with patients could be avoided by having empathy for the patient, maintaining open communications, and providing excellent customer service. If there is a pattern with one specific patient, then discuss this with a supervisor.

Health Insurance Portability and Accountability Act (HIPAA)

According to its Web site, the **Health Insurance Portability and Accountability Act (HIPAA)** of 1996 was enacted to do the following:

> . . . to improve portability and continuity of health insurance coverage in the group and individual markets, to combat waste, fraud, and abuse in health insurance and health care delivery, to promote the use of medical savings accounts, to improve access to long-term care services and coverage, to simplify the administration of health insurance, and for other purposes.

HIPAA and Pharmacy Technicians

HIPAA addresses a wide variety of procedures that a pharmacy technician may be asked to perform. Primarily, the HIPAA regulations were passed to standardize healthcare information (which includes the **patient identifiers** that can be used for identification), to standardize payment claims, and for "other purposes" such as protecting a patient's confidentiality and privacy. Any information that includes patient identifiers must not be released to anyone without the approval of the patient except in specific circumstances. Some of these circumstances include release to an insurance company for payment, release to a government agency, or release to another caregiver when that caregiver needs the information to administer proper medical care. If in doubt, the pharmacy technician should notify the pharmacist on duty prior to releasing any information with identifiers.

Patient Identifiers

Patient identifiers are unique to each patient. Patient identifiers are pieces of information utilized to match patients to correct patient records. Patient identifiers may include the following:

- Patient name
- Address and zip code
- Telephone number
- E-mail
- Date of birth
- Social security number
- Medical record number
- Account number
- Photo

Drug Insights: Anesthetics and Analgesics

In this section, you will read and learn about drugs used for anesthesia. This section also discusses drugs used as analgesics, both controlled substances and non-controlled substances. Knowledge of some terminology is essential to understanding these drugs.

Anesthetics are drugs that prevent signals from going to or returning from the brain. Some of the signals that are blocked include pain, memory, muscle control, and awareness. Anesthetics are used in medicine primarily during surgery or other invasive procedures. Surgical anesthetic drugs are available only with a prescription, and are primarily found in an institutional setting. There are also OTC anesthetics available, such as benzocaine, lidocaine, and phenol.

Analgesics are drugs that decrease, control, or eliminate pain. The public commonly refers to these types of drugs as painkillers. Analgesic drugs are available in a wide array of drug classes, strengths, and routes of administration. Some analgesic drugs may be purchased without a prescription, such as aspirin, while other analgesic drugs, such as morphine, are available only with a prescription.

The method of action for anesthetic and analgesic drugs involves the nervous system. The human nervous system is divided into two main divisions: the central nervous system (CNS) and the peripheral nervous system (PNS). An overview of each system is found in the next two sections.

What Would You Do

Question: When processing a refill request from a patient for hydrocodone with acetaminophen (Vicodin), the pharmacy technician notices that, based on the directions and the previous quantity dispensed, this refill request is 10 days early. Should the technician simply continue the refill process and produce a label for refilling?

Answer: No. The technician should notify the pharmacist on duty, as this is a controlled substance, meaning this drug has the potential for abuse and addiction. The pharmacist has the authority to determine whether the refill should be processed or stopped.

The Central Nervous System (CNS)

The central nervous system (CNS) includes the brain and spinal cord. Both the brain and spinal cord are covered by **meninges**, which are primarily for protection. The spinal cord and parts of the brain are filled with a liquid called **cerebrospinal fluid**. This fluid helps the brain maintain its normal pressure.

The CNS is the body's control center. The spinal cord contains nerve pathways called tracts that send signals from sensors in the body to the brain for interpretation. After interpretation has occurred by the brain, nerve tracts going down the spinal cord send returning signals to the body organs telling them what to do.

The signals being sent to and from the brain are electrical signals. These electrical signals stimulate chemicals to be released at many of the nerve endings. These chemicals, called **neurotransmitters**, allow the electrical signal to continue to the next nerve. Some neurotransmitters stimulate, while others inhibit, the signals. Lack of, or incorrect amounts of, these neurotransmitters can cause many different physical, mental, and emotional disorders. In the CNS, these neurotransmitters are acetylcholine, norepinephrine, dopamine, gamma-amino butyric acid (GABA), glutamate, and serotonin. Blocking or in some cases stimulating these neurotransmitters can be beneficial to the patient. Some CNS drugs stimulate these neurotransmitters, while other CNS drugs inhibit them.

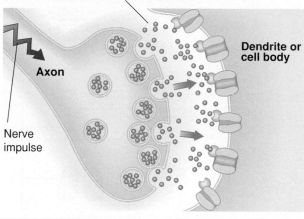

FIGURE 8.1 Neurotransmitter release.

The Peripheral Nervous System (PNS)

The **peripheral nervous system (PNS)** includes all the nerves throughout the body except those in the CNS. The PNS is divided into two groups:

- The afferent system—The **afferent system** includes all the nerves and **sense organs** such as the eyes and ears. These nerves and organs take in information and send it to the CNS.
- The efferent system—The **efferent system** includes all nerves and pathways that send information from the CNS to other organs or body systems.

The efferent system is further divided into two parts: the autonomic nervous system and the somatic nervous system, discussed next. Acetylcholine and norepinephrine are two of the many neurotransmitters in the PNS.

Autonomic Nervous System (ANS)

The **autonomic nervous system (ANS)** controls organs and body systems automatically. That means the ANS is not voluntarily controlled; rather, the brain maintains this system automatically. Some examples of functions handled by the ANS are heartbeats, digestion, the size of one's pupils, and blood sugar, just to name a few. The ANS can be further divided into two subdivisions:

- The sympathetic nervous system—The **sympathetic nervous system** is used to stimulate the body for vigorous activity, stressful situations, and emergencies. For example, imagine a person walking in the desert who suddenly sees a mountain lion. The sympathetic nervous system would immediately release neurotransmitters that would allow the person to fight or flee. The common

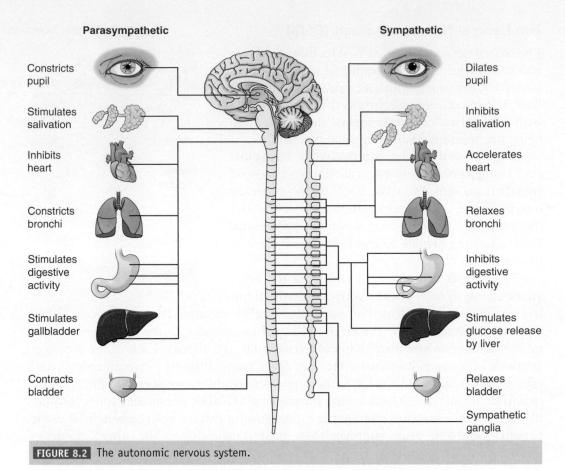

Parasympathetic

Constricts
pupil

Stimulates
salivation

Inhibits
heart

Constricts
bronchi

Stimulates
digestive
activity

Stimulates
gallbladder

Contracts
bladder

Sympathetic

Dilates
pupil

Inhibits
salivation

Accelerates
heart

Relaxes
bronchi

Inhibits
digestive
activity

Stimulates
glucose release
by liver

Relaxes
bladder

Sympathetic
ganglia

FIGURE 8.2 The autonomic nervous system.

neurotransmitters in the sympathetic nervous system include acetylcholine, norepinephrine, dopamine, glutamate, and epinephrine.

■ The parasympathetic nervous system—The **parasympathetic nervous system** returns the body to a normal state. It is the system responsible for rest and refreshment. For example, when the person is safe, the parasympathetic nervous system will return everything to the resting state. The neurotransmitter in the parasympathetic nervous system is acetylcholine.

Somatic Nervous System

The **somatic nervous system** is the nervous system that controls all the skeletal muscles in the body. The somatic nervous system is voluntary, meaning a person can decide to use a muscle or let the muscle rest. Acetylcholine is the neurotransmitter found in the somatic nervous system.

Drugs Mode of Action

Drugs that affect the nervous system affect some aspect of the neurotransmitter mechanism. Some of the drugs prevent the neurotransmitter from being destroyed by enzymes after they are released. These drugs would therefore allow the neurotransmitter to remain longer, thus prolonging the effect of that nerve transmission. An example of this would be a **monoamine oxidase inhibitor (MAOI) drug**, such as tranylcypromine (Parnate). Parnate is prescribed for depression. Some nerve-acting drugs prevent the neurotransmitter from being returned to the storage area for reuse. These drugs are called reuptake inhibitors. A reuptake inhibitor would also allow the neurotransmitter to remain longer, thus prolonging that nerve pathway's affect. Examples of these are

selective serotonin reuptake inhibitor (SSRI) drugs, such as sertraline (Zoloft). Zoloft is prescribed for depression. Both of these drug classes are discussed in Chapter 10.

Another mode of action for some drugs that affect the nervous system is for the drug to block the receptor where the neurotransmitter binds. The binding of the neurotransmitter normally allows the nerve signal to continue to the next nerve. Therefore, blocking the receptor blocks the signal transmission. An example of this type of action would be beta-blocking drugs, also called beta-blockers. A **beta-blocker** blocks norepinephrine and epinephrine, thus decreasing heart rate and lowering blood pressure. An example of a beta-blocker is metoprolol (Lopressor).

Many of the drugs used for pain control work by blocking the electrical transmission in afferent neuron pathways, thereby preventing a sensor from sending a signal to the brain. Analgesics are a special category of drugs that work via this mechanism of action. Because the pain signal is prevented from reaching the brain, the sensation of pain does not occur, as the brain has no signal to interpret. Drugs such as codeine and morphine are examples of analgesics.

Another related mode of action is for the drug to compete with the neurotransmitter for the binding site on the receptor. The neurotransmitter becomes less and less effective as more receptor sites are taken by the drug. This mode of action is common with a group of drugs that compete with acetylcholine for their binding sites. A drug that competes with a nerve-to-muscle transmission is called a **neuromuscular blocker**. This type of drug prevents skeletal muscles from being able to contract. An example of this type of drug would be rocuronium (Zemuron), which is used during surgery to relax all the patient's muscles. The discovery of drugs such as rocuronium has allowed the practice of surgery to advance significantly.

The majority of neuromuscular blockers must be refrigerated.

Extra care should be taken when dispensing a neuromuscular blocker, as a medication error could be fatal.

Surgical and Procedure Drugs

Some drugs that prevent nerve signals from going to or returning from the brain are called anesthetics. Anesthetics can prevent the patient from having a memory of an event, such as surgery. Anesthetics block the transmission of signals to muscles, thus relaxing the muscle. Some anesthetics decrease or stop the pain signal from reaching the brain, thus reducing or eliminating pain.

Anesthesia drugs can be divided into two categories, those for general anesthesia and those for local anesthesia. Major surgical procedures are performed using general anesthesia. **General anesthesia** enables doctors to place a patient in a reversible unconscious state in which there is no response to painful stimuli **TABLE 8.1**. Most general-anesthesia drugs are either in the form of a gas, and thus must be inhaled, or a sterile liquid, which must be given by the IV route. All general-anesthesia drugs are prescription only.

Local anesthesia allows for reversible loss of feeling in a specific area of the body **TABLE 8.2**. Although some local-anesthetic drugs are available without a prescription, most do require one. The local-anesthetic agents available without a prescription are usually purchased by the consumer for relief from a painful sore throat, sunburn, or minor laceration. Some anesthetic drugs can cause the patient to have no memory of an event without placing the patient in a complete unconscious state **TABLE 8.3**. A drug such as midazolam (Versed) can be placed in this class of drugs, which cause an

Table 8.1 General Anesthesia Drugs

Generic Name	Brand Name	Dosage Form	Controlled Substance
Alfentanil	Alfenta	IV	CII
Desflurane	Suprane	Gas	No
Enflurane	Ethrane	Gas	No
Etomidate	Amidate	IV	No
Fentanyl	Sublimaze	IV	CII
Isoflurane	Forane	Gas	No
Ketamine	Ketalar	Injection, IV	CIII
Methohexital	Brevital	IV	CIV
Morphine	Morphine	Injection, IV	CII
Nitrous oxide	None	Gas	No
Propofol	Diprivan	IV	No
Remifentanil	Ultiva	IV	CII
Sufentanil	Sufenta	IV	CII
Thiopental	Pentothal	IV	CIII

Table 8.2 Local Anesthetic Drugs

Generic Name	Brand Name	Dosage Form	Rx*?
Benzocaine	Americaine, others	Cream, otic, gel lozenge	No
Bupivacaine	Marcaine	Injection	Yes
Chloroprocaine	Nesacaine	Epidural	Yes
Lidocaine	Solarcaine Aloe Extra Burn Relief, others	Cream, gel, oral, ointment	No
Lidocaine	Xylocaine, Lidoderm	Injection, patch, jelly, ointment, gel	Yes
Mepivacaine	Carbocaine	Injection, IV	Yes
Procaine	Novocain	Injection, IV	Yes
Tetracaine	Cepacol, Pontocaine	Gel, ointment, liquid	No
Tetracaine	Pontocaine, Teracaine	Injection, IV, eye drop, ointment	Yes

*Rx means the drug is available only with a prescription. The drugs in Table 8.2 that do not require prescriptions are available to relieve the pain of such things as a sore throat or painful sunburn.

Table 8.3 Twilight Sleep Drugs

Generic Name	Brand Name	Dosage Form	Controlled Substance
Diazepam	Valium	Injection, IV, liquid, tablet	CIV
Lorazepam	Ativan	Injection, IV, tablet	CIV
Midazolam	Versed	Injection, IV, syrup	CIV

Table 8.4	Neuromuscular Drugs		
Generic Name	**Brand Name**	**Dosage Form**	**Refrigeration Required?**
Atracurium	Tracrium	IV	Yes
Cisatracurium	Nimbex	IV	Yes
Pancuronium	Pavulon	IV	Yes
Rocuronium	Zemuron	IV	Yes
Succinylcholine	Quelicin	Injection, IV	Yes
Vecuronium	Norcuron	IV	No

altered state of consciousness called **twilight sleep**. These drugs can be used for short procedures where general anesthesia is not required, such as a colonoscopy.

Pain

A discussion of the drugs available for pain management could not be started without a basic understanding of pain itself. Any type of tissue or cellular damage can stimulate a pain receptor. The stimulated pain receptor sends an electrical signal to the brain, which then interprets the signal. After the signal is interpreted, the patient then "feels" the pain. Two challenges associated with pain management are the ability to assess the patient's pain level and choosing the best drug to control or block that pain. Neuromuscular blockers TABLE 8.4 are used during surgery to relax the patient's muscles.

Electrical signals sent along nerve pathways must change from electrical to chemical to electrical to continue their progress to or from the brain.

To assess the patient's pain, pain has been classified into three types:

- Acute pain—**Acute pain** is the type of pain one experiences when an injury occurs, such as a burn or a cut. Acute pain is easier to manage, and usually lasts for only a short period.

- Chronic pain—**Chronic pain** usually lasts more than three months and is not caused by a malignant disease such as cancer. Chronic pain is more difficult to treat and can cause negative lifestyle changes for the patient. Often, chronic pain has no specific identifiable cause, thus making treatment even more difficult.

- Chronic malignant pain—**Chronic malignant pain** is the same as chronic pain, except that the cause is known. The cause of chronic malignant pain is a malignant disease, such as cancer, that has spread from the initial tumor. Chronic malignant pain can be difficult to treat, especially as the patient's physical condition worsens due to the underlying disease.

With all three types of pain, inadequate treatment can cause the patient to experience symptoms in addition to the pain, such as depression and a compromised immune system. This is one of the primary reasons the **World Health Organization (WHO)**, the public-health division of the United Nations, publishes an analgesic ladder (see FIGURE 8.3) for proper treatment.

Controlled Substances

As discussed in Chapter 1, a controlled substance is a drug that the Drug Enforcement Administration (DEA) has determined to have the potential for addiction

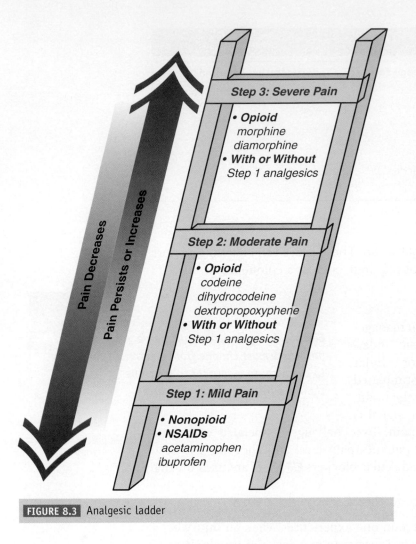

FIGURE 8.3 Analgesic ladder

and abuse. All controlled substances are classified in numbered categories, called **controlled-substance schedules (CI, CII, CIII, CIV, CV)**, based on their addiction and abuse potential TABLE 8.5. Controlled substances are listed in TABLE 8.6.

■ Schedule I controlled substances (CI) are illegal for anyone to possess except in certain institutional research facilities. CI drugs are considered by the DEA as having no current medical benefit. Two examples of CI drugs are heroin and methamphetamine.

■ Schedule II (CII) controlled substances are usually maintained by the pharmacy in a locked area. Some pharmacies may disperse CII controlled substances throughout their regular inventory, but this is not common practice. Additionally, CII controlled substances must be maintained with a continuous inventory system so the pharmacist knows at all times exactly how many of each CII drug is on hand. In some pharmacies, this inventory is maintained by the pharmacy technician with oversight by the pharmacist. CII drugs are subject to special laws that govern their prescribing and dispensing. For example, prescriptions for CII drugs may never be refilled; the patient must obtain a new prescription from the provider each time. Many CII controlled substances are made from the **opium poppy** plant. Historically, CII drugs were called narcotics, and are often still referred to as such. Some examples of CII controlled substances include morphine, codeine, and fentanyl.

■ Schedule III (CIII) through Schedule V (CV) controlled substances have different legal requirements from CII drugs with regard to inventory control, prescribing, and dispensing. For example, these drugs may be authorized by the prescriber for a maximum of five refills within a six-month time span. CIII, CIV, and CV controlled substances are not required to be kept in a locked area of the pharmacy. In addition, maintaining a continuous inventory of these controlled substances is optional, based on individual pharmacy policies. Two examples of CIII controlled substances are hydrocodone with acetaminophen (Vicodin) and acetaminophen with codeine (Tylenol with codeine) tablets. Two examples of CIV controlled substances are diazepam (Valium) and midazolam (Versed), and two examples of CV controlled substances are guaifenesin with codeine (Robitussin AC) and acetaminophen with codeine (Tylenol with codeine) cough syrups.

An old name for controlled substances is narcotics; many healthcare practitioners still use this term in practice. Many controlled substances are **opiate** based, meaning

Table 8.5 The Five Schedules Under the Controlled Substances Act

Schedule of Drug	Manufacturer's Label	About These Drugs	Examples of Drugs
I	CI	Drugs have no accepted medical use in the U.S.; highest abuse potential.	LSD, heroin
II	CII	Drugs have an accepted medical use; high abuse potential, with severe psychological or physical dependence liability; no refill allowed.	Amphetamines, methadone, opium, codeine, morphine, oxycodone
III	CIII	Drugs have an accepted medical use; moderate abuse potential (less than those in Schedules I and II); five refills allowed.	Combination narcotics such as codeine/ acetaminophen, hydrocodone/ acetaminophen and anabolic steroids
IV	CIV	Drugs have an accepted medical use; low abuse potential (less than those in Schedule III); five refills allowed.	Benzodiazepines, barbiturates
V	CV	Drugs have an accepted medical use; lowest abuse potential (less than those in Schedule IV); some drugs may be dispensed OTC if over 18 years of age in some states.	Liquid cough preparations with codeine

Table 8.6 Controlled Substances

Generic Name	Brand Name	Dosage Form	Schedule
Butorphanol	Stadol	IM, IV, nasal	CIV
Codeine	Codeine	IV, tablet	CII
Fentanyl	Duragesic, Actiq	Buccal, patch, IM, IV, tablet, transmucosal	CII
Hydrocodone*	Not available alone	Only in combination	CIII
Hydromorphone	Dilaudid	IM, IV, liquid, tablet	CII
Meperidine	Demerol	IM, IV, syrup, tablet	CII
Methadone	Dolophine	Liquid, tablet	CII
Morphine	Astramorph/PF, Kadian	Capsule, IM, IV, suppository, tablet	CII
Oxycodone	OxyContin	Capsule, liquid, concentrated solution, tablet	CII
Oxymorphone	Opana	IM, IV	CII

*Hydrocodone is available as a bulk chemical. When supplied this way, it is classified as CII. In combination with other drugs, it is classified as CIII.

Table 8.7   Controlled Substances: Common Combination Drugs

Generic Name	Brand Name	Dosage Form	Schedule
Codeine-acetaminophen	Tylenol with codeine	Liquid, tablet	CIII, CV
Hydrocodone-acetaminophen	Lortab, Vicodin, Lorcet, Norco	Capsule, liquid, tablet	CIII
Oxycodone-acetaminophen	Endocet, Percocet, Tylox	Capsule, tablet	CII
Oxycodone-aspirin	Endodan, Percodan	Capsule	CII
Oxycodone-ibuprofen	Combunox	Tablet	CII

they are manufactured from the natural alkaloids in the opium poppy plant. **Opioids** are analog drugs, either fully synthetic or semi-synthetic, that bind to the opiate receptors in the brain and are used for pain management. They are intended to mimic the effects of the natural narcotic opium alkaloid. Controlled substances are sometimes used in combination with other drugs TABLE 8.7 .

Migraine Drugs

A migraine headache is a particular type of severe headache. The throbbing pain usually occurs on one side of the head, and can be accompanied by nausea and vomiting. Migraine headaches are often preceded by an aura. An aura is a warning of the impending full migraine attack. The aura may include visual or sensory disturbances such as flashing lights, shimmering lights, flashing colors, or even partial loss of vision. The pupil of the eye, on the same side as the throbbing, may dilate. Many different drugs are used by migraine sufferers for the accompanying symptoms, such as antiemetic drugs for the nausea and opioid drugs to control the pain.

The most common drugs prescribed today for the migraine itself are selective serotonin receptor agonists called **triptans** TABLE 8.8 . The triptan drug's mode of action is to constrict the overly relaxed blood vessels in the head. Triptans are most effective if the patient takes the drug at the beginning of the aura phase, thus aborting a full attack. All of the triptan drugs are by prescription.

Patients with frequent migraines may be prescribed a routine drug-treatment regimen to prevent or lessen the frequency of the migraines TABLE 8.9 . There are multiple prophylactic treatment regimens, with medications being taken routinely, but they may not eliminate acute migraines completely. Medications for the treatment of acute migraine headaches are often prescribed in conjunction with prophylactic therapies.

Table 8.8   Migraine Drugs: Triptans.

Generic Name	Brand Name	Dosage Form
Almotriptan	Axert	Tablet
Eletriptan	Relpax	Tablet
Frovatriptan	Frova	Tablet
Naratriptan	Amerge	Tablet
Rizatriptan	Maxalt, Maxalt-MLT	Sublingual tab, tablet
Sumatriptan	Imitrex	Injection, nasal spray, tablet
Zolmitriptan	Zomig	Nasal spray, tablet

Table 8.9 Common Drugs for Migraine Prevention

Generic Name	Brand Name	Drug Class	Dosage Form
Amitriptyline	Elavil	Tricylic antidepressant	Tablet
Botulinum toxin type A	Botox	Clostridium toxin	Injection
Cyproheptadine	Periactin	Antihistamine drug	Tablet, liquid
Gabapentin	Neurontin	Anti-seizure drug	Tablet, capsule, liquid
Lamotrigine	Lamactil	Anti-seizure drug	Tablet
Propranolol	Inderal	Beta-blocker drug	Tablet, capsule, liquid, injection
Sertraline	Zoloft	SSRI drug	Tablet, liquid
Timolol	Blocadren	Beta-blocker drug	Tablet
Topiramate	Topamax	Anti-seizure drug	Tablet, capsule
Valproic Acid	Depakote	Anti-seizure drug	Tablet, capsule, liquid, injection
Venlafaxine	Effexor	SNRI drug	Tablet, capsule
Verapamil	Calan	Calcium channel blocker	Tablet, capsule, injection

The preventive drugs are prescribed by the oral route of administration with the exception of Botox, which is an injectable. They belong to several drug classes, including anti-seizure drugs. Their side effect profiles vary, but are often similar to other drugs in their class.

Tech Math Practice

Question: Working in a hospital pharmacy, the technician receives a patient order for one dose of Valium 7.5mg injection now. The pharmacy stocks Valium 5mg/mL. How many milliliters must be given to the patient?

Answer: First, establish a proportion: $\frac{5mg}{1mL} = \frac{7.5mg}{xmL}$. Cross-multiplying and solving for the unknown variable yields $xmL = \frac{(7.5mg \times 1mL)}{5mg} = 1.5mL$

Question: Working in a hospital pharmacy, the technician receives a patient order for one dose of Demerol (meperidine) 100mg injection now. The pharmacy stocks meperidine 75mg/mL. How many milliliters must be given to the patient?

Answer: First, establish a proportion: $\frac{75mg}{1mL} = \frac{100mg}{xmL}$. Cross-multiplying and solving for the unknown variable yields $xmL = \frac{(100mg \times 1mL)}{75mg} = 1.3mL$

Question: Working in a hospital pharmacy, the technician receives a patient order for Ativan 0.5mg/mL dissolved in a 100mL bag of IV fluid. The pharmacy stocks Ativan 2mg/mL in vials. How many milliliters of Ativan would you add to the 100mL bag?

Answer: First, determine the total amount of Ativan that is needed. 0.5mg × 100mL = 50mg of Ativan needed = 0.5mg/mL final concentration. Next, establish a proportion: $\frac{0.5mg}{1mL} = \frac{50mg}{xmL}$. Cross-multiplying and solving for the unknown variable yields $xmg = \frac{(50mg \times 1mL)}{0.5mg} = 100mL$.

Question: **Methadone liquid is available as 10mg/mL. The pharmacy technician receives a prescription for 15mg of methadone tid for a week. How many milliliters of methadone will need to be dispensed?**

Answer: First determine how many milligrams of methadone will be needed for the week: $^{15mg \times 3\ doses}/_{day}$ = 45mg per day needed; $^{45mg \times 7\ days}/_{week}$ = 315mg needed total for the week. Next, establish a proportion: $^{10mg}/_{1mL}$ = $^{315mg}/_{xmL}$. Cross-multiplying and solving for the unknown variable yields $x$mg = $^{(315mg \times 1mL)}/10mg$ = 31.5mL needed to dispense.

WRAP UP

Chapter Summary

- Today's pharmacy technician is a valued member of the patient-care team.
- No matter what task a pharmacy technician is performing, the technician represents the company to the public.
- The pharmacy technician should always maintain a professional appearance.
- The pharmacy technician should always behave in a professional manner.
- Being the best pharmacy technician means having a real feeling for service to others.
- Verbal communication is a practiced skill.
- Empathy, or the ability to recognize what another person feels, is a necessary communication skill.
- The pharmacy technician should use a pleasant, upbeat tone of voice when answering the telephone.
- The pharmacy technician should match his or her nonverbal communication with the verbal communication being conveyed to the patient.
- Maintaining a positive attitude is very important when working as a pharmacy technician.
- Smiling is one of the most important signs of a positive attitude.
- When gathering information from a patient, the pharmacy technician should ask open-ended questions. Open-ended questions require the patient to answer with a complete sentence.
- The pharmacy technician must maintain all patient information in a strictly confidential manner.
- Any information that could identify the patient is called a patient identifier, and is confidential.
- Discrimination and harassment should not be tolerated in the workplace.
- Rude behavior should not occur in the workplace.
- Controlled substances are drugs that the DEA has determined have the potential for addiction and abuse.

- Controlled substance drugs are divided into classes, or schedules, from I to V.
- The smaller the schedule number of a controlled substance, the more potential for addiction and abuse. Thus, Schedule II drugs have greater potential for addiction and abuse than Schedule III drugs.
- Schedule I controlled substances are illegal in the US except in certain research centers.
- Schedule II controlled substances are monitored with a continuous or perpetual inventory system.
- The central nervous system and the peripheral nervous system carry electrical signals to and from the brain.
- Neurotransmitters are chemicals that allow the electrical signals in the nervous system to travel from one nerve to the next nerve.
- Drugs that affect the nervous system affect some aspect of the neurotransmitter mechanism.
- Anesthetics are drugs that prevent signals from going to or returning from the brain.
- Analgesics are drugs that are prescribed to decrease, control, or eliminate pain by blocking signals to or from the brain.
- A migraine headache is a particular type of severe headache where blood vessels over relax.

Learning Assessment Questions

1. The pharmacy manager is interviewing candidates for a pharmacy-technician position. After the interviews, the pharmacy manager states he is hiring the female candidate because the male candidate looked gay. This is an example of which of the following?

   A. Harassment

   B. Discrimination

   C. Empathy

   D. None of the above

2. Walking into the break room in your pharmacy, you notice a new calendar hanging on the wall. The calendar features women with minimal clothing. This could be an example of which of the following?

   A. Harassment

   B. Discrimination

   C. Empathy

   D. None of the above

3. A patient hands you a prescription. Upon looking up the patient profile in the computer, you ask, "Can you explain to me which drug allergies you may have to pain medications?" This is an example of what type of question?

   A. Close ended

   B. Open ended

   C. Factual

   D. None of the above

4. Opioid drugs are derived from which of the following?

   A. Bacteria

   B. Poppies

   C. Fungus

   D. Marijuana

5. HIPAA stands for which of the following?

   A. Health Information Protection Access Act

   B. Health Insurance Portability and Accountability Act

   C. Human Information Protection and Administration Act

   D. Health Information Permission Accountability Act

6. Patient identifiers may include all but which of the following?

   A. Patient name

   B. Social security number

   C. State of residence

   D. Telephone number

7. Controlled substances are ranked into numbered categories based on which of the following?

   A. Price

   B. Amount of overall annual use

   C. The addiction and abuse potential

   D. The date the drug was approved by the FDA

8. Analgesics are drugs that do which of the following?

   A. Increase, control, or block pain

   B. Prevent signals from going to or returning from the brain

   C. Decrease, control, or block pain

   D. Increase signals going to or returning from the brain

9. Anesthetics are drugs that do which of the following?

   A. Increase, control, or block pain

   B. Prevent signals from going to or returning from the brain

   C. Decrease, control, or block pain

   D. Increase signals going to or returning from the brain

10. Meninges are primarily for which of the following?

    A. Communication of synapses

    B. Transfer of impulses

    C. Conduction of fluid

    D. Protection of brain and spinal cord

11. Neurotransmitters do which of the following?

    A. Allow the electrical signal to continue to the next nerve

    B. Allow fluid to be transmitted from organ to organ

    C. Improve hearing

    D. Decrease hearing

12. The sympathetic subdivision of the autonomic nervous system does which of the following?

    A. Relaxes the system

    B. Causes the person to fight or flee

    C. Causes the person to sleep

    D. Causes the body to release acetylcholine

13. Which of the following is a neurotransmitter in the parasympathetic system?

    A. Dopamine

    B. Norepinephrine

    C. Epinephrine

    D. Acetylcholine

14. Which of the following is an example of a selective serotonin reuptake inhibitor (SSRI)?

    A. amitriptyline (Elavil)

    B. tranylcypromine (Parnate)

    C. desflurane (Suprane)

    D. sertraline (Zoloft)

15. Which of the following is an example of a MAOI (monoamine oxidase inhibitor)?

    A. amitriptyline (Elavil)

    B. tranylcypromine (Parnate)

    C. desflurane (Suprane)

    D. sertraline (Zoloft)

16. Local anesthesia describes which of the following?

    A. A drug used to cause reversible loss of feeling in a specific area of the body

    B. A drug used to cause reversible loss of feeling in the entire body

    C. A drug used to cause irreversible loss of feeling in a specific area of the body

    D. A drug used to cause irreversible loss of feeling in the entire body

17. What is the generic name for Ativan?

    A. Midazolam

    B. Diazepam

    C. Flurazepam

    D. Lorazepam

18. Which of the following drugs is *not* a CII general anesthetic agent?

    A. Propofol

    B. Alfentanil

    C. Fentanyl

    D. Morphine

19. Which of the following drugs is *not* a local anesthetic?

    A. Benzocaine

    B. Thiopental

    C. Bupivacaine

    D. Dyclonine

20. What is the major difference between chronic malignant pain and chronic pain?

    A. The duration of the pain

    B. The intensity of the pain

    C. That the cause is known to be from cancer

    D. One pain can be treated, while the other cannot

21. With all three types of pain, inadequate treatment can cause the patient to experience all of the following *except*:

    A. Pain

    B. Lack of pain

    C. Depression

    D. Decreased immune system

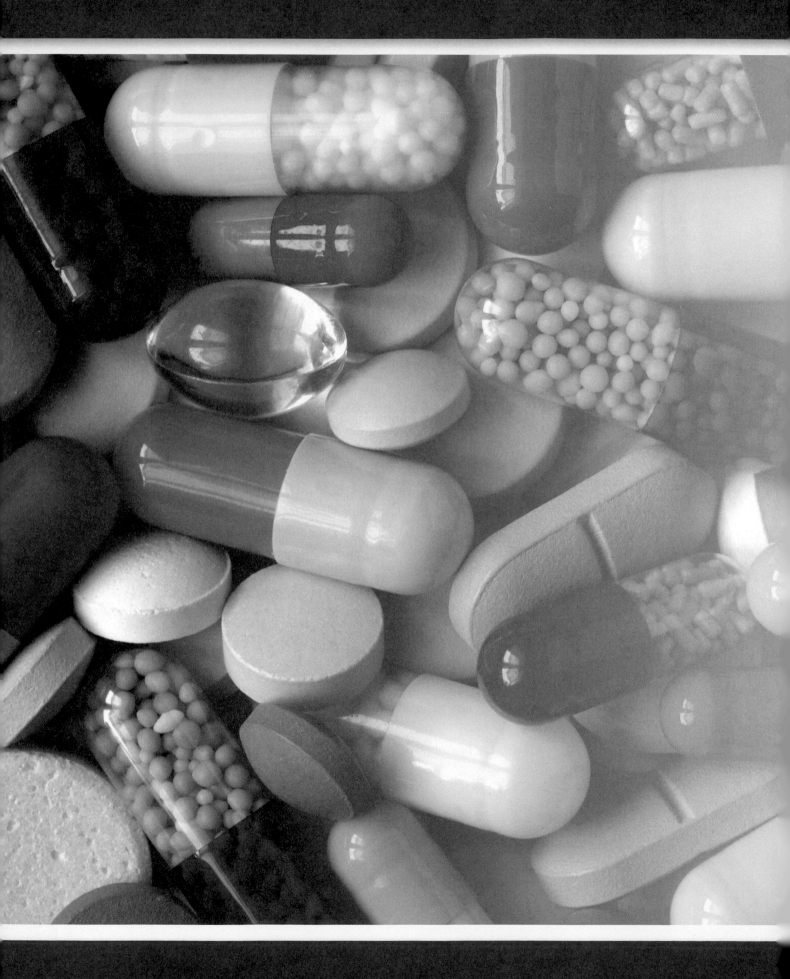

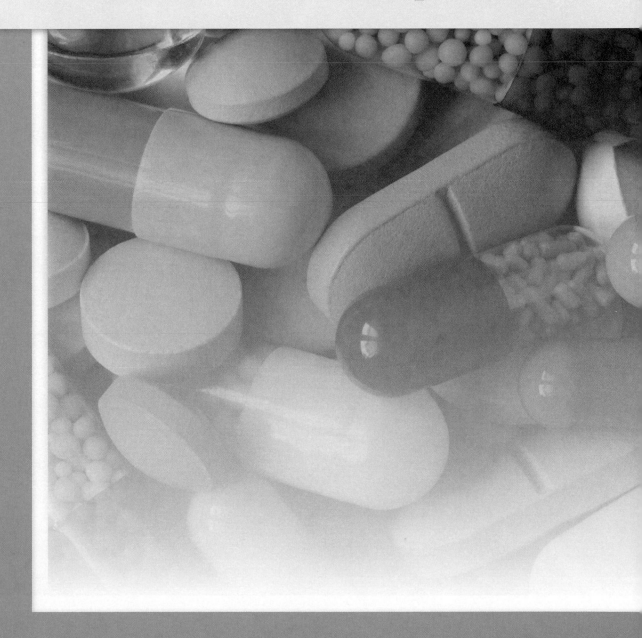

Basic Principles

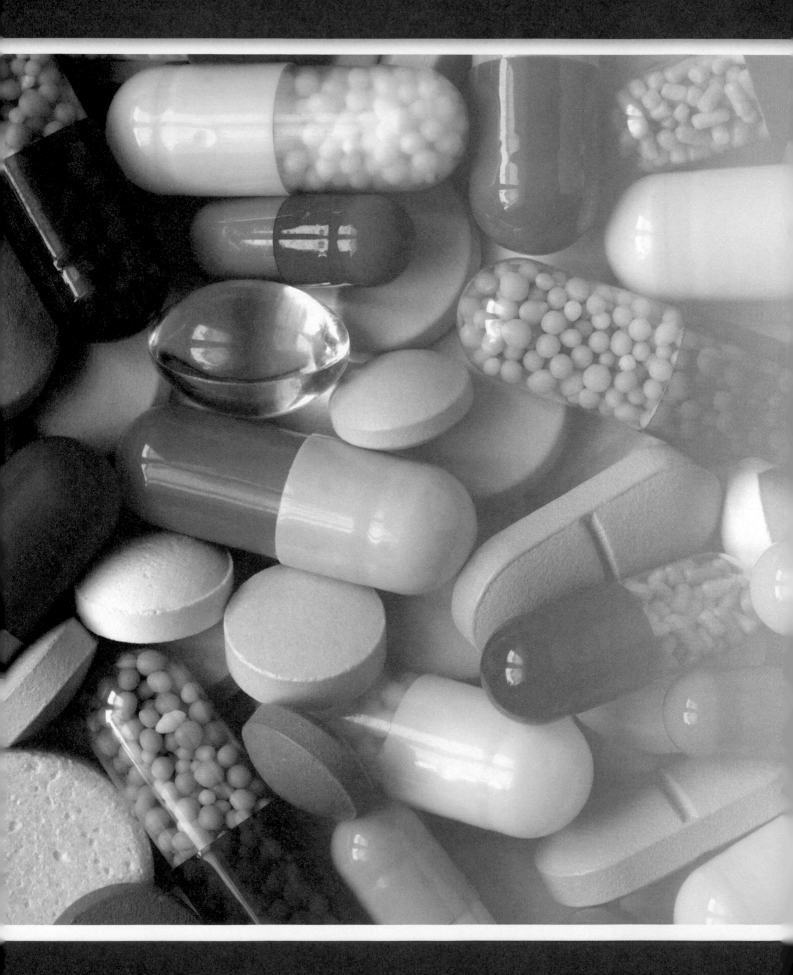

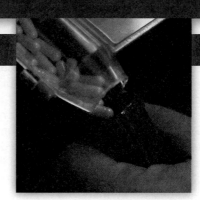

Community Pharmacy

After reading this chapter, you will be able to:

- Understand the importance of a patient profile.
- Review a patient profile form for complete and accurate information.
- Understand the types of problems that missing or inaccurate patient information can cause in the pharmacy.
- Identify strategies to resolve problems arising from incomplete patient profile forms.
- Evaluate unprocessed prescriptions for completeness and accuracy.
- Understand the additional checking steps needed when reviewing controlled-substance prescriptions.
- Compare a processed prescription to the printed label for completeness and accuracy.
- Identify practices to correct errors on printed labels generated from the processed prescription.
- Differentiate between antidepressant, antipsychotic, and anti-anxiety drugs.
- Discuss the different classes of antidepressant drugs, their uses, and their side effects.
- Discuss how lithium and other drugs are used in treating bipolar disorders.
- Discuss the drugs that prevent the side effects caused by antipsychotics drugs.
- Explain the definition and symptoms of anxiety, as well as the drugs used to treat anxiety.
- Recognize the course and treatment of panic disorders, insomnia, and alcoholism.

KEY TERMS

Alcoholism	Antipsychotic	Drug allergy
Algorithm	Benzodiazepines	Drug side effect
Anti-anxiety agent	Bipolar disorder	Drug-treatment pathway
Antidepressant	Depression	E-prescribing

Extrapyramidal symptom (EPS)	Panic attack	Schizophrenia
Gamma-aminobutyric acid (GABA)	Panic disorder	Serotonin
General anxiety disease (GAD)	Patient profile	Serotonin and norepinephrine reuptake inhibitor (SNRI) drug
Hypnotic drug	Personal digital assistant (PDA)	
Insomnia	Posttraumatic stress disorder (PTSD)	Serotonin syndrome
Legibility	Postural hypotension	Sig
Mood-stabilizing agent	Psychiatrist	Tardive dyskinesia
Norepinephrine	Psychosis	Tricyclic antidepressant (TCA) drug
NR notation	Psychotherapy	
Obsessive-compulsive disorder (OCD)	QT interval	Tyramine
	Reuptake inhibitor drug	
	Rx	

Chapter Overview

This chapter provides an overview of patient profiles, prescriptions, and labels. The ability to accurately complete a patient profile for a new patient, the ability to evaluate unprocessed prescriptions for completeness and accuracy, and the ability to compare a processed prescription label with the original prescription are three very important skills that must be mastered by every pharmacy technician working in a community pharmacy. Chapter 10 builds on this chapter by providing an opportunity for hands-on computer training in entering patient-specific data into a profile, processing the label, and processing refill requests.

This chapter will also review antidepressant, antipsychotic, and anti-anxiety drugs and their uses in the treatment of mental-health diseases.

Community Pharmacy Practice

Community pharmacy practice is an evolving practice area with pharmacists and pharmacy technicians taking on more involved roles in medication management and patient care. The community pharmacy includes retail pharmacy settings that may be a chain of retail pharmacies, an independent pharmacy owned by a sole owner or group of owners, or an ambulatory care pharmacy associated with a hospital, health-care, or health-maintenance organization. Pharmacy technicians continue to have more extended roles in the practice of pharmacy and providing patient care in the retail and community pharmacy settings.

The Patient Profile

The **patient profile** is a computerized record that contains all the information needed to accurately and safely fill a prescription for a patient. The information found on a patient profile includes the patient's personal information, such as his or her birth date, address, allergies, contact numbers, and insurance information. It also contains a list of all prescriptions that have already been filled for that patient at that location. In a chain pharmacy, the pharmacist would have access to any prescriptions filled at any of the stores in the chain. All patients should have a complete and accurate patient profile before any of his or her prescriptions can be filled. When obtaining required patient information to fill a prescription, pharmacy technicians must adhere to the

Health Insurance Portability and Accountability Act (HIPAA) to protect the privacy of the patient. HIPAA is discussed in more detail in Chapter 8.

> All patient information is confidential. Violating HIPAA regulations by sharing patient information with unauthorized parties can result in severe fines.

If a patient presenting a new prescription to the pharmacy technician does not have a profile on record, one must be created. The following is a list of common items that may be entered into a patient's computerized profile:

- Patient's full name
- Insurance information
- Prescriber
- Patient's address
- Allergies
- OTC meds being taken
- Telephone number
- Emergency contact
- Medical diagnoses
- Patient preferences
- Birth date
- Adverse drug reactions
- Special patient needs
- Gender
- Previously filled prescriptions
- Email address
- Herbal remedies being taken

In today's community pharmacy, information must be obtained from a new patient prior to filling the prescription. The pharmacy technician opens a new profile in the pharmacy computer system while the patient is available at the pharmacy window or counter to answer questions and provide information. In this scenario, the pharmacy technician must adhere to safety and privacy guidelines to ensure the patient is able to answer the questions comfortably and safely during a one-on-one discussion with the pharmacy technician. The pharmacy technician could simply ask the patient for the information needed and type it into the profile. Another method of obtaining all the required information is to give the new patient a form, which asks for all the required information. The patient could then fill out the form and return it to the pharmacy technician, after which the pharmacy technician could enter all the written information into the pharmacy computer system. An example of one of these written forms is shown in FIGURE 9.1 .

Many patients presenting a new prescription to the pharmacy technician will already have a patient profile. If a patient profile is already on file for the patient, the profile should be reviewed for accuracy, as some of the information may have changed. The pharmacy technician should first verify that the profile in the system is in fact this patient's profile. The easiest way to verify this is to ask the patient for two different patient identifiers. These two identifiers could be their birth date and address. After the profile has been verified, the pharmacy technician should update all necessary information.

PATIENT PROFILE

Patient Name

_____   _____   _____
Last   First   Middle Initial

Street or PO Box
_____

City   State   ZIP
_____

Phone   Date of Birth   Social Security No.
(__)__ ____   _____   □ Male   ___ __ _____
                               Month   Day   Year   □ Female

□ Yes, I would like medication dispensed in a child-resistant container.
□ No, I do not want medication dispensed in a child-resistant container.

Medical Insurance   Card Holder Name _____
□ Yes   □ Card Holder   □ Child   □ Disabled Dependent
□ No   □ Spouse   □ Dependent Parent   □ Full-Time Student

MEDICAL HISTORY

HEALTH   ALLERGIES AND DRUG REACTIONS
□ Angina   □ Epilepsy   □ No known drug allergies or reactions
□ Anemia   □ Glaucoma   □ Aspirin
□ Arthritis   □ Heart condition   □ Cephalosporins
□ Asthma   □ Kidney disease   □ Codeine
□ Blood clotting disorders □ Liver disease   □ Erythromycin
□ High blood pressure □ Lung disease   □ Penicillin
□ Breastfeeding   □ Parkinson disease   □ Sulfa drugs
□ Cancer   □ Pregnancy   □ Tetracyclines
□ Diabetes   □ Ulcers   □ Xanthines
Other conditions _____   □ Other allergies/reactions _____
_____   _____

Prescription Medication(s) Being Taken   OTC Medication(s) Currently Being Taken
_____   _____
_____   _____

Would you like generic medication when possible?   □ Yes □ No
Comments: _____
_____

Health information changes periodically. Please notify the pharmacy of any new medications, allergies,
drug reactions, or health conditions.

_____ Signature _____ Date   □ I do not wish to provide this information.

FIGURE 9.1 Patient profile.

Some of the common areas that must be routinely updated are the patient's address, phone number, drug allergies, and types of insurance coverage. Many pharmacies require pharmacy technicians to ask each patient with a prescription if he or she has any new drug allergies or insurance information. Even if the pharmacy does not specifically require this, a pharmacy technician should always ask the patient.

A very significant part of any pharmacy technician's routine duties is maintaining an accurate patient profile on every patient. Incorrect or incomplete allergy information could lead to a serious or life-threatening allergic reaction. Inaccurate or incomplete allergy information also prevents computer software from cross-checking other drugs that could potentially cause an allergic reaction. While drug allergies should be entered into a patient's profile, a drug side effect should not. Entering a drug side effect as an allergy in the patient's profile could prevent the patient from receiving a necessary life-saving drug in the future. A pharmacy technician must know

If, when entering information into the patient's profile, there is a doubt as to whether a drug problem is an allergy or a side effect, the pharmacy technician should ask the pharmacist on duty for assistance.

the difference between a drug allergy and a drug side effect. A **drug side effect** is any effect that the drug could routinely cause as part of the drug's method of action. For example, a patient taking a pain-killing drug such as hydrocodone and acetaminophen (Vicodin) might become constipated because one side effect of hydrocodone and acetaminophen (Vicodin) is a slowing down of the intestines. In contrast, a patient taking hydrocodone and acetaminophen (Vicodin) who develops hives or a rash is experiencing an allergic reaction, because the development of hives or a rash is not related to the drug's mode of action. A **drug allergy** is an allergic reaction to a drug. It could be manifested by itching, rash, hives, or, in the worst case, anaphylaxis and death. Drug allergies can develop at any time, even if the patient has taken a drug in the past. Many computerized patient-profile systems have a special screen in which patient-specific information such as side effects can be entered. A drug allergy and a patient's side effect to a drug are different from each other and should be documented appropriately in the profile.

Incorrect or incomplete insurance information in the patient's profile will prevent the prescription from being approved and paid for by the patient's insurance company. Issues with insurance-company approvals and payments are one of the most common problems encountered in the day-to-day activities of the community pharmacy. Additionally, issues with approval and patient insurance payments can cause some of the most annoying customer-service problems and lead to the loss of the patient as a future customer. Often, the pharmacy technician can prevent these problems by being proactive—asking the patient if any insurance information has changed and verifying that all computerized information is complete and correct. Maintaining up-to-date and accurate insurance and billing information in the patient profile is an extremely important routine duty of the community pharmacy technician. Additional information about patient prescription insurance is discussed in Chapter 11 and Chapter 12.

The New Prescription

One of the valuable services provided by a community pharmacy is the filling of prescriptions. Community pharmacies fill new prescriptions and refill prescriptions that are already on file in their computer database. New prescriptions are received in the community pharmacy through several different ways. For example, the patient might bring the new prescription into the pharmacy in person for filling, or the prescriber might call in the prescription to the pharmacist on duty. Many new prescriptions today are transmitted to the pharmacy electronically, either through E-prescribing or by fax transmission.

E-prescribing is the newest electronic method used to transmit new prescriptions to the community pharmacy. E-prescribing is an outgrowth of the move toward the use of **personal digital assistants (PDAs)** by prescribers. PDAs can provide a wealth of drug information to the prescriber with a simple click of a button. A natural evolution of this technology was the ability to use the PDA to transmit new prescription information directly to a receiving pharmacy. Although a PDA is the most mobile method of transmitting electronic prescriptions, desktop and laptop computers are also used.

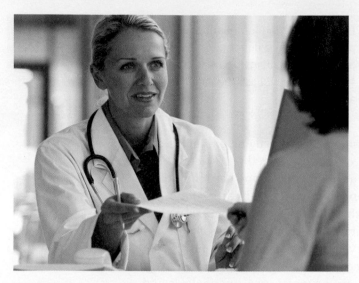

New patient prescription.

E-prescribing has many advantages, with **legibility**, or readability, being one of the most important from the point of view of the pharmacy. In addition to legibility, speed of transmission, accuracy, more efficient billing, and decreased potential for forgery are all important benefits of this newer technology. Currently, E-prescribing is legal for all prescriptions except Schedule II controlled substances. As the federal government promotes E-prescribing, some states have updated their individual state rules and regulations to allow E-Prescribing for Schedule II controlled substances. The pharmacy technician will need to be familiar with state laws that pertain to the pharmacy involved.

Regardless of the format in which the new prescription is received by the pharmacy, the same information must be presented as part of a complete prescription. A list of that information follows. Most of the information will be provided by the prescriber, with the pharmacy technician having to obtain any missing information.

- Drug name
- Drug strength
- Drug quantity to dispense
- Drug directions
- Patient's name
- Patient's address
- Patient's birthday
- Prescriber's name
- Prescriber's phone number
- Prescriber's address
- Prescriber's DEA number (for controlled substances)
- Written date of the prescription
- Number of refills
- DAW or substitution allowed

Reviewing a New Prescription

An extremely important job requirement for the pharmacy technician is reviewing a new prescription for completeness and accuracy prior to beginning the filling process. Just like all other pharmacy duties, the review of a new prescription for accuracy is completed by a pharmacy technician under the supervision of the pharmacist.

Breaking down the prescription into three information sections will help the pharmacy technician quickly verify that all needed information is noted. These three sections are as follows:

- Patient-related information
- Prescriber-related information
- Prescribed-drug information

The pharmacy technician begins by reviewing the patient related information.

Reviewing Patient-Related Information

Using the prescription shown as an example, the pharmacy technician would verify the patient's name as Jane Smith and her address as 111 Eagle Road in Mobic, Arizona, 85255. Jane's date of birth is not noted on the prescription, however, if Jane Smith were to hand the pharmacy technician this prescription, the pharmacy technician should ask for her birth date. Obtaining a correct birth date will assist the pharmacy technician in locating the correct Jane Smith in the pharmacy's computer system, thus preventing a billing error and possibly preventing a medication error in the future, which might occur if the prescription were entered into the profile of the wrong Jane Smith. Additionally, by having the patient's date of birth, the pharmacist will be able to consider the patient's age when verifying the appropriateness of the drug dosage and directions.

Reviewing Prescriber-Related Information

The next information section the pharmacy technician checks is the information regarding the prescriber. Using the prescription shown as an example, the pharmacy technician would verify the prescriber's name as John Adams MD, and his address as 1400 Professional Plaza, Phoenix, Arizona, 85200. The prescriber's phone number and DEA number are also preprinted on this prescription. Due to security concerns, however, prescriptions received by the pharmacy technician may not contain any of the prescriber's information preprinted except the name of the group practice or clinic because prescriptions are easier to forge when a prescriber's information is preprinted on the blanks. For this reason, some prescribers prefer to write in or use a stamper with their name and DEA number (if writing for a controlled substance) when writing a prescription for the patient. If there is a strong prescriber-pharmacy relationship, the pharmacist will write in the information, which is already pre-programmed in the pharmacy's computer, and it will then be recorded accurately to comply with state laws. As part of the prescriber-information check, the pharmacy technician should also verify that the prescription has been signed by the prescriber, either manually or electronically. In the prescription shown, the prescriber has signed the prescription electronically and authorized the dispensing of a generic drug based on the selection of that signature line.

Written prescriptions for covered outpatient drugs that are paid for by Medicaid must be written on a tamper-resistant prescription pad. As of October 1, 2008, prescription pads used for written prescriptions must contain all three of the following characteristics to be considered tamper-resistant:

- One or more industry-recognized features designed to prevent unauthorized copying of a completed or blank prescription form
- One or more industry-recognized features designed to prevent the erasure or modification of information written on the prescription pad by the prescriber
- One or more industry-recognized features designed to prevent the use of counterfeit prescription forms

What Would You Do?

Question: You receive a prescription, but you're not sure it meets the tamper-proof requirements. What should you do?

Answer: Have the pharmacist call the prescribing practitioner to obtain verbal confirmation of the prescription and document the confirmation appropriately. A 72-hour dose can also be filled; pharmacies can fill emergency prescriptions for 72 hours as long as they obtain the compliant prescription within 72 hours of the fill date.

Reviewing Drug-Related Information

The third section the pharmacy technician examines is the section related to the drug prescribed. In the sample prescription, the drug ordered is prednisone 10mg, with a quantity to dispense of 30, and directions of "tid" (three times a day). Examining the refill section, the pharmacy technician notes the **NR notation**, which means "no refill." If any of the essential drug information is missing, the pharmacist or pharmacy technician (depending on state law) will have to obtain the information from the prescriber prior to continuing the filling process. Two additional abbreviations appear on the sample prescription: Sig and Rx. **Sig**, from the Latin *signatura*, indicates "patient directions," while **Rx**, from the Latin "take thou," means "recipe" or "prescription."

Having verified all the necessary information, the pharmacy technician is now ready to enter the prescription into the pharmacy computer system, unless the prescription is for a controlled substance. If the prescription is for a controlled substance, additional verification of information is required.

New prescriptions for controlled substances can be divided into two categories: Schedule II (CII) prescriptions and Schedule III, IV, and V (CIII, CIV, and CV) prescriptions. Each type of controlled-substance prescription is subject to specific laws regarding refills and age of the prescription. The pharmacy technician should carefully examine the authorized refills and the date the prescription was written. Schedule II prescriptions cannot be refilled; to obtain this type of medication, the patient must present a new prescription each time the drug is prescribed. State laws vary in their requirement as to how soon a CII prescription must be filled once written by the prescriber, so the pharmacy technician must be familiar with the state law.

Schedule III and Schedule IV controlled substances prescriptions are valid for only six months from the date noted on the prescription. Additionally, CIII and CIV controlled-substance prescriptions cannot be refilled more than five times in that six-month period. Schedule V controlled substances are covered by different laws in different states. The pharmacy technician must know the laws in the state in which the pharmacy is located.

After the refills and date-written sections of the controlled-substance prescription have been checked by the pharmacy technician, the prescription itself needs to be checked for alterations. Controlled-substance prescriptions have a greater potential for abuse and addiction than non-controlled drug prescriptions. As a result, controlled-substance prescriptions are more likely to be altered or forged. The pharmacy technician should critically examine several specific areas of the controlled substance prescription for alterations.

The most commonly altered items on a controlled-substance prescription are the drug strength, the drug quantity to dispense, and the directions. A pharmacy technician receiving a new prescription for a controlled substance should be extra diligent when examining these three items on the prescription. If any of these three items are illegible, the pharmacist should be notified prior to entering the prescription into the computer system.

If the drug strength, quantity, or directions appear to be written in different-color ink, have a different style of writing, or have been changed (for example, by someone writing over an underlying word or number), the pharmacist should be notified. The pharmacy technician should examine the patient directions for the use and the quantity to dispense for alterations. For example, altering a written prescription's directions from "bid" to "tid" would allow the patient to obtain refills sooner, while changing the quantity to dispense from "10" to "20" would enable the patient to obtain extra quantities of the drug.

Question: If the pharmacy technician has concerns about the validity of the prescription, what should be done?

Answer: The pharmacy technician should ask for the pharmacist's assistance.

Lastly, the pharmacy technician should use critical-thinking skills and compare the quantity to dispense with the medical condition being treated or the type of prescriber writing the prescription. For example, receiving a prescription from a dentist for a pain drug such as hydrocodone and acetaminophen (Vicodin) with a quantity to dispense of 80, or multiple refills, should alert the pharmacy technician to the possibility that the prescription has been altered. A dentist would normally treat a patient with short-term dental pain, thus a quantity of 80 or multiple refills would be unusual.

After all information on the prescription has been determined to be complete and accurate, the pharmacy technician can begin entering the prescription information into the pharmacy computer system. When all the prescription information has been entered and approved for payment, the pharmacy computer will print a prescription label for filling. The pharmacy technician must then verify the accuracy of the prescription label with the actual new prescription.

The pharmacy technician must compare each item noted on the prescription label with the original new prescription **FIGURE 9.2**. Any incorrect items on the label must be

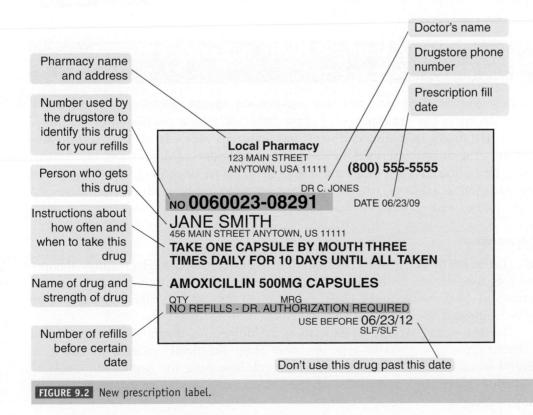

FIGURE 9.2 New prescription label.

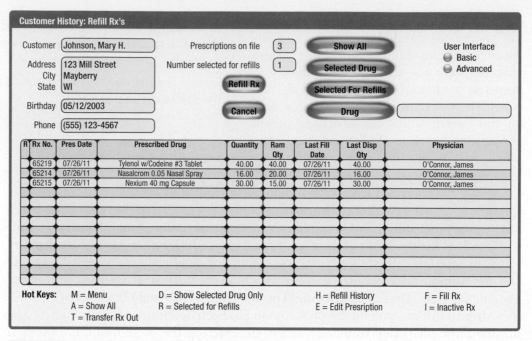

FIGURE 9.3 Electronic pharmacy patient profile.

corrected prior to the prescription and label being passed on for filling by pharmacy personnel. Any incorrect items that affect the payment for the prescription may require the reprocessing of the entire prescription. Incorrect payment information can be caused by errors involving the patient information, drug name, quantity of drug dispensed, directions for use by the patient, or amount of refills authorized **FIGURE 9.3**.

Drug Insights: Antidepressants, Antipsychotics, and Anti-Anxiety Agents

Antidepressants, **antipsychotics**, and **anti-anxiety agents** are used to treat mental-health diseases. The examination of these drugs includes a discussion of the drugs' classes, the drugs' recommended uses, and the drugs' side effects. This section also examines the drugs prescribed for mental-health diseases of depression, bipolar disorder, panic disorder, insomnia, and alcoholism. Before beginning the discussion of the drugs for each disorder, the pharmacy technician must have a basic understanding of the different diagnoses.

Depression

Depression is a mental health condition that may be accompanied by feelings of hopelessness, low self-worth, and loss of interest. It can manifest itself as many different symptoms. Depression can be transient or persist for days or years. Depression may be accompanied by drug abuse and addiction.

The American Psychiatric Association has differential diagnostic criteria for six different types of depression-type diseases. These diagnostic criteria are based on several factors, including the symptoms noted, how long the depression has been occurring, when the onset of the depression occurred, and what triggering factors may be present

Some of the most common symptoms of depression are as follows:

- Feelings of pessimism
- Constant worry
- Feelings of sadness, emptiness, or worthlessness
- Lack of motivation
- Decreasing interest in daily activities
- Eating disorders
- Sleeping disorders
- Feelings of guilt
- Weight changes
- Inability to concentrate
- Indecisiveness
- Confused thinking
- Recurrent thoughts of illness
- Recurrent thoughts of death
- Self-pity
- Suicidal thoughts or actions

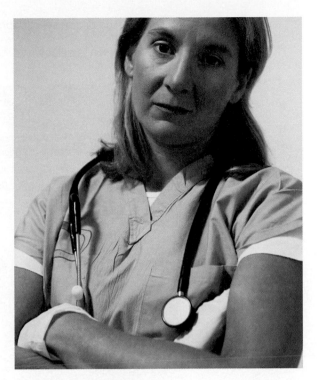

Symptoms of depression of include feelings of sadness, emptiness, or worthlessness.

Drug Therapy for Depression

Drug therapy for patients with a diagnosis of depression can be as simple as one drug or as complex as multiple drugs taken multiple times a day combined with **psychotherapy** (that is, personal counseling by a mental-health professional such as a psychotherapist or psychiatrist). Because many patients with depression need multiple therapies, many physicians and **psychiatrists** use a **drug-treatment pathway** or **algorithm** when treating this type of patient. An example of a common drug algorithm is noted in FIGURE 9.4.

Although treatment of depression usually involves the use of multiple drugs with different modes of action, the majority of drugs used for depression affect one or more neurotransmitters in the nervous system. The nervous system in the human body sends and receives signals through electrical transmissions coupled with chemical transmissions. The electrical signals stimulate the release of these chemicals, called neurotransmitters, from storage areas through the nerve pathways to and from the brain. The release of a neurotransmitter fills a space, called a synapse, in the nerve pathway that allows the signal to continue to the next nerve. Once the signal reaches the brain, the brain reads the signal and tells the body what needs to be done. This electrical-to-chemical-to-electrical pathway includes specific routes within the brain itself that require that specific neurotransmitters be released in order to function.

These brain neurotransmitters, specifically **serotonin** and **norepinephrine**, control feelings of pleasure, happiness, sadness, depression, and euphoria. Treatment of depression revolves around these neurotransmitters. Research has shown that keeping a neurotransmitter in the synapse for a longer period decreases the symptoms of depression. Chapter 8 contains a section that explains the central nervous system and the role played by neurotransmitters.

Two different drug modes of action are utilized to keep the neurotransmitter, either serotonin or norepinephrine, in the synapse for a longer period. One mode of action is to prevent the neurotransmitter from being reabsorbed, or taken back up, into the storage site. These drugs are called **reuptake inhibitor drugs**. A second mode of drug action is to prevent the neurotransmitter from being destroyed in the synapse

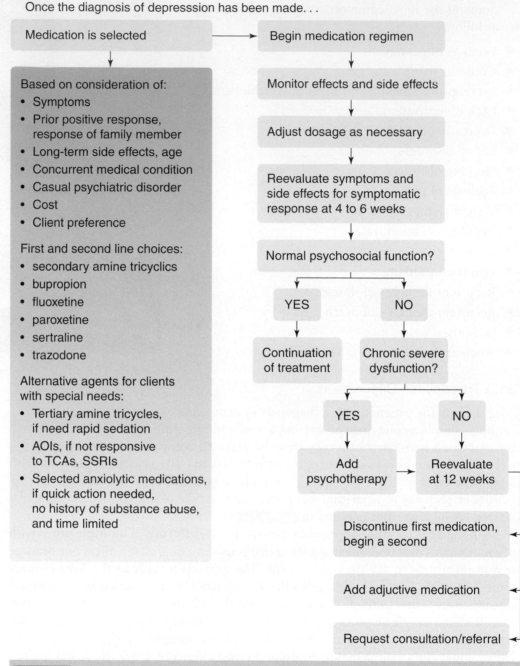

Once the diagnosis of depresssion has been made. . .

Medication is selected → Begin medication regimen

Based on consideration of:
- Symptoms
- Prior positive response, response of family member
- Long-term side effects, age
- Concurrent medical condition
- Casual psychiatric disorder
- Cost
- Client preference

First and second line choices:
- secondary amine tricyclics
- bupropion
- fluoxetine
- paroxetine
- sertraline
- trazodone

Alternative agents for clients with special needs:
- Tertiary amine tricycles, if need rapid sedation
- AOIs, if not responsive to TCAs, SSRIs
- Selected anxiolytic medications, if quick action needed, no history of substance abuse, and time limited

Monitor effects and side effects

Adjust dosage as necessary

Reevaluate symptoms and side effects for symptomatic response at 4 to 6 weeks

Normal psychosocial function?

YES → Continuation of treatment

NO → Chronic severe dysfunction?

YES → Add psychotherapy → Reevaluate at 12 weeks

NO → Reevaluate at 12 weeks

Discontinue first medication, begin a second

Add adjuctive medication

Request consultation/referral

FIGURE 9.4 Treatment algorithm for depression.

by an enzyme called monoamine oxidase. These drugs are called monoamine oxidase inhibitor (MAOI) drugs.

Based on the aforementioned mode of action, antidepressant drugs are divided in four major classes:

- Selective serotonin reuptake inhibitor (SSRI) drugs
- Serotonin and norepinephrine reuptake inhibitor (SNRI) drugs
- Tricyclic antidepressant (TCA) drugs
- Monoamine oxidase inhibitor (MAOI) drugs

Table 9.1 Common Reuptake Inhibitor Drugs

Generic Name	Brand Name	Dosage Form	Action
Citalopram	Celexa	Liquid, tablet	SSRI
Desvenlafaxine	Pristiq	Tablet	SNRI
Duloxetine	Cymbalta	Capsule	SNRI
Escitalopram	Lexapro	Liquid, tablet	SSRI
Fluoxetine	Prozac	Capsule, liquid, tablet	SSRI
Paroxetine	Paxil	Liquid, tablet	SSRI
Sertraline	Zoloft	Liquid, tablet	SSRI
Venlafaxine	Effexor	Capsule, tablet	SNRI

Selective Serotonin Reuptake Inhibitor (SSRI) Drugs

Selective serotonin reuptake inhibitor (SSRI) drugs are the most commonly prescribed drugs for depression. This class of drugs works by preventing the reuptake of serotonin. The serotonin remains longer in the nerve synapse, and the symptoms of depression are decreased. SSRI drugs have a delayed onset of effectiveness. That means the full effect of the drug may not be seen until between 10 and 21 days after starting the drug.

Serotonin and Norepinephrine Reuptake Inhibitor (SNRI) Drugs

Serotonin and norepinephrine reuptake inhibitor (SNRI) drugs arrived on the market after the SSRI drugs. SNRI drugs' mode of action is to prevent the reuptake of both serotonin and norepinephrine. Both the serotonin and norepinephrine transmitters remain in the synapse longer, and the symptoms of depression are decreased. SNRI drugs have a delayed onset of effectiveness. **TABLE 9.1** lists common SSRI and SNRI drugs.

SSRI and SNRI drugs are generally well tolerated by patients, although side effects can occur. Some of the most common side effects are insomnia, drowsiness, nervousness, and loss of appetite.

Both SSRI and SNRI drugs have the potential to cause interactions with other drugs. The pharmacy technician should be aware that a potential interaction alert may appear on the computer screen when entering these drugs as a new prescription on certain patients. A potential drug interaction alert notice should always be referred to the pharmacist before continuing to process the prescription. One of the most serious drug interactions is serotonin syndrome. **Serotonin syndrome** can occur when an SSRI or SNRI is combined with other drugs that stimulate the serotonin receptors. Serotonin syndrome is rare, but may cause excitation symptoms that, in certain cases, could be fatal. When combined with an SSRI or an SNRI, some drugs prescribed for migraine—primarily serotonin-receptor agonists, which are discussed in Chapter 8—can cause this syndrome.

Tricyclic Antidepressant (TCA) Drugs

Tricyclic antidepressant (TCA) drugs have been on the market for many years, with imipramine (Tofranil) first being synthesized in the late 1940s. The TCAs predate both the SSRI and the SNRI drugs. The exact mechanism of action of tricyclic antidepressants is not known. The believed mode of action for TCA drugs is similar to SNRI and SSRI: the prevention of either serotonin or norepinephrine from being taken up

Table 9.2   Common Tricyclic and Tetracyclic Antidepressant Drugs

Generic Name	Brand Name	Dosage Form
Common Tricyclic Drugs		
Amitriptyline	Elavil	Tablet
Clomipramine	Anafranil	Capsule
Desipramine	Norpramine	Tablet
Doxepin	Sinequan	Capsule, liquid
Nortriptyline	Pamelor, Aventyl	Capsule, liquid
Common Tetracyclic Drugs		
Maprotiline	Ludiomil	Tablet
Mirtazapine	Remeron	Tablet

back into the storage unit at the nerve synapse. Tricyclic antidepressants are effective in many patients who experience depression.

Tricyclic antidepressant drugs have more side effects than the newer drugs. Some of these side effects can be quite serious, and even fatal. Side effects can include cardiac toxicity (including the potential for arrhythmias), **postural hypotension** (a decrease in blood pressure that occurs when a person rises from a prone position), sedation, blurred vision, dry mouth, constipation, and urinary retention. Due to the potential for serious side effects, this class of drugs is usually started at a low dose and then slowly increased as needed to control depression symptoms. Maprotiline (Ludiomil) and mirtazapine (Remeron) are chemically tetracyclic drugs, but share the same drug profile and side effects with the tricyclic drugs. **TABLE 9.2** lists the most common tricyclic and tetracyclic antidepressants.

Monoamine Oxidase Inhibitor (MAOI) Drugs

Monoamine oxidase inhibitor (MAOI) drugs were one of the first classes of drugs on the market to treat depression. Although they are effective for some patients, the potential for life-threatening side effects makes them a second or third choice to treat depression, following SSRI and SNRI drugs. Although MAOI drugs are not cardiotoxic like TCAs, this entire class of drugs has a major drug interaction with certain foods. Severe and sometimes fatal hypertensive crisis can occur when a patient taking an MAOI drug eats food that contains tyramine. **Tyramine** is a chemical compound that is present in many different foods including aged cheese, pickled fish, some wines, many meat products, and broad beans, just to name a few.

The pharmacy technician should become familiar with MAOI drugs and notify the pharmacist when a prescription is received. The pharmacist will need to do additional checking on the patient's profile for possible interactions. Additionally, the pharmacist will need to counsel the patient with regard to potential food interactions. Currently, there are three common MOAI drugs on the market, as shown in **TABLE 9.3**.

Table 9.3   Common Monoamine Oxidase Inhibitor Drugs

Generic Name	Brand Name	Dosage Form
Phenelzine	Nardil	Tablet
Selegiline	Eldepryl, Emsam, Zelepar	Capsule, tablet, patch
Tranylcypromine	Parnate	Tablet

Miscellaneous Antidepressant Drugs

Two commonly prescribed drugs for depression, bupropion (Wellbutrin) and trazodone (Desyrel), do not use the modes of action of the other antidepressant drugs.

Wellbutrin's mode of action is to inhibit the uptake of dopamine. This drug does not affect serotonin, norepinephrine, or the monoamine oxidase enzyme. For the pharmacy technician, one of the most challenging issues with this drug is the different strengths available. Wellbutrin is available in three different strengths with three different dosage forms. These differences can cause confusion and a medication error if the new prescription is not clearly written or if the wrong form of the drug is entered into the pharmacy computer system. The doses available are as follows:

Question: A patient asks the pharmacy technician a question about a potential drug-and-food interaction or a drug-and-drug interaction. What should the pharmacy technician do?

Answer: The pharmacy technician should ask for the pharmacist's assistance.

- Wellbutrin tablets (three doses per day)
- Wellbutrin SR tablets (two doses per day)
- Wellbutrin XL tablets (one dose per day)

The drug bupropion (Zyban) is the same drug as Wellbutrin, but Zyban is FDA approved and usually prescribed for smoking cessation.

Desyrel's mode of action is similar to that of SNRI drugs, as this drug prevents the reuptake of both serotonin and norepinephrine. This uptake occurs through a different mechanism, however. Specifically, it is a serotonin inhibitor/antagonist. The most common side effect of Desyrel is drowsiness; for this reason, this drug should be taken at bedtime. The most common side effect of Wellbutrin is insomnia; for this reason, this drug should be taken at least two hours before bedtime.

Bipolar Disorder

Another form of depression is bipolar disorder. **Bipolar disorder** differs from depression in that patients with bipolar disorder experience a period of mania followed by a period of depression. Bipolar disorder occurs in a small percentage of the population (an estimated 1 percent).

Bipolar disorders fall into several different categories based on the frequency of the mania and the depression symptoms. For diagnostic purposes, the patient must experience three or more of the following symptoms:

- Mood swings toward elevated or expansive ideation
- Irritability
- Grandiose ideation
- Inability to control thoughts (racing ideas)
- Inability to control talking
- Distractibility
- Laughing inappropriately
- Bizarre behaviors
- Lack of need for sleep
- Inflated self-esteem
- Increased goal-directed activities

- Extensive increase in pleasurable activities without regard for consequences (sexual behaviors, shopping sprees, alcohol abuse, drug abuse, or dangerous driving)

When three of more of these symptoms are present, the patient meets the current criteria for a mania episode. The depression cycle of the bipolar disorder is diagnosed using the criteria noted previously in this chapter. A bipolar patient can have both the mania and the depression symptoms cycle within the same day. If both are occurring the same day, the patient can be diagnosed with mixed disorder bipolar disease.

Drug Treatment for Bipolar Disorder

Historically, many different drugs have been used to treat bipolar disorder. Some of these drugs, primarily anticonvulsant drugs, are still used today, usually as a second line of treatment. Drugs such as carbamazepine (Tegretol), divalproex sodium (Depakote), and valproic acid (Depakene) are some of the anticonvulsants used to treat bipolar patients. These drugs are discussed in Chapter 10. Today, the first drug of choice for treatment of bipolar disorder is lithium. Lithium is a **mood-stabilizing agent**—that is, a drug prescribed to stabilize a patient between the states of mania and depression.

Although lithium's mode of action is unknown, it is believed to decrease bipolar symptoms by indirectly interfering with the movement of sodium in nerve and muscle cells. Lithium is also known to decrease the production of certain neurotransmitters in the central nervous system while increasing the removal of norepinephrine at the nerve synapses. Lithium is available as a generic drug along with the brand-name Lithobid.

The pharmacy technician needs to take special care when entering a new prescription for lithium in the pharmacy computer system or when refilling an existing lithium prescription. If the pharmacy must change its source of lithium from one manufacturer to another, this must be explained to the patient. The patient should contact his or her provider to determine whether blood levels need to be done because small blood-level changes can have serious side effects. Serum lithium levels are drawn on a regular basis and may fluctuate somewhat when different formulations are used. The blood levels can respond to changes in the formulation of the drug that result from different manufacturers making the lithium. When this happens, the patient may experience side effects or withdrawal symptoms.

Lithium is a drug with a small therapeutic window. (A drug's therapeutic window is the range of dosages at which a drug is most effective with minimal toxicity.) Lithium has a very small effective dosage range before the drug can become very toxic to the patient. A dosing error with lithium could cause serious, potentially fatal, consequences for the patient.

One difficulty in diagnosing and treating patients with bipolar disorder is the fact that some symptoms resemble other psychotic diseases such as schizophrenia, which is discussed in the next section.

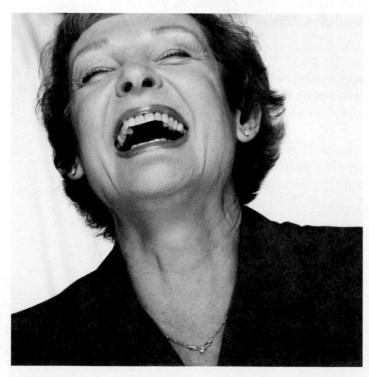

Patients with bipolar disorder experience cycles of mania, characterized by inability to control talking, distractibility, laughing inappropriately, bizarre behaviors, and lack of need for sleep, followed by depression.

Psychosis

Psychosis describes mental illnesses that dramatically interfere with a person's ability to function normally. Symptoms of psychosis include personality changes, impaired function, and a distorted sense of reality. Psychosis may appear as a symptom of some mental disorders, including personality and mood disorders.

Schizophrenia is one of the most commonly diagnosed types of psychosis. Schizophrenia is chronic, and therefore usually requires lifelong treatment. Unfortunately, drug therapy does not alter the course of schizophrenia. Instead, drug treatment decreases the patient's symptoms. The goal is for the patient to be able to function and thus improve his or her quality of life. Often, however, the patient continues to experience some symptoms even with drug treatment. Some common schizophrenia symptoms include the following:

- Delusions
- Detachment from reality
- Hallucinations
- Emotional withdrawal
- Disorganized speech
- Grossly disorganized behavior
- Flat affect
- Inability to function
- Self-care deficits
- Lack of spontaneity

Although the actual cause of schizophrenia is not yet known, scientific evidence does show several unique characteristics in the brains of patients with schizophrenia. For example, many schizophrenia patients show anatomic differences in the ventricles of their brain, while some schizophrenia patients show size differences in the frontal brain lobe. Research also shows the possibility of a neurotransmitter problem, specifically dopamine transmission. Dopamine levels are elevated in many schizophrenia patients.

Four different nerve pathways have been identified that use dopamine as their neurotransmitter. Scientists have shown that the nerve pathway involving the limbic system is the one responsible for schizophrenia symptoms. When dopamine levels become elevated in this limbic pathway, schizophrenia symptoms manifest themselves or increase in severity. The mode of action of drugs currently on the market to treat schizophrenia (the antipsychotic drugs) involves these pathways and their dopamine levels.

Antipsychotic Drug Therapy

Drugs to treat schizophrenia can be divided into two classes. One class, the older drugs, affects the dopamine levels in all four nerve pathways. The newer class of antipsychotic drugs, called atypical antipsychotic drugs, affects only the limbic-system pathway. Additionally, atypical antipsychotic drugs seem to affect the serotonin and histamine receptors. Because atypical antipsychotic drugs affect only the limbic pathway, these drugs have fewer negative side effects for the patient than the older drugs do.

Atypical Antipsychotic Drugs

Atypical antipsychotic drugs are currently the first line of treatment for schizophrenia. Although atypical antipsychotic drugs have fewer side effects than the older antipsychotic drugs, some of their side effects can be serious. Some potential side effects

Table 9.4 Common Atypical Antipsychotic Drugs

Generic Name	Brand Name	Dosage Forms
Aripiprazole	Abilify	Tablet
Olanzapine	Zyprexa	Injection, tablet
Paliperidone	Invega	Tablet
Quetiapine	Seroquel	Tablet
Risperidone	Risperdal	Liquid, tablet
Ziprasidone	Geodon	Capsule, injection

of atypical antipsychotic drugs include hyperglycemia, new onset of diabetes, weight gain, increase in lipid levels, and an increase in the **QT interval** (that is, the time it takes for an electrical signal in the heart to travel through the ventricles). Increasing the QT interval can result in arrhythmias, some of which could be life threatening.

Commonly prescribed atypical antipsychotic drugs are shown in **TABLE 9.4**. One atypical antipsychotic drug, clozapine (Clozaril), was one of the first on the market. Due to the drug's potential to cause a life-threatening reduction of white blood cells, however, this drug would no longer be considered a commonly prescribed atypical antipsychotic. Another atypical antipsychotic drug, aripiprazole (Abilify), has not been shown to increase the QT interval. Therefore, this drug may be the drug of choice among atypical antipsychotics.

Question: The pharmacy technician is presented with a new prescription for clozapine (Clozaril). What should he or she do?

Answer: The pharmacy technician should ask for the pharmacist's assistance because this drug has many special prescribing and filling requirements.

Typical Antipsychotic Drugs

Haloperidol (Haldol) is an example of a typical antipsychotic drug or first-generation antipsychotic. Other typical antipsychotic drugs are listed in **TABLE 9.5**.

Although these first-generation drugs are effective, they do have serious side effects. Just a few of the more serious potential side effects include increasing heart rate, high blood sugar, gray appearance of the skin, blindness, **extrapyramidal symptom (EPS)** (a symptom that derives from the extrapyramidal pathways in the nervous system), and **tardive dyskinesia** (involuntary repetitive body movements). Because of their potential for side effects, prescribers have moved to atypical antipsychotic drugs as their first drugs of choice in treating schizophrenia and other psychosis. If one of these

Table 9.5 Common Typical Antipsychotic Drugs

Generic Name	Brand Name	Dosage Forms
Fluphenazine	Prolixin	Injection, tablet
Haloperidol	Haldol	Injection, liquid, tablet
Loxapine	Loxitane	Capsule, liquid
Perphenazine	Trilafon	Injection, liquid, tablet
Thiothixene	Navane	Capsule, injection, liquid
Trifluoperazine	Stelazine	Injection, liquid, tablet

older drugs must be used, three drugs can currently be ordered to try to minimize the negative side effects of EPS and tardive dyskinesia. These are benztropine (Cogentin), diphenhydramine (Benadryl), and meclizine (Antivert).

As noted before, neither the atypical nor the typical antipsychotic drugs alter the course of the psychosis. Therefore, these drugs must be taken by the patient indefinitely. Both of these classes of drugs must be taken for a length of time—usually between 12 and 18 weeks—before the maximum effect will be noted. One of the accompanying disease states for some patients with schizophrenia is anxiety. Anxiety is discussed in the next section.

Anxiety

Anxiety disorders manifest themselves in many different forms, from **panic disorder**, to **posttraumatic stress disorder (PTSD)** and substance abuse–induced anxiety, to **obsessive-compulsive disorder (OCD)**. Several common symptoms of anxiety disorders include the following:

- Nervousness
- Apprehensive behavior
- Avoidance of people or places
- Feelings of losing control mentally or physically
- Fear with no known source
- Inability to concentrate
- Insomnia
- Feelings of terror
- Increased heart rate
- Feelings of powerlessness
- Religious distress
- Decreased coping skills
- Headaches
- Generalized tension

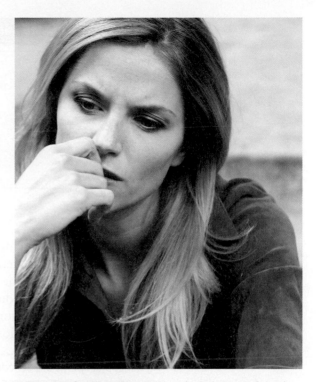

Symptoms of anxiety disorder may include: unexplained nervousness, rapid heartbeat, avoidance of people or places, feelings of losing control mentally or physically, and fear with no known source.

Like several other disorders covered in this chapter, anxiety involves neurotransmitters. With anxiety, though, the neurotransmitters involved not only include serotonin and norepinephrine, but also the inhibitory neurotransmitter **gamma-aminobutyric acid (GABA)**. The presence of GABA in the synapse of the nerve pathway prevents the rapid transmission of nerve signals, thus decreasing the symptoms of anxiety.

Anti-anxiety Drug Therapy

Many different drugs are prescribed for anxiety. These anti-anxiety drugs are composed of drugs from several different drug classes. The class called **benzodiazepines** is the most commonly prescribed anti-anxiety drug class. Two drugs from other classes include buspirone (Buspar) and venlafaxine (Effexor). Both of these drugs were originally approved for the treatment of depression. A list of commonly prescribed anti-anxiety drugs appears in TABLE 9.6.

Table 9.6   Common Anti-anxiety Drugs

Generic Name	Brand Name	Dosage Forms
Alprazolam	Xanax	Liquid, tablet
Chlordiazepoxide	Librium	Capsule
Clorazepate	Tranxene	Tablet
Diazepam	Valium	Injection, IV, liquid, tablet
Lorazepam	Ativan	Injection, IV, liquid, tablet
Oxazepam	Serax	Capsule, tablet

Benzodiazepines are important because their onset of action is quick, unlike both buspirone (Buspar) and venlafaxine (Effexor), which can take days to weeks to reach their full potential. On the negative side, benzodiazepines have several side effects, including muscle relaxation, sedation, confusion, and the potential for both physical and psychological addiction. To lessen this potential, all benzodiazepines should be prescribed at the lowest dosage for the shortest period.

All benzodiazepines are Schedule IV controlled substances.

An extreme type of anxiety is a **panic attack**. A panic attack can be overwhelming for the patient. Unlike **general anxiety disease (GAD)**, which is characterized by long-term feelings of excessive worry and anxiety, panic attacks have a specific starting point and ending point. Another difference between panic attacks and GAD is that panic attacks usually involve an overwhelming feeling of fear or apprehension. Panic attacks can cause the patient to experience chest pain, difficulty breathing, and a rapid heart rate. Frequent panic attacks can be totally disabling, as the patient becomes fearful of leaving home. Panic attacks are generally treated with the same drugs as other anxieties.

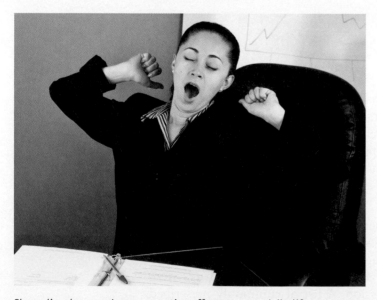

Sleep disorders can have a negative effect on your daily life.

Sleep Disorders

Sleep is a fundamental physiological function for all people. Sleeping allows the body and mind to rest and be restored. **Insomnia**, or the inability to fall asleep or sleep throughout the night, can lead to other medical conditions.

Quite a few factors can result in insomnia. These include poor sleep preparation, such as drinking caffeine or alcohol prior to going to bed. Insomnia can also be caused by stress or by medical issues such as pain or respiratory problems. Lastly, insomnia can be caused by psychiatric illnesses such as schizophrenia.

One major drug class prescribed to treat insomnia is benzodiazepines, discussed in the preceding section. Other drug groups prescribed for insomnia include barbiturates, antihistamines, and hypnotics. A **hypnotic drug** is a drug that induces sleep. **TABLE 9.7** contains a list of drugs prescribed for insomnia other than benzodiazepines.

Table 9.7	Drugs Used for Insomnia		
Generic Name	**Brand Name**	**Dosage Forms**	**Control Schedule**
Amobarbital	Amytal	Capsule, injection, IV, tablet	CII
Butabarbital	Butisol	Liquid, tablet	CIII
Secobarbital	Seconal	Capsule	CII
Diphenhydramine	Benadryl	Capsule, injection, IV, tablet	Not scheduled
Hydroxyzine	Atarax/Vistaril	Capsule, injection, tablet	Not scheduled
Chloral hydrate	Somnote	Capsule, liquid, suppository	CIV
Ramelteon	Rozerem	Tablet	Not scheduled
Eszopiclone	Lunesta	Tablet	CIV
Zaleplon	Sonata	Capsule	CIV
Zolpidem	Ambien	Tablet	CIV

Alcoholism/Alcohol Dependence

Alcoholism is a condition that makes those affected unable to stop consuming alcohol. Those suffering from alcoholism, also described as alcohol dependence, show signs of physical addiction. Alcoholism is an addiction to alcohol that affects a person for his or her entire lifetime. Alcoholism may have a genetic factor, as other members within an alcoholic's family tree are also likely to be alcoholics. Alcoholics drink for different reasons. Two common reasons include chronic pain and emotional pain.

Unlike the occasional drinker, the alcoholic is unable to stop drinking. In fact, a sudden stop in alcohol intake can result in alcohol withdrawal. Withdrawal can cause different medical problems. Some common medical issues resulting from abrupt withdrawal include mental issues, tremors, and disorientation. In some cases, the medical issues from alcohol withdrawal can be life threatening. Common life-threatening medical issues include convulsions and collapse of the blood-circulation system.

Treatment for alcoholism involves a combination of mental-health counseling, family support, and drug therapy. Drug therapy's mode of action involves using antagonist drugs. Disulfiram (Antabuse) and naltrexone (ReVia) are examples. Both drugs cause negative symptoms to appear when the alcoholic consumes any type of drink containing alcohol. These symptoms can be as mild as making alcohol consumption less pleasurable. Disulfiram (Antabuse) is an alcohol antagonist drug that exhibits effects that are more extreme, including confusion, extreme nausea, and a very hot and red-colored face, that occur with even small amounts of alcohol. This is referred to as a disulfiram-like reaction. Naltrexone (ReVia) is an opioid antagonist drug that is used to decrease the consumption of alcohol and as an aid in the treatment of alcoholism. It does not cause a disulfiram-like reaction.

The use of a drug to treat alcoholism functions as a support to prevent relapses. The most important part of treating an alcoholic is a desire on the part of the alcoholic to stop drinking. Family and psychosocial support is essential.

Tech Math Practice

Question: **You receive a prescription for citalopram 25mg oral liquid po daily. Dispense 30-day supply. It is stocked in a concentration of 10mg/5mL. How many ounces of citalopram liquid do you dispense?**

Answer: Set up a ratio proportion of $^{10mg}/_{5mL} \times {}^{25mg}/_{xmL}$. Then cross-multiply: xmL = 25mg × 5mL/10mg = 12.5mL. Next, multiply 12.5mL/day × 30 days = 375mL. Finally, calculate the following: 375mL ÷ 30mL/ounce = 12.5 ounces.

Question: **You receive a prescription for thioridazine 35mg po tid. Dispense 30-day supply. The pharmacy stocks 10mg, 25mg, and 50mg tablets. What would you dispense?**

Answer: The only way to make a 35mg dose is to use 10mg tablets and 25mg tablets. Two prescription bottles will be filled as follows.

Bottle #1:
Dispense #90 because one tablet/dose × 3 doses/day = 3tablets/day × 30 days = 90 tablets dispensed of the 10mg strength

Bottle #2:
Dispense #90 because one tablet/dose × 3 doses/day = 3 tablets/day × 30 days = 90 tablets dispensed of the 25mg strength

The label will need to instruct the patient to take the pills together to equal the total of 35mg.

Question: **You receive a prescription for alprazolam 0.25mg po. Dispense #100, Sig: 1–2 tablets every 4 hours as needed for anxiety. What is the minimum amount of time after which the patient can legally refill this medication?**

Answer: The patient could, by the prescription sig, take two tablets every four hours around the clock, for a maximum of 12 tablets per day. Therefore, you must divide the number of tablets prescribed (100 tablets) by 12: 100 tablets ÷ 12 doses maximum/day = 8.3 days. The patient could legally refill the prescription after eight days.

Question: **You receive a prescription for chloral hydrate 500mg by mouth, one dose now, and may repeat one time if necessary prior to CT scan. The prescription is for a five–year-old. The physician requests that liquid be dispensed. Chloral hydrate liquid is available in a concentration of 500mg/5mL. How many teaspoonfuls of chloral hydrate liquid will you dispense?**

Answer: The total dose will be 2 doses × 500mg/dose = 1,000mg total for dispensing, or 2 doses × 5mL/dose = 10mL. Each teaspoonful = 5mL; therefore, you will dispense 2 teaspoonfuls of chloral hydrate liquid.

Question: **You receive a prescription for amitriptyline 25mg #270 Sig: 1 tablet 3 times daily. How many days' supply is this prescription written for?**

Answer: 1 tablet/dose × 3doses/day = 3 tablets per day. 270 tablets ÷ 3 tablets/day = 90-day supply.

Question: **You receive a prescription for disulfiram 250mg #42 tablets Sig: 2 tablets daily for 2 weeks then 1 tablet daily thereafter. How many days will this prescription last?**

Answer: First, determine how many tablets will be used in the first two weeks:

2 tablets/day × 14 days (2 weeks) = 28 tablets in the first two weeks

Then, subtract the number of tablets used in the first two weeks from the total number of tablets prescribed:

42 tablets – 28 tablets = 14 tablets remaining from that prescribed

Next, determine how many days those 14 tablets will last, given that the prescription calls for one tablet per day after the first two weeks. At one per day, the 14 tablets will last 14 days.

Set up a ratio proportion for 1 tablet/day = 14 tablets/x days. Then cross-multiply: x = 14 tablets/1 tablet per day = 14 days.

Finally, add together the number of days covered by the prescription:

14 days + 14 days = 28 days.

Question: **You receive a prescription for Zolpimist (zolpidem) spray #1 canister Sig: 2 sprays at bedtime as needed. The concentration is 5mg/0.1mL/1 spray. How many milligrams of zolpidem are inhaled in two sprays of the canister?**

Answer: Set up a ratio proportion for $^{5mg}/_{1\ spray} = {}^{xmg}/_{2\ sprays}$. Then cross-multiply: $x$mg = 5mg × 2sprays/1spray = 10mg.

Question: **You receive a prescription for lorazepam 0.5mg #45 Sig: 0.25 tablet q hs. How many days' supply is this prescription for?**

Answer: The patient will be taking ½ tablet at bedtime. Therefore, 45 tablets × 2 doses/tablet = 90 doses ÷ 1 dose/day = 90 days' supply.

Question: **A patient has been stabilized on Tranxene 3.75mg po tid. What strength of Tranxene SR would be equivalent to this dose?**

Answer: 3.75mg/dose × 3doses/day = 11.25mg sustained-release product/day. When converting a therapy to a sustained-release product of the same therapy, the prescriber attempts to prescribe as close to the same total daily does as is available to maintain the patient's stabilized response to the current dosing regimen.

Question: **A prescription is presented to the pharmacy for Effexor ER 75mg daily, increase by 75mg every 4 days until max dose of 225mg/day is reached and maintain that therapy. Quantity: 30-day supply. How many 75mg capsules will you dispense?**

Answer: First, determine how many 75mg capsules are needed for the first four days of therapy, at 75mg/day:

75mg/day × 4 days × 1 capsule/75mg = 4 capsules

Next, determine how many 75mg capsules are needed for the next four days of therapy, at 150mg/day:

150mg/day × 4 days × 2 capsules/150mg = 8 capsules

Then, calculate how many days remain for the prescription:

4 days + 4 days = 8 days

30 days total − 8 days filled = 22 days remaining

Next, determine how many 75mg capsules are needed for the remaining 22 days of therapy at 225mg/day:

225mg/day × 22 days × 3 capsules/225mg = 66 capsules

Finally, add together the total number of capsules needed for the 30-day supply:

4 capsules + 8 capsules + 66 capsules = 78 capsules

Question: **Oxazepam is the suggested benzodiazepine for use in patients receiving disulfiram. You have a patient who has brought in a prescription for disulfiram 250mg Sig: 1 tablet daily, and oxazepam 15mg Sig: 1 tablet qid. How many tablets will this patient take daily if he takes only these two prescription products?**

Answer: First, determine how many disulfiram tablets the patient will take daily:

250mg/tablet × 1 tablet/dose × 1 dose/day = 1 tablet daily

Next, determine how many tablets of oxazepam the patient will take daily:

15mg/1 tablet × 1 tablet/dose × 4doses/day = 4 tablets daily

Finally, add together the number of tablets taken daily:

1 tablet disulfiram + 4 tablets oxazepam = 5 tablets daily

Question: **A patient presents with a prescription for lithium oral solution #600mL, Sig: 8mEq po qid. Lithium oral solution concentration is 8mEq/300mg/5mL. How many milligrams will the patient take daily?**

Answer: Patient is taking 8mEq, which equals 5mL, which equals 300mg po four times a day. 300mg/dose × 4 doses/day=1,200mg daily.

Question: **You have an order for diazepam 1mg IM now. The diazepam concentration is 5mg/mL. How many milliliters of diazepam injection will be administered?**

Answer: Set up a ratio proportion: $\frac{5mg}{mL} = \frac{1mg}{xmL}$. Then cross-multiply: xmL = 1mg × 1mL/5mg = 0.2mL.

WRAP UP

Chapter Summary

- The patient profile is an essential document in the pharmacy.
- All patient information is confidential.
- A drug side effect is related to the mode of action of a drug.
- A drug allergy is a hypersensitivity to a drug.
- E-prescribing or electronically sending prescriptions is increasing.
- Understanding the basic information on a prescription is essential for all pharmacy technicians.
- Controlled-substance prescriptions are for drugs assigned to controlled drug schedules based on their potential for addiction and abuse.
- Understanding all the information printed on a prescription label is essential for all pharmacy technicians.
- The drugs prescribed for anxiety, depression, and psychosis have a mode of action that affects neurotransmitters. A neurotransmitter is a chemical in the nervous system.
- Many diseases have an associated drug pathway, or algorithm. A drug pathway or algorithm is a step-by-step process for treating specific diseases.
- Anti-anxiety drugs are prescribed for all types of anxiety, including panic attacks.
- Many of the drugs prescribed for insomnia are the same drugs prescribed for anxiety.
- The most common class of drugs prescribed for anxiety is benzodiazepines. All benzodiazepines are controlled substances. As controlled substances, all benzodiazepines have the potential for addiction and abuse.
- Reuptake inhibitor drugs are prescribed for different diseases, with depression being the common reason for use.
- Reuptake inhibitor drugs prevent the destruction of a neurotransmitter by preventing reuptake of the neurotransmitter into the storage site.

- Serotonin syndrome is a potentially life-threatening side effect of excessive serotonin. Serotonin syndrome can occur when two different drugs that have the same mode of action—the prevention of the destruction of the neurotransmitter serotonin—are prescribed.

Learning Assessment Questions

1. What is a patient profile?
   A. A record that contains only the patient's address, age, and credit-card information
   B. A record that contains all the information needed to accurately and safely fill a prescription for a patient
   C. A record that contains only the patient's physician information and allergies
   D. A record that contains all the patient's allergies

2. All patient information is confidential, and a violation of HIPAA regulations can result in disciplinary action.
   A. True
   B. False

3. Common patient profile items include all but which of the following?
   A. Gender
   B. Herbal meds being taken
   C. Patient preferences
   D. Patient's children's birth dates

4. If a patient presents a new prescription to the pharmacy technician and the patient already has a computerized patient profile, the pharmacy technician should do which of the following?
   A. Say, "Thank you, your prescription will be ready in a few minutes."
   B. Ask to see the patient's prescription insurance card.
   C. Review with the patient the accuracy of the patient profile information.
   D. Have the patient complete a new patient form.

5. All but which of the following could result from a drug allergy?

   A. Anaphylaxis

   B. Hives

   C. Death

   D. Drowsiness

6. What is one of the most common problems encountered in the day-to-day activities of the community pharmacy?

   A. Computer malfunction

   B. No lunch break in an eight-hour shift

   C. Issues with insurance-company approvals and payments

   D. Patient allergies

7. What might the result of inaccurate or incomplete allergy information in a computerized patient profile be?

   A. The patient's name is spelled wrong on her prescription label.

   B. The insurance billing is rejected.

   C. There is no effect.

   D. The computer software is prevented from cross-checking other drugs against patient allergies.

8. Which of the following types of prescriptions can never be refilled without a new hard copy prescription from the physician?

   A. Schedule V

   B. Schedule IV

   C. Schedule III

   D. Schedule II

9. Which of the following have the most potential to be an altered prescription?

   A. Controlled-substance prescriptions

   B. Blood pressure prescriptions

   C. OTC prescriptions

   D. Prescriptions for a diabetic patient

10. Schedule III, IV, and V prescriptions can be refilled for how long and how many times (provided the physician has authorized the refills)?

    A. Three months, three refills

    B. Six months, five refills

    C. Four months, five refills

    D. Six months, three refills

11. Which of the following is a common abbreviation in pharmacy, and what is its meaning?

    A. Sig, meaning "Physician signature"

    B. Rx, meaning "Recipe" or "Prescription"

    C. Dr, meaning "The Dr. is a licensed MD"

    D. Quan, meaning "The number of days the patient will be taking the medication"

12. Sertraline is an example of which of the following?

    A. An SSRI with an indicated use for depression

    B. An SNRA with an indicated use for insomnia

    C. An MAOI with an indicated use for insomnia

    D. A tricyclic antidepressant with an indicated use for depression

13. What is the most common class of drugs prescribed for depression?

    A. Tricyclic

    B. MAOI

    C. SSRI

    D. SNRR

14. Which of the following describes serotonin syndrome?

    A. An understimulation of the serotonin receptors

    B. An overstimulation of the serotonin receptors

    C. An extremely common occurrence when taking SSRIs

    D. An extremely common occurrence when taking MAOIs

15. Severe and sometimes fatal hypertensive crisis can occur when a patient taking an MAOI eats food that contains tyramine. Which of the following foods contains tyramine?

    A. Potato chips

    B. Vodka

    C. Aged cheese

    D. Green leaf lettuce

16. Zyban, usually prescribed for smoking cessation, has the same generic name as which of the following drugs?

    A. Selegiline

    B. Wellbutrin

    C. Amitriptyline

    D. Clomipramine

17. Bipolar disorders fall into several different categories, based on which of the following?

    A. The frequency of the mania versus the depression symptoms

    B. The severity of the mania versus the depression symptoms

    C. The quality of the mania versus the depression symptoms

    D. The patient's suicidal tendencies

18. What brain chemical level is noted to be higher in schizophrenic patients?

    A. Norepinephrine

    B. Adrenalin

    C. Epinephrine

    D. Dopamine

19. Which of the following describes the newer class of antipsychotic drugs, called atypical antipsychotic drugs?

    A. They affect only the limbic system pathway.

    B. They affect only the serotonin pathway.

    C. They affect only the norepinephrine pathway.

    D. They affect only the dopamine levels.

20. Lithium is considered to be which of the following:

    A. An antidepressant

    B. An SSRI

    C. An SNRI

    D. A mood-stabilizing agent

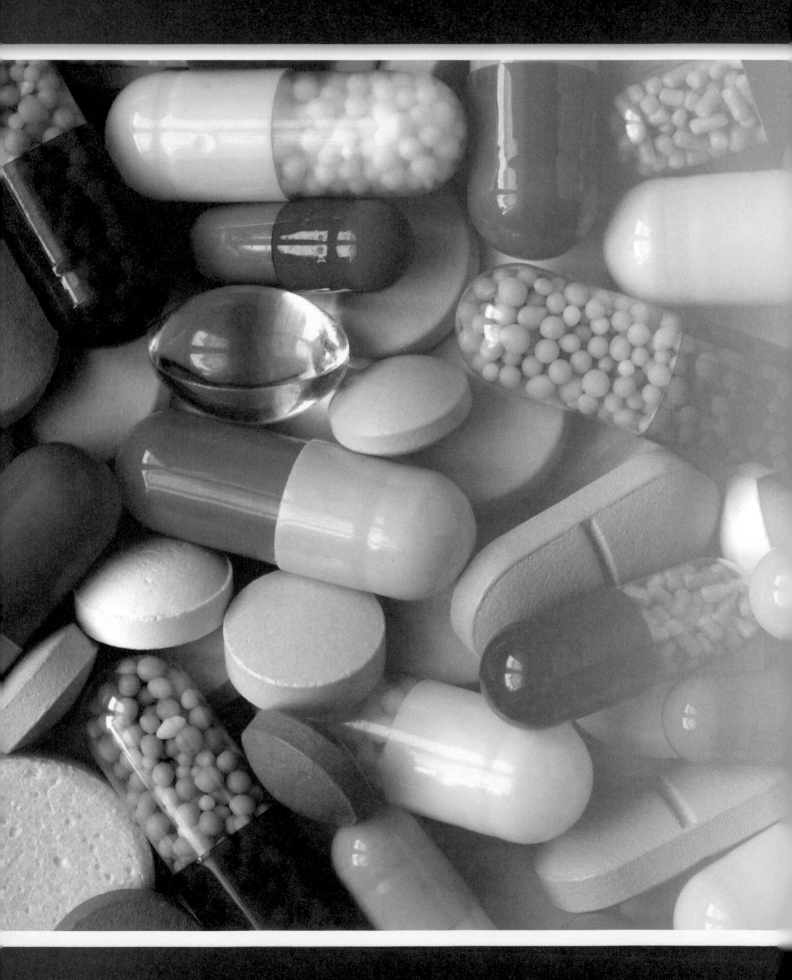

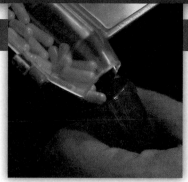

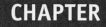
Labs for the Community Pharmacy

OBJECTIVES

After reading this chapter, you will be able to:

- Use a patient-profile software system.
- Identify standard patient-profile information and evaluate a profile for completeness and accuracy.
- Demonstrate how to process a prescription.
- Demonstrate how to process a prescription refill.
- Demonstrate how to obtain refill authorizations.
- Identify the types of seizures, the drugs used to treat them, and the goals of therapy.
- Describe Parkinson's disease and the drugs used in its treatment.
- Describe attention-deficit disorders and the goals of therapy.
- Describe Alzheimer's disease and the drugs used in its treatment.

KEY TERMS

Absence seizure
Acetylcholine
Adjunctive therapy
Alzheimer's disease (AD)
Anticonvulsants
Ataxia
Atonic seizure
Attention-deficit/
    hyperactivity
    disorder (ADHD)
Aura
Concretion
Convulsion
Diplopia

Dopamine
Dyskinesia
Epilepsy
Excitatory impulse
Gingival hyperplasia
Glutamate
Hirsutism
Hydrolysis
Inhibitory impulse
Ions
Isomer
Lymphadenopathy
Myoclonic seizure
Neurons

Nystagmus
Parathesias
Parkinson's disease (PD)
Partial seizure
Primary generalized
    seizure
Prodrug
Psychomotor
Seizure
Somnolence
Status epilepticus
Substantia nigra
Tonic-clonic seizure
Urea

Chapter Overview

This chapter addresses the pharmacy technician's role in the practice of community pharmacy. It includes several labs for tasks for which a pharmacy technician is responsible in a community pharmacy setting. These tasks may include entering patient data into a computerized patient profile, managing the patient profile system, processing new prescriptions fills, and refilling prescriptions. The drug insights section of this chapter discusses the central nervous system (CNS) and medications used to treat epilepsy, Parkinson's disease, attention deficit disorders, and Alzheimer's disease.

Lab: Entering Patient Data

The legal form a physician must fill out in order for a medication to be dispensed by a licensed pharmacist is called a prescription. Prescriptions contain all the information necessary for a pharmacist to dispense the medication and for the patient to take the medication correctly.

After a patient drops off a prescription, the pharmacy technician checks the prescription to make sure it is complete. The pharmacy technician checks to see if the patient information is already in the computer system. If it is not in the computer system, the technician enters the necessary demographic, insurance, and relevant medical and health information. All this information, along with the patient's prescription history, constitutes the patient profile **FIGURE 10.1**. A patient's profile must be updated each time he or she brings in a prescription, including the information on the patient's

---

PATIENT PROFILE

Using the brand or generic name of the drug noted by the instructor on the form, the pharmacy technician will complete all questions.

Patient Name:	**JOHN A. SMITH**
Address:	**1201 PINE VIEW LANE, NEW YORK, NY 10021**
Date of Birth:	**10/06/1969**
Gender:	**MALE**
Social Security Number:	**XXX-XX-XXXX**
Home/Work Phone:	**212-333-2121 / 212-566-2134**
Cell Phone:	**212-556-2135**
Child Resistant Container/ Easy Open Bottle:	**NO**
Insurance Company/NO:	**INSURANCE COMPANY / 000-000-000**
Medical Condition:	**EPILEPSY**
Other Prescription and OTC Medications:	**NONE**
Primary Care Physician:	**DR. JANE B. DOE**

FIGURE 10.1 The essential parts of a patient profile.

insurance card 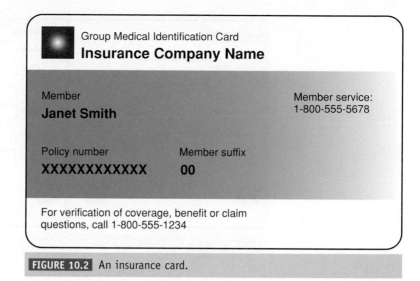. A major part of the pharmacy technician's job is to maintain the patient profile when a patient comes in to the pharmacy to get a prescription filled. If a profile for a patient already exists in the database, a patient identifier—such as the address or date of birth, in addition to the name—is used to ensure that the correct patient profile has been selected.

> The patient profile should be updated each time a patient brings in a prescription.

Group Medical Identification Card
Insurance Company Name

Member
Janet Smith

Member service:
1-800-555-5678

Policy number
XXXXXXXXXXXX

Member suffix
00

For verification of coverage, benefit or claim questions, call 1-800-555-1234

FIGURE 10.2 An insurance card.

Steps

1. After obtaining Pharmacy Rx Trainer login information from your instructor, log on to the Pharmacy Rx Trainer program. The Patient Information screen will appear **FIGURE 10.3**.
2. Type the patient's last name. For this exercise, use the information shown in Figure 10.1; enter Smith in the Last Name field. Because this is the only patient with this last name, and the patient is new to the pharmacy, no names will appear in the search results.
3. Click the Add New Patient button.
4. Enter in the following demographic information, again using Figure 10.1 as your guide: last name; first name; middle initial; date of birth; known allergies; medical condition; emergency contact's first name, last name, and phone number; address; phone number; and e-mail address. Press the Tab key to move between fields. When entering allergies, type "No Known Drug Allergies" if the patient does not have any drug allergies. As you gain proficiency with the system, you will learn the abbreviations for common drug allergies.
5. Click the Save Patient Information button.
6. Add the following information, using Figure 10.2 as your guide: insurance company name and address; pharmacy name, address, and phone number; and child-resistance safety cap information. In the insurance company and phar-

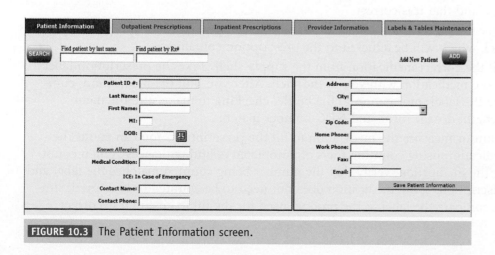

FIGURE 10.3 The Patient Information screen.

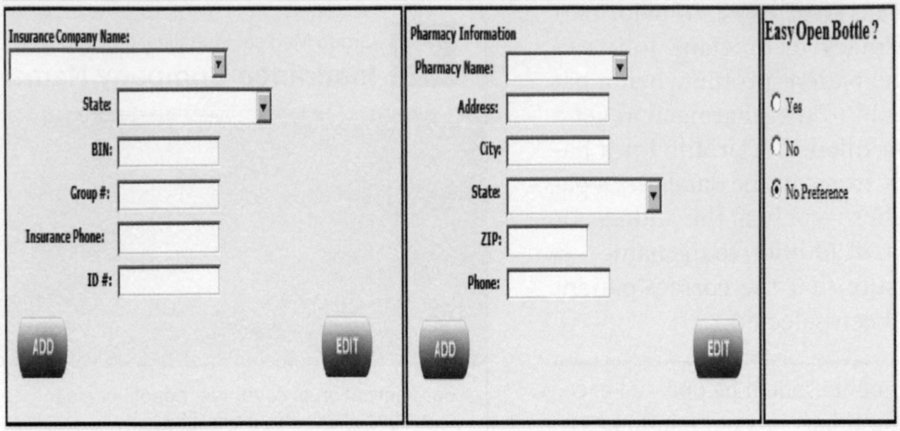

FIGURE 10.4 Insurance and pharmacy information.

macy name fields, type the name and wait to see what information populates the field. If the information is not correct, you may need to add the correct information. To add payment information, you will need the patient's insurance card.

7. Click the Save button to save this information **FIGURE 10.4**.

Lab: Processing a Prescription

In a community pharmacy, the technician usually enters the prescription orders. The technician must accurately interpret and process the prescription so that the patient receives the correct medication. The computerized label is checked against the prescription after it is filled. One label is placed on the vial for dispensing, and another label goes on the back of the original prescription. A portion of this label is also placed on a piece of paper that is signed by the patient at the time of pickup. After the prescription label is prepared, it is checked against the original prescription and is ready to be filled.

When processing a prescription, following these steps can help the pharmacy technician prevent errors:

1. Verify the prescription for completeness. The first step in processing a prescription is to verify the prescription to make sure all the necessary information is there and that it is correct.

2. Enter the prescription information into the computer system and print the label, which will be adhered to the prescription container.

3. Pull the correct medication from the supply shelf. Take the prescription label for the medication with you to the shelf. After you pull the medication, compare the label information to the bottle, checking to make sure the name, strength, dosage form, and NDC number match.

4. Count or measure the medication to fill the prescription. You can count the medication using counting trays or automated counting devices. When counting the medication, verify that the number being counted matches the label and prescription. If the medication does not need to be counted or measured, simply compare the label to the product used for the fill to ensure it is correct.

5. Select an appropriate prescription container. Choose the smallest size vial or bottle to accommodate the quantity to be dispensed. After a vial or bottle has been filled seal the container with a child-resistant lid. A patient or caregiver may request a non-child resistant lid; if this request is made, it is important to package the product accordingly for ease of use by the patient. Some pharmacies keep documentation when the patient has requested no safety caps; in most cases, this can be found on the patient profile. It is a best practice to obtain written confirmation from the patient for the safety-cap preference.

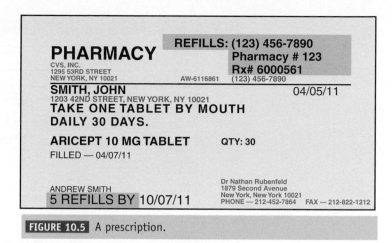

PHARMACY
CVS, INC.
1295 53RD STREET
NEW YORK, NY 10021

REFILLS: (123) 456-7890
Pharmacy # 123
Rx# 6000561
AW-6116861   (123) 456-7890

SMITH, JOHN   04/05/11
1203 42ND STREET, NEW YORK, NY 10021
TAKE ONE TABLET BY MOUTH DAILY 30 DAYS.

ARICEPT 10 MG TABLET   QTY: 30
FILLED — 04/07/11

ANDREW SMITH
5 REFILLS BY 10/07/11

Dr Nathan Rubenfeld
1879 Second Avenue
New York, New York 10021
PHONE — 212-452-7864   FAX — 212-822-1212

FIGURE 10.5 A prescription.

6. Affix the label. If the medication has been poured or counted from an original vial, place the label on the new vial, paying careful attention to keep it straight. If you are placing the label on the actual medication bottle, make sure the NDC number is not covered. All auxiliary labels must be placed in such a manner that the patient can read the instructions easily.

7. Add your initials. In some states, the pharmacy technician must initial the order after the prescription has been filled. This will communicate to the pharmacist that the prescription has been filled, and if there are errors, whom to ask. Many computer systems also keep an audit trail via the use of employee barcoding to track which employee enters, fills, and checks each prescription. However, if law or store policy requires handwritten initials, computer records may not satisfy the requirement.

8. Give the medication to the pharmacist for the final check. The last step in filling a prescription is placing the filled vial, along with the original medication container, on top of the original prescription. The pharmacist then verifies that the prescription label matches the prescription and that the medication selected by the technician matches the label **FIGURE 10.5**.

Steps

1. While logged on to the Pharmacy Rx Trainer program, click Outpatient Prescriptions in the bar at the top. The screen shown in **FIGURE 10.6** appears.
2. Click Add a New Prescription. The system prompts you to add a provider.

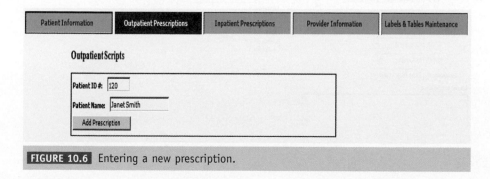

| Patient Information | Outpatient Prescriptions | Inpatient Prescriptions | Provider Information | Labels & Tables Maintenance |

Outpatient Scripts

Patient ID #: 120

Patient Name: Janet Smith

Add Prescription

FIGURE 10.6 Entering a new prescription.

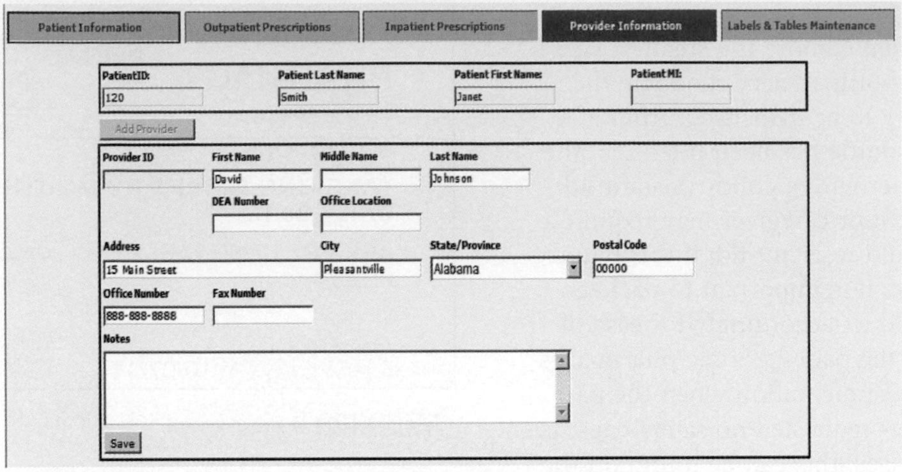

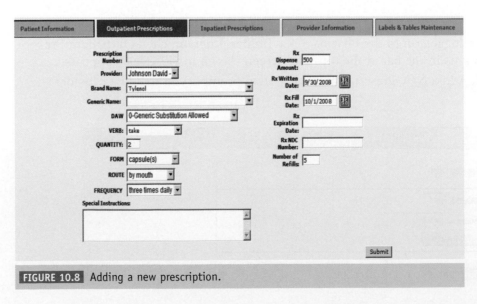

FIGURE 10.7 Adding provider information.

3. Click the Provider Information tab at the top; then click Add Provider **FIGURE 10.7**.

4. Use the information in the prescription in Figure 10.5 to enter the necessary information.

5. Add the doctor information, including the name, address, and phone number, using the information provided on the prescription in Figure 10.5.

6. Click the Save button to save the information.

7. Click Outpatient Prescriptions in the bar at the top of the screen to return to the Outpatient Prescription screen.

8. Click Add Prescription **FIGURE 10.8**.

9. Using the information in the prescription in Figure 10.5, enter the following data: doctor, drug, dispense as written information, verb, quantity, form, route of administration, frequency, quantity to dispense, the date the prescription was written, the date the prescription was filled, the expiration date of the prescription, and the number of refills permitted. For the Dispense as Written field, note that 0 = generic substitution allowed; 1 = doctor request dispense as written; 2 = patient request dispense as written; 5 = substitute brand for generic allowed; 6 = TX Medicaid only brand only; and 7 = brand drug mandated by law.

FIGURE 10.8 Adding a new prescription.

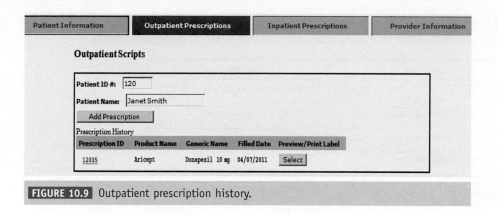

FIGURE 10.9 Outpatient prescription history.

10. Click Submit. A screen showing a history of the patient's outpatient prescriptions appears FIGURE 10.9 .

11. To view the prescription, click Prescription ID Number.

12. To view and print the label, click Preview/Print Label FIGURE 10.10 .

13. To print the label, click Select under Preview/Print Label.

14. Open the PDF file and print the label.

15. Attach one label to the bottle, vial, or bag containing the medication, and the other to the prescription for a hard copy. Print the drug monograph and make it available with the filled prescription for the pharmacist to verify that all is correct prior to dispensing.

16. Attach the drug monograph with the name of the patient showing to the pharmacy bag and place it in the bin for patient pickup.

17. To add a new drug to the formulary of drugs in the database, click the Labels and Tables Maintenance tab; then click the Add to Formulary tab FIGURE 10.11 .

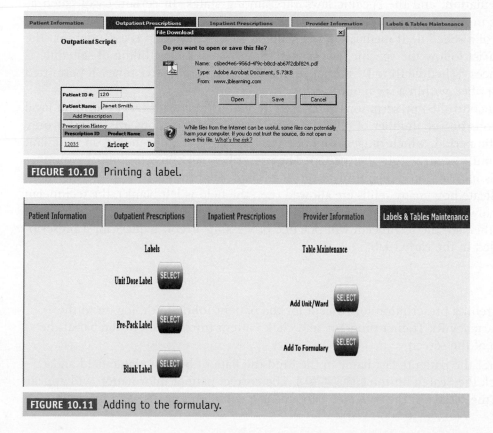

FIGURE 10.10 Printing a label.

FIGURE 10.11 Adding to the formulary.

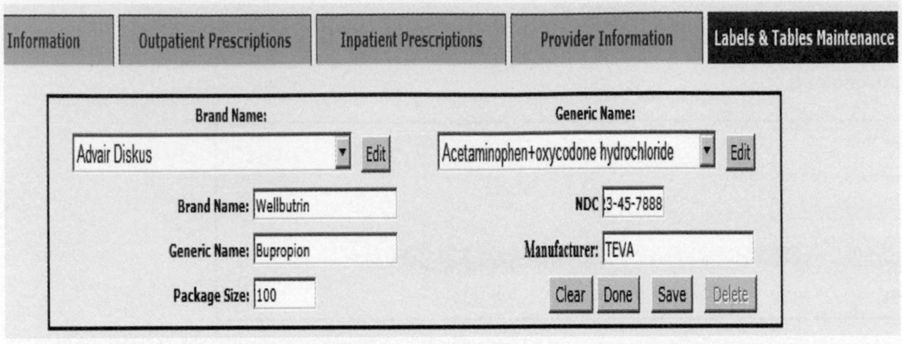

FIGURE 10.12 Saving product information to the formulary.

18. Type the brand name and generic name of the drug you are adding, the package size, the product's NDC number, and the name of the manufacturer. Then click Save FIGURE 10.12.

Repeat this same process for inpatient prescriptions.

Lab: Processing a Refill Prescription

Many patients take prescription medications over an extended period to treat ongoing medical conditions. A significant amount of a pharmacy technician's workload will involve processing requests for prescription refills.

Schedule II controlled substances cannot be refilled. A new prescription is required each time a schedule II controlled substance is dispensed. There are exceptions to this regulation, and the specific laws vary among states. In certain cases, such as hospice prescriptions and emergency situations, the pharmacist can supply a limited supply of a schedule II medication to a patient. In these cases, it is essential that the pharmacist follow the specific laws surrounding non-standard filling of schedule II substances. Schedule III to IV substances may be refilled up to five times, if permitted by prescriber, within a six-month period.

Noncontrolled prescriptions and schedule V controlled substances have no legal limitations on the number of refills. However, these prescriptions are valid for only a specific period, which ranges from one year to two years, depending on state law. Refills must occur within that period. The prescriber can chose to limit the number of refills allowed on noncontrolled or schedule V medications. If a prescriber does not indicate how many refills are allowed (i.e., the field is left blank), the technician should always assume there are no refills allowed.

In this lab, the technician will practice processing a refill request for a prescription filled in the earlier lab.

Steps

1. To refill a prescription for Aricept for the patient John Smith, log on to the Pharmacy Rx Trainer program, and click Patient Information in the bar at the top of the screen.
2. Enter the patient's last name in the Find the Patient by Last Name field and click the Search button FIGURE 10.13. The correct patient information will appear on the screen. If the patient's last name is a common one, use another unique

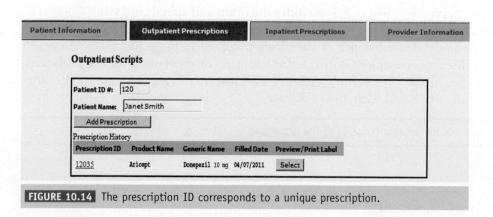

| Patient Information | Outpatient Prescriptions | Inpatient Prescriptions | Provider Information | Labels & Tables Maintenance |

SEARCH Find patient by last name Find patient by Rx#
Miller   Add New Patient ADD

Patient ID #:
Last Name:
First Name:
MI:
DOB:
Known Allergies
Medical Condition:
ICE: In Case of Emergency
Contact Name:
Contact Phone:

Address:
City:
State:
Zip Code:
Home Phone:
Work Phone:
Fax:
Email:

Save Patient Information

FIGURE 10.13 Finding the patient by last name.

patient identifier, such as the patient's date of birth, to correctly identify the patient.

3. Click Outpatient Prescriptions in the bar at the top. The patient's prescription history appears.

4. To refill a particular prescription, click the prescription ID that corresponds to the prescription **FIGURE 10.14**.

5. Enter the quantity to be dispensed and click Submit. The patient's history of outpatient prescriptions appears.

6. To view the prescription, click the prescription ID number button.

7. To view and print the label, click Preview/Print Label.

8. To print the label, click Select under Preview/Print Label.

9. Open the PDF file and print the label.

10. Attach one label to the bottle, vial, or bag containing the medication, and the other one to the prescription for a hard copy.

11. Print the drug monograph and make it available with the filled prescription for the pharmacist to verify that all is correct prior to dispensing.

12. Attach the drug monograph with the name of the patient showing to the pharmacy bag and place in the bin for patient pickup.

Repeat the same process for inpatient prescriptions.

| Patient Information | Outpatient Prescriptions | Inpatient Prescriptions | Provider Information |

Outpatient Scripts

Patient ID #: 120

Patient Name: Janet Smith

Add Prescription

Prescription History

Prescription ID	Product Name	Generic Name	Filled Date	Preview/Print Label
12035	Aricept	Donepezil 10 mg	04/07/2011	Select

FIGURE 10.14 The prescription ID corresponds to a unique prescription.

Lab: Obtaining Refill Authorizations

Often, a patient will request a refill of a medication that cannot be refilled because the prescription has expired or because the maximum number of allowable refills has been reached. Some states allow the pharmacy technician to contact the prescriber to obtain authorization for refill requests. Other states do not allow pharmacy technicians to contact the prescriber; only the pharmacist can legally obtain an authorization for a refill. For the following lab, assume that the technician practices in a state that allows him or her to contact the prescriber to obtain legal authorization for a refill request. In this lab, the pharmacy technician will simulate communication with a prescriber to obtain authorization for a refill request.

What Would You Do?

Question: A patient asks for a refill for Ritalin SR, a schedule II controlled substance that was originally filled four months ago. What would you do?

Answer: In this scenario, you would consult with the pharmacist. You would then ask the patient to return with a new prescription from the prescriber or ask the prescriber to provide a new prescription because schedule II controlled substances cannot be refilled.

Steps

1. Telephone the prescriber for the authorization request.

2. Explain to the prescriber who you are and your reason for calling. Mention the name of the pharmacy, the name of the patient, and the name of the medication(s) for which you need a refill authorization. In the case of a recorded message, provide the following information: the patient's first and last name (say it and spell it), the patient's date of birth, the medication's name (say it and spell it), the strength and quantity of the medication, the medication's instructions for use, the date of the original prescription, the date the prescription was last refilled or dispensed, the name of the prescriber, and your name and call-back number.

3. If the refill authorization is denied, make a notation of the reason for denial on the refill-authorization request form and contact the patient to notify him or her of the denial and, if available, the reason for the denial. If the authorization is granted, refill the prescription following the steps in either of the previous labs (depending on whether your pharmacy filled the original prescription).

Drug Insights: Central Nervous System Disorders

The central nervous system (CNS) includes the brain and spinal cord **FIGURE 10.15**. The brain and spinal cord serve as the main processing center that controls all the functions of the body. An imbalance of chemicals involved in these processes can result in various diseases. Treatment is directed at restoring or preventing these imbalances. Some diseases of the CNS include epilepsy, Parkinson's disease, attention-deficit/hyperactivity disorder, and Alzheimer's disease.

The central nervous system consists of the brain and spinal cord.

Epilepsy

Epilepsy is a neurological condition that is also known as a seizure disorder. It is characterized by sudden and recurring seizures. It is usually diagnosed after a person has two seizures that are unrelated to another medical disorder. **Seizures** result from an abnormal, sudden, excessive firing of a small number of **neurons**, which interferes with normal brain functioning. This abnormal electrical activity can occur in a specific area of the brain such as the outside rim of the brain, called the cortex, or can spread more extensively throughout the brain.

Seizures

All patients with epilepsy have seizures, but not all patients with seizures have epilepsy. Seizures can also be attributed to other conditions. Seizures can vary in severity, appearance, consequence, and management, and can affect different people in different ways. Patients with seizures generally have conscious periods accompanied with loss of motor control or alteration of the senses. A seizure can also result in a **convulsion**—that is, an involuntary contraction and relaxation of the muscles that causes the body to shake rapidly and uncontrollably.

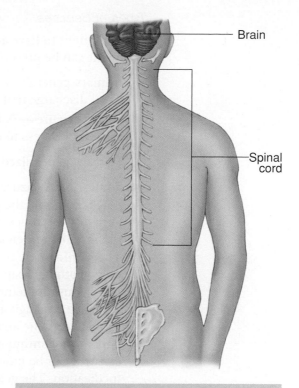

FIGURE 10.15 The central nervous system.

Neurotransmitters

Neurons are in either a resting state or a firing state. The balance between the excitatory and inhibitory impulses determines what state a neuron is in at any given time. When neurons fire uncontrollably, the excitatory impulses can lead to a seizure. Neurotransmitters bind to receptors on the cell membrane and control the movement or flow of **ions** (positive and negative) into the ion channels, and thus control whether a neuron will be in the resting or firing state. Movement of negative ions across a cell membrane inhibits a neuron from firing, while movement of positive ions induces a neuron to fire. In normal individuals, there is a balance between **excitatory impulses** (the uncontrollable firing of neurons) and **inhibitory impulses** (that is, impulses that prevent a neuron from firing). In patients with epilepsy, there is an imbalance between these impulses.

Anything that triggers an imbalance in the homeostasis of a neuron can lead to a seizure.

The two main neurotransmitters involved in seizures are **glutamate** (an excitatory neurotransmitter) and gamma-aminobutyric acid (GABA) (an inhibitory neurotransmitter). Other neurotransmitters that may play a role include **acetylcholine**, aspartate, **dopamine**, norepinephrine, and serotonin. The levels of these neurotransmitters, or the balance between glutamate and GABA, can be altered by certain conditions, which can lead to seizures. Conditions that can upset this balance include alcohol and drug abuse and withdrawal, high fever, hypoglycemia or hyperglycemia, CNS infection, brain tumor, and head injury.

Types of Seizures

It is important to have an accurate diagnosis of the type of seizure so that the correct treatment can be prescribed. Seizures can be classified into two main types:

- Primary generalized seizures—**Primary generalized seizures** begin with an electrical discharge that involves both sides of the brain and have no local origin.
- Partial seizures—**Partial seizures** are localized in a specific area of the brain, but can progress to other areas of the brain.

Primary generalized seizures are further classified as follows:

- Tonic-clonic seizures—**Tonic-clonic seizures** (formerly called grand mal seizures) combine the characteristics of tonic and clonic seizures. The seizure occurs in two phases: the tonic phase and the clonic phase. In the clonic phase, the muscles stiffen and the patient may lose consciousness and fall to the floor. The clonic phase involves muscle jerks, which may be accompanied by shallow breathing, foaming at the mouth, and loss of bladder or bowel control. Consciousness returns slowly, after which the person may be depressed, drowsy, confused, and agitated for moments or hours. These seizures generally last for between one and three minutes, except in the case of a **status epilepticus**, which is a continuous tonic-clonic seizure that lasts at least 30 minutes. These seizures can be induced by high fevers or withdrawal or noncompliance with medication. The goal of therapy with tonic-clonic seizures, and particularly status epilepticus, is to stop the convulsions and prevent brain damage.
- Absence seizures—An **absence seizure** (formerly called a petit mal seizure) is a brief episode of staring, with no convulsions, that can include changes in muscle activity. The patient may also have uncontrolled facial movements, chewing, rapid eye blinking, and twitching of the arm or leg. Absence seizures begin and end suddenly, and are usually less than 10 seconds, but can be as long as 20 seconds. The person may experience an **aura**—that is, a premonition that an attack may occur through unusual visual or sound sensations.
- Myoclonic seizures—**Myoclonic seizures** are sudden, brief muscle jerks or twitching that involve both sides of the body.
- Atonic seizures—**Atonic seizures** begin with a sudden loss of muscle strength. These seizures are also known as drop attacks because the person may suddenly drop things or fall to the ground. This seizure usually lasts less than 15 seconds.

Partial seizures can be further subdivided into simple and complex seizures. In a simple partial seizure, the patient does not lose consciousness. In a complex partial seizure, consciousness is impaired. The patient can also experience confusion and post-seizure amnesia.

Drug Therapy

Anticonvulsants, also known as antiepileptic drugs, are the drugs of choice for seizure control TABLE 10.1 . Goals of therapy are to control or reduce the frequency of seizures and to prevent behavioral and psychological changes that result from seizures. These drugs are also often indicated for other disorders.

The goal of treatment for epilepsy is to reduce the frequency of seizures and improve the quality of life.

Table 10.1	Generic and Brand Names of Commonly Prescribed Antiepileptic Drugs
Generic Name	**Brand Name**
Barbiturates	
Phenobarbital	Various
Pyrimidinediones	
Primidone	Mysoline
Benzodiazepines	
Clonazepam	Klonopin
Clorazepate	Tranxene
Diazepam	Valium
Lorazepam	Ativan
Hydantoins	
Ethotoin	Peganone
Phenytoin	Dilantin
Succinimides	
Ethosuximide	Zarontin
Other	
Carbamazepine	Tegretol
Divalproex sodium	Depakote
Gabapentin	Neurontin
Lamotrigine	Lamictal
Levetiracetam	Keppra
Oxcarbazepine	Trileptal
Tiagabine	Gabitril
Topiramate	Topamax
Valproic acid	Depakene
Zonisamide	Zonegran

To minimize the potential for drug interactions and adverse effects, treatment should begin with a single drug, increasing the dose gradually until seizures are controlled or adverse effects limit the use of the drug. If the patient does not respond adequately to one drug, additional drugs can be added. The choice of anticonvulsant will depend on the type of seizure. The need for anticonvulsant therapy should be evaluated periodically. Carbamazepine, phenytoin, and valproate stabilize the neuronal membrane and may decrease the release of excitatory neurotransmitters. Barbiturates and benzodiazepines enhance the inhibitory effect of GABA.

The choice of therapy will depend on the type of seizure.

Compared to drugs used to treat other conditions, anticonvulsants have a relatively narrow therapeutic window between the effective dose and toxicity. Drug interactions that induce or inhibit the metabolism of these drugs and cause serum concentrations of the drug to fall above or below the therapeutic index can alter their efficacy

If the therapeutic goal is not achieved with one drug, a second drug may be added or a switch to another drug can be made.

or increase the risk of toxicity. Factors that alter the pharmacokinetics of these drugs can also decrease their efficacy or increase the risk of toxicity. The American Academy of Neurology has issued a position statement recommending that generic substitutions for anticonvulsants be undertaken with caution, with the knowledge of both the prescribing physician and the patient. If possible, prescription refills should come from the same manufacturer.

All anticonvulsants have a narrow therapeutic window.

Carbamazepine (Tegretol) is available only for oral use. It is particularly effective for treatment of partial seizures and generalized tonic-clonic seizures, but may make absence or myoclonic seizures worse. Its antiepileptic effect may be related to its effect on sodium channels to limit excitatory impulses. Carbamazepine induces its own metabolism by increasing liver enzyme activity that results in its degradation. Serum concentrations often fall after a few weeks of treatment, making blood monitoring important. Therapeutic failure associated with poor bioavailability has been reported with carbamazepine, particularly when stored in humid conditions, which cause **concretion** of the tablets (that is, the tablets become harder or more solid. Carbamazepine can cause drowsiness, blurred vision, headache, dizziness, nausea, vomiting, and (although only rarely) aplastic anemia. It should be taken with food to minimize gastrointestinal disturbances.

Clonazepam (Klonopin) is a benzodiazepine used to treat myoclonic, atonic, and absence seizures resistant to treatment with other antiepileptic drugs. It is generally less effective for absence seizures than ethosuximide or valproate, and development of tolerance to its effects is common. Adverse effects of clonazepam include drowsiness and behavior disorders. Withdrawal symptoms can occur after abrupt discontinuation. The patient should avoid use of alcohol and other CNS depressants while on clonazepam therapy.

The pharmacy technician should affix a "Do Not Drink Alcohol" auxiliary label to a prescription bottle for clonazepam.

Diazepam (Valium), another benzodiazepine, is the drug of choice for treatment of status epilepticus. It can be administered through an IV or as a gel (Diastat AcuDial) available in a prefilled unit dose syringe for rectal use.

Ethosuximide (Zarontin) is recommended for treatment of uncomplicated absence seizures and is usually well tolerated. It has a long half-life, allowing for once-daily dosing, but is often divided into two doses to reduce the incidence of gastrointestinal side effects. The patient should take the dose with food. Adverse effects may include nausea, vomiting, lethargy, hiccups, headache, and behavioral changes. Patients should have a complete blood count (CBC) every four months during therapy.

Gabapentin (Neurontin) is used for **adjunctive therapy** (that is, the addition of a drug to the existing therapy) in adults and children age three and older with partial and secondarily generalized seizures. (A secondary generalized seizure starts as a partial seizure in one limited area of the brain but can spread to include the entire area of the brain and then become a generalized seizure.) Gabapentin is also effective, but not FDA-approved, as monotherapy for these same types of seizures. Like carbamazepine, gabapentin can exacerbate myoclonic seizures. Gabapentin can cause edema, weight gain, and movement disorders. Unlike some other antiepileptic drugs, gabapentin does not induce or inhibit hepatic microsomal enzymes, so it does not affect the metabolism of other drugs taken concurrently. Adverse effects include **somnolence** (sleepiness), **ataxia** (irregular muscle movements), fatigue, **nystagmus** (involuntary movement of the eyeballs), and **diplopia** (double vision). Gabapentin has also been used to treat neuropathic pain and hot flashes.

Lamotrigine (Lamictal) is FDA-approved for adjunctive therapy in adults and children age two and older with partial seizures and as monotherapy in adults with partial seizures as a substitute for carbamazepine, phenytoin, phenobarbital, primidone, or valproate. It is also FDA-approved for maintenance treatment of bipolar disorder. The most common adverse effects of lamotrigine have been dizziness, ataxia, somnolence, headache, diplopia, nausea, vomiting, rash, insomnia, and incoordination. There is a black-box warning on the package insert that recommends discontinuing lamotrigine at the first sign of rash.

Levetiracetam (Keppra) is FDA-approved as adjunctive therapy for adults and children age four and older with partial seizures, adults and children age six and older with primary generalized tonic-clonic seizures, and adults and adolescents age 12 and older with myoclonic seizures. It is available in both oral and IV formulations. Common adverse effects of levetiracetam are dizziness, somnolence, weakness, and irritability. Levetiracetam is not an inhibitor or substrate of CYP450 enzymes, and is expected to have few drug-drug interactions.

Oxcarbazepine (Trileptal) is chemically similar to carbamazepine but causes less induction of hepatic enzymes. It is approved by the FDA for treatment of partial seizures as monotherapy or adjunctive therapy in adults and children age four and older, and as adjunctive therapy in children between the ages of two and four. Like carbamazepine, oxcarbazepine is also effective in secondarily generalized seizures, but may worsen myoclonic and absence seizures. Common adverse effects of oxcarbazepine are somnolence, dizziness, diplopia, ataxia, nausea, and vomiting. Cross-reactivity with carbamazepine hypersensitivity occurs in 20 to 30% of patients. Hyponatremia is more common with oxcarbazepine than with carbamazepine. Unlike carbamazepine, oxcarbazepine does not cause induction of its own metabolism. It also decreases the effectiveness of birth-control pills. This interaction is extremely important because it may result in an unplanned pregnancy. The patient should be advised to consider using an additional form of contraception while on oxcarbazepine therapy.

Phenytoin (Dilantin) is used for treatment of partial and secondarily generalized tonic-clonic seizures. Different formulations of phenytoin may not be bioequivalent, especially at higher doses. Fosphenytoin (Cerebyx) is a water-soluble **prodrug** of phenytoin available for IV and IM use. Phenytoin is no longer considered a drug of first choice due to its complicated pharmacokinetics, inferior adverse-effect profile, and frequent drug-drug interactions. Nystagmus may occur with therapeutic serum concentrations of phenytoin and is usually present at higher concentrations. Drowsiness, ataxia, and diplopia are more likely to occur at higher serum concentrations, but can also occur at lower levels, particularly in patients with low serum albumin levels and in the elderly. **Gingival hyperplasia** (overgrowth of the gum tissue), coarsening of facial features, and **hirsutism** (excessive growth of thick dark hair in areas where there is minimal hair growth) can be troublesome. Rash may occur, usually in the first four weeks of treatment, sometimes with hepatitis, fever, and **lymphadenopathy** (enlarged lymph nodes). If rash occurs, the physician should be notified immediately, because it can progress to life-threatening Stevens Johnson syndrome. Patients should also receive routine hepatic and hematologic tests. Patients who develop hypersensitivity reactions to phenytoin are often susceptible to similar reactions with carbamazepine and phenobarbital. Phenytoin may interfere with cognitive function related to learning. Antacid and phenytoin doses should be spaced two to three hours apart. IV phenytoin should be diluted in normal saline and infused at a rate of less than 50mg/minute.

Pregabalin (Lyrica) was originally approved for the treatment of neuropathic pain associated with diabetic peripheral neuropathy and postherpetic neuralgia. It is also FDA-approved for adjunctive treatment of partial onset seizures in adults and for fibromyalgia. Among the more common adverse effects of pregabalin in clinical trials were somnolence, dizziness, ataxia, weight gain, dry mouth, blurred vision, peripheral edema, and confusion. As with gabapentin, it has no significant drug-drug interactions. Pregabalin is a schedule V controlled substance because it can cause euphoria and withdrawal.

Topiramate (Topamax) is approved for partial and primary generalized tonic-clonic seizures as monotherapy for patients age 10 and older and as adjunctive therapy in adults and children age two and older. Topiramate is also FDA-approved for migraine prophylaxis. Adverse effects of topiramate include drowsiness, dizziness, headache, and ataxia. Nervousness, confusion, **paresthesias** (the sensation of numbness or tingling on the skin), weight loss, and diplopia can occur. **Psychomotor** slowing (that is, the slowing of movement or muscular activity associated with mental processes), word-finding difficulty, impaired concentration, and interference with memory are common, particularly with rapid dose escalation and higher maintenance doses, and may require dosage reduction or stopping the drug. Topiramate is a weak carbonic anhydrase inhibitor, so it increases the risk of kidney stones. Patients should drink plenty of water to prevent the development of kidney stones.

The pharmacy technician should affix a "Drink Plenty of Water" auxiliary label to a prescription bottle for topiramate.

Valproate, which is marketed as valproic acid (Depakene) and divalproex sodium (Depakote), is approved by the FDA for monotherapy and adjunctive treatment of complex partial seizures and absence seizures and as adjunctive therapy for multiple seizure types that involve absence. The drug is also available in an IV formulation (Depacon). Because it is effective and usually well tolerated, valproate is widely used for myoclonic, atonic, and primary generalized tonic-clonic seizures. The patient should take the medication with water and should not chew or crush the tablets or capsules. Taking the dose with aspirin or aspirin products can lead to serious valproic acid toxicity. Valproate is also FDA-approved for migraine prophylaxis and bipolar disorder. Nausea and vomiting can be reduced by using the enteric-coated formulation (Depakote), by taking the drug with food, and by slow titration to an optimal dose. Weight gain is common in patients taking valproate. Serious adverse effects of the drug are uncommon, but fatal liver failure has occurred, particularly in children less than two years old taking valproate in combination with other antiepileptic drugs and in patients with developmental delay and metabolic disorders. Liver failure has also been reported in older children and adults taking valproate alone. Valproate can interfere with conversion of ammonia to **urea** (a chemical compound found in the urine that is formed from the breakdown of proteins). It can cause lethargy associated with increased blood-ammonia concentrations. The drug is contraindicated in patients with genetic defects in urea metabolism.

Valproic acid and divalproex sodium are not the same drugs.

Zonisamide (Zonegran) is a sulfonamide approved for adjunctive treatment of partial seizures in adults with epilepsy. The pharmacy technician should check for sulfa allergies when dispensing this drug. Adverse effects are usually transient and resolve on their own. They include somnolence, dizziness, confusion, anorexia, nausea, diar-

Table 10.2	First-Line Drugs of Choice for Seizure Disorders		
Seizure Type	**Generic Name**	**Brand Name**	**Available Formulation**
Partial seizures	Carbamazepine	Tegretol, Tegretol XR	Tablet, suspension
	Phenytoin	Dilantin, Dilantin-125	Capsule, tablet, suspension, injectable
	Lamotrigine	Lamictal, Lamictal CD, Lamictal ODT, Lamictal XR	Tablet
	Valproic acid	Depakene	Capsule, syrup
	Oxcarbazepine	Trileptal	Tablet, suspension
Absence seizures	Valproic acid	Depakene	Capsule, syrup
	Ethosuximide	Zarontin	Capsule, syrup
Myoclonic seizures	Valproic acid	Depakene	Capsule, syrup
	Clonazepam	Klonopin	Tablet
Tonic-clonic seizures	Phenytoin	Dilantin	Capsule, tablet, suspension, injectable
	Carbamazepine	Tegretol, Tegretol XR	Tablet, suspension
	Valproic acid	Depakene	Capsule, syrup

rhea, weight loss, agitation, irritability, and rash. Slow titration and dosing with meals may decrease the incidence of adverse effects. Zonisamide is a mild carbonic anhydrase inhibitor and may increase the incidence of symptomatic kidney stones. Patients should drink six to eight glasses of water per day to reduce the risk of kidney stones. It does not inhibit the metabolism of drugs metabolized by CYP450 isozymes.

Parkinson's Disease

Parkinson's disease (PD) is a motor-system disorder caused primarily by progressive degeneration of dopamine-containing neurons in the **substantia nigra**, which is a layer of gray substance in the brain **FIGURE 10.16**. Nerve impulses travel from the cerebral cortex to the basal nuclei and back to the cerebral cortex by electrical impulses and neurotransmitters. Normal movement requires a balance of two neurotransmitters: dopamine and acetylcholine. In healthy persons, dopaminergic neurons in the substantia nigra release enough dopamine to counterbalance the stimulating effects of acetylcholine. In PD, not enough dopamine is produced to counteract the production of acetylcholine, resulting in tremor or trembling in the hands, arms, legs, jaw, and face; rigidity; slowness of movement (bradykinesia); and postural instability.

What Would You Do?

Question: A 45 year-old patient comes into the pharmacy with a new prescription for zonisamide. While obtaining his patient information, you discover that he has a sulfa allergy. What would you do?

Answer: In this scenario, you would consult with the pharmacist and either call the physician to alert him of the sulfa allergy or ask the pharmacist to consult with the physician regarding the sulfa allergy.

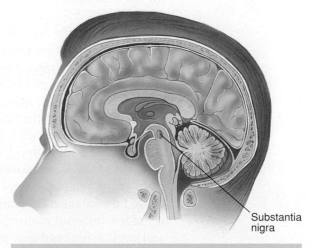

Substantia nigra

FIGURE 10.16 A cross-section of the brain.

Table 10.3   Generic and Brand Names of Commonly Used Drugs for Parkinson's Disease

Generic Name	Brand Name
M-2 Inhibitor	
Amantadine	Symmetrel
Central Nervous System Agent	
Carbidopa	Lodosyn
Central Nervous System Agent/Decarboxylase Inhibitor Combination	
Carbidopa/levodopa	Sinemet, Sinemet CR
Central Nervous System Agent/Decarboxylase Inhibitor/COMT Inhibitor Combination	
Carbidopa/levodopa/entacapone	Stalevo
MAO-B Inhibitor	
Selegiline	Eldepryl
COMT Inhibitors	
Tocapone	Tasmar
Entacapone	Comtan
Dopamine Agonists	
Bromocriptine	Parlodel
Pramipexole	Mirapex
Ropinirole	Requip
Anticholinergics	
Benztropine	Cogentin
Trihexphenidyl	Artane

Drug Therapy

There is no cure for PD. The goal of drug therapy is to provide symptomatic relief, minimize disability, and help patients maintain their quality of life. Dopamine itself cannot be used to treat PD because it does not cross the blood-brain barrier. All drugs for the treatment of PD are administered orally to reduce the incidence of side effects outside the CNS.

Levodopa, the immediate precursor of dopamine, is metabolized to dopamine in both brain and peripheral tissues. The combination of levodopa with carbidopa, a peripheral decarboxylase inhibitor, is the most effective treatment available for symptomatic relief of PD. Carbidopa prevents conversion of levodopa to dopamine in peripheral tissues, thus increasing the amount available to the CNS. For the first two to five years of treatment, levodopa produces a sustained response. As the disease progresses, however, the duration of benefit from each dose becomes shorter (the "wearing-off" effect). Still later, some patients develop sudden, unpredictable fluctuations between mobility and immobility (the "on-off" effect). After about five to eight years, the majority of patients have dose-related clinical fluctuations and dose-related **dyskinesias** (impairment of voluntary movement). As the disease progresses, levodopa-resistant motor problems (including difficulties with balance, gait, speech, and swallowing) and non-motor symptoms (including autonomic, cognitive, and psychiatric difficulties) become more pronounced. Peripheral adverse effects of levodopa, including anorexia, nausea, vomiting, and orthostatic hypotension, are prominent at the beginning of levodopa therapy. With chronic therapy, vivid dreams, hallucinations, delusions, confusion, and agitation can occur, especially in older patients with dementia. Sudden discontinuation or abrupt reduction of levodopa dosage for several days may cause a severe return of Parkinsonian symptoms. Sustained-release formulations may be beneficial for patients who experience the wearing-off phenomenon, but they can be erratically absorbed and have a slower and less-predictable onset of action.

Carbidopa/levodopa is the most effective treatment for Parkinson's disease.

Levodopa is metabolized in the periphery by two enzymes: dopa decarboxylase and catechol-O-methyl-transferase (COMT). Used in combination with levodopa, drugs that inhibit peripheral or intestinal activity of COMT prolong the half-life of levodopa and decrease Parkinsonian disability. Entacapone (Comtan) has been effective in patients with motor fluctuations resulting from the wearing-off effect. It has a short half-life and must be taken with each dose of levodopa. Entacapone is available alone and as a carbidopa/levodopa/entacapone combination (Stalevo). Tolcapone (Tasmar) is a more potent COMT inhibitor for use in patients who have not responded to entacapone. Dyskinesias, nausea, diarrhea (worse with tolcapone), and urine discoloration can occur with both COMT inhibitors. Use of tolcapone requires patient written consent and hepatic monitoring twice per month for the first six months and periodically thereafter. Because these drugs are used in combination with levodopa, the levodopa dose may have to be decreased in patients who develop dyskinesias, nausea, or hallucinations.

Amantadine (Symmetrel) is an antiviral drug that acts as an antagonist at N-methyl-D-aspartate (NMDA) receptors. Its exact mechanism of action in treating PD is unknown. It has been used alone to treat early PD or as an adjunct in later stages, usually in patients with levodopa-induced dyskinesias. Amantadine and anticholinergics may have additive adverse effects on mental function. Sudden withdrawal of amantadine may cause severe exacerbation of Parkinsonian symptoms or neuroleptic malignant syndrome and acute delirium. Taking the second dose of amantadine in the early afternoon can decrease the incidence of insomnia.

Anticholinergics such as trihexyphenidyl (Artane), benztropine (Cogentin), and biperiden (Akineton) are useful for treatment of tremor and drooling associated with PD. They balance cholinergic activity in the basal ganglia by blocking cholinergic receptors. Adverse effects include dry mouth, constipation, urinary retention, and aggravation of glaucoma. Central nervous system adverse effects, including impaired memory, confusion, and hallucinations, are particularly severe in elderly patients and generally contraindicate use of anticholinergics in this age group. Abrupt discontinuation of any of these drugs can cause severe exacerbation of symptoms.

Dopamine agonists are less effective than levodopa for motor symptoms of PD, but are less likely to cause dyskinesias or motor fluctuations. Bromocriptine (Parlodel) is an ergot-derivative dopamine agonist that improves symptoms of PD by stimulating dopamine receptors in the corpus striatum. (Ergot is a fungus that lives on rye and other grasses. Although it has been traditionally used in healing, it can also be a poison. Ergot derivatives are used to enhance the neurotransmitter dopamine.) Two oral non-ergot dopamine agonists, Pramipexole (Mirapex) and ropinirole (Requip), are used for treatment of both early (as monotherapy) and advanced disease (with levodopa). Dopamine agonists can cause nausea, somnolence, lower-extremity edema, and postural hypotension, which may limit their use. As the dosage of the dopamine agonist increases, levodopa dosage may have to be decreased. Even used alone or in low doses, dopamine agonists can cause confusion and psychosis, particularly in elderly patients. They should generally not be used in patients with dementia.

Selegiline (Eldepryl, Zelapar), an irreversible inhibitor of monoamine oxidase type B (MAO-B), inhibits the metabolism of dopamine in the brain. Selegiline's effect on symptoms is modest, but when used as monotherapy in early disease, it can delay initiation of levodopa treatment. Selegiline is available in a tablet or capsule for swallowing and in a lower-dose orally disintegrating tablet formulation (Zelapar). The disintegrating tablet formulation, which is absorbed through the oral mucosa, minimizes first-pass metabolism, increases bioavailability, and reduces serum concentrations of amphetamine metabolites.

Rasagiline (Azilect), the second MAO-B inhibitor approved for treatment of PD, also inhibits the metabolism of dopamine in the brain. Rasagiline administered early in the course of the disease may help in delaying its progression. Only rasagaline is approved by the FDA as an adjunct to levodopa for treatment of Parkinson's disease. Nausea and orthostatic hypotension may occur with MAO-B inhibitors. Unlike MAO-A inhibitors used for treatment of depression, MAO-B inhibitors at recommended doses generally do not cause hypertension after ingestion of tyramine-rich foods such as soy-based products, red wine, chocolate, aged cheese, and some fruits, including bananas, avocados, and raisins, or with concomitant levodopa therapy. Some manufacturers recommend dietary restrictions. MAO-B inhibitors can also increase levodopa adverse effects, particularly dyskinesias and psychosis in elderly patients.

Apomorphine (Apokyn), an injectable potent non-ergot dopamine agonist, is FDA-approved for treatment of immobility ("off" episodes) in patients with advanced PD. Serotonin receptor antagonists such as ondansetron are contraindicated for use with apomorphine because the combination can cause severe hypotension with loss of consciousness. Like the oral dopamine agonists, apomorphine can cause nausea, orthostatic hypotension, dyskinesias, confusion, hallucinations, and psychosis.

What Would You Do?

A patient who has been recently diagnosed with ADHD comes into the pharmacy and asks the pharmacy technician to recommend a nonstimulant medication because his current medication makes him feel "like a zombie."

In this scenario, you would tell the patient that you will get the pharmacist to speak to him.

Attention-Deficit Disorders

The majority of patients diagnosed with attention-deficit disorders are diagnosed with **attention-deficit/hyperactivity disorder (ADHD)**, which may also be referred to as attention-deficit disorder (ADD). ADHD is characterized by a persistent pattern of frequent, severe inattention and/or hyperactivity or impulsivity. The drugs used to treat both of these disorders are the same. Except for atomoxetine, guanfacine, and clonidine, all the drugs approved for treatment of ADHD by the FDA are stimulants and are classified as schedule II controlled substances by the U.S. Drug Enforcement Administration (DEA) **PHOTO 10.1**. All medications dispensed for the treatment of ADHD must include a medication guide for the patient or caretaker.

All stimulants approved for ADHD are classified as Schedule II substances by the DEA.

Drug Therapy

Atomoxetine (Strattera) is a nonstimulant, selective norepinephrine reuptake inhibitor. It has less potential for abuse than stimulants, and can be used for first-line therapy. Somnolence, nausea, and vomiting can occur, particularly when the dose is increased from initial to maximum levels within a few days. Decreased appetite can also occur, but is much less of a problem with atomoxetine than with stimulants.

Methylphenidate (Ritalin, Ritalin SR, Ritalin LA, Methylin, Methylin ER, Metadate ER, Metadate CD, Concerta, Daytrana) is the drug of choice for treatment of ADHD. It is also used for treatment of narcolepsy. The majority of methylphenidate products are mixtures of *d-* and *l-threo* enantiomers. Enantiomer is the chemical name of stereoisomers, or compounds that have the same molecular formula that are mirror images of each other. A racemic mixture contains equal amounts of the dextro- and levo-enantiomers of the same compound. Methylphenidate is available as immediate-release tablets, in controlled-release and sustained-release formulations, and as a transdermal formulation.

Concerta is the only osmotic-release methylphenidate (OROS) product currently available in the U.S. The Concerta tablet uses an osmotic delivery system to extend the duration of action of methylphenidate to up to 12 hours.

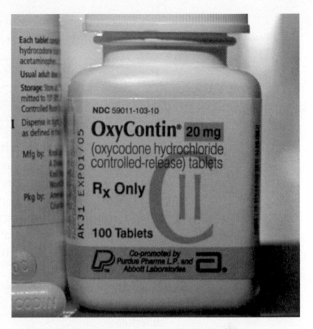

Schedule II drugs, such as methylphenidate products, feature the CII logo prominently on the label.

Daytrana is a patch formulation of methylphenidate that is worn for nine hours.

Two *d-*methylphenidate single-isomer products (Focalin and Focalin XR) are expected to have fewer side effects than methylphenidate because they contain only the pharmacologically active isomer. **Isomers** are compounds that have different structures, but contain the same number and type of atoms. Isomers are often distinguished by dextro (right) or levo (left).

Like methylphenidate, amphetamines used to treat ADHD are available as either the *d-*isomer, dextroamphetamine (Dexedrine Spansule), or as mixtures of *d-* and *l-*amphetamine (Adderall, Adderall XR). Dextroamphetamine has been as effective as methylphenidate in decreasing overactivity and inattention in children with ADHD. Some children that do not respond to methylphenidate may respond to dextroamphetamine.

Mixtures of *d-* and *l-*amphetamine are often used in patients who do not respond to dextroamphetamine or methylphenidate.

Lisdexamfetamine (Vyvanse) is a prodrug that is converted to *d-*amphetamine and *l-*lysine by enzymatic **hydrolysis**. The *l-*lysine is intended to reduce the abuse potential of dextroamphetamine.

Atomoxetine, extended-release guanfacine, and extended-release clonidine are the only non-stimulant drugs approved for ADHD.

Alzheimer's Disease

Alzheimer's disease (AD) is a degenerative disorder of the brain that leads to loss of brain function. It results in memory impairment and in loss of judgment, of decision-making ability, and of speech. It also results in changes in personality and behavior. Cognitive loss in AD is associated with depletion of acetylcholine, which is involved in learning and memory. In the early stages of the disease, the patient may experience language problems, the misplacing of items, personality changes, loss of social skills, and difficulty performing tasks that require some thought. As the disease progresses, the symptoms become worse and can interfere with normal functioning. As the disease becomes even more severe, patients with AD can no longer understand language, recognize family members, or perform basic tasks.

> The prevalence of Alzheimer's disease increases with each decade of life.

Drug Therapy

None of the treatments currently available for AD cure, reverse, or stop the progression of AD. The primary goal of therapy is to preserve patient function. Cholinesterase inhibitors increase the concentration of acetylcholine and may have beneficial effects on the symptoms of dementia, but can also cause adverse cholinergic effects such as nausea, vomiting, and diarrhea.

Tacrine (Cognex) is a cholinesterase inhibitor that has significant side effects, including hepatotoxicity. It has largely been replaced by safer, more-tolerable cholinesterase inhibitors.

Donepezil (Aricept) is a cholinesterase inhibitor approved for treatment of mild to moderately severe AD. The most common side effects are nausea, vomiting, and diarrhea.

Rivastigmine (Exelon) is another cholinesterase inhibitor approved for mild or moderate dementia from PD or AD. It is available as a solution, capsules, and patch formulation. Nausea, vomiting, and diarrhea are the most common side effects.

Galantamine (Razadyne) is the fourth cholinesterase inhibitor approved for mild or moderately severe AD. Side effects are similar to those seen with use of other cholinesterase inhibitors.

Memantine is an NMDA antagonist approved for use in patients with moderate and severe AD. Constipation, confusion, dizziness, headache, coughing, and hypertension are the most common side effects.

Tech Math Practice

Question: A prescription for immediate-release Kapvay reads, "Take one tablet two times a day," and instructs the pharmacy to dispense a 30-day supply. What quantity should be dispensed?

Answer: 2 tablets/day × 30 days = 60 tablets.

Question: A prescription for atomoxetine 80mg reads, "Take one tablet two times a day," and instructs the pharmacy to dispense a 30-day supply. The pharmacy only has 40mg tablets in stock. How many tablets should be dispensed?

Answer: Because there are only 40mg tablets in stock, each 80mg dose will require two 40mg tablets to fill. Thus, 40mg × 2 tablets = 80 mg. 2 tablets/dose × 2 doses/day = 4 tablets/day × 30 days = 120 tablets.

Question: A prescription for Dilantin oral suspension 125mg/5mL reads, "Take 125mg three times a day," and instructs the pharmacy to dispense a 30-day supply. What quantity should be dispensed?

Answer: Each dose = 5mL. 5mL/dose × 3 doses/day = 15mL/day × 30 days = 450mL.

Question: **Calculate the quantity of Parlodel to dispense for the following:**

Dispense a 14-day supply
Sig: 2 cap bid

Answer: The prescription reads 2 capsules/day × 2 doses/day = 4 capsules/day × 14 days = 56 capsules.

Question: **Calculate the quantity of Tasmar to dispense for the following:**

Dispense a 60-day supply
Sig: 1½ tab bid

Answer: The dose is 1½ tablets/dose × 2 doses/day = 3 tablets/day × 60 days = 180 tablets.

Question: **A prescription for Tegretol suspension reads, "Take 7.5mL once a day," and instructs the pharmacy to dispense a 10-day supply. What volume should be dispensed?**

Answer: 7.5mL/day × 10 days = 75mL.

Question: **A prescription for Razadyne 4mg/mL solution reads, "Take 4mg two times a day," and instructs the pharmacy to dispense a 30-day supply. What volume should be dispensed?**

Answer: The concentration is 4mg/mL with the dose being 4mg or 1mL, two times per day. 1mL × 2 doses/day = 2mL/day × 30 days = 60mL.

Question: **A prescription for a Dilantin oral suspension reads, "Take 2.5mL four times a day," and instructs the pharmacy to dispense a 30-day supply. What volume should be dispensed?**

Answer: 2.5mL/dose × 4 doses/day = 10mL/day × 30 days = 300mL.

Question: **Calculate the quantity of Comtan to dispense for the following:**

Dispense a seven-day supply
Sig: ½ tab bid

Answer: The doses = ½ tablet × 2 tablets/day = 1 tablet/day × 7 days = Seven tablets

---

Question: **Calculate the quantity to dispense for the following:**

Dispense a 30-day supply
Sig: Focalin 5mg 1½ tab qid

Answer: The dose = 1½ × 5 mg/dose = 7.5 mg/dose × 4 doses/day = 30 mg/day × 30 days = 90 tablets.

Question: **A prescription for Sinemet 10/100mg reads, "Take one tablet three times a day." How much carbidopa would the patient receive in one day?**

Answer: This Sinemet is a carbidopa 10mg/levodopa 100mg combination product. Carbidopa 10mg/dose × 3 doses/day = 30mg.

Question: **Calculate the quantity to dispense for the following:**

> Dispense a 30-day supply
> Sig: Bromocriptine 5mg tid
> The pharmacy has only 2.5mg tablets in stock.

Answer: Each dose will require two of the 2.5mg tablets to equal the 5 mg prescribed dose. So 2 tablets/dose × 3 doses/day = 6 tablets/day × 30 days = 180 2.5mg tablets.

Question: **A prescription for Namenda reads, "Take 5mg two times a day," and instructs the pharmacy to dispense a 30-day supply. The pharmacy only has a 2mg/mL solution in stock. What quantity of solution should be dispensed?**

Answer: For a dose of 5mg you must cross-multiply 2mg/mL × 5mg/x where x = 2.5mL for the dose. 2.5 mL/dose × 2 doses/day = 5mL/day × 30 days = 150mL.

WRAP UP

Chapter Summary

- A patient profile contains important personal and medical information including allergies and medication history.

- Maintaining and keeping accurate, up-to-date profiles is vital to managing a patient's medication history.

- Processing a prescription requires knowledge of how to transcribe information accurately from the prescription order.

- Controlled schedule II substances can never be refilled, except in emergency situations. Schedule III and Schedule IV controlled substances can be refilled five times within a six-month period. There are no refill limits on noncontrolled substances. These can be filled for a period of up to one year from the original date the prescription was written.

- Epilepsy is a neurologic disorder that involves an imbalance of the excitatory and inhibitory impulses in the brain that leads to seizures.

- Seizures can be classified into two main categories: generalized and partial.

- The choice of anticonvulsant will depend on the type of seizure.

- The goal of anticonvulsant therapy is to minimize the occurrence of seizures while maintaining quality of life.

- All anticonvulsants have a narrow therapeutic range. Product substitutions can result in loss of seizure control or toxicity.

- In Parkinson's disease, there is an imbalance between dopamine and acetylcholine.

- The drug of choice for the treatment of Parkinson's disease is levodopa/carbidopa.

- Most drugs used for the treatment of ADHD are stimulants and are classified as schedule II substances by the DEA.

- Atomoxetine, extended-release guanfacine, and extended-release clonidine are the only nonstimulants approved by the FDA for treatment of ADHD.

- Alzheimer's disease is a progressive degenerative disorder that leads to loss of brain function, memory impairment, and loss of judgment, of decision-making ability, and of speech.

Learning Assessment Questions

1. Seizures can be classified into which of the following two main categories?
   A. Partial and generalized
   B. Absence and partial
   C. Generalized and atonic
   D. Absence and myoclonic

2. All stimulants used for the treatment of ADHD are classified as what?
   A. Schedule II substances
   B. Schedule IV substances
   C. OTC
   D. Schedule III substances

3. Which of the following is a nonstimulant medication used for treatment of ADHD?
   A. Methylphenidate
   B. Concerta
   C. Daytrana
   D. Atomoxetine

4. Seizures are caused by an imbalance of which of the following?
   A. Calcium and sodium ions
   B. Excitatory and inhibitory impulses
   C. GABA and acetylcholine
   D. Potassium and calcium

5. Which of the following is not a cholinesterase inhibitor?
   A. Tacrine
   B. Donepezil
   C. Memantine
   D. Rivastigmine

6. Which of the following is the drug of choice for Parkinson's disease?

   A. Carbidopa/levodopa

   B. Methylphenidate

   C. Amantadine

   D. Bromocriptine

7. Which of the following is a serious seizure disorder involving tonic-clonic convulsions that last at least 30 minutes?

   A. Myclonic seizures

   B. Status epilepticus

   C. Absence seizures

   D. Partial seizures

8. Which of the following is a drug used to treat seizures?

   A. Anticonvulsant

   B. Antihistamine

   C. Antibiotic

   D. Antifungal

9. The two main neurotransmitters involved in seizure disorders are which of the following?

   A. Dopamine and acetylcholine

   B. Acetylcholine and GABA

   C. Glutamate and GABA

   D. Glutamate and dopamine

10. Loss of dopaminergic neurons in the substantia nigra leads to which of the following?

    A. Alzheimer's disease

    B. ADHD

    C. Parkinson's disease

    D. Epilepsy

11. Which of the following is a sulfonamide approved for adjunctive treatment of partial seizures in adults with epilepsy?

    A. Zonisamide

    B. Carbamazepine

    C. Phenytoin

    D. Topiramate

12. Cognitive loss in Alzheimer's disease is associated with depletion of which of the following?

    A. Dopamine

    B. Acetylcholine

    C. Norepinephrine

    D. Serotonin

13. A prescription label must have which of the following?

    A. The patient's name

    B. The name of the drug

    C. The name and address of the pharmacy

    D. All of the above

14. Which of the following is the maximum number of refills allowed for a schedule II controlled substance?

    A. 1

    B. 2

    C. 0

    D. 5

15. Which of the following is the maximum number of refills allowed for a schedule III to IV controlled substance within a six-month period?

    A. 1

    B. 2

    C. 0

    D. 5

16. When processing a refill request for a patient with a common last name, a unique patient identifier should also be used to identify the patient.

    A. True

    B. False

17. A tonic-clonic seizure was formerly known as which of the following?

    A. A petit mal seizure

    B. A grand mal seizure

    C. A post mal seizure

    D. A lateral seizure

18. An absence seizure was formerly known as which of the following?

    A. A petit mal seizure

    B. A grand mal seizure

    C. A post mal seizure

    D. A lateral seizure

19. Which of the following describes the involuntary contraction and relaxation of the muscles, which cause the body to shake rapidly and uncontrollably?

    A. Tremor

    B. Dyskinesia

    C. Convulsion

    D. Psychomotor imbalance

20. Which of the following is the only drug available in a patch formulation for the treatment of Alzheimer's disease?

    A. Namenda

    B. Razadyne

    C. Aricept

    D. Exelon

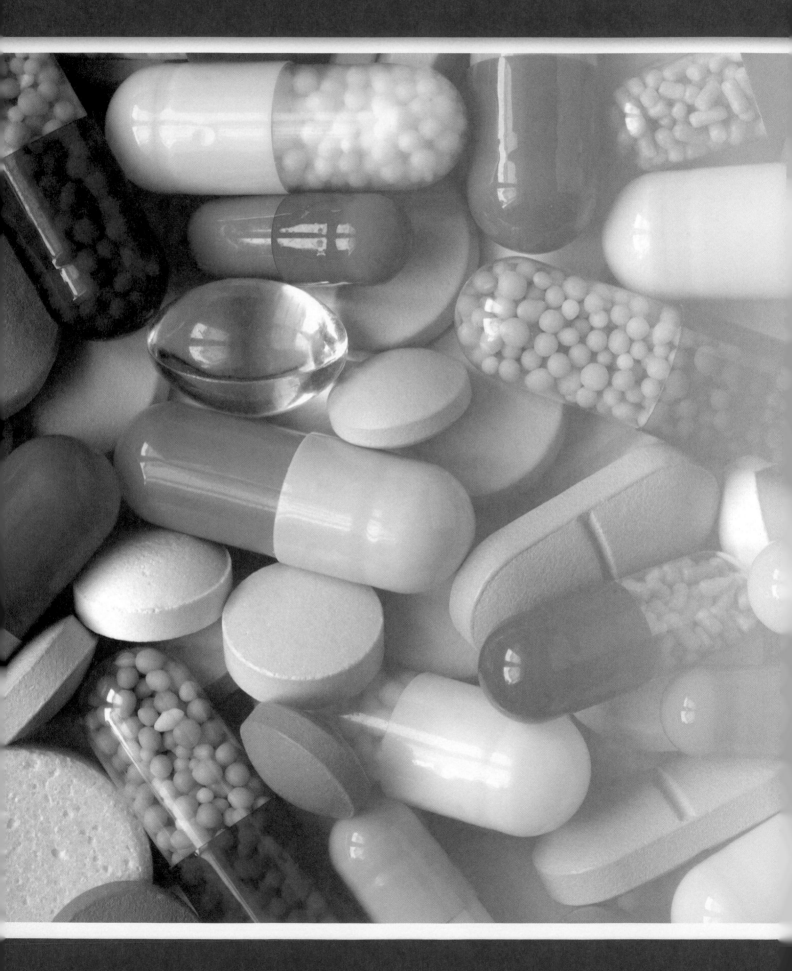

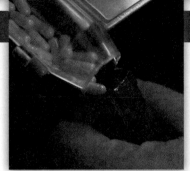

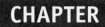

Business of the Community Pharmacy

OBJECTIVES

After reading this chapter, you will be able to:

- Describe the role of the technician in the sale of OTC medications.
- Summarize the importance of necessary cash-register management functions.
- Identify procedures for inventory management.
- Discuss drug insurance coverage.
- Define pharmacy benefits manager, tiered co-pay, and prior authorization.
- Describe how to process a workers' compensation claim.
- Identify information needed to process an online claim for a prescription drug.
- Calculate days' supply of medication for online billing.
- Resolve problems with online claims processing.
- Describe the pathophysiology and treatment of asthma.
- Describe the pathophysiology and treatment of emphysema and chronic bronchitis.
- Describe other lung-related diseases.
- Discuss the reemergence of tuberculosis and its treatment.
- Differentiate antitussives, expectorants, decongestants, and antihistamines and describe their uses.
- Describe smoking-cessation plans and supportive therapy.

KEY TERMS

Actuation	Asthma	Co-pay
Allergen	Bronchitis	Credit card
Allergy	Bronchospasm	Cystic fibrosis (CF)
Alveolar wall	Chronic bronchitis	Days' supply
Alveoli	Chronic obstructive	Debit card
Antihistamines	pulmonary disease	Decongestants
Antitussives	(COPD)	Deductible
Aspiration	Co-insurance	Dietary supplement

Discount	Markup	Pharmacy benefits
Drug diversion	Mast cells	manager (PBM)
Emphysema	Medicaid	Prime-vendor purchasing
Expectorants	Medicare	Purchasing
Fee for service	Metered dose inhaler	Receipt
Flex card	(MDI)	Receiving
Front-end merchandise	Multidrug-resistant	Respiratory distress
Group purchasing	tuberculosis	syndrome
organization (GPO)	(MDR-TB)	Rhinitis
Healthcare spending	Nebulizer	Rhinitis medicamentosa
account	Online adjudication	Rhinorrhea
Health insurance	Oral candidiasis	Spacer
Immunoglobulin E	Overhead	Tiered co-pay
Indigent	Percussion	Tuberculosis (TB)
Induration	Permeability	Want book
Inventory	Pharyngitis	Wholesaler purchasing
Inventory value	Pneumonia	Workers' compensation
Lymph	Posting	

Chapter Overview

Business functions are critical to the success of any community pharmacy. The pharmacy technician plays an important role in the sale of over-the-counter products. Knowing how to operate and manage cash-register functions is an important part of all sales. The pharmacy technician assists in inventory management and obtains all the necessary information needed to process online billing and claims. When there is a problem processing an online claim, the pharmacy technician must be able to resolve this so the claim can be processed. These skills are the focus of this chapter. This chapter also discusses common respiratory diseases and the drugs used to treat these diseases, as well as smoking-cessation plans and supportive therapy.

Over-the-Counter Medications

An over-the-counter (OTC) medication is a drug that can be sold without a prescription. The FDA approves and regulates the sale of OTC medications by ensuring that only safe, effective, and properly labeled products be sold OTC. Medications classified as OTC by the FDA generally have the following characteristics:

- Their benefits outweigh their risks.
- Their potential for abuse is low.
- They are safe and effective for a given indication when taken according to the manufacturer's labeling, and do not require monitoring by a healthcare practitioner.

OTC products include vitamins, minerals, herbal medicines, and dietary supplements.

The use of OTC products, as well as their availability, has increased over the years. In

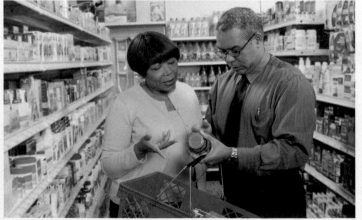

OTC products.

part, this is because buying drugs off the shelf without a prescription can result in a substantial savings for the consumer. OTC medications are generally cheaper than prescription drugs that contain the same active ingredient. Some OTC products available on the market contain the same active ingredient, with the same or lower strength, as formulations that are available by prescription only. An additional savings is incurred because doctors' appointments are not needed to obtain the medication. OTC medications are also easier to obtain than prescription medications because many stores that carry OTC medications are open longer than traditional pharmacies. Patients can obtain medications to treat everyday illnesses or symptoms without having to consult a healthcare provider, although access to a pharmacist or pharmacy technician is available when the pharmacy is open.

Patients should consider various important factors when deciding to treat themselves with an OTC product. Because there are a wide variety of products available, correctly identifying the problem or cause of the symptom is the first step in determining which product should be purchased. Manufacturers of OTC products must include on the medication's packaging all information necessary for the consumer to use the product safely and effectively. The information on the label must be clear and understandable and must include the dosage and frequency of administration for different age groups, as well as indications, precautions, and the expiration date. Many OTC medications list specific age groups that should avoid using the medication. Parents should consult with their pediatrician before giving children any OTC product. Other important factors of which consumers should be aware before buying OTC preparations include the following:

- Many OTC products contain identical ingredients. Often, branded and generic products are available and contain the same strengths and dosages of active ingredients.
- Packages of OTC products often look very similar.
- Patients who have other diseases such as hypertension or heart disease, or who are taking certain medications such as beta-blockers or ACE inhibitors, should pay careful attention when selecting an OTC product. They should look for products that may minimize the development of adverse effects.
- Proper attention should be paid to age requirements for OTC products.
- Many OTC products should be avoided if the patient is pregnant or nursing.

OTC products, just like prescription medications, may have adverse effects. In some states, some OTC products, such as those that contain dextromethorphan (Delsym, Robitussin DM) require the pharmacy technician to confirm that the consumer is more than 18 years old before allowing him or her to buy the product. Although OTC products seem harmless, they can cause serious adverse effects if taken inappropriately.

Consumers often seek the advice of the pharmacist when selecting an OTC product. They may ask the pharmacist to verify the assessment of their symptoms or ask the pharmacist to help them select a preparation if they have special needs. Pharmacy technicians may be asked to assist the customer in locating certain OTC medications or even asked specific questions about these products. Pharmacy technicians should not counsel patients on the use of OTC products. Questions regarding the use and selection of these products, indications, dosage, administration, expected side effects, and contraindications should always be directed to the pharmacist.

All questions regarding the use of over-the-counter medications should be referred to the pharmacist.

Technicians can help in the sale of OTC medications by carrying out functions such as stocking products, ordering inventory, and removing expired products from the shelf. They can show the patient where common OTC products can be found. By performing these activities, technicians help free up the pharmacist's time so that he or she can help a patient in the selection of an OTC product and counsel the patient on the correct way to safely and effectively use the product.

Schedule V OTC Drugs

Schedule V drugs are those that have a low potential for abuse and a limited potential for physical or psychological dependence. Laws for dispensing of Schedule V drugs vary from state to state. When determining which law should be followed—federal or state—the more stringent law applies. Federal law allows the dispensing of a Schedule V drug without a prescription, but requires special procedures or places limits on the sale of these drugs. Each state has specific requirements regarding the dispensing of Schedule V medications.

Pharmacies are required to adhere to the following requirements regarding Schedule V drugs that are sold over-the-counter:

- All Schedule V drugs must be stored behind the pharmacy counter. Although these drugs are considered safe enough to use without supervision of a health-care provider, most states require a signed prescription before a Schedule V product can be dispensed but others may have some Schedule V medications as OTC.
- Schedule V cough syrups sold to a single customer should be limited to a specific volume within a 48-hour period according to the state specific regulations.
- Only a pharmacist or a pharmacy technician under the direct supervision of a pharmacist can complete the sale of a Schedule V drug.
- The purchaser of a Schedule V drug must be 18 years of age or older and must have proof of age

---

All Schedule V drugs must be stored behind the counter.

The sale of an OTC Schedule V drug must be recorded in a log book along with the following information:

- Name and address of the purchaser
- Date of birth of the purchaser
- Date and time of purchase
- Product name and quantity
- Name and initials of the pharmacist or pharmacy technician completing the sale

Dietary Supplements

Dietary supplements are available OTC, but are not regulated by the FDA in the same way as OTC drugs. The manufacturer of the dietary supplement is responsible for ensuring that the dietary supplement or ingredient is safe. In general, manufacturers do not need to register their dietary product with the FDA or get FDA approval before manufacturing and selling their product. Other than the manufacturer's responsibility for ensuring the safety of the supplement, there are no rules that limit the serving size or amount of a nutrient in a dietary supplement. The FDA does not require that the dietary supplement be approved for safety and efficacy before the manufacturer can market the dietary supplement. Dietary supplements include vitamins, minerals, and herbal products. A dietary supplement is a product that is taken orally and intended to supplement the diet. The FDA requires that dietary supplements be accurately labeled. If a health claim is made regarding a dietary supplement, the claim must be approved by the FDA to ensure accuracy and that the consumer is not misled. The amount of active ingredient from one package of the same dietary supplement to another may vary in content because of inconsistencies in the manufacturing or quality control process.

The amount of active ingredient in the same dietary supplement may vary from one package to another.

Cash-Register Management

The pharmacy technician or clerk usually collects money from patients paying for their OTC medications, supplies, prescriptions, or other store merchandise. Payment can typically be made via cash, check, debit, or credit card. Procedures for collecting money may differ from one pharmacy to another. Larger pharmacies with multiple cash registers often give each technician a sign-on and password to assist in keeping track of money taken in. Most large pharmacies use barcode-scanning technology so that when a prescription or nonprescription item is scanned, the price will automatically be displayed on the screen or register. When prescription products are scanned, the pharmacy technician may be prompted to ask the pharmacist and/or patient about counseling. When certain items such as Schedule V drugs are scanned, the technician may be prompted to ask for additional information, as discussed previously, to complete the sale.

Transactions in which the customer pays by cash are relatively straightforward. The cash register usually calculates the amount of change that will need to be given to the customer. At the beginning of each day, a set amount of change is placed in the cash-register drawer. At the end of each business day, the cash is counted and balanced against the receipts.

Some patients may pay for their prescriptions or OTC medications by personal check. Procedures for accepting personal checks as a method of payment vary from pharmacy to pharmacy. Often, identification such as a driver's license may be required. The pharmacy technician should always verify the amount for which the check is made out and the signature. Larger pharmacies may have a special reader that is connected to the cash register that scans the check, accesses the customer's bank account, and alerts the technician when there are insufficient funds in the bank account to cover the amount of the check.

Some patients may prefer to pay for their pharmacy purchases by using a credit, debit, or flex card. A **credit card** is form of payment that allows people to make purchases on credit. Cardholders agree to pay the amount charged to the card at the end of each billing cycle or accrue a finance charge. A **debit card** is a form of payment in which the money is immediately deducted from the cardholder's bank account. A PIN number is required

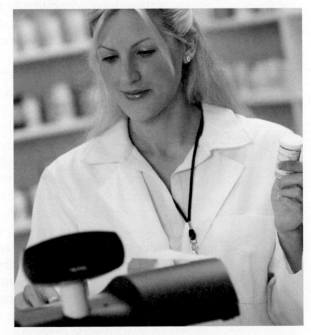

A pharmacy technician is often the final point of contact with the customer.

for a debit-card purchase. Most debit cards can also be used as a credit card. A **flex card** is a debit card that can be used to pay for out-of-pocket medical costs such as health-related items, prescription co-pays and some OTC products. A **co-pay** is the amount of money a patient must pay for healthcare services such as a prescription or doctor's visit at the time the service is rendered, with the insurer paying the rest of the costs. When a flex card is used for covered purchases, the money is automatically deducted from the individual's healthcare spending account. (A **healthcare spending account** is an account that can be used to cover medical and prescription expenses not covered under medical insurance.) This minimizes the need for submitting receipts to the insurance company and prevents delays in reimbursement. Regardless of the method of payment, a receipt should always be provided to the customer. A **receipt** is a bill of sale.

Sometimes, the purchase of a prescription or nonprescription item needs to be cancelled. When this occurs, the sale must be voided and a record of the transaction (sale and voided sale) must be kept. If the patient is supposed to receive a refund, the pharmacy technician may need to get approval from the pharmacist or store manager.

The pharmacy technician may be responsible for reconciling cash, credit-card receipts, personal checks, and voided sales with the cash-register printout at the end of each day. In large retail pharmacies, this function may be performed by the store manager. Reconciling cash, credit-card receipts, checks, and voided sales with the cash-register printout at the end of the day can also help prevent theft and drug diversion by comparing the filling with the checkout process and prescription pickups. (**Drug diversion** is the illegal distribution, abuse, or unintended use of prescription drugs.) Many pharmacies also have surveillance cameras to protect the pharmacy against theft and drug diversion.

Inventory Management

To meet the needs of all patients, a community pharmacy must be adequately stocked with or have access to nonprescription and prescription medications and supplies. All nonprescription and prescription items that are on hand for sale are known as **inventory**. It can also include **front-end merchandise**—that is, nonprescription merchandise that is sold in the front of the store. Pharmacy inventory must be carefully maintained to have an adequate supply of medications. If proper amounts of medications are not kept on hand, the pharmacy may frequently run out of a medication, causing a loss of sale, an inconvenience to the patient, or both.

The total value of all the drugs and merchandise in stock is referred to as **inventory value**. The goal of inventory management is to ensure timely purchases to maintain an adequate supply of on-hand medications. Preferably, medications are dispensed shortly after they are received in the pharmacy. This will minimize shelf space needed in the pharmacy and maximize available cash flow. Pharmacies have a considerable amount of money tied up in inventory. To minimize this cost, pharmacies aim to maintain adequate, but not excessive inventory levels. Excess inventory ties up available cash flow, utilizes shelf space, results in wastage because of expired medications, and increases the likelihood of drug diversion or theft. Most pharmacies perform an annual count of the pharmacy's inventory and a value is assigned to determine the cost of inventory and inventory turnover.

The DEA requires that a complete inventory be performed every two years for all controlled substances. An exact count or measure of contents is required for all Schedule II controlled substances and an estimated count for all Schedule III–V substances (unless the container holds more than 1,000 tablets or capsules, in which case an exact count is required). The inventory should be taken on any date within two years from the previous biennial inventory date. It can be taken exactly two years from the previous biennial inventory or any day prior to the biennial date. For all controlled substances, the inventory record should contain the name, strength, dosage form, and quantity of medication. Records for all controlled substances should be maintained for at least two years; however, most pharmacies keep these records indefinitely. Disposal of controlled substances must be recorded and witnessed by a pharmacist. Schedule II drugs are either saved until the state drug inspector can witness the destruction or sent to an authorized destruction company. Some states have more stringent requirements than the DEA; in such states, the more stringent requirement should prevail.

The DEA requires that a complete inventory be performed every two years for all controlled substances.

Other factors relating to inventory management that should be taken into account include product turnover, floor-space availability, shelf-space availability, arrangement of shelves, and available refrigerator or freezer space. The amount of inventory that should be maintained and when inventory levels should be adjusted will vary from one pharmacy to another. However, every pharmacy should employ inventory-management practices to ensure that patients have proper access to both nonprescription and prescription products.

The pharmacy technician plays an important role in managing inventory. Purchasing, receiving, stocking, and restocking inventory; locating and rotating stock; and checking for expiration dates are all functions that a pharmacy technician may perform.

The technician should designate, either by marking an X on the bottle or affixing a sticker, that a stock bottle has been opened.

Purchasing

Inventory management includes the **purchasing** or ordering of products, either to be used by the pharmacy or for sale to the consumer. The pharmacist can deal directly with a drug wholesaler or work together with other pharmacies to negotiate a discount for high-volume purchases. Working together as part of a group, called a purchasing group or **group purchasing organization (GPO)**, usually results in a better discount and more favorable contractual terms.

Wholesaler purchasing allows the community pharmacy to order and receive a variety of drug manufacturers' medications from a single source. Advantages of wholesale purchasing include lower inventory costs and faster turnaround time. Disadvantages include higher purchasing costs, supply shortages, and limitations in product availability.

Prime-vendor purchasing involves using a large distributor as the sole distributor to a pharmacy. The distributor provides medications and medical products or devices to those pharmacies that participate in the prime-vendor purchasing. With prime-vendor purchasing, the pharmacy and distributor enter into a contract that requires the pharmacy to order medications through the distributor company. Advantages of prime-vendor purchasing include lower acquisition costs and emergency delivery services.

The pharmacy technician plays an important role in the purchasing of products for the pharmacy. Pharmacies can use an automated **want book** to record inventory that needs to be reordered or software programs that automate the drug-ordering process. Usage and seasonal patterns can also play a role in the amount of inventory ordered. For example, allergy products may be purchased in larger quantities in the spring and summer months. Software programs can automatically generate a purchase order when the inventory drops to a preset minimum level. These software programs also keep track of inventory. When a prescription is dispensed or an OTC product is purchased, the system automatically calculates the remaining inventory.

The pharmacy technician may also be responsible for ordering and stocking prescription supplies such as bottles, jars, prescription containers, auxiliary labels, and measuring equipment. These supplies may not be available from a wholesaler or prime vendor and may need to be ordered directly from the manufacturer.

Receiving and Posting

The delivery and receipt of an order from a wholesaler, prime vendor, or other source is termed **receiving**. As part of the receiving process, products are carefully checked against the purchase order to ensure that the number of items received matches that on the order form. The pharmacist (for controlled substances) or pharmacy technician (for non-controlled substances) usually signs the delivery invoice, verifying that the correct number of items was delivered. When the packages, totes, or crates are opened, the contents of the shipment should be verified to make sure that the product strength, dosage form, manufacturer, NDC number, and quantity match the order form.

After the contents of the shipment have been checked, the following process occurs:

1. The invoice is reconciled.
2. The inventory is updated in the pharmacy product database.
3. The stickers that contain the pricing information and item number are affixed to the bulk bottles.

This process is known as **posting**. The products are then placed on the shelves or stored appropriately.

Drugs with earlier expiration dates should be positioned in front of those with later expiration dates so that they will be selected first.

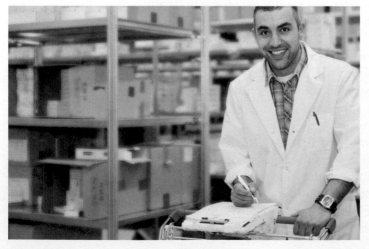

A pharmacy technician often accepts a shipment of medications or signs the delivery invoice.

Drug Returns

The pharmacy technician is usually responsible for handling drug returns to the wholesaler or prime vendor. Products that were damaged during shipment, handled improperly, outdated, recalled by the manufacturer or FDA, or incorrectly filled should be reported to the pharmacist and wholesaler immediately. Proper procedures must be followed when returning pharmaceuticals to the wholesaler.

Prescription containers that contain medication for a specific patient and are returned by the patient to the pharmacy cannot be returned to stock for dispensing to another patient once they have left the pharmacy. States have specific regulations regarding return of medications to the pharmacy. A patient may, however, return a medication for a credit if the drug has been recalled by the manufacturer or FDA. Controlled substances that are returned by the patient must be returned to the manufacturer, original supplier, or authorized reverse distributor for disposal. Credits for returned prescriptions may have to be approved by the pharmacy or store manager. Patients may be able to return unopened OTC medications in their original packaging to a pharmacy; however, this varies from one pharmacy to another. Expired non-controlled drugs that are returned to the pharmacy can be disposed of in the pharmacy through a drug waste program in which the pharmacy participates. Pharmacy protocol should be followed for disposing of returned medications.

Business Math

The pharmacy technician plays a crucial role in ensuring inventory turnover, processing insurance claims, and managing some aspects of insurance reimbursements. The technician may also price products in the pharmacy. As with all businesses, a profitable pharmacy must bring in more money in sales than it spends in expenses. Knowing how to perform business math calculations can help ensure a profitable pharmacy.

Prescription containers that are returned by the patient to the pharmacy cannot be returned to stock once they have left the pharmacy, even if they have not been opened. The medications can be disposed of by the pharmacy. Some states allow prescription containers that were dispensed in the manufacturers original container and not opened or tampered with, to be returned to stock for dispensing. Each state has specific guidelines regarding medication returns.

Markup

Markup is defined as the amount added to the cost of a particular product to cover overhead and profit. (**Overhead** is the cost of doing business. Overhead takes into account salaries, cost of equipment, operating expenses, and rent.) The selling price is calculated by adding markup to the price of acquisition. Prescription pricing may be governed by a variety of factors, including government regulations and competition within the marketplace.

Markup can be calculated using the following formula:

$$\text{Selling Price} - \text{Purchase Price} = \text{Markup}$$

The percentage markup can be calculated using the following formula:

$$(\text{Markup} \div \text{Pharmacy Cost}) \times 100 = \text{Percentage Markup}$$

Markup is the amount added to the cost of a product to cover overhead and profit.

Discount

Sometimes, a wholesaler or prime vendor offers a percentage off the original price of an item. The pharmacy then pays a lower price that reflects the percentage off the original price, or **discount**. The pharmacy may choose to pass this cost savings on to the consumer as an incentive to buy the item and to attract customers into the store. These customers not only buy the discounted item, but frequently purchase other products as well.

A discount is the percentage off the original price of a product.

Discount can be calculated using the following formula:

Purchase Price × Discount Rate = Discount

Discounted price can be calculated using the following formula:

Purchase Price − Discount = Discounted Price

Average Wholesale Price (AWP), Average Acquisition Cost (AAC), Average Manufacturer's Cost (AMP), and Other Prices

The average wholesale price (AWP) has become a controversial price point. In theory, it is the average price at which a drug is sold by the wholesaler to the pharmacy. In practice, almost no one pays the AWP, but it provides a useful benchmark. The AWP of most drugs can be found in the Medi-Span database or in *Red Book*, which is discussed in Chapter 7.

The AWP of most drugs can be found in *Red Book*.

Other prices used in pharmacy include the following:

- Average acquisition cost (AAC)—Third parties reimburse a pharmacy based on the AAC. The AAC is the average cost for a pharmacy to obtain a product.
- Maximum allowable cost (MAC)—Some states may use this to reimburse pharmacies.
- Average manufacturer's price (AMP)—The AMP is the average price paid to the manufacturer by wholesalers for drugs distributed to pharmacies. AMP was created by Congress to calculate Medicaid rebates.
- Usual and customary price—This is the amount paid by the customer without insurance.
- Wholesale acquisition cost (WAC)—The WAC is the price paid by a distributor for drugs that are purchased from a wholesaler. It is generally the price set by the manufacturer.

Prescription reimbursement may be calculated using the following formula:

Prescription Reimbursement = Average Acquisition Cost (AAC) + Markup + Dispensing Fee

Which price should be used to calculate prescription reimbursement to the pharmacy is currently a point of controversy, however, the third-party payer will not pay more than the average wholesale price, average acquisition cost, or whichever price point the pharmacy uses for the actual cost of the drug. The markup is used to cover the pharmacist and pharmacy costs for filling the prescription. Some third-party payers will also reimburse for a dispensing fee.

Health Insurance

Health insurance is medical coverage that helps protect the patient from high medical care costs associated with such things as physician visits, hospitalization, and prescriptions. A person who has health insurance is insured, while a person who does not have health insurance is uninsured. For billing purposes, the pharmacy technician must know the types of insurance coverage. In some pharmacy practice settings, the pharmacy technician must be able to differentiate between different types of insurance, determine whether a patient has prescription benefits, and be able to transmit a claim correctly. In addition, there are opportunities for pharmacy technicians to work solely in reimbursement, which requires a full understanding of the business side of pharmacy practice—especially with regard to insurance coverage.

Many people in the U.S. get their health insurance through their employers. Others may get it from state-directed programs for residents who qualify (Medicaid) or from federally administered programs for those who qualify (Medicare). Some patients are **fee for service** pay-structure patients. That is, they pay the provider for each service separately. Others are **indigent**, meaning they have no insurance, and so may fall into certain state-specific payment categories.

Types of Health Insurance

Insurance companies may outsource the administrative tasks of processing drug claims and reimbursements to outside companies. A **pharmacy benefit manager (PBM)** is a company that performs these tasks for an insurance company. Most patients pay a monthly premium for health insurance and prescription drug coverage. Private health insurance plans vary in their range of benefits, but usually include a **deductible** or a co-pay per visit or per prescription, and limits on yearly or lifetime benefits. Insurance companies try to control healthcare costs by passing some of the cost to the patient in the form of a deductible, co-pay, or **co-insurance**. (With a co-insurance plan, the patient must pay a certain percentage of the cost for medical care or for a prescription.) Some insurance companies have **tiered co-pay** systems, which have differential costs for generic drugs, preferred brands, and nonpreferred brands. For generic and preferred-brand medications, the patient pays a lower co-pay than for nonpreferred-brand medications. Insurance plans may vary in terms of how much medication can be dispensed by a particular pharmacy, but the quantity of medication ordered by the prescriber and filled by the pharmacist must be documented. Most patients receive health and drug coverage from a private insurance company through their employer or from the state (Medicaid) or the U.S. government (Medicare).

The pharmacy technician plays an important role in **online adjudication**—that is, using a computer with an Internet connection to process prescription claims. When a prescription is filled and billed to a PBM, the PBM will notify the pharmacy immediately as to the amount it should charge the patient and how much the pharmacy will be reimbursed. Note that the patient may need to meet specified criteria and the plan's deductible in order for the insurer to cover the cost of the medication, or the drug simply may not be covered under the insurance plan.

Medicare is a federal program that provides health insurance benefits for people over the age of 65, for people under the age of 65 who have certain disabilities, and people of any age who suffer from permanent kidney failure (end-stage renal failure).

Medicare part A is hospital insurance that helps pay for inpatient care. Medicare part A generally does not require payment of a monthly premium. Medicare part B is medical insurance that helps pay for medically necessary doctor's services and outpatient care. The patient must see a provider who accepts Medicare insurance, but the patient must share a percentage of the cost and has a yearly deductible. Medicare Part D offers drug-benefit coverage for an additional monthly premium. Medicare part D is not an option for Medicare patients unless the patient has drug coverage through another insurance company. Medicare part D is federally sponsored, but the actual plans are offered by non-government insurance companies who are reimbursed for services provided for Medicare Part D members. It requires the federal government to provide subsidies to those whose income is less than a certain percentage of the federal poverty limit. Some individuals are covered under both Medicaid and Medicare. These patients are known as "dual eligible." Seniors can choose from several insurance plans that are available. Each plan has its advantages and disadvantages and a different list of preferred drugs.

> Medicare is a federal program for seniors, the disabled, and dialysis patients.

Medicaid is a federal program that is managed by each individual state for low-income residents, including uninsured pregnant women. The program is funded by both the state and federal governments. It subsidizes the cost of health care for low-income and disabled citizens who meet eligibility requirements. The benefits of this program vary from state to state In general, coverage can be divided into three categories:

- The patient is not responsible for any cost and does not pay a deductible.
- The patient shares the cost in the form of a co-payment based on income.
- The patient is part of a managed care plan with which Medicaid has a contractual agreement.

If the patient is covered under Medicaid, the pharmacy technician must get a copy of the patient's insurance card, which identifies the program under which the patient is covered.

> Medicaid is a state program for low-income residents, including uninsured pregnant women.

Workers' compensation provides insurance to cover medical care and compensation from injuries suffered by employees while on the job. Coverage may be limited to a certain period, based on the extent and severity of the injury. State law requires employers to offer workers' compensation to employees. Drug and medical coverage is limited to drugs and procedures that are needed to treat the job-related injury. Workers' compensation claims are filed electronically to the insurance company. The pharmacy technician will play an important role in obtaining billing information before dispensing medications or supplies for customers with workers' compensation benefits. Many pharmacies will fill a workers' compensation prescription on a lien pending the results of the workers' compensation judgment.

> Workers' compensation provides insurance to cover the cost of medical care and compensation from injuries suffered while on the job.

Billing the Insurance Company

The pharmacy technician plays a critical role in assisting the pharmacist and the patient by processing an insurance claim. If the customer has prescription coverage, and he or she is a new customer, the technician should obtain the insurance card (see **FIGURE 11.1**) and enter all the information on the card into the patient profile. Any changes in insurance coverage for existing patients should also be entered into the pharmacy database. The technician must also enter the patient's name, the date on which a prescription is filled, the medication prescribed, the dosage, the length of therapy, the patient's date of birth, and the patient's identification number. Much of this information may be automatically added to fields in various screens in the pharmacy profile when filling a prescription. After all this information has been entered, the pharmacy receives immediate feedback from the PBM, which determines eligibility, drug coverage, and the amount of co-pay that must be collected from the patient.

If any of the information in the pharmacy database does not match the insurance company information, a claim may be rejected. If the patient does not have insurance, he or she must pay the full price for the medication unless he or she qualifies for an indigent pro-

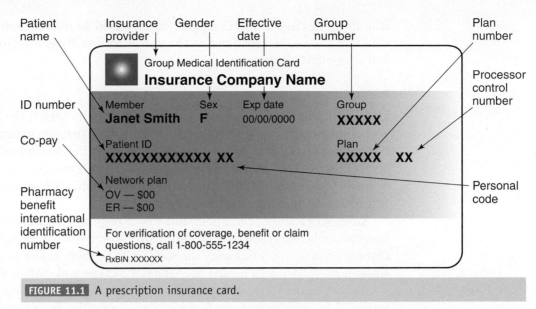

FIGURE 11.1 A prescription insurance card.

gram. A prescription may not be covered for many reasons, including the following:

- The NDC on the product may not be covered by the insurer.
- Coverage has expired.
- The maximum amount covered by the insurance company or the coverage limit has been reached.
- The patient is refilling a prescription too early.
- The prescribed duration of therapy exceeds days supply covered by patient's plan.

> The information entered into the pharmacy database must match exactly what is written on the prescription insurance card.

Often, an insurance company will pay for a medication only if a prior authorization is received. Prior authorization may be needed for a drug that is not on the formulary, or if the patient requires the use of a more-expensive treatment when a less-expensive drug is available.

Calculating Days' Supply

To process an online claim submitted from the pharmacy or to reimburse the patient, the insurer requires specific information about each prescription filled. This includes the patient's name, the date the medication is filled, the pharmacy name and address, the medication prescribed, the dosage, the patient's date of birth, and the days' supply. The **days' supply** is the length of time that a dispensed medication will last.

To calculate the days' supply, use the following equation:

$$\text{Quantity Ordered} \div \text{Quantity of Medication Used in a 24-Hour Period} = \text{Days' Supply}$$

Drug Insights: Respiratory Disorders

Many conditions affect the respiratory system. Some may be genetic; others may be due to contagious infections, smoking, or the result of environmental factors. Symptoms of respiratory illness include abnormal breathing or coughing. Asthma, emphysema, chronic bronchitis, pneumonia, cystic fibrosis, and tuberculosis and their treatment will all be discussed in this chapter. Drugs used to treat symptoms of the common cold will also be discussed in this chapter, as well as drugs used for smoking cessation and supportive therapy.

Asthma

Asthma is a chronic inflammatory airway disease in which the muscles around the bronchioles contract, narrowing the air passages so that air cannot be inhaled properly. Edema and secretion of mucus into the airway further minimizes airflow. Asthma can be precipitated by a chronic allergic reaction to substances in the environment or by exercise. Symptoms of asthma include chest tightening, wheezing, difficulty breathing, and coughing that lead to airway obstruction.

FIGURE 11.2 shows the upper and lower respiratory tract through which oxygen flows and where oxygen is exchanged with carbon dioxide. In patients with asthma or chronic obstructive pulmonary disease (COPD), there is less oxygen available or the amount of surface area for the exchange of oxygen and carbon dioxide is reduced.

In asthmatic patients, **mast cells**, which are rich in histamine and heparin, are activated by **immunoglobulin E**, which are antibodies found in the lungs, skin, and mucous membranes. Mast cells are also activated by exercise, cold weather, and allergens. (An **allergen** is any substance that elicits an allergic reaction.) Activation of mast cells leads to airway obstruction caused by smooth-muscle contractions, mucus secretion, and increased vascular permeability. (**Permeability** refers to the ease with which a liquid or gas is able to pass through a membrane.) During an asthma attack, release of histamine and other mediators from mast cells results in mucus production

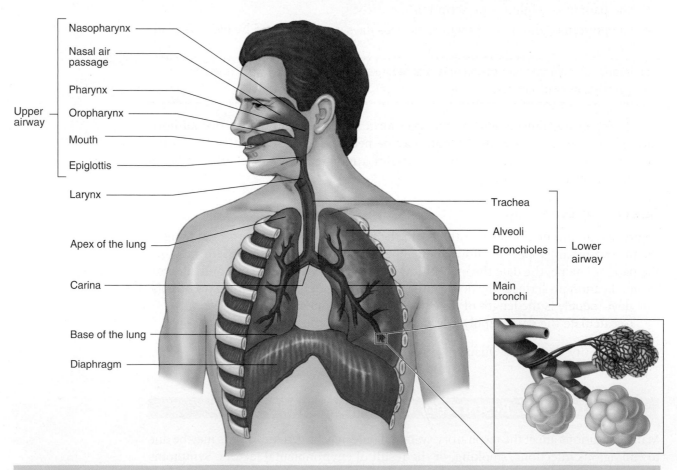

FIGURE 11.2 Upper and lower respiratory tract.

and **bronchospasm** (that is, spasmodic contraction of the bronchial smooth muscles). After this phase, the airway becomes more sensitive because of bronchoconstriction with delayed, sustained reactions that cause inflammation.

Using prophylaxis medications, most asthma attacks can be avoided. Avoiding triggers can help prevent the onset of an attack. Goals of asthma therapy include the following:

- Maintaining a normal level of functioning
- Sleeping well every night
- Freedom from wheezing and coughing
- Tolerating medicines well
- Limiting exposure to irritants or triggers

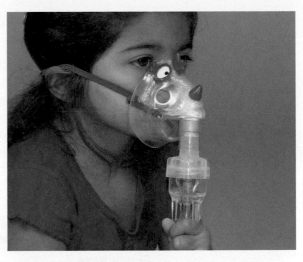

A child uses a nebulizer to deliver asthma medication.

Medications can prevent or reverse asthma attacks. Two types of medications are used in asthma patients: those used to prevent an attack and those used to treat an attack. Long-term medications include corticosteroids, beta-agonists, mast cell stabilizers, methylxanthines, and leukotriene receptor antagonists. Short-acting anticholinergics and beta-agonists are used for acute asthma attacks.

Asthma medications are often administered to children via a nebulizer. A **nebulizer** is a device that creates a fine mist, which the patient inhales through a mouthpiece or mask. For adults, asthma medications are often delivered by a **metered dose inhaler (MDI)**, which contains medication and compressed gas. An MDI delivers a specific amount of medication with each actuation that is fine enough to penetrate into the lungs. **Actuation** describes the release of medication while taking a slow, deep breath. An MDI may be used with a spacer. A **spacer** helps the patient breathe in the mist at a slower rate, providing better penetration of the drug into the lungs. Spacers are especially useful in patients who have difficulty using an inhaler alone.

Some MDIs use hydrofluoroalkane (HFA) as the propellant. Others use a dry powder in which a pellet is placed in the inhaler and crushed. All MDIs should be primed before use. Priming refers to the process of getting the inhaler ready for use by spraying the inhaler once into the open air.

The steps for using an HFA MDI are as follows:

1. Prime the MDI. (Shake it for five seconds before actuation.)
2. Exhale.
3. Place the mouthpiece between the lips.
4. Press down on the inhaler and breathe in slowly.
5. Hold breath and count to 10.
6. Exhale slowly.

The steps for using a dry-powder MDI are as follows:

1. Activate the inhaler.
2. Prime the inhaler.
3. Exhale.
4. Place the mouthpiece between the lips.
5. Inhale quickly.

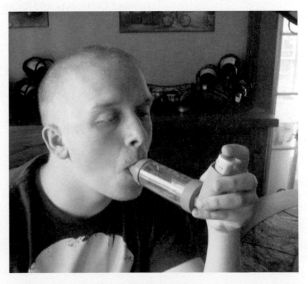

A spacer is useful for patients who have difficulty using an inhaler alone.

6. Hold breath and count to 10.

7. Exhale slowly.

If more than one puff is required, wait for one minute after the first puff and repeat the preceding steps. Clean the mouthpiece after each use as recommended by the manufacturer. If the inhaler contains a corticosteroid, rinse the mouth after each use to prevent dryness, throat irritation, and oral fungal infections.

TABLE 11.1 lists common drugs used in the treatment of asthma.

Corticosteroids produce smooth muscle relaxation and lessen the constriction of the bronchial tubes by inhibiting inflammatory cells. If inhaled, corticosteroids may

Table 11.1   Common Drugs Used in the Treatment of Asthma

Generic Name	Brand Name	Available Formulations
Inhaled Corticosteroids		
Beclomethasone dipropionate	QVAR, Beconase AQ	MDI
Budesonide	Pulmicort Flexhaler, Pulmicort Respules	Dry-powder inhaler, suspension for nebulization
Ciclesonide	Alvesco	MDI
Flunisolide	AeroBid	MDI
Fluticasone propionate	Flovent Diskus, Flovent HFA	Dry-powder inhaler, MDI
Mometasone furoate	Asmanex Twisthaler	Dry-powder inhaler
Triamcinolone acetonide	Azmacort	MDI
Inhaled Short-Acting Beta-2 Agonists (Bronchodilators)		
Albuterol	ProAir HFA, Proventil HFA, Ventolin HFA	Solution for nebulization, MDI
Levalbuterol	Xopenex, Xopenex HFA	Solution for nebulization, MDI
Pirbuterol	Maxair Autohaler	MDI
Inhaled Long-Acting Beta-2 Agonists (Bronchodilators)		
Salmeterol	Serevent Diskus	Dry-powder inhaler
Formoterol	Foradil Aerolizer	Dry-powder inhaler
Inhaled Corticosteroid/Long-Acting Beta-2 Agonist		
Fluticasone/salmeterol	Advair Diskus, Advair HFA	Dry-powder inhaler, MDI
Budesonide/formoterol	Symbicort HFA	MDI
Leukotriene Receptor Antagonists		
Montelukast	Singulair	Chewable tablets, oral granules
Zafirlukast	Accolate	Tablets
Zileuton	Zyflo CR	Tablets
Mast-Cell Stabilizer		
Cromolyn sodium	Crolom, Nasalcrom	Solution for nebulization or nasal spray
Methylxanthine		
Theophylline	Theo-24	Extended-release capsules and tablets, elixir
Anti-IgE Antibody		
Omalizumab	Xolair	Powder for subcutaneous injection

cause **oral candidiasis** (fungal infection), irritation and burning of the nasal mucosa, reflex cough, bronchospasm, and hoarseness. To minimize the incidence of these adverse effects, patients should be instructed to rinse the mouth thoroughly with water after use of a corticosteroid inhaler.

Long-acting bronchodilators are recommended for chronic prophylaxis of asthma and are used in conjunction with inhaled corticosteroids. The bronchodilator helps open the airway and allows for more of the steroid to reach its site of action. Side effects of this class of drugs include headache, nasal congestion, dizziness, sore throat, and hoarseness.

Theophylline (Theo-24) reverses bronchospasm associated with antigens by causing relaxation of airway smooth muscle and dilation.

Leukotriene receptor antagonists block the synthesis of or response to leukotrienes, blocking the inflammatory response. Common side effects of these drugs include headache and cough.

Mast-cell stabilizers protect mast-cell membranes from rupture caused by antigens. They work by stabilizing mast cells. A bronchodilator must be administered first to open up the airway. Side effects include hoarseness, stuffy nose, bad taste in mouth, drowsiness, cough, and throat irritation.

All MDIs should have the auxiliary label "Shake Well."

Anti-IgE antibody is a recombinant monoclonal antibody that prevents IgE from binding to mast cells, thereby preventing release of inflammatory mediators after allergen exposure. It is approved by the FDA for adjunctive use in patients at least 12 years old with well-documented specific allergies and moderate to severe persistent asthma that is not well controlled on an inhaled corticosteroid with or without a long-acting beta-2 agonist. Side effects include pain at the injection site and bruising.

Combination drugs usually combine a short- and long-acting drug. These drugs are designed to decrease exacerbations or acute attacks and control symptoms. The side effects of these drugs are similar to those seen with the individual components.

Chronic Obstructive Pulmonary Disease

Any long-term condition that can damage the lungs can cause **chronic obstructive pulmonary disease (COPD)**. Chronic bronchitis and emphysema are two types of diseases that cause COPD.

Bronchitis is an inflammation of the lining of the bronchial airways, which leads to obstruction of airflow upon exhalation. It is usually characterized by a productive cough that may contain pus or blood, shortness of breath, and excess mucus production. Acute bronchitis is usually self-limiting, although antibiotics may be used to prevent or treat bacterial infections. **Chronic bronchitis** is a more serious form of bronchitis. Cigarette smoke; exposure to pollution, dust, and irritants; and bacterial infection can all contribute to the development of chronic bronchitis.

Emphysema is a disorder characterized by destruction of the **alveolar walls** and **alveoli** that eventually leads to a loss of lung elasticity. The alveoli lose their ability to expand and contract and their ability to remove carbon dioxide. This condition worsens as the surface area of the lungs becomes further reduced. Patients with emphysema may have a difficult time walking even short distances.

Emphysema and chronic bronchitis often occur together. Some of the treatments used for asthma are also effective for the management of COPD. Antibiotics (penicillins, cephalosporins, tetracyclines) may be needed if the sputum is green or pus-like or if a fever is present, as these are signs of an infection. Expectorants such as guaifenesin (Mucinex) are used to stimulate secretions and make a cough productive. Water helps

Table 11.2 Common Drugs Used for Treatment of COPD		
Generic Name	Brand Name	Available Formulations
Inhaled Corticosteroid/Long-Acting Beta-2 Agonists		
Fluticasone/salmeterol	Advair Diskus, Advair HFA	Dry-powder inhaler, MDI
Budesonide/formoterol	Symbicort HFA	MDI
Inhaled Long-Acting Beta-2 Agonists		
Formoterol	Perforomist	Inhalation
Arformoterol	Brovana	Inhalation
Methylxanthine		
Theophylline	Theo-24	Extended-release capsules and tablets, elixir
Inhaled Anticholinergic/Short-Acting Beta-2 Agonist		
Ipratropium/Albuterol	Combivent	Inhalation
Anticholinergic		
Tiotropium	Spiriva	Capsule for inhalation
Mucolytics		
Acetylcysteine	Mucomyst	Solution for inhalation, IV, oral liquid
Dornase alfa	Pulmozyme	Inhalation

break up the mucus and helps the patient cough up secretions. **TABLE 11.2** lists drugs commonly used in the treatment of COPD.

Water is the expectorant of choice.

Inhaled long-acting beta-2 agonists are used for the long-term treatment of COPD. These medications should be assigned a "use by" date, which can be either four months after the dispensing date or the product expiration date, whichever comes first. These products must be stored in the refrigerator until dispensed.

Patients with COPD should be advised to get yearly influenza and pneumococcal vaccinations.

Patients allergic to peanuts and peanut products may have a cross-sensitivity to ipratropium-albuterol (Combivent, DuoNeb) because the propellant is based on soy lecithin. (Patients with peanut allergies may have a cross sensitivity to soy lecithin.)

Anticholinergics inhibit the action of the neurotransmitter acetylcholine, thus relaxing the smooth muscle of the bronchioles. Tiotropium is used for long-term treatment of bronchospasms associated with COPD. Dry mouth is a common side effect of this drug.

Mucolytics such as acetylcysteine (Mucomyst) and dornase alfa (Pulmozyme, which is only available as a generic drug for inhalation) work by thinning mucus secretions, allowing for easier removal of the secretions.

Other Lung Diseases

Transmission of infection can occur when a person comes into contact with fluids or droplets that contain bacteria, viruses, or fungi. Avoiding smoking, secondhand smoke, and air pollution; frequent hand washing; and influenza and pneumococcal vaccinations are several measures to help prevent or minimize the risk of lung disease.

Pneumonia

Pneumonia is an infection of one or both lungs. Pneumonia may be contracted by breathing in droplets from a cough or sneeze that contain the causative organism or bacteria or viruses that are normally present in the mouth, throat, or nose and inadvertently enter the lungs via **aspiration** during sleep. The most common bacterial organisms causing pneumonia are *Streptococcus pneumoniae* and *Streptococcus aureus*. These organisms settle in the air sacs and airways of the lungs, causing the lung to become filled with pus and fluid. Persons with a weak immune system or heart disease and alcoholics are at higher risk for developing pneumonia. If the pneumonia is caused by a bacterial organism, the choice of which antibiotic to use will be based on the isolated or suspected organism.

Cystic Fibrosis

Cystic fibrosis (CF) is an inherited disease that involves the secretory glands, including the glands that make mucus and sweat. In patients with CF, the mucus becomes thick and sticky and builds up in the lungs. This buildup blocks the airways of lungs and makes it easy for bacteria to grow. The mucus also blocks the bile ducts in the pancreas, leading to a deficiency in digestive enzymes.

Patients with CF experience a lack of oxygen and difficulty breathing. Treatment includes respiratory therapy and antibiotic therapy. Nebulizers are used to liquefy pulmonary secretions. **Percussion**, a tapping movement to induce cough and expectorate mucus, is also used.

Treatment may include acetylcysteine, dornase alfa, or a bronchodilator (refer to **TABLE 11.3**) to liquefy secretions.

Respiratory Distress Syndrome

Respiratory distress syndrome is a breathing disorder that occurs in newborns. It is more common in premature infants because their lungs are unable to make an adequate amount of surfactant. Surfactant lowers the surface tension between the air and alveolar sacs. Without surfactant, the lungs collapse, making it harder for the infant to breathe.

Treatment of respiratory distress syndrome involves replacement of surfactant. These lung surfactants are supplied as a suspension for intratracheal administration. They prevent the alveoli from collapsing by lowering the surface tension between the air and alveolar sacs. Table 11.3 lists drugs commonly used to treat respiratory distress syndrome.

Tuberculosis

Tuberculosis (TB) is a common, highly contagious bacterial disease that is characterized by an infection within the lining of the lungs. It is caused by the bacterium *Mycobacterium tuberculosis*. TB is transmitted by droplets infected with the bacteria. Once inhaled, the bacteria spread throughout the body in the blood and lymph. (**Lymph** is a

Table 11.3 Common Drugs Used for Treatment of Respiratory Distress Syndrome

Generic Name	Brand Name	Available Formulations
Beractant	Survanta	Intratracheal suspension
Calfactant	Infasurf	Intratracheal suspension
Poractant alfa	Curosurf	Intratracheal suspension

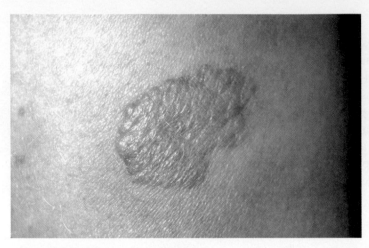

A positive TB skin test.

type of interstitial fluid, which bathes tissue in the body.) The bacteria need oxygen to survive, and the lungs provide an environment that is extremely oxygenated. The bacteria may also occur in bone and kidney tissue.

Tuberculosis is generally seen in alcoholics, those living in confined spaces such as prisons, the immunocompromised, and the elderly. TB generally develops slowly and may take a long time to present. Once exposed, patients have a risk of reactivity for the remainder of their life.

Persons who have been exposed to TB may have a positive TB skin test. A TB skin test contains a purified protein derivative (PPD) that is injected intradermally. Persons who have the disease or who have been exposed to the bacteria will develop an **induration**, or a hardened circular area of tissue, within 48 to 72 hours at the injection site. A chest X-ray is taken if the skin test is positive to determine the presence of active disease.

Goals of TB therapy include the following:

- Prompt initiation of therapy
- Conversion of sputum culture from positive to negative
- Cure without relapse
- Prevention of emergence of drug-resistant strains

Active tuberculosis is treated with a combination of drugs. Prophylaxis therapy includes only one drug to minimize the development of drug-resistant bacteria. For patients with no symptoms, isoniazid is generally preferred. Risk factors include failing to complete therapy, being prescribed inappropriate drugs, and recurrence of TB. A strain that is resistant to current drugs and is difficult to treat is **multidrug-resistant tuberculosis (MDR-TB)**. MDR-TB can be treated with capreomycin and cycloserine. The drugs used to treat TB are bactericidal. The treatment of TB depends on the patient's symptoms. Rifampin plus pyrazinamide is used to treat active TB. Examples of drugs used to treat TB are given in TABLE 11.4.

Table 11.4   Common Drugs Used for Treatment of Tuberculosis

Generic Name	Brand Name	Available Formulations
Capreomycin	Capastat	Injectable
Ciprofloxacin	Cipro	Injectable, tablet, liquid
Ethambutol	Myambutol	Tablet
Ethionamide	Trecator-SC	Tablet
Isoniazid (INH)	N/A	Injectable, tablet, liquid
Isoniazid-pyrazinamide-rifampin	Rifater	Tablet
Isoniazid-rifampin	Rifamate	Capsule
Ofloxacin	Floxin	Tablet, injectable
Pyrazinamide	N/A	Tablet
Rifampin	Rifadin	Capsule, injectable
Rifapentine	Priftin	Tablet

Patients must be instructed to complete the entire course of therapy to eradicate the bacteria completely from their system.

Rifampin (Rifadin, Rimactane) may discolor urine, tears, sweat, and other body fluids, turning them a reddish-orange. It can also permanently discolor soft contact lenses. It should be taken on an empty stomach.

Rifapentine (Priftin) has a longer duration of action than rifampin, but a similar adverse effect profile. Unlike rifampin, it should be taken with food.

Female patients taking oral contraceptives and rifampin should be instructed to use alternative forms of birth control.

Rifampin should be taken on an empty stomach, while rifapentine should be taken with food. Advise patients to avoid alcohol consumption when being treated with anti-tuberculosis medications.

Cough, Cold, and Allergy

Many conditions such as genetic causes, contagious infections, smoking, and environmental factors can affect the respiratory system. Although the causes of upper respiratory tract infections (URIs or URTIs) can vary, similar types of medication such as antitussives, expectorants, decongestants, and antihistamines are used to treat them. Upper respiratory tract infections are those that originate in the nose, sinuses, pharynx or larynx.

The most common form of an upper respiratory tract infection is the common cold. The common cold is usually caused by a rhinovirus and is generally self-limiting. Symptoms of a common cold include cough, congestion, sneezing, and fever, as well as **rhinitis** (stuffy nose), **pharyngitis** (inflammation of the pharynx), and **rhinorrhea** (runny nose). Common symptomatic treatments for a common cold include decongestants, antihistamines, antitussives, and expectorants. Getting lots of rest and drinking lots of water can also help fight a cold.

Some of the symptoms of allergies such as sneezing, a runny nose, or itchy eyes are the same as for a cold. The common cold is viral, while an allergy is the result of an immune response to a particular antigen. Both colds and allergies can be treated with some of the same medications.

Antitussives

Coughing is a mechanism for clearing the airways of foreign bodies. **Antitussives** are medications that suppress or reduce the frequency of coughing.

Hydrocodone-chlorpheniramine (Tussionex) is prescribed for cough and upper respiratory symptoms. It is addictive and has a high street value. It is classified as a Schedule III controlled substance. Side effects include

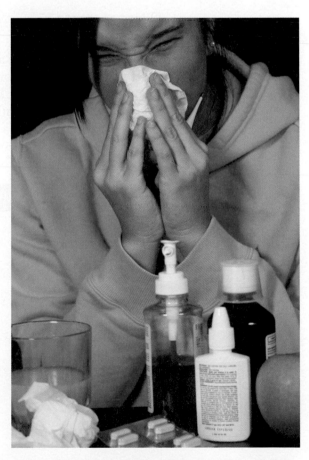

Many cough, cold, and allergy products are available OTC.

dose-related respiratory depression, sedation, drowsiness, dryness of the pharynx, and rash.

Benzonatate (Tessalon) works by anesthetizing stretch receptors in the airways, lungs, and membranes that line the thoracic cavity. Frequently observed side effects include headache and dizziness. The capsules should not be chewed.

Dextromethorphan (Delsym) is a nonopioid derivative of morphine. It is similar to codeine in efficacy, but without the analgesic properties of codeine. In most states, the purchaser must show identification and proof of age because it is a popular recreational drug. Side effects include dizziness, nervousness, confusion, and stomach upset.

Expectorants

Expectorants are drugs that break up thick mucus secretions so they can be expelled through coughing. They decrease the thickness and viscosity of the mucus so it is easier to cough it out. Expectorants should be taken with lots of water to help liquefy mucus. Water is also an expectorant.

Guaifenesin (Mucinex) is the most commonly used expectorant. It loosens mucus and thins bronchial secretions to make a cough more productive. It is often available in combination with antitussives or decongestants. Side effects of guaifenesin include nausea, GI upset, and drowsiness.

Potassium iodide (Lugol's Solution) is an expectorant that has been used, but is not FDA-approved, in patients with CF. The dose is diluted with a glass of water or fruit juice. Side effects include iodide or potassium toxicity, but do not generally occur when used as instructed. **TABLE 11.5** lists common antitussives, expectorants, and decongestants.

Decongestants

Decongestants stimulate the adrenergic receptors of the vascular smooth muscle, causing vasoconstriction and a decrease in mucus production. They also promote nasal sinus drainage. Decongestants should be used with caution in patients with high blood pressure, diabetes, hyperthyroidism, prostatic hypertrophy, or cardiovascular disease. They are frequently combined with antihistamines to offset the drowsiness caused by antihistamines.

Table 11.5   Common Antitussives, Expectorants, and Decongestants

Generic Name	Brand Name	Available Formulations	Type of Drug
Benzonatate	Tessalon	Capsule	Antitussive
Codeine	Robitussin A-C	Liquid	Antitussive
Dextromethorphan	Delsym	Capsule, liquid	Antitussive
Guaifenesin	Mucinex, others	Tablet, liquid	Expectorant
Guaifenesin-dextromethorphan	Robitussin DM	Liquid	Expectorant/antitussive
Guaifenesin-codeine	Robitussin A-C	Liquid	Expectorant/antitussive
Guaifenesin-pseudoephedrine	Mucinex D	Liquid	Expectorant/decongestant
Hydrocodone-chlorpheniramine	Tussionex	Liquid	Antitussive/decongestant
Hydrocodone-guaifenesin	Hycotuss Expectorant Syrup	Liquid	Antitussive/expectorant

Decongestants are used to relieve nasal congestion due to upper respiratory allergies and the common cold. Decongestants can be administered topically or orally. Decongestants used topically for a prolonged period can result in a phenomenon called **rhinitis medicamentosa**, or rebound nasal congestion due to the extended use of topical nasal decongestants. Use of a topical nasal decongestant should be limited to three days to prevent the development of this rebound nasal congestion.

Pseudoephedrine (Sudafed) is the most commonly used decongestant. It is also combined with other drugs such as ibuprofen, codeine, naproxen sodium, and some antihistamines. Pseudoephedrine is a derivative of ephedrine and can be made into methamphetamine. Because of the illegal production of methamphetamine, there are legal limits on the amount of pseudoephedrine that can be purchased at one time. (The limits placed on the amount of pseudoephedrine that can be purchased vary from state to state. This is discussed in more detail in Chapter1.) Pseudoephedrine-containing products are kept behind the counter. Identification is required to purchase these products. Common side effects include drowsiness, constipation, headache, nausea, nervousness, and dizziness.

Phenylephrine (Sudafed PE, Neo-Synephrine) has largely replaced pseudoephedrine because it cannot be made into methamphetamine. There are no legal limits placed on the sale of phenylephrine. Phenylephrine is often used in eye drops or nasal sprays for the treatment of allergy.

Common side effects of oral decongestants include CNS stimulation, dizziness, increased blood pressure and heart rate, and tremor. Common side effects of topical decongestants include dry mouth, stinging or burning sensation, and rhinitis medicamentosa. **TABLE 11.6** lists commonly used decongestants.

Antihistamines

An **allergy** is an immune response to a foreign substance. Histamine is released during an allergic reaction. Histamine induces capillary permeability, increases gastric acid secretion, and increases heart rate. There are two types of histamine receptors: H_1 and H_2. Antihistamines block H_1 receptors in the respiratory tract, while H_2 blockers block histamine receptors in the gastrointestinal tract. Drugs that block the activity of H_1 receptors are known as antihistamines; drugs that block the activity of H_2 receptors are known as H_2 blockers or antagonists.

Antihistamines are used to block the effects of histamine on the respiratory tract. They can be used to treat a variety of conditions including allergies, rashes, insomnia, hay fever, nausea and vomiting, vertigo, and extrapyramidal side effects of antipsychotics. Antihistamines are also used for the treatment of hypersensitivity reactions.

First-generation antihistamines include diphenhydramine, promethazine, and meclizine. Second-generation antihistamines include cetirizine, clemastine, desloratadine, fexofenadine, levocetirizine, and loratadine. First-generation antihistamines cause more drowsiness than second-generation antihistamines. Some second-generation antihistamines cause little or no sedation. Common side effects of first-and second-generation antihistamines include dry mouth, constipation, urinary retention,

Table 11.6 Commonly Used Decongestants

Generic Name	Brand Name	Available Formulations
Pseudoephedrine	Sudafed	Capsule, tablet, liquid
Phenylephrine	Many brand names	Many dosage forms
Oxymetazoline	Afrin	Nasal spray

Table 11.7   Commonly Used Antihistamines.

Generic Name	Brand Name	Available Formulations
Azelastine	Astelin, Optivar	Nasal spray, ophthalmic
Brompheniramine	Brovex, Dimetane	Liquid
Cetirizine	Zyrtec	Liquid, tablet
Chlorpheniramine	Chlortrimeton	Tablet
Clemastine	Tavist Allergy	Liquid, tablet
Desloratadine	Clarinex	Liquid, tablet
Diphenhydramine	Benadryl	Capsule, liquid, tablet, injectable
Fexofenadine	Allegra	Capsule, tablet
Hydroxyzine	Atarax, Vistaril	Capsule, liquid, tablet, injectable
Levocetirizine	Xyzal	Tablet
Loratadine	Claritin	Liquid, tablet
Meclizine	Antivert	Tablet, capsule
Promethazine	Phenergan	Tablet, suppository

hyperactivity in children, dizziness, and sedation. **TABLE 11.7** lists commonly used antihistamines.

Nasal Corticosteroids

Nasal corticosteroids are used to treat rhinitis caused by colds, allergens, pollution, or strong odors, or irritants such as tobacco smoke. Common symptoms of rhinitis include runny and itchy nose, sneezing, and congestion. Adverse effects of these drugs include local irritation and bleeding. Patients who use nasal corticosteroids long term may also be at increased risk for *Candida abicans* infections. **TABLE 11.8** lists commonly used nasal corticosteroids.

Smoking Cessation

Cigarette smoking can increase the risk of lung cancer; cancers of the mouth, larynx, pharynx, esophagus, cervix, and kidney; heart disease; COPD; and stroke. Second-hand smoke also poses a significant threat to health because it contains all the chemicals and carcinogens found in inhaled smoke. Children living in homes of smokers

Table 11.8   Commonly Used Nasal Corticosteroids

Generic Name	Brand Name	Available Formulations
Beclomethasone	Beconase AQ	Nasal spray
Budesonide	Rhinecort Aqua	Nasal spray
Ciclesonide	Omnaris	Nasal spray
Fluticasone furoate	Veramyst	Nasal spray
Fluticasone propionate	Flonase	Nasal spray
Mometasone	Nasonex	Nasal spray
Triamcinolone	Nasacort AQ	Nasal spray

have a higher risk of respiratory infections and asthma than children who live with nonsmokers.

Nicotine is the addictive chemical found in tobacco that is readily absorbed in the lungs and the oral or nasal mucosa. Chronic nicotine ingestion can lead to physical and psychological dependence. Nicotine can cause increases in blood pressure, heart rate, and cardiac output. Nicotine can induce liver enzymes that are responsible for the metabolism of some drugs. Smoking cessation can result in improved health and self-esteem. It can also result in a huge economic savings. Smoking increases alertness, improves cognitive performance, and produces pleasure, making it hard to quit. Smoking-cessation therapy involves behavior modification, social support, and nicotine-replacement therapy. The key to quitting is abstinence.

Patients on smoking-cessation therapy should be advised to stop smoking to avoid excessive nicotine levels. Signs of excess nicotine levels include dizziness, perspiration, confusion, and headache. **TABLE 11.9** lists common drugs used in smoking-cessation therapy.

Bupropion (Zyban) helps to reduce the craving for smoking and withdrawal symptoms of nicotine. It should be started one to two weeks before quitting and taken for seven to 12 weeks after stopping smoking. Commonly reported side effects include dry mouth, difficulty sleeping, and seizures, with a higher rate in patients who have a history of seizures.

Nicotine nasal spray (Nicotrol) most closely resembles the effects of cigarette smoking due to its rapid absorption after nasal administration. Adverse effects of the nasal spray include nasal irritation, throat irritation, runny nose, sneezing, and cough. The gum (Nicorette, Thrive) is most often used for smoking cessation in users of smokeless tobacco. Adverse effects include jaw ache and hiccups. Nicotine gum should be "puckered," not chewed like regular gum, because molecules of nicotine are gradually dislodged from the resin in the gum and then absorbed into the bloodstream through the membranes that line the inside of the mouth. Nicotine gum also contains a buffer that maintains an acidity level that ensures the nicotine will be absorbed at a steady rate. Nicotine lozenges (Commit, Nicorette) should be sucked and moved side to side in the mouth until dissolved. Nicotine patches should be applied to a dry, non-hairy part of the upper body. The most common adverse effect of the patch is irritation at the site of application.

Varenicline (Chantix) reduces the craving and withdrawal symptoms of nicotine. It should be started one week before quitting and continued for 24 weeks. Common side effects include nausea and vivid dreams.

Table 11.9	Common Drugs Used for Smoking Cessation	
Generic Name	**Brand Name**	**Available Formulations**
Bupropion	Zyban	Tablet
Nicotine	Nicorette, Habitrol, Nicoderm CQ, Nicotrol, Thrive	Gum, lozenge, patch, nasal spray, inhaler
Varenicline	Chantix	Tablet

Tech Math Practice

Question: A patient enters your pharmacy with a prescription for terbutaline 5mg tablets with the following sig: "Take one tablet twice daily Quantity: 40." What is the days' supply?

Answer: Use the following equation to determine the days' supply: 40 tablets ÷ 2 = 20 days' supply.

Question: A patient has a prescription for vancomycin 250mg with the following sig: "Take one capsule twice daily for 21 days." How many capsules of vancomycin should be dispensed for a 21-day supply?

Answer: To calculate the quantity to dispense, use the following formula:

   Quantity of Medication Used in a 24-hour Period × Days' Supply = Quantity to Dispense

So, 2 capsules/day × 21 days = 42 capsules of vancomycin for a 21-day supply.

Question: A patient has a prescription for tetracycline 250mg with the following sig: "Take one capsule twice daily for 6 weeks." How many capsules of tetracycline should be dispensed for a six-week supply?

Answer: To calculate the answer, use the following equation: 2 capsules/day × 42 days (6 weeks × 7 days/week = 42 days) = 84 capsules of tetracycline for a 42-day supply.

Question: Suppose the maximum inventory level for zafirlukast 20mg tablets is 1,000 capsules, and that the minimum inventory level at which the drug is automatically reordered is 700 tablets. At the end of the business day, the inventory level is 635 tablets. How many tablets should be ordered?

Answer: To calculate the answer, use the following equation: 1,000 tablets – 635 tablets = 365 tablets should be ordered.

Question: A 30-day supply of rifapentine sells for $80. It costs the pharmacy $55. What is the markup?

Answer: To calculate the markup, use the following formula:

   Selling Price – Purchase Price = Markup

So, $80 – $55 = $25 is the markup.

Question: Using the information from the preceding question, what is the percentage markup?

Answer: To determine the percentage markup, use the following formula:

   (Markup ÷ Cost) × 100% = Percentage Markup

So, ($25 ÷ $55) × 100% = 45% percentage markup.

Question: A wholesaler offers a 10 percent discount on the purchase if the balance of an invoice is paid in full within 15 days of the date the inventory was delivered. What is the total discounted purchase price of three cases of albuterol, which cost $125/case.

Answer: First, calculate the total purchase price using the following equation:

Quantity of Product × Cost Per Unit = Total purchase price

So, 3 cases × $125/case = $375 is the total purchase price.

Next, calculate the discount using the following formula:

Total Purchase Price × Discount Rate = Discount

So, $375 × 0.10 (10% = 0.10) = $37.50 is the discount.

Then, calculate the discounted purchase price using the following formula:

Total Purchase Price – Discount = Discounted Purchase Price

So, $375 – $37.50 = $337.50 is the discounted purchase price.

Question: Ciprofloxacin 250mg is available in a bottle that contains 100 tablets. The AWP of ciprofloxacin is $75. The pharmacy purchases the drug from the wholesaler at AWP minus 12 percent. How much does the pharmacy purchase the drug for?

Answer: First, calculate the amount of the discount the pharmacy would receive using the following equation: $75 × 0.12 = $9 is the discount the pharmacy would receive.

Next, using the discount the pharmacy would receive, calculate the purchase price of the drug: $75 – $9 = $66 would be the purchase price of 100 tablets of ciprofloxacin 250mg after the discount.

Question: A patient brings in a prescription for albuterol sulfate 2mg/5mL solution with the following sig: "Give ½ teaspoonful twice daily for 10 days." What is the total volume of albuterol sulfate needed to complete a 10-day course of therapy?

Answer: To calculate the days' supply, first calculate the volume taken in each dose by converting ½ teaspoonful to milliliters. 1 tsp = 5mL, so ½ tsp/dose × 5mL = 2.5mL/dose.

Next, calculate the amount of drug prescribed per day: 2 doses/day × 2.5mL/dose = 5mL/day.

Finally, calculate the total volume needed for a 10-day supply: 5mL/day × 10 days = 50mL.

Question: A patient brings in a prescription for Cipro 250mg/5mL with the following sig "Give 1 teaspoonful twice daily for 10 days." Medicaid insurance does not cover this strength, but will cover Cipro 500mg/5mL. If the substitution to the covered strength is made, what will the new sig be?

Answer: First, calculate the volume of Cipro 500mg/5mL needed to provide the 250mg dose. To do so, use the ratio-proportion method: $^{xmL}/_{250mg} = {}^{5mL}/_{500mg}$. Then cross multiply: $xmL = 2.5mL$. The new sig should be, "Take ½ teaspoonful twice daily for 10 days."

Question: **Using the information in the preceding question, calculate the total volume of medication needed to complete a 10-day course of therapy.**

Answer: First, calculate the volume of medication needed per day: 2.5mL/dose × 2 doses/day = 5mL/day. Then calculate the volume of medication needed for 10 days: 5mL/day × 10 days = 50mL.

Question: **A large and extremely busy pharmacy has the following overhead expenses:**

- Salaries: $5,000,000
- Rent: $1,000,000
- Utilities: $500,000
- Computer maintenance: $1,000,000
- Software subscriptions: $1,000,000
- Insurance: $12,000,000
- Drug inventory: $950,000

If an 18 percent profit is desirable, what must the pharmacy's income be to meet this goal?

Answer: In this case, the profit is to be 18%. First, determine the percentage rate to use as a multiplier to solve for profit. $18\% = \frac{18}{100} \times 100\% = 0.18$. Put another way, Profit = Overhead × 0.18. Next, you must calculate overhead by determining the sum of the aforementioned expenses: $5,000,000 + $1,000,000 + $500,000 + $1,000,000 + $1,000,000 + $12,000,000 + $950,000 = $21,450,000.

So, profit = $21,450,000 × 0.18 = $3,861,000. To calculate the total income needed, add the overhead to the profit: $21,450,000 + $3,861,000 = $25,311,000.

WRAP UP

Chapter Summary

- The pharmacy technician has an important role in the sale of OTC medications.

- The pharmacy technician must understand all cash-register management functions including cash, check, credit-card, debit-card, and flex-card transactions.

- A variety of private and government-based healthcare plans provide medical and prescription coverage.

- The technician plays an important role in the purchasing, receiving, and returning of drugs.

- All information must be entered correctly and accurately into the pharmacy database to avoid rejection of a drug claim by a PBM.

- The pharmacy technician must understand basic calculations involving markups, discounts, AWP, and days' supply.

- Asthma is a chronic inflammatory airway disease in which the muscles around the bronchioles contract, narrowing the air passages so that air cannot be inhaled properly.

- Medications can prevent or reverse asthma attacks.

- Asthma medications are often delivered by a metered dose inhaler (MDI) that contains medication and compressed gas.

- Short-acting anticholinergics and beta-agonists are used for acute asthma attacks.

- Long-term medications include corticosteroids, long-acting bronchodilators, leukotriene receptor antagonists, cromolyn, theophylline, nedocromil, and immunomodulators.

- Corticosteroids produce smooth muscle relaxation and lessen the constriction of the bronchial tubes by inhibiting inflammatory cells.

- Long-acting bronchodilators are recommended for chronic prophylaxis of asthma and are used in conjunction with inhaled corticosteroids.

- Theophylline reverses bronchospasm associated with antigens by causing relaxation of airway smooth muscle and dilation.

- Leukotriene receptor antagonists block the synthesis of or response to leukotrienes, blocking the inflammatory response.

- Mast-cell stabilizers protect mast-cell membranes from rupture caused by antigens.

- Anti-IgE antibody is a recombinant monoclonal antibody that prevents IgE from binding to mast cells, thereby preventing release of inflammatory mediators after allergen exposure.

- Any long-term condition that can damage the lungs can cause chronic obstructive pulmonary disease (COPD). Chronic bronchitis and emphysema are two types of diseases that cause COPD.

- Bronchitis is an inflammation of the lining of the bronchial airways, which leads to obstruction of airflow upon exhalation.

- Emphysema is a disorder characterized by destruction of the alveolar walls and alveoli that eventually leads to a loss of lung elasticity.

- Pneumonia is an infection of one or both lungs. Pneumonia may be contracted by breathing in droplets from a cough or sneeze that contain the causative organism or bacteria or viruses that are normally present in the mouth, throat, or nose and inadvertently enter the lungs via aspiration during sleep.

- Cystic fibrosis (CF) is an inherited disease that involves the secretory glands, including the glands that make mucus and sweat. In patients with CF, the mucus becomes thick and sticky and builds up in the lungs.

- Respiratory distress syndrome is a breathing disorder that occurs in newborns. It is more common in premature infants because their lungs are unable to make an adequate amount of surfactant, which lowers the surface tension between the air and alveolar sacs.

- Tuberculosis (TB) is a common, highly contagious bacterial disease that is characterized by an infection within the lining of the lungs. It is caused by the bacterium *Mycobacterium tuberculosis*.

- The most common form of an upper respiratory tract infection is the common cold.

- Antitussives are medications that suppress or reduce the frequency of coughing.

- Expectorants are drugs that break up thick mucus secretions so that they can be expelled through coughing.

- Decongestants stimulate the adrenergic receptors of the vascular smooth muscle, causing vasoconstriction and a decrease in mucus production. They also promote nasal sinus drainage.

- Decongestants used topically for a prolonged period can result in a rebound phenomenon called rhinitis medicamentosa.

- Antihistamines are used to block the effects of histamine on the respiratory tract. They can be used to treat a variety of conditions including allergies, rashes, insomnia, hay fever, nausea and vomiting, vertigo, and extrapyramidal side effects of antipsychotics.

- Nasal corticosteroids are used to treat rhinitis caused by colds, allergens, pollution, or strong odors.

- Cigarette smoking can increase the risk of lung cancer; cancers of the mouth, larynx, pharynx, esophagus, cervix, and kidney; heart disease; COPD; and stroke.

- Smoking-cessation therapy involves behavior modification, social support, and nicotine-replacement therapy.

Learning Assessment Questions

1. A PBM is which of the following?

   A. A prime vendor

   B. A manufacturer

   C. An insurance company

   D. A company that contracts to perform certain tasks for an insurance company

2. A drug that can be sold without a prescription is called which of the following?

   A. OTC drug

   B. Legend drug

   C. Schedule II substance

   D. Schedule III substance

3. OTC drugs are regulated by which of the following?

   A. The DEA

   B. The individual state board of pharmacy

   C. The FDA

   D. OSHA

4. Which of the following describes the total value of all the drugs and merchandise in stock?

   A. Inventory value

   B. Front-end merchandise

   C. Back-end merchandise

   D. Maximum value

5. Medicaid covers all but which of the following?

   A. Women who are pregnant

   B. Disabled persons

   C. Persons with low income

   D. Persons with high income

6. Which of the following is the amount a pharmacy sets for a particular product that includes overhead and profit, in addition to the cost to acquire the product?

   A. Markup

   B. Discount

   C. AWP

   D. None of the above

7. Which of the following describes insurance to cover medical care and compensation from injuries suffered by employees while on the job?

   A. Medicaid

   B. Medicare

   C. Workers' compensation

   D. Tricare

8. AWP is an acronym for which of the following terms?

   A. Acquisition wholesale price

   B. Average wholesale price

   C. Allowable wasted product

   D. Average cost to the patient

9. Patients with asthma should avoid which of the following?

   A. Beta-blockers

   B. Montelukast

   C. Albuterol

   D. Corticosteroids

10. Drugs used for the treatment of asthma include which of the following?

    A. Leukotriene receptor antagonists

    B. Bronchodilators

    C. Corticosteroids

    D. All of the above

11. The disorder characterized by destruction of alveoli of the lungs is known as which of the following?

    A. Chronic bronchitis

    B. Emphysema

    C. Rhinitis

    D. Respiratory distress syndrome

12. Drugs used for the treatment of tuberculosis include which of the following?

    A. Isoniazid

    B. Rifampin

    C. Rifapentine

    D. All of the above

13. Rhinitis medicamentosa can occur with the use of which of the following?

    A. Topical decongestants

    B. Antitussives

    C. Antihistamines

    D. Expectorants

14. Which of the following is the most commonly used expectorant?

    A. Codeine

    B. Guaifenesin

    C. Dextromethorphan

    D. Pseudoephedrine

15. Side effects of antihistamines include which of the following?

    A. Dry mouth

    B. Urinary retention

    C. Constipation

    D. All of the above

16. Drugs used for smoking cessation include which of the following?

    A. Varenicline

    B. Phenylephrine

    C. Benzonatate

    D. Rifapentine

17. Which of the following is a Schedule II controlled substance used to relieve cough?

    A. Diphenhydramine

    B. Codeine

    C. Dextromethorphan

    D. Zyban

18. Antihistamines can be used to alleviate which of the following?

    A. Vertigo

    B. Insomnia

    C. Nausea and vomiting

    D. All of the above

19. Replacement of endogenous surfactant is used for the treatment of which of the following?

    A. Emphysema

    B. Chronic bronchitis

    C. Respiratory distress syndrome

    D. Cystic fibrosis

20. Agents that break up thick mucus secretions so that they can be expelled through coughing are called which of the following?

    A. Cough drops

    B. Expectorants

    C. Antitussives

    D. Decongestants

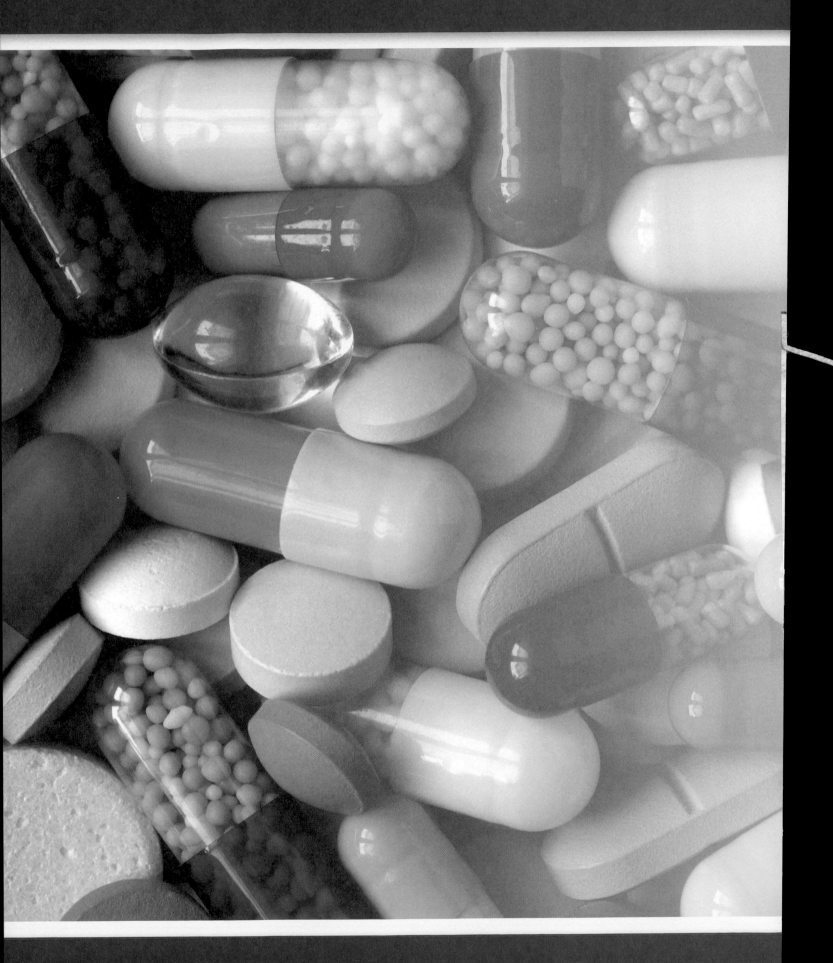

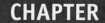
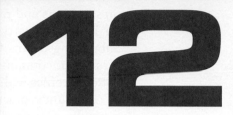

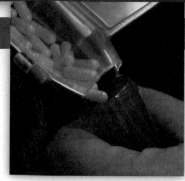

Labs for Business of the Community Pharmacy

OBJECTIVES

After reading this chapter, you will be able to:

- Summarize the process for filing third-party or insurance claims.
- Cite the reasons that third-party claims are often rejected and the steps needed to resolve these problems.
- Identify the reasons for cash pricing of prescriptions.
- Explain how an audit log is prepared using pharmacy management software.
- Describe the role of the pharmacy technician in pharmacy administration.
- Identify common drugs for gastrointestinal diseases and conditions.
- Understand the prevention and treatment of malaria.
- Understand the prevention and treatment of hepatitis.

KEY TERMS

Abuse
Capture
Cash price
Chemoreceptor trigger zone (CTZ)
Chemosensory organ
Constipation
Crohn's disease
Diarrhea
Emesis
Erosions
Extreme obesity
Fiber
Fraud

Gastric emptying time
Gastritis
Gastroenteritis
Gastroesophageal reflux disease (GERD)
Gastrointestinal (GI) system
Gastroparesis
Hepatitis
Inflammatory bowel disease (IBD)
Irritable bowel syndrome (IBS)

Malaria
Nausea
Obesity
Overweight
Peptic ulcer
Peptic ulcer disease
Probiotics
Third-party adjudication
Transit time
Ulcerative colitis (UC)
Vomiting
Waste

Chapter Overview

Pharmacy technicians are routinely involved in transactions such as payments for prescriptions and reimbursement for pharmacy services. Most prescriptions are paid for by a third party, such as a government health plan or private health insurance. Submitting claims for proper payment, following up and obtaining additional information, communicating with the patient about insurance benefits, and updating patient profiles with insurance information are primary roles of pharmacy technicians in community practice. In hospitals and other institutional settings, this process is generally completed outside the pharmacy department. However, in some hospital, institutional, and home healthcare settings, pharmacy technicians are responsible for insurance verification and processing billing information.

Correct processing of claims is critical to ensure efficient, timely care. Understanding the features and nuances of common insurance plans and software systems enables technicians to accurately submit claims, verify pricing, and resolve issues related to prescription payments. Errors in submission may result in delayed care, patient frustration, incorrect payments to the pharmacy, incorrect copayment amounts, and even allegations of fraud.

Business of the Community Pharmacy

Insurance companies and government health providers are considered "third parties." They move payment from the patient (the "first party") to the pharmacy (the "second party").

Every pharmacy has its own specific software that aids in prescription processing and claim submission. Pharmacy technicians will receive site-specific training in a community practice. With countless third-party plans available, a detailed explanation of each plan is impractical. Instead, this chapter explains the general principles behind third-party prescription claims, cash pricing of medications, and audit logs related to drug dispensing and payment. Once in practice, you will become familiar with the coverage plans that are popular in your community.

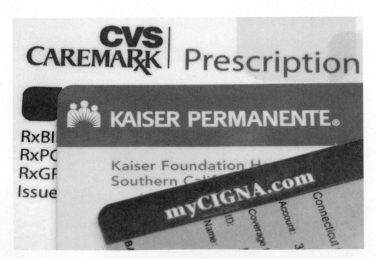

Pharmacy technicians should become familiar with the information provided on insurance cards and the documentation required for processing prescription claims.

Insurance Cards

Information about prescription coverage is indicated on an insurance card, which the patient produces for the pharmacy. This card will contain the patient's name, identification number, group number for the coverage plan, benefit identification number (BIN), and the responsible party or code denoting the primary person insured. The primary account holder is usually person 1 or 01, and the spouse or secondary dependent is 2 or 02. Subsequent dependents will be consecutively numbered, often from oldest to youngest.

Not all insurance companies require the same information, so pharmacy technicians should become familiar with common insurance cards. Verifying the required information will expedite claim submission. Always ensure that patients present their most current insurance card, and that their demographic information is correct in the computer system.

Practical Exercise

Identify the following information on these insurance cards:

Patient code

Prescription coverage identification number

Prescription coverage group number

BIN number

Phone number for pharmacies to call with claims questions

Third-Party Claims

More than half of Americans are covered by private health insurance. Additionally, more than 100 million people receive healthcare services through government-sponsored plans such as Medicare, Medicaid, Tricare, the Veterans Administration, and the Indian Health Service.

Most public and private insurance plans and services provide some type of prescription coverage. In such cases, when a patient presents a prescription to a pharmacy for processing, the pharmacy is responsible for submitting a claim to the coverage provider. Pharmacies rarely interact in a direct relationship with the actual third parties, but instead deal with companies called pharmacy benefit managers (PBMs). PBMs adjudicate claims on behalf of the health plans. The PBM will approve or reject a claim based on parameters defined by the health plan. Refer to Chapter 11 for more in-depth discussion on these topics.

To accurately submit a claim to a third party or PBM, the pharmacy must take care to keep accurate and up-to-date patient information. The pharmacy staff must then accurately input all required information.

Once approved, the third party pays the pharmacy for the prescription on behalf of the patient.

The first step in the claim-submission process is to ensure accurate entry of the prescription into the pharmacy's computer software. Third-party processing relies on accurate patient information. Take care to verify the patient's personal information; an error could result in a claim rejection and delay of care. The third party will use the information entered into the computer such as the patient information, prescriber, medication, frequency of administration, duration of therapy, quantity, and refills to make a judgment as to whether the prescription will be paid for by the insurance company and, if so, at what cost. This process of making a coverage decision is known as **third-party adjudication**. Most of the time, this process occurs through online or electronic communication, or online adjudication.

All providers and insurers are required to have comprehensive training programs in place to ensure that claims are submitted and processed correctly. These programs also include processes to detect, correct, and prevent fraud, waste, and abuse. Fraud *is an intentional act of deception, misrepresentation, or concealment by a person that could result in an unauthorized medical benefit to that or another person.* Waste *is the overutilization of services or other practices that result in the misuse of resources.* Abuse *refers to healthcare provider practices that are inconsistent with sound fiscal, business, and medical practices that will result in unnecessary costs or financial loss. The Centers for Medicare and Medicaid Services (CMS) provide guidance for the development and implementation of these plans. Employees are to be trained on the fraud, waste, and abuse directives as directed by CMS.*

If a particular product is not covered by an insurance provider, ask the pharmacist to contact the PBM or prescriber for an alternative medication that is covered.

The amount reimbursed to the pharmacy by the insurance company is based on the cost of the drug plus a dispensing fee. The cost of the drug is usually the average acquisition cost minus any discounts available from the wholesaler or distributor. The third-party plan remits payment to the pharmacy electronically, directly depositing funds into a bank account.

Claims Rejections

Third-party adjudication will result in a payment (also called a **capture**) or a rejection. Rejections commonly occur for the following reasons:

- The drug is not covered by an insurance plan (often noted by the National Drug Code number or Drug Generic Code Number, also referred to as the GCN)—If a drug is not covered by the insurance company, a patient will need to pay cash for the prescription in order to have it filled as written. Alternatively, the pharmacist may contact the prescriber and suggest an equivalent substitution that is covered by the insurance company. Advise the patient that this process may take some time, as prescribers do not often respond immediately to prescription-related messages. It is impossible and impractical for pharmacy staff to memorize the formulary of drugs that are covered by each insurance company; resolving coverage issues takes time, because it requires communication among the pharmacist, the prescriber, the insurance company, and the patient.

- Prior authorization is required—In some cases, prior authorization may be required before an insurance company will allow payment for a particular drug. In such cases, the insurance company requires more information before processing the claim, such as documentation from a physician as to why a certain drug was prescribed. This process can take several days to resolve. A patient can choose to wait for authorization or pay cash immediately for the medication. In this case, the patient can file a claim for reimbursement from his or her insurance provider. Alternatively, the insurer will pay the healthcare provider, which will in turn reimburse the patient. If a patient is covered by a government program, cash up front is not an acceptable form of payment. In this case, the claim is submitted to the insurer first.

Any prescription may include directions to use "as needed" or "as directed." In the case of insulin prescriptions, most computer systems default to a 30-day supply or the actual days' supply, whichever is less. When processing an insurance claim for insulin, verify how much insulin the patient usually uses to determine when he or she should be permitted to refill the prescription. Defaulting to a 30-day supply will not allow the patient to refill his insulin prescription if he or she uses the vial in less time.

- The drug has already been dispensed—In duplicate-therapy cases, the insurance company has already paid for a similar drug and will not approve payment again. If a patient received two similar prescriptions from two different prescribers who were unaware of other prescriptions, then such a rejection is legitimate. It may be, however, that a patient's condition was uncontrolled with one medication and a second was added under the guidance of the original prescriber. If this happens, it may be necessary to verify with the pharmacist and prescriber that two similar medications are both necessary. It will then be necessary to resolve the rejection by calling the insurance company or PBM and obtaining authorization.

- The patient's health plan does not cover certain pharmacy services—If a rejection occurs because a patient is not covered, begin the resolution by verifying that the patient provided his most up-to-date insurance card. Often, insurance benefits change or patients receive new cards, and they fail to provide this information to the pharmacy. Review the patient's profile and verify the information. If the patient does not have valid prescription coverage according to the information provided, advise the patient to provide proof of prescription coverage. This may entail some research on the part of the pharmacy technician. Some states have specific protocols for handling rejections for patients receiving government-sponsored prescription coverage. Remain up to date on state-specific laws governing the dispensing of medications in these circumstances.

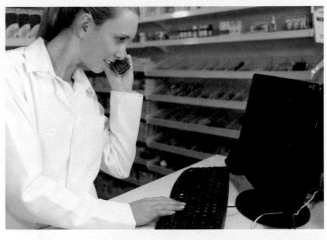

It is often necessary to verify the patient and prescription information entered in the online adjudication system and call the insurance provider to resolve claim rejections.

- A refill is ordered to soon—Each insurance company has its own specific requirements as to how soon a prescription may be refilled, based on the days supplied and sometimes even the instructions provided for taking the medication. To resolve an error of this type, first verify that the days' supply was entered correctly for the original prescription; this is a common source of errors, particularly for ointments, creams, and drops. If a patient simply forgot that he has a sufficient supply already, the prescription claim may be cancelled and the patient will be able to refill the prescription at a later date. If the patient lost a prescription or it was stolen, an override is often available by calling the insurance company. Such overrides for these specific situations are available on a limited basis, allowing approval when it would otherwise be too early. Overrides are sometimes available when a patient will be on vacation or unavailable to refill a prescription at a later time. If no overrides are available and a patient still wishes to refill a prescription, he must pay cash for the refill.

Patients should always be instructed to use medication exactly as prescribed. Taking more or less of a medication than ordered is not only unsafe, but may result in fraudulent insurance claims if a patient knowingly takes medication differently than directed in an effort to deceive the third-party payer.

A rejection might also occur if the prescription is entered incorrectly or patient information is inaccurately entered in the computer. Patients can easily become frustrated if they are unfamiliar with their coverage plans or do not understand the process of third-party adjudication. A different drug might be indicated for the same condition or need to be used first based upon a protocol the insurer uses to determine coverage. In some cases, the patient's deductible may not be met and thus the claim is rejected. After a rejection has occurred, it is usually the job of the pharmacy technician to resolve the claim and com-

Maintain communication with patients throughout the process of submitting claims, resolving rejections, and obtaining a capture. If delays occur or follow-up is needed, patients may be able to provide information that will assist the pharmacy technician. Patients may become especially frustrated if there are delays or problems with payment and they are not informed about what is happening.

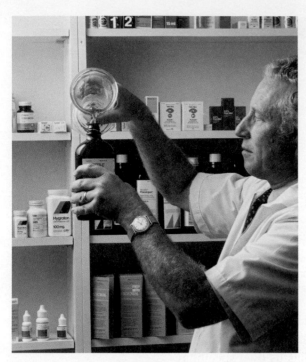

Pharmacy technicians should be able to identify information on stock bottle labels.

municate the outcome with the patient. The first step is to review the reason for rejection and correct any submission errors if possible.

Practical Exercise

Identify the following information on these stock bottle labels:

Brand name of drug

Generic name of drug

NDC or GCN number

Lot number

Expiration date

Manufacturer

Dosage form

Strength

Cash Pricing

When a patient does not have prescription insurance coverage or he or she wishes to pay for a prescription without filing an insurance claim, a pharmacy technician must verify the **cash price** of the medication. The cash price for a particular medication may vary from pharmacy to pharmacy, so patients may often ask pharmacy technicians to verify the price prior to filling the prescription. Assist patients with obtaining this information, as well as investigating prescription assistance programs for uninsured and under-insured individuals to promote affordable health care.

Pharmacy software will contain a searchable database of drug-pricing information. This information will often by classified by drug name or description and NDC number. The database will often provide the pharmacy's cost for the drug, the markup, patient-specific discounts available, the profit, and the price that should be quoted to the patient.

When verifying cash pricing, take care to choose the correct drug or product from the database. Many manufacturers make several similar products in different strengths or dosage forms, and these can vary markedly in price. Also, verify the quantity that the patient wishes to purchase.

Audit Logs

Pharmacy software is integral to the organized and economical operation of a pharmacy. Comprehensive software allows for efficient processing of prescriptions, maintenance of patient profiles, accurate record keeping, and prompt payment from insurance providers. In today's pharmacies, pharmacy technicians are taking on a larger role in managing these day-to-day operations and assuming larger administrative responsibilities.

What Would You Do?

Question: A patient enters your pharmacy with a prescription for Lipitor 20mg daily, quantity of 30. He states that his physician instructed him to take only half of a tablet daily, but that by filing the insurance claim with these instructions, he will get twice as many tablets paid for by his healthcare plan. How do you file the claim?

Answer: Knowingly entering fraudulent information for third-party billing is unprofessional, unethical, and unlawful. Your pharmacy might incur fines from the insurance company if the company audits payment or processing history. Additionally, the prescriber and the patient could be held liable and dismissed from participation in the coverage plan. Fraudulent insurance claims harm the healthcare system and lead to increased costs for all parties. In this case, ask the pharmacist to verify the correct dose, quantity, and directions with the prescriber and use that information to file a claim.

Accurate record-keeping is required, not only for reporting business statistics, but also for adhering to regulatory requirements. Most pharmacy software programs can easily generate reports that detail drug-usage patterns, including prescriber practices, HIPAA compliance, dispensing of controlled substances, inventory management, and price logs. A daily audit log can be produced that details a list of pharmacy staff who logged in or out of the software system, the number of prescriptions filled by each staff member, an overview of all prescriptions filled, a summary of sales, and a cost-analysis according to payment plan.

The information provided in a daily audit log helps pharmacy management estimate profits, losses, future sales, and scheduling needs. Pharmacy technicians—particularly those with advanced experience or in supervisory roles—are increasingly responsible for preparing and presenting logs and reports of pharmacy resources to pharmacy management.

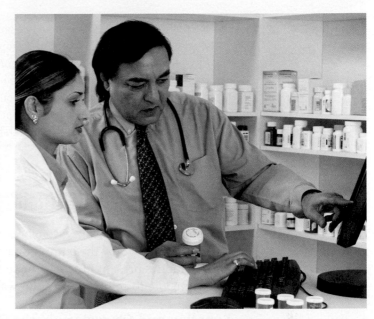

Pharmacy software enables the pharmacy to operate efficiently, manage resources, and process payments.

The use of pharmacy software allows for workload management and resource allocation. Pharmacy technicians support these administrative roles and allow pharmacists to spend more time on direct patient care and on activities related to the management of medication therapy.

Practical Exercise: Think Like a Technician

Use the information you learned about processing insurance claims to answer the following questions:

1. What key pieces of information must you have in order to correctly process a prescription, from receipt through online adjudication?
2. A patient asks you to refill her prescription at your community pharmacy for her blood pressure medicine. She is compliant with her medication and always obtains a 30-day supply with her refill. Her insurance is valid and you have the most up-to-date information. Her last refill of her blood-pressure medicine was filled seven days ago. She also takes aspirin daily and an inhaled corticosteroid for allergies, though she is not refilling any other prescriptions today. What is a potential reason that this claim might be rejected? What questions would you ask the patient, and how might you resolve the rejection?
3. A patient enters your community pharmacy with prescriptions for atenolol 50mg by mouth daily, fluticasone two sprays per nostril once daily, and famotidine 20mg by mouth twice daily. You note on his profile that he recently filled prescriptions for carvedilol 25mg twice daily and telithromycin 800mg once a day for seven days. The patient presents a valid insurance card and you have his most up-to-date information. What is a potential reason that this claim might be rejected? What questions would you ask the patient, and how might you resolve the rejection?
4. A father enters your community pharmacy with a prescription for amoxicillin 900mg daily for 10 days for his five-year-old son. The father does not have insurance coverage to pay for prescription drugs and worries about the cost of the medication. How will you process this prescription and how can you help the father understand his payment options?

5. A patient has been taking home IV therapy with Vancomycin 1.5 gram every 12 hours for six weeks. After the first week of therapy, the patient develops a reaction known as "Red Man's Syndrome" and it cannot be resolved by changing the rate of administration to infuse the antibiotic more slowly. The prescriber has changed the prescription to Daptomycin 600mg IV daily to complete the course of therapy. What does the pharmacy technician need to do prior to filling this prescription? When entering the prescription into the system, how many more weeks of therapy are needed for the Daptomycin?

Drug Insights: Gastrointestinal and Related Diseases

The **gastrointestinal (GI) system** breaks food down into small compounds that can be absorbed and used by the body. Primarily controlled by the autonomic nervous system and hormones present in saliva, the stomach, the pancreas, and the liver, the GI system is responsible for eliminating solid waste products from the body **FIGURE 12.1**.

Function and Physiology of the Gastrointestinal System

The GI tract, a major part of the GI system, is made up of a long tube that begins in the mouth, travels through the pharynx, esophagus, stomach, and small and large intestines, and ends at the anus. Propulsive movements and contractions of the GI tract move food in one direction through the system.

Chewing food initiates the secretion of saliva and begins the digestive process. Next, the stomach receives food, and mixes and churns it into smaller compounds. The pancreas produces digestive enzymes and bicarbonate to neutralize gastric acid.

The GI tract is lined with a mucous membrane that protects it from damage from harsh enzymes and an acidic environment.

The liver produces bile salts, which promote the digestion and absorption of fat. The GI tract also contains normal microbial flora that aid in digestion and prevent the overgrowth of fecal bacteria.

The stomach delivers food to the small intestine, where most absorption takes place. Nutrients, vitamins, minerals, and fluids are absorbed for use by the body's cells. Products that are not absorbed by the small intestine pass to the large intestine. The large intestine dehydrates these waste products, producing a firm fecal mass. This mass is eliminated from the body through defecation.

The cells throughout the gastrointestinal system produce and secrete fluids to aid in digestion and absorption of food. In the average adult, the gastrointestinal system produces a total of 7 to 10 liters of fluid a day.

GI **transit time** refers to the time it takes for food to pass through the GI tract. This can vary depending on the amount of food consumed, the amount of fat consumed, smoking, and various diseases and medications. A component of GI transit time, **gastric emptying time**, is the time it takes for food to pass through the stomach. Reduced transit time or rapid gastric emptying can lead to a decreased absorption of

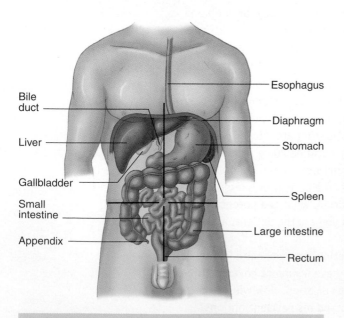

Bile duct
Liver
Gallbladder
Small intestine
Appendix

Esophagus
Diaphragm
Stomach
Spleen
Large intestine
Rectum

FIGURE 12.1 The human gastrointestinal system.

nutrients. Increased transit time or delayed gastric empty-ing, also known as **gastroparesis**, can lead to increased absorption of nutrients, but may also cause uncomfortable or irritating symptoms such as nausea, vomiting, lack of appetite, bloating, abdominal pain, and heartburn.

Gastrointestinal Diseases and Conditions

Common GI symptoms include heartburn, abdominal pain or discomfort, nausea, vomiting, diarrhea, consti-pation, and bleeding from ulcers, gastritis, and various other conditions. More significant signs and symptoms of GI disorders include anemia, weight loss, and difficulty swallowing.

Gastroesophageal Reflux Disease (GERD)

Gastroesophageal reflux disease (GERD), often referred to as heartburn, is a common problem, but it is most com-monly seen in patients over 40 years of age in Westernized countries. GERD results in damage to the mucosa of the GI tract caused by an abnormal reflux of stomach contents into the esophagus. If this reflux occurs for a prolonged period, the highly acidic contents of the stomach can cause permanent damage to the esophagus, and can also lead to the development of several forms of cancer.

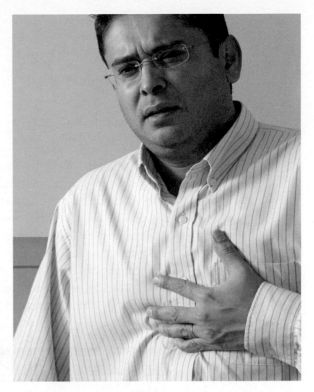

The symptoms of GERD are often described as a burning sensation in the abdomen.

One in five Americans experiences symptoms of GERD on a weekly basis.

The most common complaint associated with GERD is a warm or burning sensa-tion rising from the abdomen toward the neck. The symptoms vary in frequency and intensity but often include chest pain, sore throat, nausea, cough, bad breath, and earaches.

Following are several behaviors, foods and drinks, and medications that precipitate or worsen symptoms of GERD:

- Eating quickly
- Eating late at night
- Overeating
- Smoking
- Alcohol
- Caffeine
- Citric acid
- Garlic
- Gas-producing foods
- High-fat foods
- Onions
- Peppermint and spearmint
- Spicy foods
- Tomato juice
- Aspirin
- Barbiturates

- Estrogen
- Nitrates
- NSAIDs
- Potassium chloride
- Progesterone
- Theophylline
- Tetracycline

The goals of GERD treatment are to relieve the symptoms of heartburn, prevent the return of symptoms, and promote the healing of the esophageal mucosa. Therapies may include a combination of lifestyle modifications and pharmacological therapy.

There are over-the-counter and prescription drugs available to treat GERD. Persistent GERD, lasting longer than two weeks, should not be treated without supervision from a healthcare provider. **TABLE 12.1** lists common medications used to treat symptoms of GERD.

Antacids neutralize the acidic contents of the stomach. Antacids do not prevent reflux, but do help prevent irritation of the esophagus if reflux occurs. Antacids must

Table 12.1 OTC and Prescription Treatments for Symptoms of GERD

Class	Generic name	Brand name
OTC products		
Antacids	Aluminum hydroxide	AlternaGel
	Aluminum hydroxide-magnesium carbonate	Gaviscon Extra Strength
	Aluminum hydroxide-magnesium hydroxide-simethicone	Mylanta
	Magnesium hydroxide	Phillips Milk of Magnesia
Histamine II receptor antagonists	Cimetidine	Tagamet HB
	Famotidine	Pepcid AC
	Nizatidine	Axid AR
	Ranitidine	Zantac
Proton pump inhibitors	Omeprazole	Prilosec OTC
Combination products	Calcium carbonate-famotidine-magnesium hydroxide	Pepcid Complete
Prescription-strength products		
Histamine II receptor antagonists	Cimetidine	Tagamet
	Famotidine	Pepcid
	Nizatidine	Axid
	Ranitidine	Zantac
Proton pump inhibitors	Esomeprazole	Nexium
	Omeprazole	Prilosec
	Pantoprazole	Protonix
	Rabeprazole	Aciphex
Coating agent	Sucralfate	Carafate
Prostaglandin E analog	Misoprostol	Cytotec
Promotility agents	Metoclopramide	Reglan

be dosed frequently and can cause GI disorders of their own, including diarrhea and constipation, depending on the product. Patient compliance is a barrier to effective therapy.

Histamine receptor antagonists (H2RAs) block the action of histamine H_2, which effectively lowers gastric acidity. Histamine stimulates the secretion of gastric acid and pepsin in the stomach, so blocking the histamine receptors prevents the secretion of these acidic agents. All H2RAs available for GERD are available in OTC and prescription-only formulations. The OTC products contain lower doses than the prescription products. They are indicated for short-term use unless otherwise prescribed by a healthcare provider for longer term maintenance regimens. The onset of action of H2RAs is relatively slow, but the duration of action is longer than other acid-reducing therapies. Of note among the H2RAs are the drug interactions related to cimetidine (Tagamet). Cimetidine (Tagamet) is a potent inhibitor of the CYP450 family of hepatic enzymes, so drug-drug and drug-food interactions are likely.

Proton pump inhibitors (PPIs) block the secretion of gastric acid in the stomach. PPIs are more effective than H2RAs at producing long-term relief of GERD symptoms. PPIs must be administered daily to ensure relief.

Combination products, which contain multiple acid-reducing therapies, are available to target several principles of GERD therapy. Combination products may increase patient compliance but are not more effective than single-agent treatments.

NSAIDs are prostaglandin antagonists. Because prostaglandins promote mucosal defense and protect the gastrointestinal mucosa from damage, NSAIDs increase the susceptibility to injury. Therefore, chronic NSAID therapy can lead to the formation of gastric ulcers and GERD symptoms. Misoprostol (Cytotec) replaces prostaglandins destroyed by NSAIDs. Misoprostol can cause diarrhea and abdominal pain. Pregnant women must not handle or come in contact with misoprostol because it can induce labor.

Promotility agents are often used in conjunction with acid-reducing therapy for patients with a GI motility dysfunction, such as delayed gastric emptying or an incompetent LES, pressure of the LES, maintaining its closure and preventing reflux. Metoclopramide (Reglan) speeds gastric emptying time.

GERD treatment should continue until relief of symptoms. Some patients will experience a recurrence of symptoms after discontinuation of therapy or lowering of a dose, and maintenance therapy may be required for these cases. Long-term therapy with low-dose PPIs is safe, and long-term therapy with H2RAs is useful for patients with mild disease. On-demand or as-needed therapy is not recommended for GERD maintenance, although some patients decide to administer OTC medications this way to reduce the costs associated with daily treatment.

Ten percent of Americans will suffer from a peptic ulcer at some point during their lives.

Peptic Ulcer Disease (PUD)

Acid-related disorders of the upper GI tract include the following:

- Gastritis—**Gastritis** is a widespread inflammation of the lining of the stomach caused by excess acid production.
- Erosions—**Erosions** are superficial degradations of the GI mucosa.
- Peptic ulcers—**Peptic ulcers** usually extend deeper into the mucosal lining of the GI tract than gastritis or erosions. The three most common types of peptic ulcers include *H. pylori*-associated, NSAID-induced, and stress-related.

Peptic ulcer disease (PUD) is characterized by a frequent recurrence of peptic ulcers. At least 60 percent of ulcers return within one year of initial healing.

Causes of peptic ulcers include the following:

- *H. pylori* infection
- NSAIDs
- Critical illness
- Corticosteroids
- Alcohol
- Potassium chloride
- Methotrexate
- Iron
- Smoking

The goal of PUD treatment is to relieve pain and discomfort associated with the ulcer, heal the ulcer, and prevent its recurrence. Common drug regimens include antimicrobial therapy to eliminate *H. pylori* infections and acid-reducing agents to decrease the symptoms of PUD. **TABLE 12.2** lists common antimicrobial agents used to treat *H. pylori* infections. A more detailed discussion of their mechanisms of action, as well as side effects and precautions, is presented in the "Drug Insights" section of Chapter 6. Most antimicrobials are administered for seven to 14 days for the initial treatment of *H. pylori* infections.

H2RAs and PPIs used to treat GERD are also used to treat PUD. H2RAs are preferred over PPIs for PUD, however, because H2RAs accelerate healing and provide longer symptom relief. Lifestyle modifications are also important in PUD. Eliminating aggravating foods from the diet, reducing stress, and smoking cessation will promote ulcer healing and reduce pain.

Inflammatory Bowel Disease (IBD)

Inflammatory bowel disease (IBD) includes **ulcerative colitis (UC)** and **Crohn's disease**.

UC is an inflammation of the rectum and colon. UC causes continuous lesions and affects the mucosa and submucosa.

Crohn's disease is not confined to a specific portion of the GI tract and results in discontinuous lesions throughout the tract. Nutritional deficiencies are common with Crohn's disease, because nutrient absorption is altered due to inflammation and damage in the small intestine.

The goals of IBD treatment depend on the type of disease present and the severity of disease. Common agents used to treat IBD are presented in **TABLE 12.3**. Treatment may be short-term, requiring only a few weeks of treatment before IBD remits, or maintenance of remission may require years of therapy.

Table 12.2   Antimicrobial Treatments for *H. pylori* Infections

Generic Name	Brand Name
Amoxicillin	Amoxil, Trimox
Clarithromycin	Biaxin
Metronidazole	Flagyl
Tetracycline	Sumycin

Table 12.3 Common Treatments for IBD		
Class	**Generic Name**	**Brand Name**
Immunosuppressants	Azathioprine	Imuran
	Mercaptopurine	Purinethol
	Cyclosporine	Neoral, Sandimmune
	Methotrexate	Rheumatrex, Trexall
Antimicrobials	Metronidazole	Flagyl
	Ciprofloxacin	Cipro
Anti-inflammatory agents	Sulfasalazine	Azulfidine
	Mesalamine	Rowasa, Asacol, Pentasa, Lialda, Canasa
	Olsalazine	Dipentum
	Balsalazide	Colazal
	Budesonide	Entocort

Nausea and Vomiting

Nausea is defined as the feeling of imminent vomiting. **Vomiting**, or **emesis**, is defined as the expulsion of gastric contents through the mouth. Vomiting is triggered by impulses to a section of the medulla known as the vomiting center, which are received from the **chemoreceptor trigger zone (CTZ)**. The CTZ is a **chemosensory organ** (a structure that receives input relating to the perception of chemicals) for emesis. Its stimulation is associated with chemical-induced vomiting. Antiemetic agents decrease or prevent nausea and vomiting. **TABLE 12.4** lists common antiemetics.

Antihistaminic-anticholinergic agents are effective for the treatment of simple nausea and vomiting caused by a variety of factors.

Phenothiazines are the most commonly prescribed antiemetic agents. They block dopamine receptors in the CTZ.

Butyrophenones block dopamine receptors in the CTZ. While effective, these agents are not first-line therapy for nausea and vomiting due to potential cardiotoxicity.

Corticosteroids are effective at reducing chemotherapy-induced and postoperative nausea and vomiting.

Approximately 90 percent of the serotonin present in the body is located in the GI tract. A majority of the remaining serotonin is located in the central nervous system.

Serotonin receptor antagonists block presynaptic serotonin receptors in the wall of the GI tract. These agents are used for chemotherapy-induced and postoperative nausea and vomiting. SSRIs are often used in combination with dexamethasone to prevent chemotherapy-induced nausea and vomiting.

Substance P is a neurotransmitter that mediates chemotherapy-induced nausea and vomiting. Aprepitant is currently the only available substance P antagonist.

Diarrhea

Diarrhea is a gastrointestinal discomfort that affects virtually every person at some point during his or her life. Diarrhea is defined as an increased frequency and decreased consistency of fecal matter compared with an individual's normal bowel habits.

Table 12.4 Common Antiemetic Agents

Class	Generic Name	Brand Name	Availability
Antihistamine-anticholinergic agents	Dimenhydrinate	Dramamine	OTC
	Hydroxyzine	Vistaril	Rx
	Meclizine	Bonine, Antivert	OTC and Rx
	Scopolamine	Transderm Scop	Rx
	Trimethobenzamide	Tigan	Rx
	Chlorpromazine	Thorazine	Rx
Phenothiazines	Prochlorperazine	Compazine	Rx
	Promethazine	Phenergan	Rx
	Dronabinol	Marinol	Rx
Cannabinoids	Nabilone	Cesamet	Rx
	Haloperidol	Haldol	Rx
Butyrophenones	Droperidol	Inapsine	Rx
	Dexamethasone	Various	Rx
Corticosteroids	Prednisone	Sterapred	Rx
	Alprazolam	Xanax	Rx
Benzodiazepines	Lorazepam	Ativan	Rx
	Dolasetron	Anzamet	Rx
Serotonin-receptor antagonists	Granisetron	Kytril	Rx
	Ondansetron	Zofran	Rx
	Palonosetron	Aloxi	Rx
Substance P receptor antagonists	Aprepitant	Emend	Rx

Diarrhea can be a sign or symptom of a systemic condition.

Diarrhea can be caused by a number of bacterial or viral organisms, but may also be caused by other disease states, conditions, medications, or food intolerances. Most cases of diarrhea, although inconvenient and uncomfortable, are self-limiting and short-lived. Acute diarrhea is defined as diarrhea lasting less than 14 days. Persistent diarrhea lasts more than 14 days, and chronic diarrhea lasts more than 30 days.

Diarrhea accounts for 7 percent of all adverse drug events. Of these, 25 percent are caused by antibiotics.

Common drug-related causes of diarrhea include the following:

- Laxatives
- Magnesium-containing drugs
- Antineoplastic agents
- Antibiotics
- Antihypertensives
- Cholinergics
- Cardiac agents
- NSAIDs

- Misoprostol
- Colchicine
- PPIs
- H2RAs

> *Polycarbophil absorbs up to 60 times its weight in water. It is used to treat both diarrhea and constipation.*

Diarrhea decreases transit time through the GI tract. Therefore, it leads to altered absorption of nutrients. Diarrhea can be dangerous when it occurs as a chronic condition or leads to dehydration. Management of diarrhea focuses on maintaining hydration and electrolyte balance as well as treating the underlying cause of diarrhea, if identifiable. Common drugs used for treating diarrhea are presented in **TABLE 12.5**.

Antimotility agents are opioid derivatives. These agents slow GI transit time, which improves absorption, decreases the frequency of bowel movements, and increases the consistency of bowel movements. Normally, opioids and related compounds cause constipation as a side effect, so using them to treat diarrhea is an example of using a drug's side effect to treat another condition. Many of these drugs may cause drowsiness, as well as addiction or dependence with long-term use.

Adsorbent agents provide symptom relief for acute diarrhea. These agents are nonspecific in their mechanism of action, meaning they do not target a specific drug or substance, so they adsorb all types of fluid, nutrients, and drugs from the GI tract. Adsorbents do not affect GI transit time. Adsorbents are appropriate for short-term self-management of diarrhea. If diarrhea symptoms persist for more than 24 hours, patients should seek medical advice. Due to limited systemic absorption, most adsorbent agents have few side effects. Infrequent side effects include constipation, bloating, and a feeling of fullness.

Bismuth subsalicylate is the only nonprescription bismuth product available in the United States. Patients who are sensitive to salicylates (for example, those with an aspirin allergy) should not use bismuth subsalicylate products. Also, bismuth subsalicylate may induce attacks of gout in patients with salicy-

What Would You Do?

Question: A patient approaches your pharmacy counter to pick up a prescription. He also presents a bottle of Pepto-Bismol for purchase and casually mentions that he has had "an upset stomach" recently. You recall that his prescription profile notes an aspirin allergy. Would you sell him the Pepto-Bismol?

Answer: Bismuth subsalicylate, the active component in Pepto-Bismol and other generic OTC products, is structurally related to aspirin (acetylsalicylic acid). Therefore, patients with an allergy or sensitivity to aspirin should not use bismuth subsalicylate. Make sure the pharmacist warns the patient about this contraindication and offer to get the pharmacist to help the patient choose a more suitable product based on his symptoms and medical history.

Table 12.5   Common Treatments for Diarrhea

Class	Generic Name	Brand Name	Availability
Antimotility agents	Diphenoxylate-atropine	Lomotil	Rx
	Loperamide	Imodium, Imodium AD	OTC and Rx
	Paregoric (opium tincture)	N/A	Rx
	Difenoxin-atropine	Motofen	Rx
Adsorbents	Kaolin-pectin mixture	Kaopectate	OTC
	Polycarbophil	FiberCon	OTC
	Bismuth subsalicylate	Pepto-Bismol	OTC
Enzymes	Lactase	Lactaid, Dairy Ease	OTC

The BRAT Diet for Diarrhea

The BRAT diet (bananas, rice, apple-sauce, and toast) is commonly pre-scribed for the management of acute diarrhea and vomiting, particularly among children, due to the bland nature of the food. However, this diet is falling out of favor because it provides insufficient calories, fat, and protein. The BRAT diet is no longer recommended by the American Academy of Pediatrics. Even so, pharmacy technicians should be familiar with it as it is still recommended by some clinicians.

late-induced gout. Children and teenagers with viral illnesses should not use bismuth subsalicylate due to the risk of Reye's syndrome. Bismuth subsalicylate should not be used by people taking tetracyclines, or those with a history of GI bleeding or blood co-agulation disorders.

Lactase is the enzyme that digests lactose, the sugar in milk and other dairy products. Without lactase, patients will experience diarrhea and other uncomfortable GI symptoms after consuming products containing lactose. If the enzyme lactase, available in many OTC preparations, is consumed with a meal containing lactose, the GI symptoms will be avoided.

Dietary management of diarrhea is also important to maintain fluid and electrolyte balance. A normal diet is recommended for most patients, because bowel rest is not necessary after acute episodes of diarrhea that do not result in dehydration. In general, a diet rich in complex carbohydrates (found in rice, potatoes, breads, and cereals), yogurt, lean meats, fruits, and vegetables is appropriate. Patients should avoid foods and drinks high in fat, simple sugars, and caffeine, because these ingredients can worsen diarrhea.

Acute diarrhea may be also caused by alterations in the balance of fecal and normal flora. This is commonly caused by antibiotics, which kill normal flora and allow the overgrowth of microorganisms in fecal matter. Agents that restore normal flora are called **probiotics**. These can be purchased as OTC supplements to restore the normal GI flora and promote healthy digestion. Although many patients report relief of common GI complaints with probiotics, these supplements are not regulated by the FDA and not approved for the treatment of diarrhea. No benefit has consistently been shown among probiotic research. Flora-restoring microorganisms are also present in yogurt, some cheeses, and some soy-based products.

When diarrhea is caused by an infection of a parasite or protozoan, a bacterium, or a virus, eradicating the causative microorganism is critical. **Gastroenteritis** is an inflammation of the gastrointestinal tract. It is most often caused by a virus, but may be caused by bacteria. Food-borne transmission is a common mode of spreading infectious agents. Viral gastroenteritis generally causes mild diarrhea, while bacterial gastroenteritis leads to more severe cases of diarrhea.

Constipation

Constipation is the decreased frequency of bowel movements or difficulty defecating. Constipation is not a disease, but can be a symptom of an underlying issue. The most effective treatment of constipation begins by determining and treating the cause. The two most common causes of constipation are a lack of dietary fiber and drug-induced constipation. In the case of drug-induced constipation, the offending

Analogy: Pathogens in the GI Tract

Imagine an area of Yellowstone National Park that is high in the mountains, far from human interference. In remote areas, animals occupy territories, or niches. This is similar to the territory occupied by normal flora in the GI tract. Wolves, for example, live in harmonious groups and roam across area that is theirs. They mark their territory with urine, so that other wolves from outside the group will stay away. If something happens to the family group, such that they become sick or are killed, a new group of wolves or a different predator species will move into their space. In the case of gaps in the normal flora of the GI tract, the new group is often pathogenic.

agent should be discontinued if possible. If it cannot be discontinued, a lower dose may relieve the constipation, but dietary management or pharmacological therapy may be necessary.

Common drug-related causes of constipation include the following:

- ACE inhibitors
- Antacids
- Anticholinergics
- Antihistamines
- Benzodiazepines
- Beta-blockers
- Calcium channel blockers
- Clonidine
- Iron preparations
- Non-potassium-sparing diuretics
- NSAIDs
- Opioid analgesics

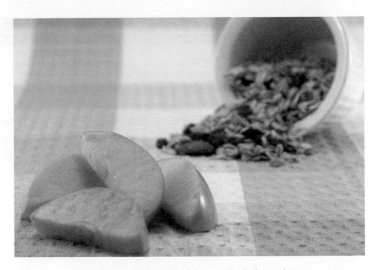
Fiber can be found in fruits, vegetables, and whole grains.

Dietary modification relieves a majority of cases of constipation. **Fiber**, the indigestible portion of plant-based foods, increases stool bulk, helps retain water in the stool, and increases transit time through the GI tract. According to the American Dietetic Association, patients should consume 25 to 30g of fiber in their diets daily to maintain healthy bowel function; most Americans consume only half this amount.

Fiber is found in fruits, vegetables, cereals, and bran. When dietary modification alone does not improve constipation, fiber or bulk-forming agents may be added to the diet with products like psyllium (Metamucil, Fiberall). Improvement in constipation may take up to one month with a high-fiber diet. The primary side effects of high-fiber diets include bloating and excessive gas, but these subside after a few weeks.

If low fiber intake is not the cause of constipation, pharmacological treatment may be necessary to increase the frequency or decrease the difficulty of bowel movements. Several classes of products are available to treat constipation, and they are presented in TABLE 12.6.

Osmotic laxatives draw water into the colon and encourage defecation. Taken orally, these agents cause stool softening in one to three days. Glycerin suppositories can result in a soft stool in as little as one hour. They can be used safely with few side effects, and are frequently given to children. Saline laxatives also draw water into the colon. These agents generally result in a soft or semisolid stool in six to 12 hours. Abdominal cramping, excessive diuresis, nausea, vomiting, and dehydration are rare side effects of laxatives. The magnesium present in saline laxatives may be absorbed by the body and cause serious adverse effects in patients with impaired renal function.

Bisacodyl stimulates contraction of the entire colon, encouraging defecation. The onset of action of bisacodyl is rapid—15 to 60 minutes—and a soft stool is generally produced in six to 12 hours after oral administration or 15 to 60 minutes after rectal administration. Stimulant laxatives should be used for no more than one week without the advice of a healthcare provider. Abdominal cramping, nausea, and vomiting are possible side effects of stimulant laxatives.

Surfactants are also known as emollient laxatives. They are anionic surfactants that improve the wetting efficiency of the fluid in the intestine, helping to mix water and fatty substances to make fecal matter. The onset of action is generally 24 hours,

Table 12.6	Common Agents to Treat Constipation		
Class	**Generic Name**	**Brand Name**	**Availability**
Osmotic laxatives	Glycerin suppository	Fleet	OTC
	Lactulose	Enulose	Rx
	Polyethylene glycol 3350	MiraLax	OTC
Saline laxatives	Magnesium hydroxide	Phillips Milk of Magnesia	OTC
	Magnesium sulfate (Epsom salts)	N/A	OTC
Stimulant laxatives	Bisacodyl	Dulcolax	OTC
Surfactants	Docusate	Colace, Ex-Lax	OTC
	Docusate-senna	Senokot-S	OTC
Bulk-forming agents	Psyllium	Fiberall, Metamucil	OTC
Anti-gas	Aluminum hydroxide-magnesium hydroxide-simethicone	Mylanta	OTC
	Calcium carbonate-simethicone	Maalox	OTC
	Simethicone	Gas Aid, Mylanta Maximum Strength, Mylicon Drops	OTC
Bowel evacuants	Polyethylene glycol 3350 and electrolytes	GoLYTELY, HalfLytely	Rx
Miscellaneous	Lubiprostone	Amitiza	Rx

and the effects of surfactants last up to 72 hours. A soft stool is generally produced in one to two days. Surfactants may be used for up to one week without the advice of a healthcare provider. Surfactants may cause mild abdominal cramping and diarrhea.

Anti-gas agents are available to decrease bloating and distension associated with excess gas related to constipation. The onset of action of these agents is rapid, causing relief in just a few minutes in some cases. Simethicone (Gas-X, Mylanta, Mylicon) is also safe for use in infants.

Lubiprostone (Amitiza) is the first drug approved for chronic idiopathic constipation. Headache, diarrhea, and nausea are the most common side effects of lubiprostone (Amitiza). This drug is not approved for use in children.

Irritable Bowel Syndrome (IBS)

Irritable bowel syndrome (IBS) is a GI syndrome that includes chronic abdominal pain and altered bowel habits. It is not associated with any specific cause, but is the most commonly diagnosed GI condition. IBS may affect any age group or gender, but younger female patients are the most likely to be diagnosed with IBS. Although no particular cause has been identified for IBS, new research points toward altered levels of serotonin in IBS sufferers.

IBS is either diarrhea-predominant or constipation-predominant. It often includes lower abdominal pain, altered defecation, and bloating. In general, the treatment of IBS depends on the type and severity of symptoms present. Often, common treatments for diarrhea and constipation are sufficient to control IBS symptoms. In severe IBS, serotonin receptor agonists, including tegaserod (Zelnorm), and SSRIs are treatment options.

Obesity

Nearly 100 million American adults are overweight or obese, and the proportion of children and adolescents who are overweight or obese is increasing rapidly. Both conditions are associated with serious health consequences, such as cardiovascular diseases, pulmonary disorders, metabolic dysfunction, and psychological conditions.

Body mass index (BMI) is traditionally used to quantify healthy body weight. It is calculated by dividing a patient's weight in kilograms by the square of his height in meters:

$$BMI = weight\ (kg) \div height^2\ (m^2)$$

A BMI between 19 and 25 is considered a healthy body weight. **Overweight** is defined as a BMI of 25 or greater, and **obesity** is defined as a BMI of 30 or greater. A BMI of 30 is roughly equal to being 30 pounds over a healthy body weight. **Extreme obesity** is defined as a BMI of 40 or greater.

BMI is a reliable indicator of body fatness for most adults, and it serves as a thorough guideline for assessing weight-related disorders. However, BMI is not appropriate for every patient. For example, BMI may be overestimated for people who have a high proportion of muscle mass; they may be considered overweight in spite of having a healthy percentage of body fat. Edema also affects BMI measurements, as do muscle-wasting syndromes or extremely short stature. In these cases, clinical judgment and a complete medical history and physical exam must be used together to determine whether a weight-related disorder exists.

One BMI unit is equivalent to approximately 7 pounds in men and 6 pounds in women.

Additionally, BMI is not effective in determining weight status in children, adolescents, or young adults less than 20 years of age, because body composition and body fat proportions change during growth and development. For these patients, BMI is calculated using the standard formula, but then converted to a percentage based on height- and weight-for-age charts, resulting in BMI-for-age guidelines. Children who fall under the 5th percentile of BMI-for-age are considered underweight; those between the 5th and 85th percentiles are healthy weight; those between the 85th and 95th percentile are overweight; and those above the 95th percentile are obese.

Childhood obesity is a serious public-health crisis. It leads directly to adult obesity and its resultant health consequences.

Alternatively, waist circumference can be used to identify overweight and obese individuals. A patient may have excess body fat if the waist circumference is equal to or greater than 35 inches in women or 40 inches in men.

When patients are determined to be overweight or obese, dietary management and behavior modification are the first steps to losing excess body fat. Lifestyle choices that support sustained weight loss are essential to main-

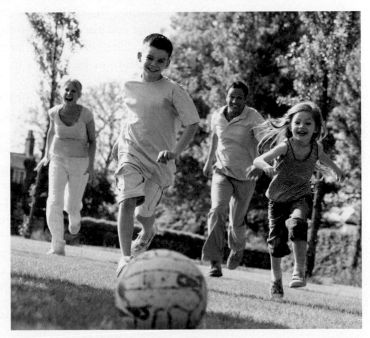

Regular physical activity helps to maintain a healthy weight and avoid the negative health consequences of overweight and obesity.

Table 12.7	Drugs Used to Encourage Weight Loss		
Class	**Generic Name**	**Brand Name**	**Availability**
Lipase inhibitors	Orlistat	Xenical, Alli	Rx, OTC
Stimulants	Phentermine	Fastin, Obytrim, Adipex-P	Rx
	Diethylpropion	Tenuate	Rx

taining a healthy body weight and avoiding the health consequences associated with obesity. A well-balanced diet containing proteins, fats, and carbohydrates, along with regular physical activity, are the most effective weight-control methods available. Severely calorie-restricted diets or extremely limited food choices do not show long-term benefit in health status or weight loss. If six months of dietary and behavior modifications are not effective in reducing body weight, pharmacological therapy may be initiated. These agents should be reserved for patients with a BMI of 30 or greater. In the presence of other complicating disease states, weight-loss agents may be used in patients with a BMI of 27 or greater. Common weight-loss aids are presented in TABLE 12.7.

Orlistat is a gastrointestinal lipase inhibitor that is available as both a prescription product and an OTC product. (The OTC product, Alli, is half the dose of the prescription Xenical.) Orlistat (Alli, Xenical) inhibits the action of gastric and pancreatic lipase in the stomach and small intestine. Therefore, fat from the diet is not metabolized or absorbed, but it is simply excreted from the body. However, fat-soluble vitamins are not absorbed, either, which means that patients who take orlistat should be advised to take a daily multivitamin. Orlistat (Alli, Xenical) is indicated for long-term weight control, and patients should be advised to consume a healthy diet low in fat while taking orlistat (Alli, Xenical). Fecal urgency, fecal incontinence, fatty or oily stools, and flatus with discharge are side effects associated with orlistat (Alli, Xenical).

Stimulants are commonly used for short-term weight loss. They should be used to initiate weight loss in obese patients while lifestyle changes are introduced. Dextroamphetamine (Dexedrine) and methamphetamine (Desoxyn) are amphetamine stimulants that can also be used to treat ADHD. The abuse potential of these agents is high, as is the risk of cardiovascular complications. Withdrawal symptoms, including tremor, confusion, or headaches may occur upon discontinuation of amphetamines after long-term use.

Diethylpropion (Tenuate) and phentermine (Fastin, Obytrim, Adipex-P) are structurally related to amphetamines, but offer less CNS stimulation and less potential for abuse. These agents enhance transmission of norepinephrine and dopamine. This stimulation leads to appetite suppression, which results in decreased caloric intake and weight reduction. Amphetamine-like stimulants may cause cardiovascular side effects including hypertension, increased heart rate, and arrhythmias. These agents should not be administered within 14 days of an MAO inhibitor.

No herbal products or supplements are approved by the FDA for the treatment of being overweight or obesity. The content, safety, and effectiveness of such products cannot be guaranteed, and patients should be advised to use caution with these agents.

Weight loss of as little as 5 percent of total body weight significantly reduces the cardiovascular and metabolic risks associated with being overweight or obese.

Table 12.8	Agents Used to Treat Hepatitis B
Generic Name	**Brand Name**
Interferon alfa-2b	Intron A
Peginterferon alfa-2a	Pegasys
Lamivudine	Epivir
Telbivudine	Tyzeka
Adefovir	Hepsera
Entecavir	Baraclude

Hepatitis

The three most common types of viral **hepatitis** are A, B, and C. These infections cause damage to the cells of the liver, and cause the liver to become swollen and tender. Permanent liver damage may occur if not treated properly.

Hepatitis A virus (HAV) is transmitted through blood and body fluids, usually by the fecal-oral route. It is most prevalent among populations with poor sanitation and hygiene. Hepatitis A occurs most commonly in children. Hepatitis A is rarely fatal. Two inactive HAV vaccines are available in the United States: Havrix and Vaqta.

Hepatitis B virus (HBV) can cause either acute or chronic infections. Acute infections are usually short-lived and self-limiting, but chronic infections can lead to permanent liver damage and death. HBV is transmitted sexually, parenterally, and perinatally. Infants and children are at the highest risk for HBV infections and complications. Two HBV vaccines are available: Recombivax HB and Energix B. Antiviral therapy can also be used to treat HBV infections. These agents are listed in TABLE 12.8 .

Long-term treatment with antiviral therapy is often required for chronic HBV infections. This induces antimicrobial resistance to antiviral agents.

Hepatitis C virus (HCV) is a blood-borne pathogen and may be either acute or chronic, but most infections lead to long-term complications. Acute HCV infections may not cause symptoms, and the infection is often not diagnosed until significant disease progression has occurred. HCV infections may occur in users of illegal injectable drugs, patients who received blood transfusions prior to 1992, patients who received clotting factors prior to 1987, chronic hemodialysis patients, patients infected with HIV or other sexually transmitted diseases, or people who received tattoos with contaminated instruments. Healthcare workers who are routinely in contact with blood or blood products are also at risk for HCV infection.

No vaccine is available for HCV. Avoidance of contact with infected blood products is the most effective prevention for hepatitis C. Combination treatment with peginterferon (Pegasys) and the antiviral ribavirin (Copegus, Rebetol) is first-line therapy for HCV infections. Ribavirin is only effective in combination with peginterferon; it should never be used as monotherapy. Side effects of ribavirin limit patient compliance and often require discontinuation of therapy. Extreme fatigue, flu-like symptoms, anemia, and psychiatric symptoms, including severe depression and suicidal behaviors, have been associated with ribavirin.

Malaria

Malaria is an infection of the blood caused by the parasite *Plasmodium spp.*, which is transmitted by an infected *Anopheles* mosquito. Malaria may also be transmitted through contact with infected blood products, such as with injectable drug use or via

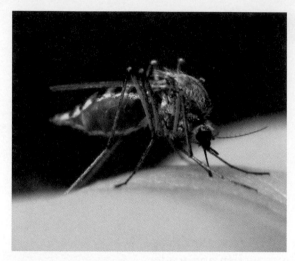

The parasite that causes malaria is transmitted to humans by infected mosquitoes.

a blood transfusion. Although uncommon in the United States, nearly 500 million new cases of malaria are reported annually throughout the world; of these, 1 to 2 million cases will lead to death.

Travelers to areas where malaria is prevalent are at the highest risk for contracting the disease. Chemoprophylaxis prior to departure, and continuing during and after travel, is effective for the prevention of malaria. Chloroquine (Aralen) 300mg once weekly, beginning one week prior to travel and continued for four weeks after leaving an endemic area, is an appropriate prophylaxis against all *Plasmodium* infections for most adults. Chloroquine may also be used to treat infections of malaria. However, chloroquine-resistant *P. falciparum* are emerging; the combination of atovaquone and proguanil (Malarone) may be used to treat infections caused by this parasite. It is well-tolerated and poses few side effects. A combination of atovaquone and proguanil is also a suitable alternative to chloroquine chemoprophylaxis against *P. falciparum* infections. For prophylaxis, it should be taken once daily beginning one to two days prior to travel and continued for one week after leaving malaria-endemic areas.

Plasmodium spp. *reproduce sexually in mosquitoes, but asexually in humans.*

Quinine (Qualaquin) has been used for several centuries to treat malaria, and it is still used in combination with an antibiotic such as doxycycline (Adoxa, Doryx, Vibra-Tabs, Vibramycin) to treat chloroquine-resistant malaria infections. Quinine (Qualaquin) can cause blood disorders, hearing loss, cardiac abnormalities, visual disturbances, and, in high doses, death. Primaquine is also an effective chemoprophylaxis against *P. vivax* and *P. falciparum* malaria. Doxycycline (Vibramycin) may also be used for malaria prophylaxis and treatment of chloroquine-resistant infections in non-pregnant adults and children eight years of age and older. Clindamycin (Cleocin) is an alternative for these patients.

Tonic water contains small amounts of quinine.

Tech Math Practice

Question: A brand-name drug costs $120 for 100 tablets. The generic equivalent costs $34 for 100 tablets. Calculate the cost difference for a 30-day supply between the brand and generic products if three tablets are taken daily.

Answer: Tablets required: 3 tablets/day × 30 days = 90 tablets

Cost of brand-name product: $120/100 tablets × 90 tablets = $108
Cost of generic product: $34/100 tablets × 90 tablets = $30.60
Cost difference: $108 – $30.60 = $77.40

Question: The AWP of a medication is $80. If the wholesaler offers a 10 percent discount when the account is paid in full within 15 days, what is the pharmacy's purchase price?

Answer: Amount of discount: 10% = 0.10

$80 × 0.10 = $8

Purchase price: $80 − $8 = $72

Question: **A pharmacy purchases an ointment for $25. The pharmacy adds a markup of 5 percent to all prescriptions dispensed, plus a dispensing fee of $2.50. What is the total cash price for one tube of ointment?**

Answer: Markup price per tube = 5% = 0.05

$25 + ($25 × 0.05) = $26.25

Final prescription price = $26.25 + $2.50 = $28.75

Question: **The AWP of a bottle of 200 tablets is $198. The pharmacy receives a 20 percent discount off AWP. The insurance company reimburses the pharmacy at the purchase price plus 3 percent. What is the total amount that the pharmacy will be reimbursed by the insurance company if 30 tablets are dispensed? What is the total profit made by the pharmacy on the 30-tablet prescription?**

Answer: Discount: 20% = 0.20

$198 × 0.20 = $39.60

Pharmacy purchase price = $198 − $39.60 = $158.40

Price per tablet = $158.40/200 = $0.79

Reimbursement for 30 tablets = 3% = 0.03

30 × ($0.79 + ($0.79 × 0.03)) = $24.41

Profit = Reimbursement price − purchase price = $24.41 − 30 × ($0.79) = $0.71 total profit

---

Question: **An inhaled medication has an AWP of $87. The pharmacy receives a 15 percent discount on the purchase price. The pharmacy sells the prescription for $99. What is the markup rate on the drug?**

Answer: Purchase price: $87 × 0.15 = $13.05 discount

$87 − $13.05 = $73.95

Markup = Sale price − Purchase price = $99 − $73.95 = $25.05

Markup rate = $25.05/$73.95 × 100 = 33.87%

Question: **A patient presents a prescription for cephalexin 125mg/5mL 200mL, with directions to take 250mg by mouth four times daily. Calculate the days' supply that will be dispensed.**

Answer: 250mg × 5mL/125mg = 10mL

10mL × 4 times/day = 40mL/day

200mL/40mL/day = 5 days

Question: A patient presents a prescription for one 10mL vial of Lantus insulin (U-100) 25 units subcutaneously every morning. Calculate the days' supply available in one vial of insulin.

Answer: 25 units × 1mL/100 units = 0.25mL daily

1 day/0.25mL × 10mL/vial = 40 days

Question: A patient presents a prescription for Humalog 75/25 insulin (U-100) 30 units subcutaneously every morning and every evening. What volume of insulin is needed to achieve a 30-day supply?

Answer: 30 units × 2 times/day × 1mL/100 units = 0.6mL daily

0.6mL/day × 30 days = 18mL

Question: A patient wants to pay cash for a 90-day supply of NPH insulin. He administers 65 units every evening. Calculate the volume of insulin needed by this patient.

Answer: 65 units × 1mL/100 units = 0.65mL daily

0.65mL/day × 90 days = 58.5mL

Insulin is only available in 10-mL vials, so the volume dispensed must be rounded to 60mL.

Question: Referring to the previous problem, your pharmacy purchases each vial of insulin for $47.85. If the pharmacy adds a 20% markup and a $4 dispensing fee, what is the total cash price of this patient's prescription.

Answer: $47.85/vial + ($47.85 × 0.2) = $57.42/vial

$57.42 × 6 vials + $4 = $348.52

Question: Your pharmacy pays $123.89 for the Combivent inhaler. The markup rate on the product is 45%. What is the cash price for the inhaler?

Answer: Markup = $123.89 × 0.45 = $55.75

Total purchase price = $123.89 + $55.75 = $179.64

Question: A mother does not have prescription insurance coverage and wants to pay cash for her child's antibiotic prescription: amoxicillin 250mg by mouth twice daily for 10 days. The pharmacy pays $37.72 for a bottle of 100 250mg tablets and adds a 35% markup to the price. Calculate the total price for this patient's prescription.

Answer: Dose: 2 tablets/day × 10 days = 20 tablets

Pharmacy cost per tablet: $37.72/100 tablets = $0.38/pill

Markup per tablet = $0.38 + ($0.38 × 0.35) = $0.51

Total cash price = $0.51/tablet × 20 tablets = $10.20

WRAP UP

Chapter Summary

- Most prescriptions are paid for by insurance companies or government health providers. Pharmacy technicians are responsible for processing claims with these third parties and resolving claim rejections.

- Claim rejections may occur because a drug is not covered, a patient is not covered, or a refill is ordered too soon. Communication among the patient, the pharmacist, the prescriber, and the coverage provider is often necessary to resolve claim rejections and disputes. This process may be time-consuming. Pharmacy technicians must maintain positive communication with the patient throughout the resolution.

- If a patient does not have insurance coverage or his or her prescription is not covered, he or she may pay cash for a medication. The cash price of a medication can be verified in most pharmacy software systems. The cash price is often based on the average acquisition cost or pharmacy purchase price along with any discounts, markups, or fees that are associated with a medication.

- Pharmacy software is used to manage the resources and promote efficient operations within a pharmacy. Patient profiles, regulatory records, and business statistics are maintained using pharmacy software. Audit logs detailing drug usage patterns, pharmacy compliance, and inventory management can be easily generated by pharmacy technicians. These reports help to predict future pharmacy activity and allocate resources and manpower within the pharmacy.

- The gastrointestinal (GI) system digests food, absorbs nutrients, and eliminates waste from the body. The GI tract is one long tube, beginning at the mouth and ending at the anus. Disorders and diseases of the GI system cause significant morbidity and mortality.

- Gastroesophageal reflux disease (GERD) occurs when stomach contents reflux into the esophagus. This condition may cause discomfort and decreased quality of life, and may also lead to damage to the esophagus over a long period. GERD treatment focuses on relieving the symptoms of heartburn, preventing the return of symptoms, and healing the esophagus. This may be accomplished through pharmacological therapy that decreases the acidity of stomach contents, improves gastric emptying, increasing the pressure of the lower esophageal sphincter, and protects the esophageal mucosa. Antacids, histamine receptor antagonists (H2RAs), and proton pump inhibitors (PPIs) are the mainstays of GERD treatment.

- Peptic ulcer disease (PUD) is characterized by the chronic recurrence of ulcers in the upper GI tract. Peptic ulcers may be related to stress, medication use, or bacterial infection. Antibiotic therapy is appropriate for bacterial-associated peptic ulcers, and PPIs and H2RAs may be added for symptom relief.

- Crohn's disease and ulcerative colitis are types of inflammatory bowel disease (IBD). UC causes inflammation and lesions in the colon and rectum. Crohn's disease causes widespread damage to the GI tract. Anti-inflammatory agents, antimicrobials, and immunosuppressants are used to treat the underlying causes of IBD.

- Nausea and vomiting are common GI-related complaints. The chemoreceptor trigger zone (CTZ) incites nausea and vomiting when stimulated by toxins, pathogens, or numerous other neurotransmitters. Agents that block multiple receptor types associated with vomiting prevent or decrease nausea and vomiting. Agents for simple nausea and vomiting are available as OTC products, but chemotherapy-induced and postoperative nausea and vomiting must be treated with prescription products.

- Diarrhea and constipation are frequent, common GI complaints that signal the presence of an underlying condition.

- Diarrhea may be caused by numerous infectious agents, medications, disease states, or food intolerances. Most cases are self-limiting and not serious, but dehydration and electrolyte imbalances are possible consequences of chronic diarrhea.

- Constipation is usually caused by low fiber in the diet, but may also be caused by medication or disease states. Increasing dietary fiber intake resolves most cases of constipation, but laxatives may be necessary for severe cases.

- Irritable bowel syndrome is a chronic GI syndrome that results in abdominal pain and altered bowel habits. It may be either diarrhea-predominant or constipation-predominant.

- Overweight and obesity are conditions that are defined as the presence of excess body fat, which is usually measured by the body mass index. A BMI of 25 or greater is considered overweight, and a BMI of 30 or greater is considered obese. Weight loss with a balanced diet and regular physical activity is the most effective treatment for people who are overweight or obese. Pharmacological treatment options are available to stimulate weight loss in patients who do not achieve weight loss with lifestyle modification alone.

- Hepatitis is a viral infection of the liver. Hepatitis A virus is transmitted by contact with contaminated food, blood, or body fluids. Hepatitis B virus is transmitted sexually, parenterally, or perinatally. Hepatitis C virus is transmitted through contaminated blood products. Vaccines are available to prevent hepatitis A and B. Antiviral therapy can be used to treat hepatitis B and hepatitis C.

- Malaria is an infection of the blood caused by a parasite of the genus *Plasmodium*. Chemoprophylaxis prior to, during, and after travel to malaria-endemic areas is effective prevention for most cases of malaria. If an infection occurs, malaria may be treated with numerous antimicrobial agents. However, antimicrobial resistance is emerging among malaria, limiting available treatment options.

Learning Assessment Questions

1. Prescriptions are most often paid for by whom?
   A. A third-party insurance provider
   B. The patient
   C. The pharmacy
   D. The manufacturer

2. Which of the following is not a common cause of rejection of a prescription claim by a third party?
   A. Duplicate therapy
   B. Refill too soon
   C. Patient not covered
   D. Duration of therapy written clearly on the prescription

3. Which of the following is an important role of the pharmacy technician related to pharmacy administration?
   A. Negotiating discounts with wholesale providers
   B. Projecting future pharmacy profits and losses
   C. Producing and reporting audits of pharmacy workload and resources
   D. Participating in medication therapy management

4. What are the symptoms of gastroparesis?
   A. Obstruction, perforation, or bleeding of the GI tract
   B. Altered bowel habits, blurred vision, arthritis, and hemorrhoids
   C. Nausea, vomiting, bloating, abdominal pain, and lack of appetite
   D. Anemia, weight loss, and dysphagia

5. Which of the following factors does not aggravate GERD symptoms?
   A. Eating late at night
   B. Consuming citric acid
   C. Chronic aspirin therapy
   D. Avoiding alcohol

6. Which agent used for the treatment of GERD presents a high risk of drug interactions?

   A. Cimetidine

   B. Misoprostol

   C. Cisapride

   D. Lansoprazole

7. Which agent can be used to treat GERD and urinary retention?

   A. Nizatidine

   B. Aluminum hydroxide

   C. Bethanechol

   D. Calcium carbonate

8. Peptic ulcers may be caused by all but which of the following?

   A. Chemotherapy

   B. Radiation therapy

   C. NSAID use

   D. *Giardia lamblia* infections

9. Which agent or class of agents is the treatment of choice for NSAID-induced peptic ulcers when the NSAID cannot be discontinued?

   A. H2RAs

   B. PPIs

   C. Celebrex

   D. Clarithromycin

10. What is the maximum concentration of promethazine allowed for intravenous administration?

    A. 7 percent

    B. 100mg/L

    C. 25mg/mL

    D. 10g/mL

11. Which class of antiemetics blocks dopamine receptors in the chemoreceptor trigger zone?

    A. Butyrophenones

    B. Corticosteroids

    C. Substance P receptor antagonists

    D. SSRIs

12. Which of the following is not a common cause of diarrhea?

    A. Laxative use

    B. Antibiotic use

    C. Lactase deficiency

    D. Calcium-containing medications

13. Which of the following agents can be used to treat both diarrhea and constipation?

    A. Bismuth subsalicylate

    B. Polycarbophil

    C. Paregoric

    D. Polyethylene glycol 3350

14. Which of the following microbes is a common cause of infectious protozoal diarrhea?

    A. *Plasmodium* spp.

    B. *Salmonella* sp.

    C. *Entamoeba histolytica*

    D. *E. coli*

15. What is the recommended daily intake of fiber?

    A. 10 to 15g

    B. 100mg

    C. 25 to 30g

    D. 1 to 2g

16. How long does it take for docusate to produce a soft stool?

    A. 15 to 60 minutes

    B. Six to 12 hours

    C. 72 hours

    D. One to two days

17. Pharmacological weight-loss agents should generally be reserved for which patients?

    A. Patients with a BMI of 30 or greater

    B. Children above the 85th percentile of BMI-for-age

    C. People with diabetes

    D. People who have failed at weight loss with herbal supplements

WRAP UP

18. What is the mechanism of action of phentermine?

A. Increases carbohydrate metabolism

B. Enhances transmission of norepinephrine and dopamine, which leads to appetite suppression

C. Inhibits the reuptake of serotonin, which increases thermogenesis

D. Prevents the digestion and absorption of dietary fats

19. Which hepatitis A virus vaccine is preservative-free?

A. Ribavirin

B. Energix

C. Vaqta

D. Havrix

20. Which agent is effective chemoprophylaxis for most types of malaria among adults?

A. Chloroquine

B. Doxycycline

C. Quinine

D. Atovaquone

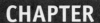

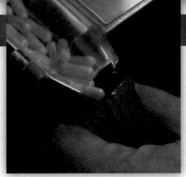

Non-sterile Compounding

OBJECTIVES

After reading this chapter, you will be able to:

- Define the term "compounding" and describe common situations in which compounding is required.
- Identify examples of non-sterile compounding.
- Describe and demonstrate good compounding practices in the pharmacy.
- Identify quality standards for non-sterile compounding contained in USP-NF Chapter 795, including product selection and beyond-use or expiration dates.
- Compare the components and purpose of a master control record with those of a compounding log.
- Calculate common mathematical problems that occur in a compounding pharmacy.
- Identify and describe the equipment used for weighing, measuring, and compounding pharmaceuticals.
- Define "percentage of error" and understand how it relates to accuracy in the compounding pharmacy.
- Explain the common methods used for combining and blending pharmaceutical ingredients.
- Discuss how solutions, suspensions, ointments, creams, powders, suppositories, and capsules are prepared.
- Explain the steps that are necessary in the compounding process.
- Identify references used for compounding.
- Describe the renal system and explain how it works.
- Identify the parts of the renal system.
- Identify the drugs used to treat renal disease.
- Identify the causes and treatment of urinary tract infections.
- Understand the classes of diuretics and explain how they work.

KEY TERMS

Anticipatory compounding	Forceps	Pill tile
Beyond-use date	Graduated cylinders	Pipette
Blending	Immunosuppressant	Pulverization
Class II balance	Levigation	Pyelonephritis
Class III balance	Manufactured products	Renal (urinary) system
Comminution	Master control record	Sifting
Component	Material safety data sheet (MSDS)	Spatulas
Compounded preparations	Meniscus	Spatulation
Compounding log	Mortar and pestle	Sterile compounding
Cystitis	Non-sterile compounding	Trituration
Diluent powder	Oleaginous	Tumbling
Diuretic	Percentage error	Urethritis
Expiration date	Pharmaceutical Compounding Centers of America (PCCA)	Urinary tract infection (UTI)
Extemporaneous compounding		

Chapter Overview

The practice of compounding dates back thousands of years. As more and more pharmaceuticals were manufactured on a large scale by drug companies, the need for individual compounding by pharmacists has decreased.

Compounding is the process of preparing a prescribed medication, from bulk ingredients, that is not commercially available. Compounding may be sterile or non-sterile. **Sterile compounding** refers to compounding of medications, such as parenterals or ophthalmic preparations (discussed in detail in Chapter 18) that must be free from microorganisms or particulate matter. Sterile compounding usually occurs in a hospital pharmacy. **Non-sterile compounding** is performed in a non-sterile environment. It is used for medications such as ointments, pastes, creams, capsules, solutions, suspensions, and tablets.

Dosage forms and dosages made by drug manufacturers are not adequate for everyone. With the advent of personalized medicine, it is increasingly apparent that being able to individualize medication dosages is important. In this chapter, the renal system, common kidney diseases, urinary tract infections, and the drugs used to treat these diseases will be explained.

Non-sterile Compounding

Non-sterile compounding, also called **extemporaneous compounding**, is an important part of pharmacy practice. Capsules, creams, ointments, powders, suppositories, solutions, and suspensions are examples of preparations that can be compounded in a pharmacy.

Non-sterile compounding is required in the following circumstances:
- When a product is not commercially available
- When a specialized dosage form or strength is needed
- When the medication requires flavoring to make it easy for patients to take
- When the patient is allergic to a preservative, dye, or additive
- When combining several medications will increase compliance
- When the patient cannot take the available dosage form

Non-sterile compounding refers to compounding of two or more ingredients by a licensed pharmacist in a non-sterile environment. The equipment, techniques, standards, regulations, and laws for compounding are different from those for other pharmacy practices. According to the FDA, reconstituting an antibiotic powder per the directions on the label is not compounding. However, pharmacy technicians routinely reconstitute antibiotic powders, and it is a necessary job function.

Some reasons why preparations must be compounded by the pharmacy include the following:

- A specialized dosage strength is needed—For patients who have special needs, pharmacists may have to compound a preparation if the strength of medication required is not commercially available.

- A different dosage form is needed—For patients who have difficulty swallowing a tablet or capsule, pharmacists may need to make a liquid formulation from the available solid dosage form.

- The product is not commercially available—Veterinary patients may require a pharmacist to compound a veterinary preparation prescribed by a veterinarian for an animal. Specialty care dermatology patients may require pharmacists to compound topical products. Patients receiving hormonal therapy that must be customized to specific hormone levels may require the pharmacist to prepare patient-specific topical, vaginal, or rectal compounds.

- Medication requires flavoring to make it taste better and easier to take—Taste can affect compliance. To ensure compliance, pharmacists often prepare a more palatable preparation.

- Patient cannot take the available dosage form—For a patient who is allergic to an inert ingredient in a commercially available product, pharmacists may have to prepare a product with the same active ingredient and other inert ingredients.

The FDA requires that non-sterile compounded products adhere to standards of the United States Pharmacopeia-National Formulary (USP-NF) Chapter 795. State Boards of Pharmacy regulate compounding pharmacies, and many require pharmacists to comply with these standards. Pharmacists must also develop guidelines, quality-control standards, and documentation practices, and follow all federal laws, regulations, and standards related to compounding.

The FDA requires compounded products adhere to the USP-NF Chapter 795 standards.

Many community pharmacies do not have the capability, time, space, or staff necessary to prepare compounded preparations. As a result, there are pharmacies that specialize in compounding that have the necessary equipment, space, and knowledge to prepare compounded preparations safely. These are called compounding pharmacies. There are basic types of compounding that a pharmacy technician will need

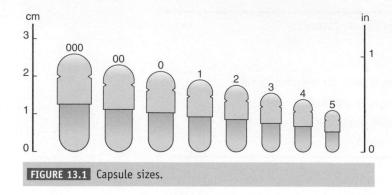

FIGURE 13.1 Capsule sizes.

to know even if he or she does not work in a compounding pharmacy, such as how to compound capsules, creams and ointments, powders, suppositories, solutions, and suspensions. In addition, the pharmacy technician may help the pharmacist by ordering the proper ingredients and maintaining a clean workspace.

Capsules

Capsules can be used to provide commercially unavailable doses of powder, granules, or liquids. Hard gelatin shells consist of a body, which is the larger part of the capsule and an end or cap, the smaller part of the capsule. Capsule sizes range from 5, the smallest, to 000, the largest **FIGURE 13.1**. For more information about capsules, see Chapters 4 and 14.

Creams and Ointments

Ointments, creams, and lotions are often requested by dermatologists and gynecologists to individualize treatment for their patients. The properties of these semisolid dosage forms are discussed in Chapter 4. Bases used in compounding these formulations vary in their degree of water washability, absorption, and occlusiveness.

Powders

Powders are single entities or mixtures of drugs or chemicals that vary in size (extremely fine to very coarse). The powder size is a number designation that refers to the amount of powder that can pass through sieves of various sizes. Historically, powders were prepared in bulk, weighed into individual doses, and then placed into separate pieces of paper (usually a wax paper), which were folded and then dispensed to the patient. Today, some powder products are still available commercially as individual powder doses, such as BC Powder (used for treatment of headaches, arthritis, and body pain).

Suppositories

Suppositories come in a variety of sizes (up to 5g) depending on the type of the material that makes up the suppository mold. Suppository molds can be composed of many materials such as aluminum, plastic, and rubber. Suppositories are used to administer medications rectally, vaginally, or urethrally. They can be prepared by hand-rolling, compression, or fusion-molding. The base used to make a suppository provides a medium to carry the medication and also allows the medication to be released. The bases used can be **oleaginous** (that is, greasy or oily), such as cocoa butter, or water-soluble, such as polyethylene glycol or glycerinated gelatin.

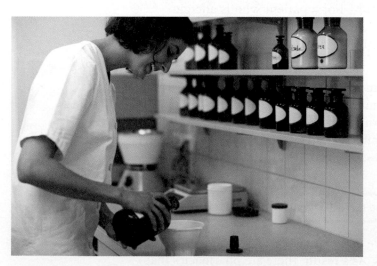

A pharmacy technician makes a compounded preparation.

Suppositories can be prepared by hand-rolling, compression, or fusion-molding.

Solutions

As discussed in Chapter 4, solutions are homogenous liquids in which the active ingredient or solute is dissolved in a liquid vehicle or solvent. A solution can be prepared by dissolving the solute in a liquid or by further diluting an already-made solution. Often, coloring or flavoring agents are added to the solution to make the solution more palatable. Syrup NF is used commonly for compounding preparations. It is made by dissolving 85g of sucrose in 100mL of purified water.

Suspensions

As discussed in Chapter 4, a suspension is a mixture in which solid medication is dispersed in a liquid vehicle. A suspending agent is added to ensure the medication does not easily settle. All suspensions must be shaken well before dispensing, as over time all of the active ingredient will sink to the bottom of the mixture. In addition, flavoring agents are added to make the suspension taste better, or for palatability. Some drugs that are available in only tablet form can be compounded into a suspension. This involves proper trituration, or grinding of the tablet into a powder. Always follow the formula because the order and rate at which the ingredients are mixed is crucial. The formula will also indicate proper storage and stability information. Not all solid oral dosage forms can be compounded into liquid dosage forms. It is imperative that the pharmacy have a formula for each compound prepared.

All suspensions should have an auxiliary label that reads "Shake Well."

Laws, Regulations, and Standards for Compounding

Federal and state laws and regulations and national standards address issues of quality by requiring the adoption of certain practices regarding compounding. A compounding pharmacy must be licensed by the state board of pharmacy and, if it is compounding controlled substances, the federal government and the DEA.

The Food and Drug Administration established guidelines to evaluate the safety and effectiveness of products for the consumer. In a compounding pharmacy, this means the adoption of good compounding practices (GCPs) to ensure a quality preparation. The United States Pharmacopeia (USP) has developed a uniform set of guidelines for pharmacists to follow for both non-sterile and sterile compounding **TABLE 13.1**. For the most up-to-date information on good compounding practices, see the most recent edition of the *Pharmacists' Pharmacopeia*.

The pharmacist can prepare a compounded preparation in anticipation of a prescription, called **anticipatory compounding**, as long as it is prepared according to the history of prescriptions prepared by the pharmacy. These preparations must be labeled or contain documentation with the following: a complete list of ingredients or preparation name, dosage form, strength, preparation date, name and address of the compounder, inactive ingredients, lot number, and assigned beyond-use date.

Pharmacies that directly supply compounded preparations in bulk in advance to other pharmacies or healthcare professionals must apply to the FDA for a manufacturing license and follow good manufacturing practice (GMP) guidelines. These guidelines require quality-control checks and inspections, and are more stringent than good compounding practice guidelines.

Table 13.1	USP Good Compounding Practices
Categories of GCP	**Standards**
Compounding process	Must follow step-by-step process with a final check performed by the pharmacist.
Facilities	Must have adequate space for storage of equipment and materials. Must have a clean, orderly, well-ventilated, separate work area for sterile compounding.
Equipment	Must have proper equipment that is stored to prevent contamination. Equipment used for compounding must be cleaned, calibrated, and routinely inspected.
Containers	Must be stored and sterilized properly. Selection should not alter the strength, purity, or quality of the product.
Controls	Must have quality programs and written procedures in place.
Labeling	Should contain all the necessary information required by law.
Records and reports	Must maintain hard copy of the prescription with formulation and compounding records.
Personal	Must possess education, training, and knowledge, and be familiar with applicable federal and state guidelines.
Component selection	Must attempt to use USP-NF drug substances or those manufactured by a facility registered with the FDA.
Labeling of excess product	Must label with the formula, control number, and beyond-use date.
Patient counseling	Must provide information on how to take and store the preparation.

A prescription for a compounded prescription is received by the pharmacy. The patient asks you how long it would take to fill the prescription. Advise the patient that this is a prescription for a medication that requires compounding and that it may take some time to prepare.

USP Chapter 795

The *United States Pharmacopeia* (USP) has developed and published practice standards for compounding in the USP-NF. These standards, under federal law, are the official standards of the United States. The USP-NF contains several general chapters. Chapter 795 provides procedures and requirements for non-sterile compounding. The guidelines for compounding of sterile preparations are outlined in Chapter 797, and are stricter than those for non-sterile compounding.

In the USP-NF, **manufactured products** are products that are manufactured by a pharmaceutical company, whereas **compounded preparations** refer to those that are prepared in a compounding pharmacy.

Chapter 795 defines what constitutes good manufacturing practices and provides general information on how to compound preparations of acceptable strength, quality, and purity. The pharmacy must also meet minimum standards for training and education of personnel, procedures and documentation, facilities, equipment, component selection, packaging, compounding controls, patient counseling, and records and reports.

Component Selection

Proper selection of quality ingredients is important to prepare a high-quality product. The pharmacist usually makes the decision about what source is used to obtain ingredients. Chapter 795 specifies that only USP-NF drug substances manufactured in an FDA-registered facility be used. A **component** is any ingredient that is used in the compounding of a drug product, but might not appear on the labeling of the product. If the components are not available from an FDA-registered facility, components of high quality such as those that are chemically pure, analytical reagent grade, American Chemical Society certified, or Food Chemicals Codex grade may be used. Many compounding pharmacies use their membership with **Pharmaceutical Compounding Centers of America (PCCA)** as a source for obtaining ingredients because it provides information and research on compatibility and stability. Pharmacists should have more than one source for obtaining products in case of a shortage, drug recall, or back order. Technicians commonly order the ingredients for a compounding pharmacy. A **material safety data sheet (MSDS)** contains important information on the properties of chemicals and includes information on their hazards and safe use. An MSDS should be filed for all bulk ingredients or drug substances. Every pharmacy is required to have an MSDS binder with information about all chemical products and how to handle accidental contact.

The pharmacy technician should check the expiration dates of all ingredients prior to making any compounded preparation.

Beyond-Use Dating

Chapters 795 and 797 specify requirements for beyond-use dating. Manufactured products have an **expiration date** (a date after which the product should no longer be used), whereas compounded preparations have beyond-use dating.

The **beyond-use date** is the date after which the compounded preparation is not to be used. It is based on the date on which the preparation is compounded, not the date on which it is dispensed. Legally, the date given cannot be beyond the expiration date of any of the ingredients in the product. Beyond-use dates may be assigned based on criteria that are different from those used by a manufacturer to assign expiration dates. Drug-specific and general-stability literature, the proper container for packaging, expected storage conditions, and intended duration of therapy should be taken into consideration when assigning a beyond-use date. When stability information is not available for a specific drug or preparation, the following maximum beyond-use dates are recommended:

- For non-aqueous liquids or solutions—If the manufactured drug product is the source of the active ingredient, the beyond-use date is no later than 25% of the time remaining until the product's expiration date or six months, whichever is earlier. If the USP or NF substance is the source of the active ingredient, the beyond-use date is no later than six months. If the dates differ between ingredients, the earliest date is always used.

- For water-containing formulations—The beyond-use date is not later than 14 days for liquid preparations stored between 2°C and 8°C.

- For all other formulations—The beyond-use date is not later than whichever comes first: the intended duration of therapy or 30 days.

If other beyond-use dating is used, the integrity of the final compound must be verified by scientific research. If the PCCA has data that extends the beyond-use date past that recommended by USP-NF Chapter 795, that date can be used.

Documentation of Non-sterile Compounding

Documentation of all ingredients used, calculations performed, and instructions followed for compounding are necessary to comply with good compounding practices, federal and state laws, and USP-NF Chapter 795 guidelines.

Compound Title
ketoprofen 10% and ibuprofen 2.5% in pluronic lecithin organogel

Compound Ingredients
ketoprofen...10 g
ibuprofen..2.5 g
lecithin: isopropyl palmitate 1:1 solution ....22 mL
Pluronic F127 20% gel qs to total.................................100 mL

Compound Procedure
Mix the ketoprofen and ibuprofen powders with propylene glycol to form smooth paste. Incorporate the lecithin:isopropyl palmitate solution and mix well. Add sufficient Pluronic F127 gel to volume and mix using high-shearing action until uniform. Package and label.

FIGURE 13.2 A master control record.

Master Control Record

Compounding a medication requires mixing ingredients by following a formula or recipe. A **master control record** contains the instructions or recipe for making a compounded preparation **FIGURE 13.2** . This record can be kept in the pharmacy's database or as a hard copy on recipe cards. The master control record is prepared and reviewed by the pharmacist or provided by a compounding service such as the PCCA. The master control record contains the name of each drug or ingredient, strength, dosage form, and quantity, and the instructions for compounding. It also includes storage requirements and beyond-use dates.

Compounding Log

A **compounding log** is filled out for each compounded preparation. It is like the master control record, but is specific for each individual prescription. The compounding log contains all the calculations necessary to make the preparation, and the equipment the technician will need when preparing the compound. It contains the same information as the master control record, but also includes the date of compounding and the assigned lot number, as well as the manufacturer, NDC number, and expiration date of each ingredient. The pharmacy technician who compounds a preparation and the pharmacist who signs off also initial the compounding log. Each step of the compounding process is checked and initialed by both the technician and the pharmacist. A prescription record is kept for each specific prescription that is dispensed from the compounded preparation documented in the compounding log. The prescription record is stored either using a paper system or electronically and can be used for refills on that prescription. In the case of compounding controlled substances, special procedures and record keeping should be followed.

Equipment for Measuring, Weighing, and Compounding

Pharmacies have equipment to measure, weigh, and compound ingredients. The minimum required equipment list is provided by each state board of pharmacy. Personal protective equipment including gloves, goggles, masks, and gowns may be worn to ensure sterility of the preparation.

Measuring Devices

Graduated cylinders are used to measure liquids. They are available in a various sizes (1mL to 1L), shapes (conical and cylindrical), and types (glass and plastic). Cylindrical graduated cylinders are more accurate, but conical graduates are easier to clean. Other measuring instruments include pipettes, syringes, and beakers. A **pipette** is a hollow, long, thin tube with a suction device used to transfer

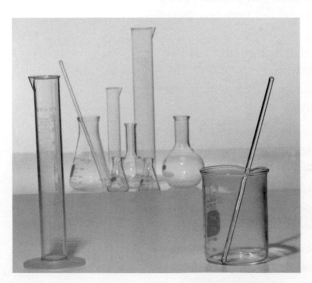

Various measuring devices can be found in a pharmacy.

volumes less than 1.5mL. Beakers are used when an exact measurement is not required.

Weighing Equipment

Scales differ in style and in the amounts they can weigh. A **class III balance** is a two-pan torsion balance used for weighing small amounts of material. It employs counterbalance to determine the weight of the substance being measured. It uses special weights in a range of milligrams and grams. Typical metric sets contain 1, 2, 5, 10, 20, 50, and 100g weights. Weights are used to measure ingredients and to calibrate scales. Ingredients and weights placed on a class III balance should always be placed on weighing or powder paper to avoid contamination of the trays.

A **class II balance** (also called an electronic balance) is more accurate than a class III balance. It has a digital readout of the weight. No weights are used with this type of balance.

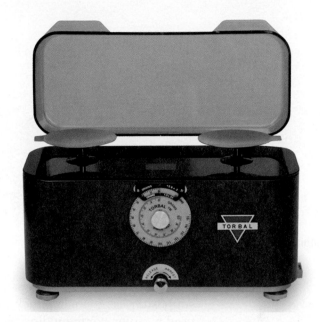

A class III prescription balance is used to weigh small amounts of material.

A class II balance is more accurate than a class III balance.

Compounding Equipment

Various types of compounding equipment are necessary, depending on the types of ingredients to be prepared. A **mortar and pestle** is used to crush solids and for grinding and mixing. Glass mortar and pestles are used for preparing liquids such as solutions and suspensions, and porcelain ones are used to blend powders or to grind crystals or granules.

Glass mortar and pestles are used to prepare liquids.

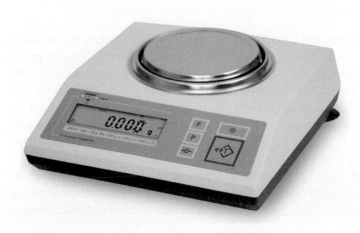

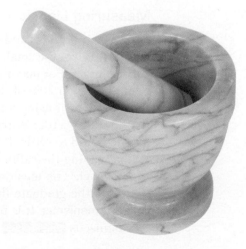

A class II prescription balance.

A mortar and pestle.

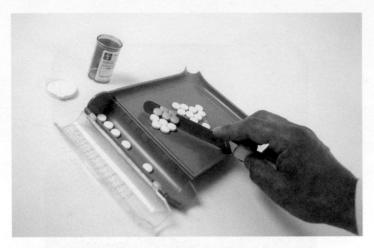

Spatulas are used for a variety of functions.

Forceps are instruments used to pick up and transfer pharmaceutical weights. **Spatulas** are used to prepare ointments and creams and to transfer ingredients to weighing pans. They can be stainless steel, plastic, or rubber.

A rubber spatula is used for corrosive materials.

Compounding parchment paper is a disposable non-absorbent paper that is ideal for mixing compounds. A compounding slab is a flat ground glass plate that is used to mix compounds.

Additional equipment and supplies can also be found in a compounding pharmacy. These include freezers and refrigerators to store ingredients and compounded preparations. Various suppository molds are used to prepare suppositories. A single-punch tablet press, pellet press, and capsule machine are also used by some compounding pharmacies.

Techniques for Measuring, Weighing, and Compounding

Following the correct techniques for measuring, weighing, and compounding can minimize errors that could result in serious consequences, and can help to ensure a high-quality product.

Personal Requirements

The requirements for non-sterile compounding are not as stringent as those for sterile compounding. Regardless of the type of compounding in which the pharmacy technician will be engaged, he or she should tie long hair back or wear a hair net, and wear clean protective clothing, a lab coat, and gloves to reduce contamination of a product and to protect themselves from the ingredients with which they are compounding. Eye goggles, a mask, and double gowning may also be needed. Hands should be washed with a liquid antimicrobial soap for at least 15 seconds and dried with a paper towel prior to and after compounding.

Measuring Liquids

Volumes of liquids can be measured using beakers, graduated cylinders, syringes, or pipettes. Select the smallest container or device that holds the required volume to ensure accuracy. For maximum accuracy, use the 20% rule. The volume measured should be no less than 20% of the total capacity of the graduate. Pour the liquid slowly into the container if using a beaker, graduated cylinder, or similar container and wait for the liquid to settle. Withdraw the liquid if using a syringe or pipette and again wait for the liquid to settle. If the liquid is viscous, pour toward the center of the graduate. When reading the calibrations of a beaker or graduated cylinder, bring the container to eye level. The tension of liquid will create a moon shape in a graduate, and the narrower the graduate the more pronounced this shape will be. This moon shape is called a **meniscus**. It is important that the level of the liquid is read at the bottom of the meniscus **FIGURE 13.3**.

When measuring liquid volumes, always read the level of the liquid at eye level. Measurements should be read at the bottom of the meniscus.

Weighing Ingredients

All balances should be placed on a level, non-vibrating surface. If needed, the balance can be leveled using its adjustable legs. Each balance has an arrest knob or button that locks the scale in place when it is not being used or is being moved. A balance should also be placed in an area where there is minimal airflow. Although a class III balance is often used for compounding, a class II balance is preferred in most cases. The class II balance should be warmed up and calibrated prior to use. Some electronic balances produce a printout that can be attached to the compounding log.

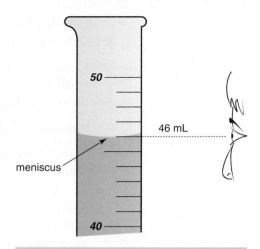

FIGURE 13.3 The meniscus is the level at the bottom at which liquids are measured.

To use a class II balance (electronic balance), follow these steps:

1. Place the balance on a level surface or adjust the legs on the balance to level it.
2. Locate the zero point (include the weight of the weighing paper).
3. Using a spatula, place a near precise amount of the chemical or drug to be weighed onto the weighing paper on the pan.
4. A small amount of drug or chemical can be added by lightly tapping the spatula to place a small amount onto the weighing paper while the balance is unlocked.
5. Read the digital weight measurement.
6. Unlock the balance before removing the measured chemical or drug.

To use a class III balance, follow these steps:

1. Place the balance on a level surface or adjust the legs on the balance to level it.
2. Place weighing papers on both sides of the balance.
3. Zero the balance to prevent the weight of the paper from being included in the measurement.
4. Place a counterweight on the right side of the balance.
5. Set the balance to the proper weight.
6. Verify that the weight is accurate and specifically what is called for in the compounding formula.
7. Using a spatula, place the substance to be measured on the left side of the balance.
8. Lock the balance and remove the substance.

Compounding Drugs

The master control record contains the recipe or set of instructions for compounding a particular preparation. If no recipe is available, the pharmacist will prepare the set of instructions for compounding. Before compounding, gather all the necessary equipment and ingredients, as well as the compounding log and master control record.

When measuring liquids, choose the container size closest to the volume required; the calibrations will be more accurate than in larger containers. For maximum accuracy, use the 20% rule. For example, if 80mL of solution is needed, use a 100mL graduated cylinder (20%). If a 250mL graduated cylinder were to be used, the measurement would not be accurate (32%).

Learning how to prepare a compound includes knowing the best techniques for properly mixing the ingredients:

- Comminution—**Comminution** is the process of reducing solid substances to small fragments such as powders.
- Blending—**Blending** is the process of combining two substances.

Processes used for comminution and blending include the following:

- Trituration—**Trituration** is the process of grinding a substance into fine particles, usually with a mortar and pestle.
- Levigation—**Levigation** is the process of grinding a solid into powder. It is typically used during the preparation of an ointment. A liquid levigating agent is added to the powder to form a paste, and the paste is then triturated and added to an ointment base.
- Pulverization—**Pulverization** is the process of reducing the particle size of a solid by mixing or dissolving the solid in a substance in which it is soluble, such as alcohol. The solvent evaporates so that it is not part of the final compound.
- Spatulation—**Spatulation** is the process of combining ingredients using a spatula.
- Sifting—**Sifting** is the process of combining powders using a sieve.
- Tumbling—**Tumbling** is the process of combining powders by placing them into a sealable container and tumbling or shaking the contents.

Preparing Solutions

Solutions are prepared through the dissolution of the solute in a solvent or by mixing two liquids together. When making a solution, it is important to measure the ingredients accurately and mix them thoroughly. If the solute is soluble in the solvent, a solution or syrup can be made. If the solute is not soluble in the solvent, a suspension or emulsion can be made.

Preparing Reconstitutable Suspensions

Reconstitution of a prepackaged suspension involves mixing a liquid (usually sterile water) into a powder to form a suspension. Many pediatric antibiotic suspensions are reconstituted at the time of dispensing because they have limited stability (usually 10 to 14 days). When reconstituting a suspension, the technician must read and follow the directions which indicate the proper amount of sterile water, or vehicle, to be mixed with the powder. When reconstituting a suspension, follow the manufacturer's instructions. Often, two thirds of the total volume of diluent is added first, the bottle is shaken, and then the remaining amount is added and the suspension is shaken again. After reconstitution, the expiration date must be calculated based on the date of preparation and then be

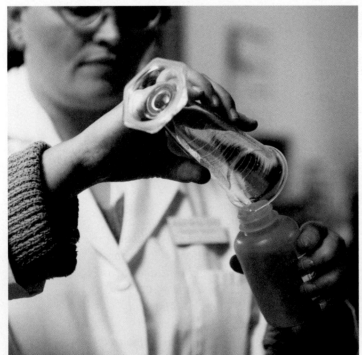

A technician reconstitutes an antibiotic suspension.

marked clearly on the product. All suspensions must be shaken before administration to evenly distribute the powder.

When reconstituting a suspension, add only half the water first.

In compounding, "qs" means to add a quantity sufficient to reach a certain final volume.

Compounding Ointments and Creams

Gynecologists and dermatologists often tailor therapy to the individual patient and prescribe strengths of medication that are not commercially available. Most ointments and creams are prepared by levigation, mixing, blending, and spatulation. In some cases, a powder is triturated and added to a cream or ointment base. When adding a powder to a cream or ointment base, gradually add small amounts of powder and blend with a spatula or mortar and pestle. When adding more than one ingredient to a base, add each ingredient sequentially and mix thoroughly before adding in the next ingredient.

When adding more than one ingredient to a cream or ointment base, add each ingredient sequentially, mixing thoroughly before adding the next ingredient.

Compounding Powders

Powders can be combined by trituration, spatulation, sifting, or tumbling. Powders can also be added to a liquid levigating agent to form a paste and then added to an ointment base. Powders can also be used to fill capsules and make suspensions and solutions. To make pediatric doses from commercially available tablets, tablets are triturated to a powder form using a mortar and pestle. This powder can then be added to a **diluent powder** and used to make tablets or capsules.

Compounding Capsules

Capsules mask the taste of medications in powder form, and are easy to swallow. After the powder is prepared in the proper proportions, it is gathered and compressed using a spatula to approximately ¼ to ½ of the height of the capsule body on a clean, flat surface. Using the punch method (described in Chapter 14), the body of the capsule is punched into the powder until the capsule is full. When the body of the capsule is full, it is attached to the end of the capsule and weighed to make sure each capsule contains the same amount of drug. USP-NF Chapter 795 standards require that capsules not weigh—less than 90% or more than 110% of the calculated weight for each unit.

Preparing Suppositories

Suppositories are used to administer medications rectally, vaginally, and urethrally (into the urethra). They can be prepared by hand-rolling, compression, and fusion-molding.

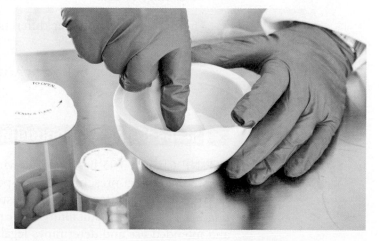

A technician compounds a powder using a mortar and pestle.

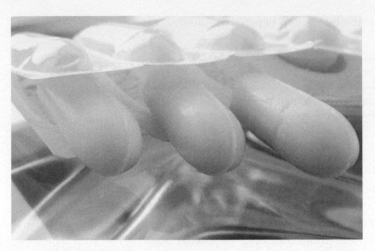

A suppository mold is used to make suppositories.

The hand-rolling method is the oldest and simplest process for molding suppositories. To prepare suppositories using the hand-rolling method, triturate grated cocoa butter with the active ingredient in a mortar. Roll the suppository into a cylinder using a **pill tile** (a slab used for mixing medicines with a spatula) or spatula and cut it into suppository segments. Roll one end to form a conical shape. The suppository is prepared by using the hands to shape the material and thus mold it into the suppository. It is then placed on wax paper or a tray to harden. It is often put in the refrigerator to complete this process and hold the mold of the suppository. This is dependent on the ingredients in the mixture. It does not require heat.

The compression process involves a mechanical approach but also avoids heat in the molding of the suppository. The compounded preparation is forced into a mold using a press or a cold-compression machine. The pressure from the machine forces the mixture into the suppository molds and thus the suppositories are formed.

If suppository molds are used, the formulation is poured in the mold cavity just before it reaches its congealing point in a slow, steady manner. This is the fusion-molding method. If the formulation is poured too soon after heating, it can result in a hole in the top of the suppository. The mold is filled slightly over the top, and can be removed with a heated metal spatula. The shells may be filled either by pouring or by using a syringe. Metal or rubber molds require a lubricant so that the suppositories can be easily removed from the molds. The molds must be kept at room temperature to prevent the suppositories from breaking during rapid cooling or refrigeration.

Calculating Percentage Error

Measurements are not always accurate. When a liquid is measured or a solid is weighed, two quantities are important: the apparent weight or volume measured and the possible excess or deficiency in the actual quantity obtained. **Percentage error** is the maximum potential error divided by the quantity desired, multiplied by 100%:

Percentage of Error = (Maximum Potential Error/Quantity Desired) × 100%

The amount of error is the difference between the actual amount and the quantity desired.

Amount of Error = Actual Amount − Quantity Desired

Steps in the Compounding Process

USP-NF Chapter 795 lists the following compounding steps to minimize errors and ensure the correct prescription is dispensed to the patient. Following these steps will help prevent medication errors and ensure the preparation of a high-quality product. The pharmacist judges the suitability of the prescription to be compounded in terms of safety and intended use and determines legal limitations, if any, that may be applicable.

1. The pharmacist performs necessary calculations to determine the quantity of ingredients needed.

2. The pharmacist identifies the necessary equipment needed for the technician to compound the preparation.

3. The pharmacy technician wears protective clothing and washes his or her hands properly.

4. The pharmacy technician cleans the area and equipment needed.

5. Only one prescription should be compounded at a time in the compounding area. This prevents potential errors by the pharmacy technician preparing the compound and the pharmacist checking it.

6. The pharmacy technician gathers all ingredients needed to compound the prescription.

7. The pharmacy technician compounds the preparation according to the recipe or master control record.

8. The pharmacy technician assesses the weight variation, adequacy of mixing, clarity, odor, color, consistency, and pH of the formulation.

9. The pharmacy technician fills out the compounding log and initials it.

10. The pharmacy technician prepares the label. The prescription container is labeled with the following information: name of the compound prepared, internal identification number, beyond-use date, initials of the compounder who prepared the preparation, storage requirements, and other information required by state law.

11. The pharmacist signs and dates the prescription and verifies that the preparation was filled according to the instructions. The pharmacy technician and pharmacist initial the prescription and compounding log.

12. The technician cleans the compounding equipment and area and stores the ingredients, equipment, preparation, and excess preparation properly.

13. This compounded preparation can now be dispensed to the patient in part or in whole using the dispensing process in place in the pharmacy.

References for Non-sterile Compounding

As discussed earlier in this chapter, the *United States Pharmacopeia* sets standards for compounding that are recognized by the FDA. These standards can be found in Chapter 795. The *United States Pharmacopeia* includes monographs and guidelines for compounding preparations. PCCA provides USP- and NF-grade ingredients, classes and seminars, and master control records for compounding. Local hospital pharmacies can also provide information regarding formulas and recipes as well as best practices for safe compounding. The International Academy of Compounding Pharmacists is an association of pharmacists and pharmacy technicians that focuses on the specialty practice of compounding.

Drug Insights: Renal-System Drugs

The **renal (urinary) system** FIGURE 13.4 performs many functions that are important in maintaining homeostasis, which is a state of equilibrium that produces a constant internal environment throughout the body. The renal system does the following:

- Maintains the body's balance of water, salts, and acids by removing excess fluids from the body or reabsorbing water as needed.

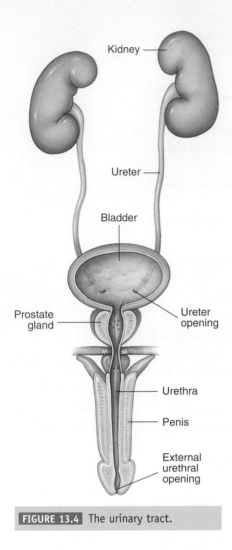

Kidney

Ureter

Bladder

Prostate gland

Ureter opening

Urethra

Penis

External urethral opening

FIGURE 13.4 The urinary tract.

- Filters the blood to remove urea and other waste products from the bloodstream. Urea is the major waste product of protein metabolism.
- Converts these waste products and excess fluids into urine in the kidneys and excretes them from the body via the urinary bladder.

The kidneys maintain homeostasis through the formation of urine.

Renal Disease

Accidents, toxic agents, and illnesses can lead to acute or chronic renal failure. As the kidney ages, it is harder for it to compensate for fluid imbalances in the body. As renal failure progresses, there is a buildup of wastes and an imbalance of fluids. This imbalance can result in a toxic syndrome in which the organs shut down, resulting in bone weakness and coma.

Drug Therapy for Renal Disease

Renal disease is diagnosed by clinical signs and symptoms and by lab measurements. Evaluations of blood pressure, skin turgor, temperature, color, weight loss, and edema are used to assess the extent of renal disease. Glomerular filtration rate (the flow rate of filtered fluid through the kidney), urine volume, electrolyte concentrations, serum creatinine, and blood urea nitrogen values are also used to determine the extent renal disease.

The goal of renal therapy is to restore homeostasis by treating the primary problem and reestablishing fluid volume and blood pressure. Drugs that may be used to treat renal disease include diuretics, antihypertensives, and corticosteroids.

The doses of some drugs may need to be adjusted for patients with renal impairment.

When a patient receives a kidney transplant, that patient must take drugs for his or her entire life to prevent the body from rejecting the new organ. Mycophenolic acid is an **immunosuppressant** that is given with cyclosporine to prevent rejection. (Note that immunosuppressants may also increase the risk of infection.) Mycophenolate (CellCept) is another immunosuppressant.

Drugs for Urinary Tract Infections

A **urinary tract infection (UTI)** is a bacterial or fungal infection of any part of the urinary tract. The most common UTI is caused by *Escherichia coli*. The infection usually starts in the urethra and bladder and can progress to the ureters and kidneys.

UTIs are classified based on their location. If the infection occurs in the urethra, it is called **urethritis**. If the infection is in the bladder, it is called **cystitis**. If it is in the kidney, it is called **pyelonephritis**. Symptoms can vary with the type of infection, but may include pain and burning with urination, fever, and cloudy or bloody urine. Urinary tract infections can also be classified as complicated or uncomplicated. Complicated urinary tract infections are the result of another abnormality or obstruction.

Table 13.2 Common Drugs for Renal Disease

Generic Name	Brand Name	Indication	Dosage Forms Available
Cinacalcet	Sensipar	Secondary hyperparathyroidism Hypercalcemia in patients with parathyroid carcinoma Severe hypercalcemia in patients with primary hyperparathyroidism Lowers parathyroid hormone, calcium, and phosphorus levels in the blood to prevent some bone disease	Tablet
Darbepoetin alfa	Aranesp	Anemia with chronic renal failure Anemia with non-myeloid malignancies due to chemotherapy	IV or SC
Epoetin alfa	Epogen and Procrit	Anemia with chronic renal failure Anemia in zidovudine-treated HIV patients Treatment of anemia from chemotherapy Reduction of allogeneic blood transfusion in surgery patients	IV or SC
Methoxy polyethylene glycol-epoetin beta	Mircera	Anemia with chronic renal failure	IV or SC
Vitamin D	Ergocalciferol	Vitamin D replacement therapy, given to patients on dialysis	Capsule, oral solution
Iron dextran	INFeD	Iron deficiency anemia in patients who cannot take oral formulations	IV or IM
Folic acid	N/A	Folic acid supplementation administered to patients on dialysis Helps in the formation of red blood cells	Tablet, injection
Iron sucrose	Venofer	Iron deficiency anemia in patients on dialysis Helps replenish iron stores in the body	IV
Sevelamer	Renagel	Control of serum phosphorus in patients with chronic kidney disease on dialysis Prevents the absorption of phosphorus	Tablet
Mycophenolate	CellCept	Prophylaxis of organ rejection	Capsule, tablet, suspension, IV

Uncomplicated UTIs are isolated to the bladder and involve no other diseases or other infectious processes.

Antibiotics are usually the drugs of choice for treatment of UTIs. Which agent to use depends on the pathogen responsible for the infection. Cystitis can be treated with a three-day course of oral trimethoprim/sulfamethoxazole, a three-day course of a fluoroquinolone such as ciprofloxacin or levofloxacin, or a seven-day course of nitrofurantoin. Pyelonephritis can often be treated with a seven- to 10-day course of ciprofloxacin or levofloxacin.

Drugs frequently used for the treatment of urinary tract infections include the following:

- Amoxicillin (Amoxil) and amoxicillin-clavulanate (Augmentin) are penicillin antibiotics frequently used to treat UTIs.
- Ampicillin (Principen) is another penicillin antibiotic; it should be taken on an empty stomach.
- Cephalexin (Keflex, Keftab) is a cephalosporin antibiotic used to treat uncomplicated UTIs. It should be taken with food or milk.

- Ciprofloxacin (Cipro) is a fluoroquinolone that should not be taken with antacids, warfarin, magnesium, or calcium. It can be taken with a meal that contains dairy or calcium, but do not take it alone with a dairy product, like milk or yogurt or calcium-fortified juice.
- Methenamine (Hiprex) is an anesthetic and antibiotic. It should not be taken with antacids, sulfonamides, or alkaline foods.
- Sulfamethoxazole-trimethoprim (Bactrim, Bactrim DS) is a sulfa drug that should be taken with lots of water.
- Nitrofurantoin (Macrodantin, Macrobid) should not be given with alcohol. It may turn the urine brownish.
- Phenazopyridine (Pyridium) is a local anesthetic used for relief of burning, itching, and urgency. It turns the urine orange and has no antibacterial properties.

Diuretics

A **diuretic** is a drug that increases the amount of urine excreted. Diuretics are the first-line agents used to treat hypertension and edema. They increase urine output and reduce overall fluid volume in the body, which reduces the work of the heart. Diuretics also reduce sodium levels, which is critical in lowering blood pressure.

There are several classes of diuretics:

- Thiazide diuretics—Thiazide diuretics are named based on their chemical structure. They work by blocking the reabsorption of sodium and chloride into the blood from the distal tubule, decreasing the amount of sodium in the blood, and decreasing vasoconstriction. Side effects of thiazide diuretics include hypokalemia (decreased potassium levels), hypomagnesemia (low magnesium levels), hypercalcemia (elevated calcium levels), and hyperglycemia (higher glucose levels). Hydrochlorothiazide is an example of a thiazide diuretic. Chlorthalidone is a thiazide-like diuretic. It works in the ascending loop of Henle and inhibits reabsorption of sodium and chloride.
- Loop diuretics—A loop diuretic works in the ascending loop of Henle and inhibits the reabsorption of sodium and chloride. The effects and side effects of loop diuretics are similar to those of thiazide diuretics. Furosemide (Lasix), bumetanide (Bumex), and torsemide (Demadex) are examples of a loop diuretic.
- Potassium-sparing diuretics—A potassium-sparing diuretic blocks the exchange of potassium from the blood with sodium from the urine. Side effects of these drugs include hyperkalemia, which can lead to life-threatening arrhythmias. Due to additive hyperkalemic effects, these drugs should be used with caution in patients taking ACE inhibitors. Amiloride (Midamor), eplerenone (Inspra), and spironolactone (Aldactone) are examples of potassium-sparing diuretics.
- Carbonic anhydrase inhibitors—A carbonic anhydrase inhibitor increases urine volume and increases its pH by inhibiting the reabsorption of bicarbonate in the proximal tubule. Acetazolamide (Diamox) and methazolamide (Neptazane) are examples of carbonic anhydrase inhibitors.
- Osmotic diuretics—An osmotic diuretic inhibits the tubular reabsorption of water and increases urinary output by increasing osmotic pressure. Mannitol (Osmitrol) is the only osmotic diuretic commercially available.

Mannitol works to draw water into the urine much like salt works to draw water out of a snail. The high concentration of solute (the salt and the mannitol) draws fluid across the concentration gradient in order to even out the concentration of solute.

Table 13.3 Common Diuretics

Class	Generic Name	Brand Name	Dosage Forms Available
Thiazide diuretics	Hydrochlorothiazide	Oretic, Hydrodiuril	Tablet
Loop diuretics	Furosemide	Lasix	Tablet, injectable
	Bumetanide	Bumex	Tablet, injectable
	Torsemide	Demadex	Tablet, injectable
Potassium sparing diuretics	Amiloride	Midamor	Tablet
	Eplerenone	Inspra	Tablet
	Spironolactone	Aldactone	Tablet
Carbonic anhydrase inhibitors	Acetazolamide	Diamox	Tablet, capsule, injectable
	Methazolamide	Neptazane	Tablet
Osmotic diuretics	Mannitol	Osmitrol	Injectable

Often, diuretics are combined with antihypertensives to improve compliance. Atenolol-chlorthalidione (Tenoretic) is a beta-blocker combined with a diuretic. Lisinopril-hydrochlorothiazide (Zestoretic) is a combination of an ACE inhibitor and a thiazide diuretic. Losartan-hydrochlorothiazide (Hyzaar) is a combination of an angiotensin receptor blocker and a thiazide diuretic.

A patient complains that he has muscle cramps and explains that he is taking hydrochlorothiazide. The technician gets the pharmacist to speak with the patient. The pharmacist explains that hypokalemia, or low potassium levels, is a side effect of hydrochlorothiazide, and that the patient should eat bananas and citrus fruits, and drink orange juice. The patient is also advised to contact his doctor.

Tech Math Practice

Question: **An elderly patient cannot swallow a 125mg tablet, so the pharmacist needs to compound a suspension of the medication that will have a final concentration of 125mg/5mL. The final volume will be 360mL. How many tablets are needed to prepare this suspension?**

Answer: Use the following proportion to calculate the total amount of the drug that is needed:

x mg/360mL = 125mg/5mL

x mg = (125mg $\times$ 360mL)/5mL = 9,000mg

Next, divide the total dose needed by the strength of the individual tablet:

9,000mg/125mg = 72 tablets

Question: **A prescription is received to prepare a cream using 20g of lidocaine 3% and 40g of ketoprofen 10%. How much of each ingredient is needed, and how should the compound be prepared?**

Answer: Use the following equation to calculate the amount of lidocaine needed:

3% $\times$ 20g = 0.03 $\times$ 20g = 0.6g $\times$ 1,000mg/1g = 600mg of lidocaine

Use the following equation to calculate the amount of ketoprofen needed:

10% $\times$ 40g = 0.1 $\times$ 40g = 4g $\times$ 1,000mg/1g = 4,000mg of ketoprofen

Next, weigh the amounts of each ingredient needed. Then mix these powders and add a sufficient amount of propylene glycol to dissolve them. Add this mixture to a base to make the 60g final product.

Question: **A prescription is received to prepare a compound in a ratio of 1:2:6 = 90g. How much of each ingredient is needed?**

Answer: You can answer the question by setting up a ratio, but using it with the given unit of measurement—in this case, a gram. Thus, the ratio 1:2:6 would become 1g:2g:6g. In this equation, the ratio equals 90 grams, so each ratio component would be multiplied by 10 to achieve 10g:20g:60g = 90g.

Question: **A prescription is received for 150mL of drug A to be prepared in a 1:15 solution. How much of drug A is needed to fill this order?**

Answer: Starting with $\frac{1}{15} = \frac{x}{150}$, cross multiply for x: $15x = 150g$, or $x = 10g$ of drug A. Measure 10g of drug A and add a sufficient quantity (qs) of sterile water to end up with a final volume of 150mL.

Question: **The pharmacy technician receives a prescription for sevalemer (Renagel) 800mg po tid with a 30-day supply. The pharmacy only has 400mg capsules in stock. How many 400mg tablets are to be dispensed to this patient?**

Answer: 180 tablets. Each tablet contains 400mg. To obtain a dose of 800mg, two tablets are required per dose × 3 doses/day = 6 tablets per day. Six tablets/day × 30 days = 180 tablets.

Question: **A dry powder must be reconstituted prior to administration. The label states that the dry powder occupies 0.5mL. The final volume is 10mL. What is the diluent volume?**

Answer: When preparing a solution, the space that the powder occupies is referred to as powder volume (pv). The powder volume is the difference between the final volume (fv) and the volume of the diluent (dv): pv = fv – dv. Use this formula to calculate the volume of the diluent: dv = fv – pv. So if fv = 10mL and pv = 0.5mL, the answer is 9.5mL.

Question: **The label states that 8.3mL of diluent is added to 1g of dry powder to make a final solution of 100mg/mL. What is the powder volume?**

Answer: To calculate powder volume, use the following formula: pv = fv – dv. First, calculate the final volume using the ratio-proportion method:

xmL/1,000mg = 1mL/100mg.

xmL = 1,000mg × 1mL/100mg = 10mL

Then apply the aforementioned formula for calculating powder volume (pv = fv – dv): pv = 10mL – 8.3mL = 1.7mL.

Question: **An order to prepare 100mL of iodine solution is received by the pharmacy. How much of each ingredient will you need? The solution's formula is as follows:**
- **Iodine: 30g**
- **Sodium iodide: 25g**
- **Purified water qs ad: 1,000mL**

Answer: Based on this formula, the volume of the final preparation is 1,000mL. Because 100mL/1,000mL = 1/10, to fill the prescription, you will need $^1/_{10}$ of each ingredient. Divide each ingredient by 10:

- Iodine: 30g ÷ 10 = 3g
- Sodium iodide 25g ÷ 10 = 2.5g
- Purified water qs ad: 100mL

Question: **A cream is formulated with two ingredients on April 30, 2011, with the following source drugs and expiration dates:**

Drug	Source	Expiration Date
Drug A	Bulk	December 2011
Drug B	Bulk	January 2012

Using this information, what should the beyond-use date be?

Answer: The labeled beyond-use date should be June 30, 2011. This is 25% of the eight months that elapse from April 30, 2011 (date the cream was compounded) to December 31, 2011 (the date of expiration for drug A).

Question: **A liquid water-containing preparation is combined with a flavoring agent on June 30, 2011, with the following source drugs and expiration dates:**

Drug	Source	Expiration Date
Drug A	Manufacturer	November 2011
Drug B	Bulk	December 2011

Using this information, what should the beyond-use date be?

Answer: The labeled date should be July 14, 2011. It is 14 days after the date of preparation and should be stored between 2°C and 8°C.

Question: **A prescription calls for 900mg of substance A. After weighing this amount on a balance, the pharmacist weighs it again on a more sensitive balance. It weights 700mg. What is the percentage of error?**

Answer: To determine the percentage of error, you must first determine the amount of error by subtracting the actual amount from the quantity desired: 900mg – 700mg = 200mg. Then divide the amount of the error by the quantity desired and multiply by 100%: 200mg/900mg × 100% = 22.2%.

WRAP UP

Chapter Summary

- Non-sterile compounding can be used to prepare doses that are not commercially available, need to be in a more palatable form, or need to be prepared in a different strength or dosage form.

- Compounds are prepared according to the master control record.

- The standards for non-sterile compounding are found in USP-NF Chapter 795. These standards are required by the FDA.

- The beyond-use date is the date after which the compounded preparation expires or should not be used. It is based on the date on which the preparation is compounded, not the date on which it is dispensed.

- The master control record and compound log must be filled out for all compounded preparations.

- Tools used for compounding include balances, weights, spatulas, forceps, graduated cylinders, pipettes, beakers, weighing paper, mortar and pestles, and beakers.

- Proper technique should be followed to ensure a high-quality preparation.

- Following the steps required by USP-NF Chapter 795 will maximize the quality and efficacy of the preparation.

- The renal system is composed of the kidneys, bladder, and urethra.

- Renal disease is divided into stages based on the glomerular filtration rate.

- Antibiotics are generally drugs of choice for the treatment of uncomplicated urinary tract infections.

- Urinary tract infections are classified by the site of infection.

- Diuretics are classified by how and where they work. They are used to treat hypertension and edema.

Learning Assessment Questions

1. To crush or grind powders using a mortar and pestle is called which of the following?
   A. Mixing
   B. Levigation
   C. Trituration
   D. Spatulation

2. Which balance is most accurate?
   A. Class II balance
   B. Class I balance
   C. Class III balance
   D. Torsion balance

3. Which of the following describes a meniscus?
   A. The weight of a compound
   B. The lowest level of liquid used to determine the volume
   C. A type of graduated cylinder
   D. The amount of solute in a mixture

4. Which of the following is true of beyond-use dates?
   A. They are dates assigned by the pharmacy for compounded preparations.
   B. They are expiration dates assigned by the manufacturer.
   C. They are the expiration dates of bulk chemicals.
   D. They are always one year.

5. The FDA requires that non-sterile compounded products adhere to the USP-NF standards found in which of the following chapters?
   A. 797
   B. 795
   C. 21
   D. 11

WRAP UP

6. Which of the following describes the function of the arrest knob on a balance?

   A. It locks the balance in place.

   B. It is used to measure the compound.

   C. It adjusts the feet of the balance.

   D. It contains weights used for weighing objects.

7. Which of the following are reasons a preparation must be compounded?

   A. A specialized dosage strength is needed

   B. The medication requires flavoring to make it easy to take

   C. The product is not commercially available

   D. All of the above

8. The punch method is used to fill which of the following?

   A. Suppository molds

   B. Syringes

   C. Capsules

   D. Graduated cylinders

9. All suspensions should have an auxiliary label that says which of the following?

   A. "Shake Well"

   B. "Take with Food"

   C. "Avoid Sunlight"

   D. "May Cause Drowsiness"

10. Which of the following is not found on the master control record?

    A. Doctor's name

    B. Mixing instructions

    C. Name of the ingredients

    D. Beyond-use date

11. USP good compounding practices include which of the following?

    A. Designating a separate area for sterile compounding

    B. Using only high-grade chemicals

    C. A final check by the pharmacist

    D. All of the above

12. Types of diuretics include which of the following?

    A. Carbonic anhydrase inhibitors

    B. Beta-blockers

    C. ACE inhibitors

    D. Cephalosporins

13. Most urinary tract infections are caused by which of the following?

    A. *E. coli*

    B. *S. Pyogenes*

    C. *H. Pylori*

    D. Streptococcus

14. Which class of diuretics inhibits reabsorption of sodium and chloride in the ascending loop of Henle and distal renal tubule?

    A. Thiazide diuretics

    B. Loop diuretics

    C. Potassium-sparing diuretics

    D. Carbonic anhydrase inhibitors

15. Common side effects of potassium-sparing diuretics include which of the following?

    A. Headache

    B. Visual disturbances

    C. Hyperkalemia

    D. Hypoalbuminemia

16. Which of the following is the process in which substances are pulled back into the blood after waste products have been removed?

    A. Reabsorption

    B. Distribution

    C. Elimination

    D. Metabolism

17. A urinary tract infection that occurs in the bladder is termed which of the following?

    A. Nephritis

    B. Kidneitis

    C. Cystitis

    D. Urethritis

WRAP UP

18. Products that are manufactured by a pharmaceutical company are called which of the following?
    A. Manufactured products
    B. Compounded preparations
    C. Intravenous solutions
    D. Bulk preparations

19. Tumbling combines powders by which of the following methods?
    A. Mixing them in a blender
    B. Trituration
    C. Spatulation
    D. Placing them in a bag and shaking it

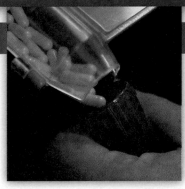

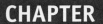

Labs for Non-sterile Compounding

OBJECTIVES

After reading this chapter, you will be able to:

- Calculate and reconstitute powders.
- Compound capsules.
- Perform the procedures and understand the rationale for creating oral suspensions from tablets and capsules.
- Prepare creams, ointments, gels, and pastes.
- Recognize common cardiovascular diseases and drugs.

KEY TERMS

Angina pectoris
Arrhythmia
Atherosclerosis
Cardiac cycle
Cardiac output
Cholesterol
Diastole
Deep vein thrombosis
Gastrostomy tube
Heart failure
Hypertension

Infarction
Ischemic heart disease
Myocardial infarction
 (MI)
Nasogastric tube
Orthostatic hypertension
Prehypertension
Pulmonary embolism
 (PE)
Reconstitute

Sinus rhythm
Stable angina
Stroke
Systole
Thrombus
Transient ischemic
 attack (TIA)
Triturate
Unstable angina
Variant angina

Chapter Overview

Before the mass-production of pharmaceutical products, most medications were individualized and prepared based on an order from a physician. This process of compounding included making tablets, creating suspensions, and filling capsules from raw ingredients. Today, products that are not commercially available must still be compounded, including oral dosage forms, suppositories, capsules, lozenges, creams, ointments, gels, and pastes. The FDA does not allow compounding if the final product is essentially a copy of a commercially available product. Sometimes, compounding is necessary to prepare a product in a strength that is not commercially available, or to prepare a product to meet a patient's unique needs, such as allergies or dietary restrictions.

As in all aspects of pharmacy, safety, accuracy, and record-keeping are essential to proper compounding. Maintain a clean workspace free of distractions, and wear proper personal protective equipment to maintain your safety and the integrity of the compounded product. Double-check all calculations and measurements, and keep a compounding log that records the process and ingredients used for each compounded product.

Lab: Reconstituting Powders

Often, liquids and oral suspensions are supplied by the manufacturer as powders that must be reconstituted. To **reconstitute** a powder, add distilled water or another fluid (as directed by the manufacturer) to the powder containing the active drug. It is essential to accurately measure the amount of fluid to be added to the powder to ensure the correct concentration of the final product.

Powders are advantageous compared to liquids because they are more stable. Powders are also easier to store and transport than liquids.

For some patients, oral suspensions are preferred to solid dosage forms because those patients are unable to swallow tablets or capsules. Also, oral suspensions are preferred in infants and children, as well as patients with nasogastric tubes. A **nasogastric tube** is a plastic tube that is inserted through the nose, past the throat, and directly into the stomach. A **gastrostomy tube**, or G-tube, is a plastic tube that is inserted directly into the stomach through the abdomen. Both the nasogastric tube and the gastrostomy tube are used for feeding or administering medications to patients who are unable to take nutrition by mouth.

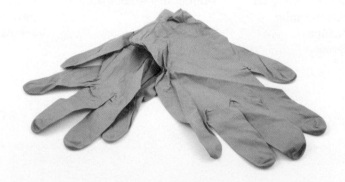

Latex, vinyl, or nitrile disposable gloves are recommended during compounding to protect the safety of both the person doing the compounding and the patient, and to maintain the integrity of the final product.

In this lab, you will reconstitute Augmentin powder for oral suspension. You will measure the distilled water, add it to the Augmentin powder, and prepare it for dispensing.

Equipment Needed

- Gloves
- 100mL graduated cylinder, Reconstitube, or similar device
- Distilled water
- 100mL bottle of Augmentin (amoxicillin/clavulanic acid) oral suspension (125mg/5mL) to be reconstituted
- Medication label
- Auxiliary labels

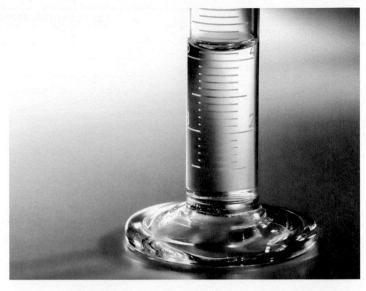

When measuring liquid in a graduated cylinder, make sure the water is at eye level. Measure the volume at the lowest point of the curvature of the water within the cylinder.

Steps

1. Gather the necessary supplies and place them at a clean workstation.
2. Wash your hands using appropriate hand-washing technique and put on gloves.
3. Fill a graduated cylinder or a Reconstitube with a sufficient amount of water (qs) to equal the desired final amount.
4. Ask an instructor or pharmacist to double-check this volume.
5. Tap the Augmentin bottle gently against your palm or the countertop until the powder flows freely.
6. Remove the cap from the Augmentin bottle. Add approximately two-thirds of the total water (about 60mL) to the Augmentin powder. Shake vigorously to suspend the powder.
7. Add the remaining water to the bottle; then shake vigorously again.
8. Inspect the bottle. Verify that all the powder has been suspended, and that no powder is stuck to the bottom or sides of the bottle. Continue shaking until all the powder is dissolved.
9. Affix the patient medication label to the bottle of Augmentin. Also attach auxiliary labels: "Shake Well" and "Refrigerate."
10. Complete the compounding log in **FIGURE 14.1** as directed by your instructor. Log the ingredient and final product details, as well as your name, the date, expiration date, and other required information.

Proper hand-washing technique requires wetting the hands with warm water; scrubbing with soap to cover the hands, fingernails, and wrists for at least 30 seconds; rinsing with warm water; and drying with a clean paper towel. Use a towel to turn off the faucet after your hands are clean and dry.

The manufacturer will order the correct volume of water to add to a powder for reconstitution. The volume will be presented on the bottle itself or in the package insert.

All oral suspensions require a "Shake Well" auxiliary label.

COMPOUNDING/PREPACK LOG							
Pharmacy Name				Date Compounded			
Compound/Prepacked Name and Strength				Compound/Prepacked Serial Number			
Procedure for Compounding/Prepacking							
Ingredients	Procedures						
Ingredient Detail							
Ingredient	Strength	Manufacturer	Lot Number	Exp Date	Qty Used	Tech	Pharmacist
Prepared By			Final Product Verification				
Name	Signature		Name			Signature	

FIGURE 14.1 A compounding log.

▌ Lab: Filling Capsules

Capsules are solid dosage forms in which the drug is enclosed within a hard or soft soluble container or shell. Most capsules are made from gelatin, although some are made of starch or other substances. Hard-shell capsules for human use range in size from 000 (the largest) to 5 (smallest). The largest capsules have a volume of approximately 1.36mL, while the smallest have a volume of approximately 0.13mL. Larger capsules are available for use in veterinary medicine.

Hard-shell capsules have two telescoping pieces: a cap and a body. In compounding, the body, the larger section of the capsule, is filled and the cap is placed over the body. Today, filling capsules by hand is not common practice in most pharmacies. However, it is still done to make specialty products or capsules for people who are allergic to certain excipients or are unable to take certain dosage forms. An excipient is an inactive ingredient that is added to a drug product to act as a carrier or delivery system for the active ingredient.

Hard-shell capsules offer a customized dosage form that can be easily and conveniently prepared.

When filling capsules, always make enough powder for at least one extra capsule, because some powder will be lost in the trituration and filling process.

A commonly used method of filling capsules by hand is the punch method. Using this method, powder is packed into a level cake and the open capsule is punched into the powder. This process requires accuracy and precision. Each capsule must contain the same amount of active ingredients and excipients.

In this lab, a mortar and pestle will be used to **triturate**, or break and grind, the tablets into a fine particulate powder before filling the capsules with the punch method. Then, small amounts of powder must be weighed and reweighed until the capsules contain the required amount of drug. Assume that 500mg of drug is needed in each capsule per a prescription or medication order.

Equipment Needed

- Gloves
- Bulk bottle of 500mg placebo powder
- Counting tray and counting spatula
- Mortar and pestle
- Glass ointment slab
- 8- or 10-inch stainless-steel spatula
- Six empty gelatin capsules, size 0
- Digital balance or scale
- Clean, dry gauze pad or cloth
- Weighing paper
- Prescription vial

Steps

1. Gather the necessary supplies and place them at a clean workstation. Make sure all equipment is clean and dry. Wash your hands and put on gloves.

2. Use the counting tray and spatula to count out 10 tablets from the stock bottle. Place them in the mortar, and then use the pestle to triturate, or break and grind, them into a fine powder. Use a back-and-forth grinding motion rather than a stirring or pounding motion.

3. Pour the powder from the mortar onto the ointment slab, scraping the sides of the mortar with the spatula to get as much powder as possible onto the slab. Form the powder into a compact, level cake, approximately half the height of the unfilled capsule body **FIGURE 14.2**.

4. Remove the capsule cap (the smaller section of the capsule) from five empty capsules. Set the caps aside. Place the bodies on the ointment slab.

5. Hold one empty capsule body between the thumb and forefinger, open side down. Punch or press the open end of the capsule into the powder until the open mouth of the capsule touches the ointment slab **FIGURE 14.3**.

6. Gently rotate the capsule and slightly pinch its open end. Then lift the capsule straight up out of the powder **FIGURE 14.4**.

7. Repeat the punching process for the capsule body until it is completely filled.

8. After the capsule body is completely filled with the powder, carefully invert the capsule so the open end is facing up. Then place the capsule cap back on the capsule body **FIGURE 14.5** and set the capsule aside.

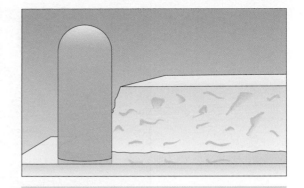

FIGURE 14.2 The cake of powder should be half the height of the capsule body.

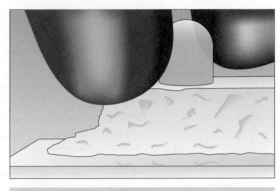

FIGURE 14.3 Punch the capsule straight down into the powder.

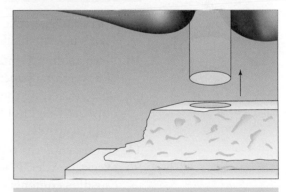

FIGURE 14.4 Lift the capsule straight up out of the powder.

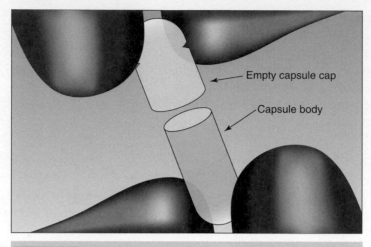

FIGURE 14.5 Replace the cap on the body of the capsule.

You will complete the punching process twice with each capsule body. This should sufficiently fill the capsule body with powder. If the capsule body is not filled after the second punch, repeat the punching process again.

Some capsules have a ridge in the center that acts as a locking mechanism between the capsule body and its cap. When replacing the cap, do not close or lock these capsules too tightly or they may be hard to reopen without damaging them.

9. Ensure the balance is on a flat surface. Then, following instructions in the scale's user manual, turn it on and allow it to zero.

10. Place an empty, intact capsule (the sixth capsule) on the weighing pan on top of a weighing paper and allow the balance to register a reading. Press Tare or Re-zero, setting the balance to zero. Now, when the filled capsules are weighed, only the weight of the contents will be displayed by the balance. Remove the empty capsule.

11. Gently wipe the outside of the filled capsule with gauze or cloth to remove excess powder. Place the capsule on the balance and obtain the weight of the capsule's contents.

12. If the weight is greater than 500mg, carefully open the capsule and gently tap some of the powder out onto the cake of powder on the ointment slab. Reseal, clean, and weigh the capsule again. If the weight is less than 500mg, carefully open the capsule and repeat the punching process as described in steps 7 through 9. Reseal, clean, and weigh the capsule again. Repeat this process until the capsule contains 500mg of powder. An error rate of 1 or 2mg is acceptable for the purposes of this lab.

Do not use a scooping motion when filling capsules. Punch straight down and lift straight up.

13.   Reshape the powder into a cake and repeat the punching and weighing process (steps 5–13) for the remaining four capsules.

14. When all five capsules contain 500mg of powder, gently wipe the exterior of the capsules again. Ask an instructor to verify the weight of each capsule.

15. Once the weights are verified, place the five capsules into a prescription vial.

16. Wash, dry, and put away all supplies and clean your workstation.

17. Complete the compounding log as directed by your instructor.

If the amount of drug required to compound a capsule is less than the minimum amount weighable on the balance or is too small to fill an entire capsule, inert ingredients such as cornstarch or lactose may be added to add weight or bulk to the capsules.

Lab: Creating Suspensions from Tablets

Oral suspensions may be administered to patients by a spoon, oral syringe, or dosing cup. They are useful for patients who cannot take solid dosage forms, such as pediatric or geriatric patients. Often, powders for oral suspension are available from the manufacturer and simply require reconstitution before dispensing to a patient. However, not all mediations are available as oral suspensions, so compounding one may be necessary for a particular patient or medication order.

In this lab, you will begin with the original medication in tablet form. You will triturate the tablets, making a fine powder, and then suspend the powder in a liquid vehicle to be taken orally. Assume that a final concentration of 500mg/5mL is required per a prescription or medication order; a total quantity sufficient for "500mg qid×10 days is required."

Equipment Needed

- Gloves
- Calculator
- Counting tray and counting spatula
- Bulk bottle of 500mg placebo tablets
- Two weighing boats
- Syrpalta 200mL or equivalent liquid vehicle
- Beaker or Erlenmeyer flask, 250mL or larger
- Digital balance or scale
- Mortar and pestle
- Compounding spatula
- Stirring rod
- Amber bottle, 8 oz or larger
- Auxiliary labels

Steps

1. Gather the necessary supplies and place them at a clean workstation. Make sure all equipment is clean and dry. Wash your hands and put on gloves.

2. Complete calculations to determine the number of tablets required to prepare the entire medication order:

Amount of medication needed for one day:
500mg/dose × 4 doses/day = 2,000mg
Number of tablets needed for one day:
2,000mg × 1 tablet/500mg = 4 tablets
Number of tablets needed for entire regimen:
4 tablets/day × 10 days = 40 tablets

3. Using the counting tray, count out the total number of tablets needed to compound the entire prescription. Place the tablets into a weighing boat and set aside.

In practice, technicians should have a pharmacist verify work during the compounding process after all the ingredients have been counted, weighed, or measured, but before they have been mixed.

4. Pour 200mL Syrpalta or other suspending vehicle into a beaker. Set aside.

5. Ensure the balance is on a flat surface. Using the scale's user manual, turn it on and allow it to zero.

6. Place an empty weighing boat on the weighing pan and allow the balance to register a reading. Press Tare or Re-zero, setting the balance to zero.

7. Remove the empty weighing boat from the balance and place the weighing boat containing the tablets on the balance. Record the weight. This weight will be the total amount needed for the final compounded product.

8. Have an instructor verify the weight and quantity of tablets.

9. Remove the weighing boat from the scale and empty the tablets into the mortar.

10. Using the counting tray and spatula, count an additional three tablets from the stock bottle and add them to the mortar. This addition will allow for the loss of powder that occurs during the compounding process.

11. Using the mortar and pestle, triturate the tablets into a fine powder. Use a back-and-forth grinding motion rather than a stirring or pounding motion.

12. Place an empty weighing boat on the balance and again tare the balance. Use the spatula to pour powder from the mortar into the weighing boat. You need the same weight as that recorded in step 7. If the weight is greater than the weight recorded, remove some of the powder from the weighing boat back into the mortar. If the weight is less than the weight recorded, add some more powder from the mortar. The margin of error for this laboratory exercise is ±5%, though this is not an appropriate margin of error for all compounded products.

13. Have an instructor verify the weight of your powder, as well as the volume of your Syrpalta.

14. Use the spatula to transfer a small amount of powder from the weighing boat into the Syrpalta. With the stirring rod, stir the suspension until the small amount of powder is suspended.

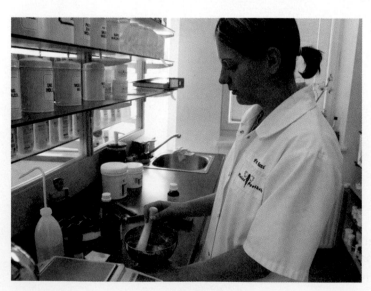

Use a back-and-forth grinding motion to triturate the tablets in the mortar and pestle.

15. Gradually add the rest of the powder in small batches to the Syrpalta. Stir continuously to ensure uniform consistency. Scrape all the powder from the weighing boat into the beaker to confirm the final concentration of the suspension.

16. After all the powder has been added to and suspended in the Syrpalta, transfer this liquid to an amber bottle. Swirl the beaker as you gradually pour the suspension into the bottle.

17. Label the product according to your instructor's directions and place a "Shake Well" auxiliary label on the bottle. Present the product to your instructor for a final check of the compounded suspension.

18. Wash, dry, and put away all supplies and clean your workstation.

19. Complete the compounding log as directed by your instructor.

Lab: Creating Suspensions from Capsules

Creating suspensions from capsules is similar to creating suspensions from tablets, as completed in the previous lab exercise. In this lab, you will compound a suspension of amoxicillin 250mg/5mL. A total quantity sufficient for amoxicillin 250mg qid×10 days is required. (Note that in practice, this product would not be compounded, as it is already prepared commercially. However, this product represents a good example for learning basic compounding skills.)

Equipment Needed

- Gloves
- Calculator
- Counting tray and counting spatula
- Bulk bottle of 250mg amoxicillin capsules
- Weighing boat
- Syrpalta 200mL or equivalent liquid vehicle
- Beaker or Erlenmeyer flask, 250mL or larger
- Stirring rod
- Amber bottle, 8 oz or larger
- Auxiliary labels

Steps

1. Gather the necessary supplies and place them at a clean workstation. Make sure all equipment is clean and dry. Wash your hands and put on gloves.

2. Complete calculations to determine the amount of capsules required to prepare the entire medication order:

Amount of medication needed for one day:
250mg/dose × 4 doses/day = 1,000mg
Number of capsules needed for one day:
1,000mg × 1 capsules/250mg = 4 capsules
Number of capsules needed for entire regimen:
4 capsules/day × 10 days = 40 tablets

If the powder inside the capsules is not fine and uniform, open the capsules, empty the contents into a mortar and pestle, and triturate the powder before adding it to the suspending liquid. Weigh the powder before and after trituration. You may need to break open additional capsules to make up for the loss of powder that occurs during trituration.

3. Using the counting tray, count out the total number of capsules needed to compound the entire prescription. Place the tablets into a weighing boat and set aside.

4. Pour 200mL Syrpalta or other suspending vehicle into a beaker. Set aside.

5. Have an instructor verify the quantity of capsules and the volume of Syrpalta.

6. Carefully open one capsule and empty its contents into the beaker of Syrpalta. Examine the capsule to ensure all the powder has been dislodged from the capsule. If necessary, gently tap the capsule against the beaker to free the remaining powder. Use the stirring rod to mix the suspension until the powder is dissolved.

7. Repeat step 6 with remaining capsules until the contents of all the capsules have been emptied into the beaker of Syrpalta.

8. With the stirring rod, stir the suspension until all the powder is dissolved and the mixture is uniform.

9. Transfer the liquid to an amber bottle. Swirl the beaker as you gradually pour the suspension into the bottle.

10. Label the product, according to your instructor's directions and place a "Shake Well" auxiliary label on the bottle. Present the product to your instructor for a final check of the compounded suspension.

11. Wash, dry, and put away all supplies and clean your workstation.

12. Complete the compounding log as directed by your instructor.

Lab: Preparing Creams, Ointments, Gels, and Pastes

Creams, ointments, gels, and pastes are preparations for topical use. Most topical preparations are readily available, but some need to be compounded for specific strength preparations or based on individual patient needs. In this case, an inert base ingredient is combined with the medication or active ingredient. An example is a topical formulation being created with a specific base to delivery drugs transdermally in veterinary medicine. Compounding a semisolid dosage form will use an ointment slab and a method called spatulation, in which the flat side of a spatula is used to mix ingredients against the ointment slab.

A complete discussion of dosage forms is located in Chapter 4. The following information briefly reviews dosage forms that are relevant to this lab exercise.

A cream is a semisolid dosage form that is either an oil-in-water or a water-in-oil emulsion. Most creams are water soluble. Creams can be prepared and used topically on the skin, as well as vaginally and rectally.

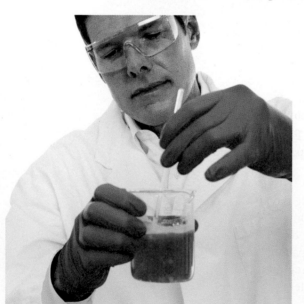

Mix the powder into the suspending agent until all the powder is dissolved.

An ointment is a semisolid dosage form that has a hydrocarbon base. Most ointments are not water soluble. Ointments are useful as protectants, lubricants, and emollients. They can be administered topically to the skin or mucous membranes.

A gel is a semisolid dosage form that contains small or large molecules dispersed throughout an aqueous base that contains a gelling agent. Gels can be applied topically to the skin, in the eyes, nasally, vaginally, or rectally.

A paste is a semisolid dosage form intended for topical application to the skin. Pastes are thicker than ointments and often less greasy. Pastes are stiff and remain in place after application, so they can be used to absorb secretions from the skin or to provide protection to areas of the skin.

In this lab exercise, you will compound an aspirin gel for topical application. The gel strength will not be calculated as the purpose of this exercise is to learn compounding technique.

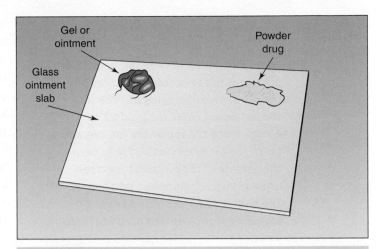

FIGURE 14.6 Place base and active ingredients on opposite corners of the ointment slab.

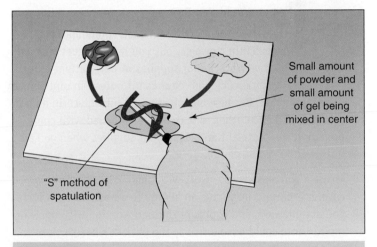

FIGURE 14.7 Mix the ingredients in the center of the ointment slab, scraping the flat surface of the spatula against the slab and pulling it though the ingredients in a back-and-forth "S" pattern.

Equipment Needed

- Gloves
- Counting tray and counting spatula
- Bulk bottle of 325mg aspirin tablets
- Mortar and pestle
- Digital balance or scale
- Two weighing boats
- Two compounding spatulas
- One tube of surgical lubricant, 15 grams or larger
- Ointment slab
- Small ointment jar

Steps

1. Gather the necessary supplies and place them at a clean workstation. Make sure all equipment is clean and dry. Wash your hands and put on gloves.

2. Using the counting tray and counting spatula, count out ten 325mg aspirin tablets. Place them in the mortar. Triturate the tablets using the mortar and pestle. Use a back-and-forth grinding motion.

3. Ensure the balance is on a flat surface. Using the balance's user manual, turn it on and allow it to zero.

4. Place an empty weighing boat on the weighing pan and allow the balance to register a read-

Because no particle-size reduction occurs during spatulation, the powder needs to be fine and uniform in size before mixing

When filling an ointment jar, pack the product into the bottom and sides of the jar to avoid trapping air. The size of the jar should allow the product to almost reach the top of the jar, but not touch the lid when closed. Try to keep the outside of the ointment jar clean when transferring product into the jar. The final product, inside and out, should appear clean and presentable to a patient.

What Would You Do?

Question: You recently finished compounding amoxicillin capsules, but you have not yet cleaned your workstation or supplies. A new patient enters the pharmacy and requires nitroglycerin ointment to be compounded. Because amoxicillin and nitroglycerin do not interact with each other, is it correct to proceed with compounding the ointment and clean your supplies when you are finished?

Answer: You must always work with clean supplies. In this case, the patient may have an allergy to amoxicillin of which you are unaware, and exposure through working with unclean instruments could pose a risk to the patient's health. Take the time to maintain a clean workstation and supplies in order to maintain patient health and safety.

ing. Press Tare or Re-zero, setting the balance to zero.

5. Add 2.5 grams of the aspirin powder into the empty weighing boat using the first compounding spatula to scrape it out of the mortar.

6. Repeat step 4 with the second empty weighing boat. Add 10 grams of the surgical lubricant into this weighing boat using the second compounding spatula.

7. Have your instructor verify the weights of both the aspirin and the lubricant.

8. Place both ingredients—the lubricant and the aspirin powder—on separate parts of the ointment slab. Use the first compounding spatula to scrape the powder from the first weighing boat onto an upper corner of the ointment slab. Next, use the second spatula to scrape the lubricant from the second boat onto the opposite upper corner of the slab.

9. Begin mixing the base ingredient and the active ingredient by using a spatula to scrape a small amount of powder (approximately one-fifth of the total) to the center of the slab. Next, pull a small amount of the lubricant (again, approximately one-fifth of the total) to the center of the slab.

10. Mix the ingredients using the spatulation method: Move the flat surface of the spatula through both ingredients against the flat surface of the slab. Apply downward pressure and move the spatula back-and-forth in an "S" pattern **FIGURE 14.7**. Continue to mix the small amounts of ingredients until the texture and consistency are uniform.

11. Drag another small portion of each ingredient to the center of the slab using your spatula. Using the "S" pattern of mixing, gradually incorporate the ingredients into the product that you already mixed. Mix until a uniform consistency is achieved.

12. Repeat step 11 until all the ingredients have been incorporated into the final product. Mix until the texture is smooth and uniform.

13. Have your instructor check the consistency of the final product.

14. Use the compounding spatula to scrape all the final product off the ointment slab and place it in an ointment jar.

15. Wash, dry, and put away all supplies and clean your workstation.

16. Complete the compounding log as directed by your instructor.

Drug Insights: Cardiovascular Diseases

The cardiovascular system includes the heart and blood vessels. The heart consists of two pumps (the right heart and the left heart) that drive the unidirectional flow of blood through the blood vessels of the pulmonary system, where the exchange of oxygen, nutrients, and hormones takes place **FIGURE 14.8**. Each side of the heart possesses one ventricle and one atrium. Each beat of the heart, or **cardiac cycle**, involves several coordinated events, including the electrical activation of the atria and ventricles and the contraction (**systole**) and relaxation (**diastole**) of the atria and ventricles. Also, cardiac valves open and close to allow the atria and ventricles to fill with blood and then empty as the heart pumps blood to the rest of the body. The electrical activation of the heart begins in the sinoatrial node and spreads rapidly to the atrial muscle. Next, the atrioventricular node is activated, followed by the ventricular muscle. The entire process takes approximately 0.2 seconds. The rate of activation can be affected by nerves in the sinoatrial node, hormones, calcium concentration in the heart muscle cells, and body temperature.

The heart receives oxygen-poor blood from the vena cavae into the right atrium. The blood passes through the tricuspid valve to the right ventricle, and then flows through the pulmonary arteries to the lungs to receive oxygen. Oxygen-rich blood returns to the heart through the pulmonary veins into the left atrium. Blood then flows through the mitral valve into the left ventricle, then through the aortic valve. The blood enters the aorta, and then flows to the rest of the body.

Diseases of the cardiovascular system are a leading cause of death in the United States. Many of these deaths occur without prior history of cardiovascular disease. Still, more than 70-million people in the United States are affected by cardiovascular disease. Non-modifiable risk factors for cardiovascular disease are those that cannot be changed or controlled and include advanced age, male gender, race (with African-American and Hispanic people being at higher risk), and family history. Modifiable risk factors are those that can be controlled or changed by a person and include tobacco exposure, excessive alcohol consumption, obesity, high blood pressure, high blood cholesterol, and physical inactivity. A diagnosis of diabetes mellitus also puts patients at increased risk for cardiovascular disease. A healthy lifestyle is crucial for preventing and managing cardiovascular diseases, but drug therapy can augment lifestyle modifications to achieve optimal results.

Every second, one person dies from cardiovascular disease.

Angina

Angina pectoris (or, simply, angina) is chest pain caused by a diminished supply of oxygenated blood to the heart. Although angina can cause significant pain, it does not cause irreversible damage to the heart or blood vessels. Angina is the hallmark symptom of **ischemic heart disease**. Ischemic heart disease is a condition in which the muscle of the heart receives a decreased supply of blood.

There are three distinct types of angina:

- Stable angina—**Stable angina** is chest pain due to exertion or exercise. The pain is relieved with rest and is usually predictable.

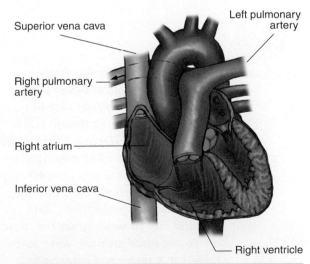

Superior vena cava

Left pulmonary artery

Right pulmonary artery

Right atrium

Inferior vena cava

Right ventricle

FIGURE 14.8 Cross-section of the human heart.

- Unstable angina—**Unstable angina** is pain that occurs with increasing frequency and diminished response to treatment. Unstable angina may signal an oncoming myocardial infarction.
- Variant angina—**Variant angina** is chest pain caused by coronary artery spasm. This pain is not predictable and is not stress-induced.

Most episodes of angina involve severe chest discomfort or pain. Angina episodes may also involve sweating, dizziness, and shortness of breath. Angina pain is usually brief.

The goals of angina treatment are to reduce symptoms and prevent the occurrence of a heart attack. Three main drug classes are used to treat angina: nitrates, beta-blockers, and calcium channel blockers. **TABLE 14.1** lists common angina treatment options.

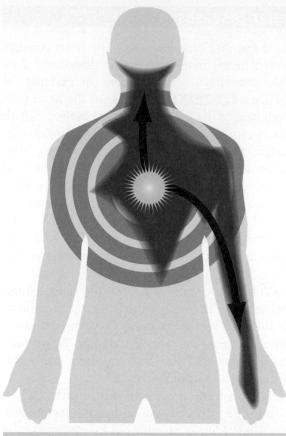

FIGURE 14.9 Angina pain usually radiates up to the neck and jaw or through the left shoulder and arm.

Chest pain due to angina is often described as heaviness, pressure, tightness, choking, or a squeezing sensation.

Patients should not take nitrates together with medications to treat erectile dysfunction (ED) such as sildenafil (Viagra), vardenafil (Levitra), or tadalafil (Cialis). Nitrates and ED treatments are often prescribed by different physicians, and patients may not inform their prescribers that they are taking both medications. Both nitrates and ED medications can cause decreased blood pressure; when taken together, a severe and potentially life-threatening drop in blood pressure could occur.

Nitrates

Nitrates are the most commonly prescribed drugs for angina. They relieve angina symptoms by relaxing vascular smooth muscle and dilating coronary vessels, allowing blood to distribute to areas of the heart that need oxygen.

Nitroglycerin is the drug of choice for acute angina attacks. It is administered sublingually, as a tablet or a spray, and the pain usually subsides within five minutes. The patient should be advised that if the pain does not subside after nitroglycerin administration, the patient must call 911. The patient must not take more than three doses, one every five minutes, over 15 minutes. Nitroglycerin may also be used to prevent an angina attack when taken a few minutes before an activity known to precipitate chest pain.

Nitroglycerin can cause severe headaches or orthostatic hypertension when first used. (**Orthostatic hypertension** is an increase in blood pressure when moving to an upright position.) Nitroglycerin tablets should always be dispensed in the original amber

Table 14.1	Common Drugs Used to Treat Angina Pain		
Class	**Generic Name**	**Brand Name**	**Dosage Forms Available**
Nitrates	Nitroglycerin	Minitran, Nitro-Bid, Nitro-Dur, Nitrostat	Capsule, IV, injection, tablet, ointment, transdermal patch
	Isosorbide mononitrate	Imdur	Tablet, IV
	Isosorbide dinitrate	Isordil	Capsule, tablet
Beta-blockers	Acebutolol	Sectral	Capsule
	Atenolol	Tenormin	Tablet
	Bisoprolol	Zebeta	Tablet
	Carvedilol	Coreg	Tablet
	Labetolol	Normodyne, Trandate	IV, tablet
	Metoprolol	Lopressor, Toprol-XL	IV, tablet
	Propranolol	Inderal	Capsule, IV, oral liquid, tablet
Calcium channel blockers	Amlodipine	Norvasc	Tablet
	Diltiazem	Cardizem, Dilacor XR	Capsule, IV, tablet
	Felodipine	Plendil	Tablet
	Nicardipine	Cardene	Capsule, injection
	Nifedipine	Procardia	Capsule
	Verapamil	Calan, Covera HS, Isoptin, Verelan	Capsule, IV, tablet

glass vial; it should never be repackaged. Nitroglycerin tablets lose potency when exposed to moisture, heat, and air. Patients should receive new nitroglycerin tablets every three months, even when stored properly. Nitroglycerin for infusion adheres to plastic and becomes ineffective when stored or dispensed in plastic.

Nitroglycerin is also available as a transdermal patch. To prevent tolerance, leave the patch on for 12 to 14 hours, then remove it for 10 to 12 hours prior to applying the next patch. This allows for a drug-free interval to help prevent nitrate tolerance and/or a reduction in effectiveness. Other nitrates include isosorbide mononitrate and isosorbide dinitrate, which are often used for angina prophylaxis. Angina prophylaxis is indicated when patients are participating in activities that are known to precipitate chest pain, or when angina occurs on a frequent and routine basis.

For storage and stability reasons, patients should not mix nitroglycerin tablets with other medications.

Beta-Blockers

Beta-blockers are used to treat angina pain because they slow the heart rate and lower blood pressure. If taken regularly, beta-blockers reduce the severity and frequency of angina attacks. Beta-blockers are also used to treat hypertension and arrhythmias. Slowed heart rate is the primary side effect of beta-blockers, but they also mask, or cover up, the symptoms of low blood sugar and decreased thyroid function.

Calcium Channel Blockers

Calcium channel blockers reduce the heart's demand for oxygen and relax coronary smooth muscle, dilating coronary blood vessels. Overall, oxygen supply to the heart is increased. Calcium channel blockers are routinely used to treat hypertension and arrhythmias. The most common side effects of calcium channel blockers include slowed heart rate, low blood pressure, nausea, constipation, fatigue, and dizziness.

Arrhythmia

An **arrhythmia** is a variation of a normal heart rate or rhythm. The heartbeat may be too slow or too fast, or the contractions of the ventricles and atria may not be synchronized.

A normal heart rate is approximately 70 to 80 beats per minutes (bpm), and the normal rhythm of the heart is coordinated by the sinoatrial node. Arrhythmias may result from ischemia, **infarction** (the death of heart tissue to due a sudden decrease in blood supply), or alterations of body chemicals. These abnormalities in the contractions of the heart lead to tachycardia (high heart rate), atrial flutter, or atrial fibrillation. Symptoms of arrhythmias include palpitations, syncope (loss of consciousness), light-headedness, visual disturbances, pale complexion, weakness, sweating, chest pain, and decreased blood pressure.

Several classes of medications are available to treat arrhythmias by restoring the normal heart rate and rhythm. They work through different mechanisms and action at different areas within the heart. Examples of the most common drugs available to treat arrhythmias are listed by class in **TABLE 14.2**.

> Antiarrythmic agents are divided into classes based on their mechanism or site of action.

Class I Antiarrhythmic Agents

Membrane-stabilizing agents are considered Class I antiarrhythmics. These agents reduce the movement of sodium ions into the cardiac cells, weakening the ability of the heart to trigger abnormal rates and rhythms. Disopyramide should be avoided in patients with heart failure. It is an anticholinergic agent, so dry mouth, urinary retention, constipation, and blurred vision are common side effects of disopyramide. The side effects of flecainide are dizziness, blurred vision, tremor, nausea, and vomiting.

Table 14.2   Common Antiarrhythmic Agents

Class	Generic Name	Brand Name	Dosage Forms Available
Membrane-stabilizing agents	Disopyramide	Norpace	Capsule
	Flecainide	Tambocor	Tablet
	Lidocaine	Xylocaine	IV
	Procainamide	Pronestyl	Capsule, injection, IV, tablet
	Quinidine	None	Injection, IV, tablet
Potassium channel blockers	Amiodarone	Cordarone	IV, tablet
	Dofetilide	Tikosyn	Capsule
Miscellaneous antiarrhythmic agents	Atropine	None	Injection, IV, tablet
	Digoxin	Lanoxin	Capsule, IV, tablet
	Isoproterenol	Isuprel	IV

Lidocaine is most effective in reducing abnormalities in the ventricles, but has little effect on the atria. Quinidine slows electrical conduction through the heart. Its side effects include decreased production of blood platelets, headache, blurred vision, ringing in the ears, confusion, and nausea. Procainamide is similar in mechanism and function to quinidine, and the two drugs are often used interchangeably.

Class III Antiarrhythmic Agents

Class III antiarrhythmics are potassium channel blockers. These agents block the flow of potassium ions across the cell membranes of the heart muscle. This prevents the generation of an abnormal heart rate or rhythm. Amiodarone is a very effective drug for arrhythmias that originate in the atria or the ventricles, but it is not considered a first-line agent due to potentially fatal toxicities. It should be used for patients who do not respond to treatment with other antiarrhythmic agents, and should not be used in patients with congestive heart failure. Hypotension is a significant side effect of amiodarone. When given intravenously, amiodarone must be mixed in dextrose 5% in water (D_5W) and administered from a glass bottle or bag made of polyolefin, a synthetic plastic made of polymers of hydrocarbon chains. Polhyethylene and polypropylene are examples of polyolefin.

Dofetilide is used only in patients who have already been converted to a normal **sinus rhythm**, or normal beating of the heart. Dofetilide may actually induce arrhythmias itself, so monitoring is critical. It must be initiated in a hospital setting that uses continuous monitoring systems and has resuscitation equipment available. Dofetilide may only be dispensed from a community pharmacy setting by pharmacies and prescribers who have completed specialized training and education, and documentation must be maintained regarding the initiation of the drug therapy.

Atropine is an anticholinergic agent that decreases parasympathetic activity and increases sympathetic activity. It is used to treat heart rates below 60bpm. Atropine doses that are too low can decrease the heart rate, while high doses can cause fast heart rates. Atropine can cause dry skin, urinary retention, constipation, dry throat and mouth, and dry eyes and blurred vision. Isoproterenol dilates coronary vessels, reducing heart rate and contractility.

Digoxin, a digitalis derivative, is one of the most commonly used drugs to manage atrial flutter and atrial fibrillation. It does not result in a normal sinus rhythm, but slows ventricular rates and decreases ventricular response to stimulation. Digoxin does pose a risk of toxicity, especially in elderly patients. Symptoms of digitalis toxicity include nausea, vertigo, general weakness, and visual disturbances, including seeing yellow-green halos around objects. Toxicity may also include arrhythmias. If toxicity occurs, digoxin should be discontinued. Digoxin-immune Fab (DigiFab) is available as an antidote to digitalis toxicity.

Heart Failure

Heart failure is a syndrome in which the heart cannot pump enough blood to meet the oxygen and metabolic needs of the rest of the body. Simply, the heart pumps out less blood than it receives. Heart failure can be caused by a disorder or condition that reduces the filling of the ventricles, or one that reduces the contraction of the heart muscle. Approximately five-million Americans have heart failure, including 10% of people over the age of 75 years. Heart failure ac-

Dutch artist Vincent Van Gogh is believed to have been treated for epilepsy and mental disorders with extracts from the foxglove plant—a digitalis derivative similar to digoxin. Although only a theory, many believe that he suffered from digitalis toxicity, and his extensive use of the color yellow and his painting of halos around objects are a direct result of the visual disturbances apparent in digitalis toxicity.

counts for approximately 300,000 deaths per year owing to a progressive failure of the heart or sudden cardiac death.

In heart failure, blood accumulates in the heart and stretches the walls of the heart. Because the kidneys, along with the rest of the body, do not receive enough blood or oxygen, they retain water and electrolytes, leading to increased blood volume and fluid retention in the body's tissues and organs. Therefore, the terms "heart failure" and "congestive heart failure" (CHF) are used interchangeably. Heart failure that is isolated to the left side of the heart leads to fluid accumulation in the lungs; heart failure of the right side results in accumulation of fluid in the extremities.

Hypertension and coronary artery disease are the leading causes of heart failure. Secondary causes include high salt intake, kidney failure, stress, infection and inflammation, cigarette smoking, and obesity. All these conditions, both primary and secondary causes, require the heart to work harder than it should have to. Therefore, the muscles of the heart become enlarged and thickened due to overwork and overstimulation.

The goals of CHF therapy are to prolong survival, prevent disease progression, relieve symptoms, and improve quality of life. Usually, a combination of drugs is required to meet these goals. Angiotensin-converting enzyme (ACE) inhibitors and beta-blockers are first-line agents. A diuretic, an antiplatelet or anticoagulant agent, and digoxin are often added to CHF regimens. When used in combination, these drugs slow disease progression, improve symptoms, and reduce morbidity and mortality associated with CHF. Common drugs used to treat CHF are listed in **TABLE 14.3**. Beta-blockers are presented in Table 14.1. Digoxin is presented in Table 14.2.

Vasodilators

Vasodilators are effective in CHF treatment because they dilate the blood vessels, decreasing the amount of work the heart muscle needs to do. Milrinone dilates the blood vessels and increases the contraction of the heart muscle. It is usually used for short-term IV therapy for CHF. The combination of isosorbide-hydralazine is commonly used to supplement CHF therapy in African Americans. Both drugs are vasodilators, using the production of nitrous oxide to relax blood vessels. This drug may cause headaches and dizziness. It is usually used in patients with decreased renal function or those who cannot tolerate ACE inhibitors.

BiDil (isosorbide dinitrate-hydralazine) was the first drug approved by the FDA for a specific race.

Table 14.3   Common Drugs Used to Treat Heart Failure

Class	Generic Name	Brand Name	Dosage Forms Available
Vasodilators	Milrinone	Primacor	IV
	Nitroprusside	Nitropress	IV
	Isosorbide-hydralazine	BiDil	Tablet
ACE inhibitors	Benazepril	Lotensin	Tablet
	Captopril	Capoten	Tablet
	Enalapril	Vasotec	IV, tablet
	Lisinopril	Prinivil, Zestril	Tablet
	Quinapril	Accupril	Tablet
	Ramipril	Altace	Capsule

ACE Inhibitors

ACE inhibitors prevent the conversion of the enzyme angiotensin I to angiotensin II, which leads to less constriction of the blood vessels. This reduces the resistance to blood flow and lowers blood pressure. Lower blood pressure, in turn, allows the heart to work more efficiently. ACE inhibitors preserve potassium in the body, so a patient may develop an elevated potassium level (hyperkalemia) while on ACE-inhibitor therapy, especially when combined with other potassium-sparing agents. Potassium levels should be monitored in patients at risk for hyperkalemia.

ACE inhibitors may cause a persistent dry cough. Although not dangerous in itself, the cough is largely annoying to many patients and noncompliance becomes an issue. Angioedema, a swelling of the face and tongue, is the most serious side effect of ACE inhibitors. Angioedema may occur a few hours after treatment is initiated, or several years into therapy. ACE inhibitors may also cause dizziness and orthostatic hypotension, especially in the first few days of treatment.

Hypertension

Blood pressure is defined as the product of cardiac output and total peripheral resistance. **Cardiac output**, the amount of blood pumped by the heart in one minute, is the product of stroke volume and heart rate. Each of these parameters is influenced by a variety of factors, including blood viscosity, blood volume, and nerve controls.

A blood-pressure measurement is expressed as the systolic blood pressure (the pressure when the heart ejects blood) over the diastolic blood pressure (the pressure when the heart relaxes and fills with blood). A normal blood pressure is a systolic blood pressure less than or equal to 120mm Hg over a diastolic blood pressure of less than or equal to 80mm Hg (commonly expressed as 120/80mm Hg). Complications of high blood pressure are usually associated with a blood pressure greater than 140/90, so most people are advised to maintain a blood pressure below this level. Individual blood-pressure goals are based on comorbid disease states, personal and family medical history, and concomitant drug therapy.

Hypertension is defined as a systolic blood pressure over 140mm Hg or a diastolic blood pressure over 90mm Hg. A systolic blood pressure between 120 and 139mm Hg or a diastolic blood pressure between 80 and 89mm Hg is classified as **prehypertension**. Patients with prehypertension are still at risk for diseases and conditions associated with elevated blood pressure, and for developing hypertension. Approximately one-third of American adults have blood pressure that is greater than or equal to 140/90mm Hg.

The risk of morbidity and mortality related to hypertension is directly related to elevated blood pressure. Untreated hypertension can lead to a variety of devastating diseases, including a host of cardiovascular diseases and events, kidney dysfunction, whole-body edema, and fluid accumulation in the lungs. Hypertension management begins with lifestyle modifications such as decreasing sodium intake, losing weight, increasing physical activity, decreasing alcohol consumption, controlling stress, and quitting smoking.

If lifestyle modifications do not effectively lower blood pressure, drug therapy is usually initiated, especially for people with substantial cardiovascular risks. Antihypertensive agents reduce the risks of cardiovascular events and death associated with hypertension. The most commonly used antihypertensive agents are listed in **TABLE 14.4**. ACE inhibitors, beta-blockers, and calcium channel blockers are first-line agents for treating hypertension, and have been listed previously in Tables 14.1 and 14.3.

Table 14.4   Common Antihypertensive Agents

Class	Generic Name	Brand Name	Dosage Forms Available
Diuretics	Hydrochlorothiazide	Esidrex	Tablet
	Methyclothiazide	Enduron	Tablet
	Chlorthalidone	Hygroton	Tablet
	Bumetanide	Bumex	Injection, tablet
	Ethacrynic acid	Edecrin	Injection, tablet
	Furosemide	Lasix	Injection, IV, oral, liquid, tablet
	Torsemide	Demadex	IV, tablet
	Amiloride	Midamor	Tablet
	Eplerenone	Inspra	Tablet
	Spironolactone	Aldactone	Tablet
	Triamterene	Dyrenium	Capsule
	Acetazolamide	Diamox	Capsule, injection, IV, tablet
	Methazolamide	Neptazane	Tablet
	Mannitol	Osmitrol	IV
	Indapamide	Lozol	Tablet
	Metolazone	Zaroxolyn	Tablet
Angiotensin receptor blockers	Candesartan	Atacand	Tablet
	Irbesartan	Avapro	Tablet
	Losartan	Cozaar	Tablet
	Olmesartan	Benicar	Tablet
	Telmisartan	Micardis	Tablet
	Valsartan	Diovan	Capsule, tablet
CNS agents	Clonidine	Catapress, Catapress-TTS, Duraclon	IV, tablet, transdermal patch
	Guanfacine	Tenex	Tablet
	Methyldopa	Aldomet	IV, tablet
Alpha-blockers	Alfuzosin	Uroxatrol	Tablet
	Doxazosin	Cardura	Tablet
	Prazosin	Minipress	Capsule
	Terazosin	Hytrin	Capsule, tablet
Vasodilators	Eproprostenol	Flolan	IV
	Fenoldopam	Corlopram	IV
	Hydralazine	Apresoline	IV, tablet
	Minoxidil	Loniten	Tablet
Direct renin inhibitors	Aliskiren	Tekturna	Tablet

Many antihypertensive agents are available in combination with each other. Often, more than one drug is needed to control blood pressure, and one dosage form that contains two or more active ingredients improves compliance. There are countless combination drugs used to treat hypertension, which are not listed here. Individually, the drugs work with the same mechanism of action and achieve the same effectiveness as single-drug agents listed in Table 14.1.

Diuretics

Diuretics are the first-line agents used to treat hypertension. They increase urine output and reduce overall fluid volume in the body, which reduces the amount the heart has to work. They also reduce sodium levels, which is critical in lowering blood pressure. Different classes of diuretics are discussed in more detail in Chapter 13.

Angiotensin Receptor Blockers

ACE inhibitors, calcium channel blockers, or angiotensin receptor blockers (ARBs) may be used as first-line antihypertensive agents in patients without indications to such treatment. Unless there is a compelling indication for the use of beta-blockers as first-line therapy, beta-blockers do not usually reduce the risk of cardiovascular events as much as these other three classes. ARBs work in the renin-angiotensin system, just like ACE inhibitors. Rather than inhibiting the production of angiotensin II, however, ARBs block the action of angiotensin II at its receptors. Because they work in the same system, ACE inhibitors and ARBs are rarely used together. ARBs are generally well-tolerated and do not cause the cough associated with ACE inhibitors.

Central Nervous System Agents

If first-line antihypertensive therapy does not lower blood pressure to the desired range, then alternative agents may be added to the drug regimen to provide additional blood-pressure lowering. Central nervous system (CNS) agents reduce sympathetic activity (activity that controls the body's internal organs) and increase parasympathetic activity (activity that maintains homeostasis), resulting in a decreased heart rate, decreased cardiac output, and decreased peripheral resistance. CNS agents may cause drowsiness and fatigue. Clonidine is the only antihypertensive agent available in a transdermal system.

Alpha-Blockers

Alpha-blockers are peripheral acting agents, blocking the constriction of blood vessels. This action leads to vasodilation and decreased blood pressure. The most significant side effect of most alpha-blockers is orthostatic hypotension. It is most severe with the first dose. Patients should be advised to take alpha-blockers at bedtime to reduce the risks associated with falling and dizziness due to orthostatic hypotension.

Vasodilators

Vasodilators relax the smooth muscles of the arteries, which reduces peripheral resistance. Some vasodilators are used to treat other cardiovascular conditions, while others are preferred for use in hypertension treatment. Hypotension, headache, flushing, and nausea are common side effects of many vasodilators.

Direct Renin Inhibitors

Aliskiren exerts its action in the renin-angiotensin system by inhibiting the action of renin. The absorption and effectiveness of this medication is affected by high-fat foods, so this drug should not be taken with meals.

Myocardial Infarction

A **myocardial infarction (MI)** is more commonly known as a heart attack, and causes significant morbidity and mortality throughout the world. An MI occurs after a long period of decreased oxygen delivery to the heart muscle, which causes the cells of the heart to die. If the vessels leading to the heart are occluded, reducing oxygen delivery, the likelihood of an MI increases substantially. To prevent an MI, many lifestyle modifications may be initiated, including quitting smoking, reducing blood pressure, exercising regularly, maintaining an ideal body weight, decreasing alcohol consumption, reducing cholesterol levels, and controlling diabetes. Drug therapy may be needed to achieve these measures.

Once an MI has occurred, treatment promotes normal healing of the heart while reducing the risk of death or recurrent MI. Beta-blockers, presented in Table 14.1, and daily 81mg aspirin are often prescribed to reduce the heart's workload and prevent clot formation.

Blood Clots

A **thrombus** is a blood clot transported in the blood. A thrombus may result from abnormal coagulation, altered blood flow, increased platelet adhesion, or damaged blood vessels. A blood clot is potentially life threatening.

Blood clots may be present but undiagnosed, representing a serious risk to patient health and life. A **pulmonary embolism (PE)** occurs when a piece of a blood clot breaks off and travels to the lung. This leads to a sudden block of the pulmonary artery. A **deep vein thrombosis (DVT)** is a thrombus that occurs in veins deep within the body, most often the legs. A DVT that is located at or above the knee is the most serious type of DVT and is the most likely to be fatal. Risk factors for DVT include age over 40 years, extended periods of immobility or limited mobility, high-dose estrogen therapy, estrogen therapy combined with nicotine exposure, major illness, obesity, pregnancy, previous DVT, surgery, trauma, and varicose veins.

Anticoagulant and antiplatelet agents are the drugs of choice to prevent the formation of blood clots in patients at risk of a thrombus. Commonly used anticoagulant and antiplatelet agents are presented in **TABLE 14.5**.

Anticoagulants

Anticoagulant therapy is typically initiated with IV heparin, a naturally occurring anticoagulant. IV anticoagulant therapy requires intense monitoring via laboratory tests and observation of patient signs and symptoms. Therapy should be switched to an oral form of anticoagulant therapy, often warfarin, when patients are stable and prepared for discharge from the hospital. The most significant risk of anticoagulant therapy is bleeding. Patients receiving any type of anticoagulant therapy should be educated about the signs and symptoms of bleeding, and when to contact a physician or emergency services.

Heparin may not be appropriate for or tolerated by all patients, so alternative injectable anticoagulants are available, including lepirudin, bivalirudin, and fondaparinux. Low-molecular weight heparins

Patients receiving long-term anticoagulant therapy with warfarin should be directed to wear an alert bracelet or carry a wallet card that identifies the fact that they are on such therapy in the case of an emergency.

Table 14.5 Common Anticoagulant and Antiplatelet Agents

Class	Generic Name	Brand Name	Dosage Forms Available
Anticoagulant agents	Bivalirudin	Angiomax	IV
	Fondaparinux	Arixtra	Injection
	Heparin	None	Injection, IV
	Lepirudin	Refludan	IV
	Warfarin	Coumadin	Tablet, injection
	Dalteparin	Fragmin	Injection
	Enoxaparin	Lovenox	Injection
	Tinzaparin	Innohep	Injection
Antiplatelet agents	Aspirin	Various	Tablet
	Clopidogrel	Plavix	Tablet
	Ticlopidine	Ticlid	Tablet
	Abciximab	ReoPro	IV
	Eptifibatide	Integrilin	IV
	Tirofiban	Aggrastat	IV

(LMWHs) are alternatives to heparin and have become the standard of care for clot-formation prophylaxis after many types of surgeries. Compared to heparin, LMWHs provide more reliable responses, reduced bleeding, predetermined dosing, and no need for monitoring. LMWHs include enoxaprin, dalteparin, and tinzaparin.

Antiplatelet Agents

Antiplatelet agents prevent platelets from becoming sticky. Aspirin is the most commonly used antiplatelet agent, but clopidogrel and ticlopidine are also available. Patients may experience gastrointestinal upset due to regular aspirin therapy, and patients with a history of gastrointestinal bleeding or other bleeding disorders should not take aspirin. Clopidogrel also presents an increased risk of bleeding. Ticlopidine should be used in patients who cannot tolerate aspirin or clopidogrel; it can cause diarrhea, nausea, and rash, as well as blood and platelet disorders.

Glycoprotein antagonists act as antiplatelet agents by preventing platelet aggregation. These agents, including abciximab, eptifibatide, and tirofiban, are used in acute coronary syndrome and during invasive surgical procedures to prevent artery closure.

Fibrinolytic Agents

Once a clot has formed, anticoagulant agents and antiplatelet agents cannot break up or dissolve the clot. Therefore, treatment with fibrinolytic agents is indicated. These agents dissolve clots by binding to the protein in the clot. The most common fibrinolytic agents are presented in TABLE 14.6.

All fibrinolytic agents are supplied by the manufacturers as powders that must be reconstituted prior to administration. The reconstituted solution should be gently swirled, never shaken, to maintain the integrity of the chemical structure of the drug. Additionally, most solutions have very specific storage and administration requirements. Take care to read the manufacturer's instructions carefully for fibrinolytic agents. The risk of bleeding is high with all fibrinolytics.

Table 14.6   Common Fibrinolytic Agents

Generic Name	Brand Name	Dosage Forms Available
Alteplase	Activase	IV
Reteplase	Retavase	IV
Tenecteplase	TNKase	IV
Urokinase	Abbokinase, Kinlytic	IV

High Cholesterol

Cholesterol is found naturally in foods of animal origin, but not plant origin. It is necessary for the proper functioning of several organs and body systems. The liver is responsible for processing cholesterol consumed from food and for making cholesterol when more is needed. The liver packages molecules of cholesterol together with lipids bound to proteins (lipoproteins). Most of the lipoproteins in the body are either high-density lipoproteins (HDL) or low-density lipoproteins (LDL). HDL is referred to as good cholesterol and is attached to approximately 20 to 30% of total cholesterol. LDL is referred to as bad cholesterol and is attached to 60 to 70% of the total cholesterol.

Triglycerides are fats synthesized from carbohydrates and release free fatty acids into the blood. Triglycerides circulate with cholesterol, and represent one of the three major classes of lipids in the body.

LDL circulates through the body, bringing cholesterol to body parts that need it. LDL is not used by many cells, so it is, instead, deposited in the walls of arteries, which may eventually clog the blood vessel **FIGURE 14.10**. This narrowing of arteries is known as **atherosclerosis** and can result in stroke or MI. It can also lead to poor circulation and the eventual loss of limbs due to gangrene. Elevated levels of LDL increase the risk of atherosclerosis. HDL returns cholesterol to the liver, so elevated levels actually lower the risk of atherosclerosis.

Lipoprotein levels are influenced by genetics, and a strong family history of premature atherosclerosis and high lipoprotein or cholesterol levels is a significant risk factor for the development of high cholesterol. Other risk factors include diabetes, obesity, alcohol consumption, hypothyroidism, liver disease, kidney disease, and age.

High cholesterol is a risk factor for several other cardiovascular diseases and events. Lowering and managing cholesterol levels are, therefore, important parts of cardiovascular health. Ideally, total cholesterol levels should be maintained below 200mg per 100mL blood, or 200mg per deciliter (mg/dL). LDL cholesterol should be less than 100mg and HDL greater than 60mg. Triglycerides should be less than 150mg/dL. A low-fat diet and healthy lifestyle modifications, including regular physical activity, smoking cessation, and weight loss (if needed), can be effective in maintaining optimal cholesterol levels. Drug therapy can also be added to help achieve these goals. Common lipid-lowering agents are presented in **TABLE 14.7**. Each class of agents works differently and has varying effects on LDL, HDL, and triglyceride levels. Often, a combination of agents from different classes is required to optimize all

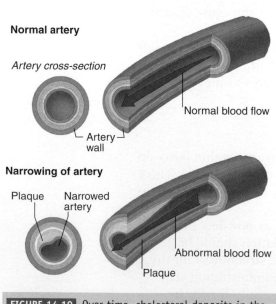

Normal artery

Artery cross-section

Normal blood flow

Artery wall

Narrowing of artery

Plaque   Narrowed artery

Abnormal blood flow

Plaque

FIGURE 14.10 Over time, cholesterol deposits in the blood vessels impede the circulation of blood.

Table 14.7	Common Cholesterol-Lowering Agents		
Class	**Generic Name**	**Brand Name**	**Dosage Forms Available**
HMG-CoA reductase inhibitors	Atorvastatin	Lipitor	Tablet
	Fluvastatin	Lescol	Capsule, tablet
	Lovastatin	Altocor, Mevacor	Tablet
	Pravastatin	Pravachol	Tablet
	Rosuvastatin	Crestor	Tablet
	Simvastatin	Zocor	Tablet
Fibric acid derivatives	Fenofibrate	TriCor	Tablet, capsule
	Gemfibrozil	Lopid	Tablet
Bile acid sequestrants	Cholestyramine	Questran	Powder for suspension
	Colesevelam	WelChol	Tablet
	Colestipol	Colestid	Granules for suspension, tablet
Miscellaneous agents	Ezetimibe	Zetia	Tablet
	Niacin	Niacor, Niaspan	Tablet
	Psyllium	Fiberall, Metamucil	Powder for suspension, capsule, chewable bar
	Fish oil omega-3 fatty acid	Lovaza	Capsule

lipoprotein levels. There are several combination products available, which increases patient compliance, but they are not listed here.

HMG-CoA Reductase Inhibitors

HMG-CoA reductase inhibitors are commonly known as statins. These drugs inhibit the enzymatic process of cholesterol formation in the liver. Gastrointestinal upset and headache are the most common side effects of statins, but usually improve over time. Unexplained muscle pain or weakness should be reported to a physician, as it may be a sign of a serious adverse effect. Cholesterol levels, as well as liver-function tests, should be routinely monitored for patients receiving statin therapy.

Statins are substrates of the cytochrome P450 family of enzymes, and, therefore, may present a risk of drug interactions.

Fibric Acid Derivatives

Fibric acid derivatives increase the excretion of cholesterol in bile. Therefore, the body must produce more bile acids. Because bile acids are synthesized from cholesterol, more cholesterol is used by the body, lowering LDL levels.

These drugs may increase the risk of gallstones. As with statins, unexplained muscle pain or weakness should be reported immediately. Gastrointestinal upset is the most common side effect of most fibric acid derivatives.

Bile Acid Sequestrants

Bile acid sequestrants form a complex with bile acids in the intestine, preventing their absorption from the intestines into the blood stream. The excess bile acids are excreted in the stool. As with fibric acid derivatives, the body must use cholesterol to make more bile acid, resulting in lower LDL levels. Constipation is the most common side effect of bile acid sequestrants.

Miscellaneous Cholesterol-Lowering Agents

Niacin is available OTC and by prescription as vitamin B_3. It lowers LDL and triglyceride levels. Niacin commonly causes extreme flushing when first taken, but this can be avoided by aspirin prophylaxis 30 minutes prior to niacin administration. It can also cause gastrointestinal upset and increased uric acid levels, which precipitates gout.

Psyllium, available in over-the-counter preparations, lowers cholesterol by forming a complex with soluble fiber from the diet and excreting it from the body. Because the body absorbs less cholesterol, it must use more of its own to produce hormones and other compounds, effectively lowering LDL levels. Eating a high-fiber diet has the same effect as taking daily fiber supplements.

Ezetimibe inhibits the absorption of cholesterol in the small intestine, thereby decreasing the amount of cholesterol delivered to the liver.

If patients want to purchase omega-3 fatty acid supplements without a prescription, help determine that the supplement is a fish-derivative and is a USP grade product.

Omega-3 fatty acids in the form of fish oil help lower triglyceride levels. Some omega-3 fatty acid products can be purchased over the counter, but they are also available as a prescription product. Compliance can be an issue with fish-oil capsules because large doses are often prescribed, and a fishy smell can actually permeate the skin of patients taking the supplements.

Stroke

A **stroke** occurs when oxygen supply to a localized area of the brain is interrupted. This may be a result of obstructed blood flow or hemorrhage. Strokes that result from occluded blood flow are called ischemic strokes and account for roughly 90% of all strokes. Alternatively, hemorrhagic strokes, or cerebral hemorrhages, occur when a weakened blood vessel in the brain ruptures, causing blood to spill out of the blood vessels into the space within the brain.

Ischemic strokes can be caused by blood clots or emboli within the blood vessels of the brain. Atherosclerosis is a cause of most ischemic strokes. A **transient ischemic attack (TIA)** is similar to an ischemic stroke, but lasts less than 24 hours—often less than 30 minutes. TIAs require urgent intervention to prevent the occurrence of a stroke.

Hemorrhagic strokes are most often caused by hypertension. Modifiable risk factors for stroke include cigarette smoking, coronary artery disease, diabetes, excessive alcohol consumption, high cholesterol, hypertension, obesity, and physical inactivity. Advanced age, male gender, family history of stoke, African-American race, and previous stroke are also risk factors for stroke. The reasons for the increased risk of stroke among African-Americans are not well-defined, but the risk is significant; African-Americans are more likely to suffer from and have long-term morbidity and mortality related to stroke.

Stroke prevention includes treatment with antiplatelet and anticoagulant therapy to prevent clot formation, fibrinolytic therapy to break up an already-formed clot, and surgical prevention. Lifestyle modification and drug therapy to control modifiable risk factors are also appropriate stroke prevention. These drug classes are discussed in Tables 14.1, 14.3, 14.4, and 14.7.

After a stroke, therapy to prevent a recurrent stroke depends on the type of stroke that occurred initially. The cause of a stroke should be unequivocally confirmed before therapy is started. For example, administering antiplatelet, anticoagulant, or fibrinolytic agents after a hemorrhagic stroke could be fatal.

A few drugs are available for stroke prevention that have not been discussed previously among the other classes of cardiovascular drugs. Dipyridamole (Persantine) inhibits platelet aggregation and is often used in combination with warfarin to prevent a variety of thromboembolic disorders and to maintain vessel patency after surgery. Dipyridamole is also available in a combination capsule with aspirin (Aggrenox). It is used to prevent a recurrent stroke or TIA. Pentoxyfilline (Trental) improves blood flow by increasing the flexibility of red blood cells and reducing the viscosity of blood. It is available as a time-release tablet and must be taken with food.

Tech Math Practice

Question: **A brand-name drug costs $51.30 for 100 tablets. The generic equivalent costs $18.50 for 100 tablets. Calculate the cost difference for a 30-day supply between the brand and generic products if two tablets are taken daily.**

Answer: Tablets required: 2 tablets/day × 30 days = 60 tablets

> Cost of brand name product: $51.30/100 tablets × 60 tablets = $30.78
> Cost of generic product: $18.50/100 tablets × 60 tablets = $11.10
> Cost difference: $30.78 – $11.10 = $19.68

Question: **The pharmacy's price to purchase a medication is $175. If the wholesaler offers a 15% discount when the account is paid in full within 15 days, what is the pharmacy's purchase price?**

Answer: Amount of discount: $175 × 0.15 = $26.25

> Purchase price: $175 – $26.25 = $148.75

Question: **A pharmacy purchases a bottle of 100 pills for $67.50. The pharmacy adds a markup of 40% to prescriptions dispensed. What is the prescription price for a quantity of 30 tablets?**

Answer: $67.50/100 = $0.675/tablet

> Markup price per tablet = $0.675 + ($0.675 × 40%) = $0.945
> Price of 30 tablets = $0.945 × 30 = $28.35

Question: **A pharmacy maintains an average inventory of $35,000. The pharmacy's annual sales total $175,000. What is the turnover rate?**

Answer: Turnover rate = annual sales/average inventory = $175,000/$35,000 = 5

Question: **The pharmacy's price to purchase a prescription ointment is $38.75 per tube. The pharmacy receives a 10% discount off their purchase price. The insurance company reimburses the pharmacy at their purchase price plus 2%, plus a $2.50 dispensing fee. If the pharmacy sells 15 prescriptions for this ointment, how much profit was made?**

Answer: Discount: $38.75 × 10% = $3.88

Pharmacy purchase price = $38.75 – $3.88 = $34.87

Reimbursement = $38.75 + ($38.75 × 2%) + $2.50 = $40.03

Profit = Reimbursement price – purchase price = $5.16 per prescription

Profit per 15 prescriptions = $5.16 × 15 = $77.40

Question: **An injectable drug costs a hospital $9.56 per 5mg vial. The drug is administered at a rate of 0.2mg/kg/hr for 24 hours. What is the daily cost to the hospital of the drug for a 165-pound patient?**

Answer: Amount of drug needed: 165lbs × 1lb/2.2kg = 75 kg

75kg × 0.2mg/kg/hr × 24 hr = 360 mg per day

Number of vials needed: 360mg × 1 vial/5mg = 72 vials

Cost of drug = $9.56/vial × 72 vials = $688.32

Question: **An inhaled medication has a pharmacy purchase price of $23.65. The pharmacy receives a 15% discount on the purchase price. The pharmacy sells the prescription for $33.50. What is the markup rate on the drug?**

Answer: Purchase price: $23.65 × 0.15 = $3.55 discount

$23.65 – $3.55 = $20.10

Markup = Sale price – Purchase price = $33.50 – $20.10 = $13.40

Markup rate = $13.40/$20.10 × 100 = 66.67%

WRAP UP

Chapter Summary

- Non-sterile compounding may be required to prepare a product that is not commercially available or to meet the unique needs of a patient.

- When compounding, have a pharmacist check the calculations, weights, and measurements before mixing ingredients.

- Maintain an accurate compounding log of the steps completed and ingredients used for each prescription compounded.

- To reconstitute powders for oral suspension, add a quantity of water or other liquid to the bottle of powder, as directed by the manufacturer. Shake vigorously to mix, and apply a "Shake Well" auxiliary label to the dispensed prescription.

- Capsules are simple and easy dosage forms to prepare when customized doses are required. Filling capsules requires weighing and reweighing of the filled capsules to ensure accurate and precise dosing.

- To create an oral suspension from tablets or capsules, triturate the solid dosage form or powder and add it to a syrup or liquid vehicle for oral use. Oral suspensions are administered by a spoon, oral syringe, or dosing cup, and are useful for patients who have difficulty swallowing solid dosage forms.

- Several types of semisolid dosage forms are available for topical use. Creams, ointments, gels, and pastes can be used as protectants, lubricants, emollients, or moisturizers. To blend an active ingredient into an inert semisolid base, use the spatulation method, in which small amounts of base and active ingredient are successively added and thoroughly blended using a spatula on an ointment slab.

- Diseases of the cardiovascular system affect 70-million people in the United States. Modifiable risk factors for preventing cardiovascular disease include smoking, excessive alcohol consumption, obesity, high blood pressure, high cholesterol, and physical inactivity. When lifestyle changes do not control the risk factors, drug therapy can be initiated to decrease the occurrence of cardiovascular diseases or events.

- Angina pectoris is chest pain caused by a decreased oxygen supply to the heart. Nitroglycerin is the drug of choice for acute angina attacks. Beta-blockers and calcium channel blockers reduce the severity and frequency of angina attacks.

- An arrhythmia is a variation in the normal rate and/or rhythm of the heart. Class I antiarrhythmic agents are membrane destabilizing agents. Beta-blockers are Class II antiarrhythmic agents. Potassium channel blockers are Class III antiarrhythmic agents, and calcium channel blockers are Class IV antiarrythmic agents.

- Heart failure is a condition in which the heart cannot pump enough blood to meet the demands of the body. Hypertension and coronary artery disease are the leading causes of heart failure. Heart failure causes the body to retain fluid and electrolytes and is also referred to as congestive heart failure. First-line treatment for heart failure includes an ACE inhibitor or a beta-blocker; an antiplatelet agent or anticoagulant, a diuretic, and digoxin are added to most heart-failure regimens.

- Hypertension is a blood pressure over 140/90mm Hg. The extent of hypertension is directly related to the risk of morbidity and mortality. Several classes of antihypertensive agents are available that may be used alone or in combination: ACE inhibitors, beta-blockers, calcium channel blockers, diuretics, ARBs, central nervous system agents, alpha-blockers, vasodilators, and direct renin inhibitors.

- A myocardial infarction is also known as a heart attack and occurs after prolonged oxygen deprivation to the heart. Lifestyle modifications are crucial to preventing an MI, but controlling risk factors, including hypertension, high cholesterol levels, and diabetes, may require drug therapy.

- Blood clots can cause significant morbidity and mortality. Blood clots result from abnormal coagulation, altered blood flow, increased platelet adhesion, or damaged blood vessels. A blood clot can flow through the blood stream and cause sudden blockages of vital arteries. Anticoagulants and antiplatelet agents prevent the formation of clots. Fibrinolytic agents dissolve clots that have already formed.

- High cholesterol is a risk factor for other cardiovascular diseases. Lifestyle modifications are essential to reducing excess cholesterol in the body, but many drug classes are available that may be used alone or in combination to decrease lipid levels: HMG-CoA reductase inhibitors, fibric acid derivatives, bile acid sequestrants, and miscellaneous agents.

- A stroke occurs when oxygen supply to the brain is interrupted. An ischemic stroke may occur as the result of a blood clot in a vessel leading to the brain. A hemorrhagic stroke may occur as a result of a ruptured blood vessel, often caused by hypertension. Controlling risk factors, as well as preventing clot formation, are imperative in stroke prevention.

Learning Assessment Questions

1. The final volume of Augmentin for oral suspension is 125mg/5mL. If the prescribed dose is Augmentin 125mg four times daily, how much of this solution will be needed for a seven-day supply?
   A. 500mL
   B. 700mL
   C. 140mL
   D. 125mL

2. If the volume required for reconstituting a powder for oral suspension is 75mL, approximately what volume of water should be added first?
   A. 50 mL
   B. 25 mL
   C. 75 mL
   D. 5 mL

3. What does it mean to triturate?
   A. To use a scoop and fill technique for filling capsules
   B. To break and grind a solid tablet into a fine powder
   C. To reconstitute powder for an oral suspension
   D. To sterilize instruments prior to compounding IV medications

4. The height of the powder cake used for filling capsules should be approximately equal to _____.
   A. The height of the entire capsule body
   B. One-third of the height of the capsule cap
   C. Half the height of the capsule body
   D. The total amount of powder divided by the number of capsules to be made

5. If a suspension was compounded using thirty 250mg tablets and 200mL of liquid, what is the concentration of the final product?
   A. 37.5mg/mL
   B. 30 mg/5mL
   C. 1.25mg/mL
   D. 0.8mg/mL

6. An oral suspension can be administered by all of the following devices except _____.
   A. A medication spoon
   B. An oral syringe
   C. An insulin syringe without the needle
   D. A dosing cup

7. Gloves are important in non-sterile compounding for all of the following reasons except _____.
   A. To maintain the integrity of the medication and supplies that may be affected by oil from the technician's hands
   B. To keep the technician's hands warm so his body temperature does not affect the final compounded product
   C. To protect the technician from exposure to medication
   D. To protect the patient from potential contamination

8. When should a pharmacist check the technician's work during the compounding process?

   A. The pharmacist should check the technician's work after the product has been placed in its container for dispensing, but before the patient medication label has been affixed to the prescription bottle.

   B. The pharmacist should check the technician's work after the technician has gathered all the supplies and ingredients, but before they have been weighed.

   C. The pharmacist should check the technician's work after the ingredients have been measured, counted, or weighed, but before they have been mixed.

   D. The pharmacist only needs to check the compounding log after the supplies have been put away, but before the medication is dispensed.

9. A common method of compounding creams, ointments, gels, and pastes is _____.

   A. Spatulation

   B. Trituration

   C. Emulsion

   D. Suspension

10. What is the best way to mix an active ingredient into a base ingredient?

    A. Mix the entire quantity of each directly in the ointment jar.

    B. Mix half of the active ingredient into all of the base ingredient.

    C. Mix all of the active ingredient into a small amount of the base ingredient.

    D. Mix a small amount of each ingredient at a time.

11. Non-sterile compounding might be necessary in all of the following situations except _____.

    A. A patient does not like the packaging on the manufacturer's cream.

    B. A geriatric patient is unable to swallow tablets and must take an oral liquid.

    C. A physician orders an ointment in a strength that is not manufactured.

    D. A patient is allergic to one of the ingredients in the manufacturer's gel.

12. Compounding lozenges would not be appropriate in which of the following circumstances?

    A. An adult patient has a sore throat and requires localized pain relief.

    B. A pediatric patient is unable to swallow solid oral dosage forms.

    C. A drug that is unstable in high heat needs to be administered to the oral mucosa.

    D. A geriatric patient has a fungal infection of the mouth and requires localized treatment.

13. When compounding lozenges, solutions containing sugar should not be heated above what temperature?

    A. 300°C

    B. 212°F

    C. 149°F

    D. 155°C

14. How many people in the United States are affected by cardiovascular disease?

    A. Five million

    B. 70 million

    C. 10% of the population

    D. 300,000

15. Which of the following is not a type of angina?

    A. Stable angina

    B. Unstable angina

    C. Variant angina

    D. Congestive angina

16. Which of the following is considered a normal heart rate?

    A. Less than 60 bpm

    B. 120 to 139 bpm

    C. 70 to 80 bpm

    D. Greater than 90 bpm

17. Which set of side effects is common with anticholinergic agents?

    A. Hypoglycemia and hypothyroidism

    B. Palpitations, syncope, sweating, and weakness

    C. Dry mouth, urinary retention, constipation, and blurred vision

    D. Headache, confusion, and nausea

18. Which set of symptoms is consistent with digitalis toxicity?
    A. Nausea, vertigo, weakness, and visual disturbances
    B. Dizziness, orthostatic hypotension, and swelling of the face and tongue
    C. Rash, diarrhea, and blood disorders
    D. Headache, muscle pain or weakness, and gastrointestinal upset

19. All of the following drug classes may be used as first-line therapy for treating hypertension except _____.
    A. ACE inhibitors
    B. Beta-blockers
    C. Calcium channel blockers
    D. Angiotensin receptor blockers

20. What is the most significant risk associated with anticoagulant therapy?
    A. Bleeding
    B. Nausea
    C. Blood clots
    D. Hypertension

21. Which of the following sets of drugs or classes of drugs could contribute to stroke prevention?
    A. A fibrinolytic, digoxin, and aspirin
    B. A cholesterol-lowering drug, an antihypertensive, and warfarin
    C. A nitrate and a beta-blocker
    D. Pentoxyfilline and a calcium channel blocker

22. Which of the following statements about cholesterol is true?
    A. It occurs naturally in foods from plant sources, but not in foods from animal sources.
    B. It is necessary for the proper functioning of certain body systems.
    C. The kidney is responsible for metabolizing cholesterol consumed from the diet.
    D. An ideal total cholesterol blood level should be greater than 200mg/100mL.

23. Which laboratory tests should be routinely monitored in patients taking an HMG-CoA reductase inhibitor?
    A. Total cholesterol and liver function tests
    B. Blood pressure and triglycerides
    C. Cardiac output, hemoglobin, and hematocrit
    D. Vitamin B3 and glomerular filtration rate

24. Which of the following sets of lifestyle modifications can contribute to a decreased risk of cardiovascular diseases and events?
    A. Smoking cessation, increased alcohol consumption, and periods of immobility
    B. High-salt diet and family history
    C. Weight loss, increased physical activity, and decreased stress
    D. Low-fat diet, increased fiber intake, and nitrate prophylaxis

25. Which of the following is true regarding antiplatelet therapy?
    A. Ticlopidine is the preferred antiplatelet agent due to its high tolerability and low risk of side effects.
    B. Low molecular weight heparins are reliable antiplatelet agents.
    C. Antiplatelet agents prevent platelets from sticking to each other and forming clots.
    D. Clopidogrel poses no increased risk of bleeding.

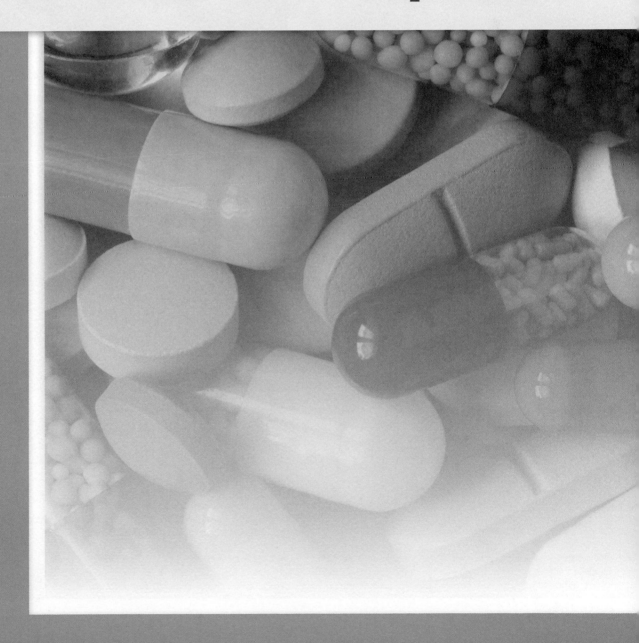

Advanced Principles

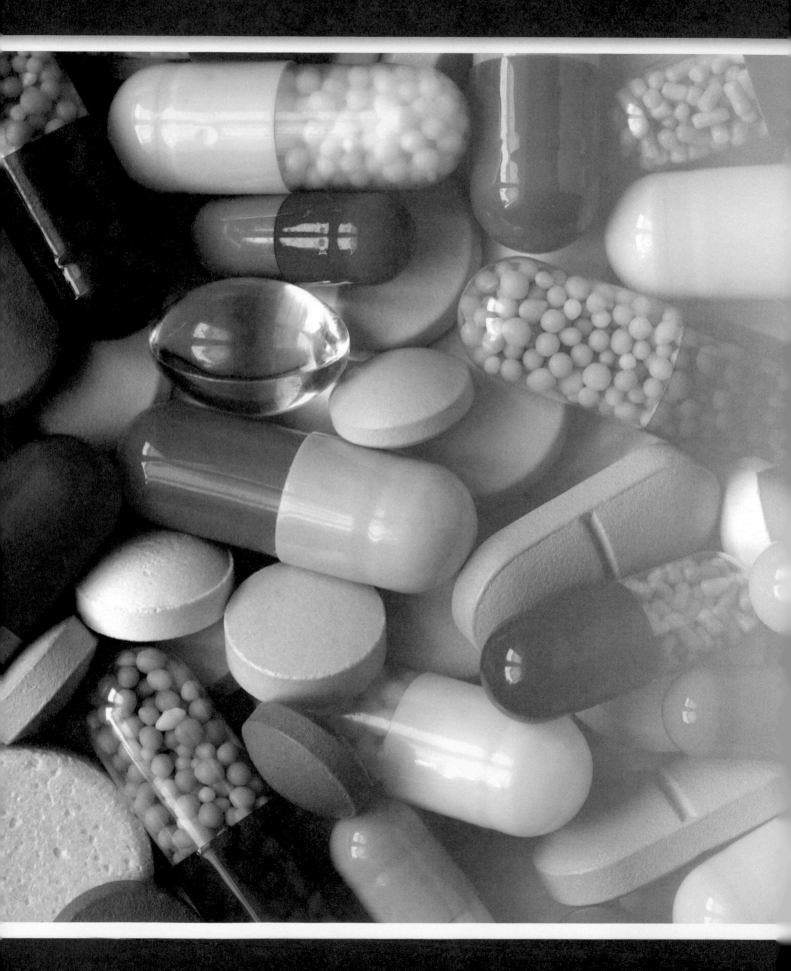

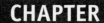

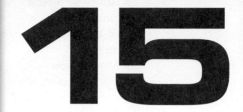

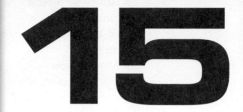

CHAPTER 15

Institutional Pharmacy

OBJECTIVES

After reading this chapter, you will be able to:

- Describe the classifications and functions of a hospital and the role of the director of pharmacy.
- Identify services that are unique to a hospital pharmacy.
- Contrast a medication order with a unit-dose profile.
- Identify the advantages of a unit dose drug-distribution system.
- Explain the proper procedures for repackaging medications.
- Identify the process of dispensing and filling medication in a hospital pharmacy.
- Discuss the advantages of an automated floor stock system for medication, including narcotics.
- Describe specialty services such as intravenous admixtures and total parenteral nutrition.
- Describe a medication administration record (MAR).
- Define muscle relaxants.
- Identify muscle relaxants and their mechanisms of action.
- Identify non-narcotic analgesics and describe their uses and mechanisms of action.
- Explain autoimmune diseases.
- Identify agents used to treat arthritis, rheumatoid arthritis, and gout, and discuss their usage and side effects.

KEY TERMS

Admitting order
Antipyretic
Arthritis
Autoimmune disease
Bursitis
Cart-fill list

Cartilaginous joint
Chart
Continuation order
Cyclooxygenase I (COX-1)
Cyclooxygenase II
   (COX-2)

Director of pharmacy
Disease-modifying
   antirheumatic drugs
   (DMARDs)
Fibrous joint
Floor stock

Good manufacturing practices (GMPs)	Mixed analgesic	Tophi
Gouty arthritis	Muscle relaxants	Total parenteral nutrition (TPN)
Hospital	Nonsteroidal anti-inflammatory drugs (NSAIDs)	Total parenteral nutrition (TPN) service
IV admixture service		
Joint	Nutritional support	Tumor necrosis factor (TNF)
Medication administration record (MAR)	Osteoarthritis	
	Pyrogens	Unit dose
Medication order	Rheumatoid arthritis	Unit-dose profile
Medication profile	Stat order	
	Synovial joint	

Chapter Overview

This chapter outlines the functions of a hospital pharmacy, the responsibilities of the director of pharmacy, and the expanded role of a pharmacy technician in a hospital pharmacy setting. The increase in patient volume and need for pharmacy evaluations for patients have changed the demands on a hospital pharmacist. As a result, pharmacy technicians have assumed control of some of the tasks that had been performed by pharmacists in the past. Services that are unique to a hospital pharmacy will be discussed in this chapter. Drug-distribution systems, automation, and specialty services provided by hospital pharmacies are also reviewed in this chapter. In addition, drugs used to treat disorders involving the muscles and joints are discussed.

Organization of a Hospital

A **hospital** is a complex organization with many departments, all working together to provide emergency, medical, trauma, and surgical care to the community. Hospitals serve many functions. These include providing treatment, diagnosis and testing, providing education and support programs, training health professionals, and researching to advance medical knowledge. Depending on the function of the hospital, patient populations can vary. Hospitals can be classified by the number of beds available for patient use; the services they provide; their capability for diagnosis, surgery, and outpatient services; their affiliation with a university or academic center; whether they are for profit or nonprofit; and length of stay (short-term versus long-term). An acute care hospital provides care for patients with short lengths of stay. These hospitals require a special license and must maintain a certain level of care. The Joint Commission is an organization that accredits and certifies healthcare organizations that meet certain performance standards.

The organization of a hospital can vary depending on the number of beds and the services it provides. Usually, a president, chief executive officer (CEO), or chief medical officer (CMO) runs the hospital and reports to the board of directors. Heads of each department report directly to the president, CEO, or CMO. Some hospitals are subdivided into medical and surgical specialties and further subdivided into specific surgical subspecialties (cardiac surgery, emergency surgery) or medical subspecialties (cardiology, gastroenterology). The president, CEO, or CMO usually oversees the departments responsible for clinical services, pharmacy, laboratory, radiology, medical records, and social services.

The Director of Pharmacy

The functions of a hospital pharmacy can vary depending on the functions of the hospital. The **director of pharmacy** is the pharmacist responsible for all of the hospital's pharmacy services. The director of pharmacy usually reports to the president, CEO, or CMO and works closely with the director of nursing and the heads or chiefs of medicine and surgery.

The director of pharmacy is responsible for staffing the pharmacy, including hiring and firing all pharmacy personnel. He or she is also responsible for managing the pharmacy budget, developing policies and procedures, and complying with hospital policies, federal and state regulations, and regulatory boards. The State Board of Pharmacy requires that the director of pharmacy be responsible for all pharmaceutical services provided in the hospital. In a larger hospital, there may also be assistant directors or supervisors that help the director oversee the daily functions of the pharmacy. They report directly to the director of pharmacy.

The director of pharmacy is responsible for overseeing all the functions of a hospital pharmacy, such as outpatient pharmacy services, drug information, inpatient drug distribution, types of medications provided, and clinical services. This includes determining the availability and types of services that will be offered by the pharmacy.

The director of pharmacy is responsible for creating, submitting, and maintaining a budget. Maintaining a budget is a difficult task because newer, more expensive drugs constantly enter the marketplace. Some hospital pharmacies may outsource certain services that it provides by contracting with an outside company to help maintain its budget. The director of pharmacy may choose to contract with a company that provides nutrition services, clinical services, or outpatient services. These services can be provided off premises and can be delivered to the hospital.

The director of pharmacy is also responsible for making sure all pharmacy personnel and services comply with federal and state laws, regulations, and standards. The director develops written policies and procedures relating to all of the pharmacy services it provides.

Services of a Hospital Pharmacy

The services provided by a hospital pharmacy are similar to those provided by a community pharmacy, but hospital pharmacies also dispense oral medications, parenteral medications, biologics, and chemotherapy that are often not provided by a typical community pharmacy.

Hospital pharmacy services include the following:

- Filling a 24- to 72-hour supply of medication orders
- Dispensing unit-dose packaging
- Delivering medications to the floor for emergency or routine use
- Maintaining automated floor stock system
- Preparing intravenous medications
- Properly handling and disposing of biological and hazardous materials
- Providing drug-information services
- Preparing and maintaining a formulary
- Conducting drug-utilization reviews
- Maintaining patient-medication histories
- Monitoring patient response to therapy
- Counseling patients at time of discharge
- Providing clinical services and rounding with physicians
- Participating in research studies

- Providing specialty services such as **nutritional support** (artificial feeding for people who cannot get enough nourishment by eating or drinking)

Hospital Orders

In a hospital, when the doctor writes a prescription for a patient, it is in the form of a medication order **FIGURE 15.1**. A **medication order** is equivalent to a prescription that is given to a patient to bring to a community pharmacy, but is processed differently. The order is written on a physician's order sheet and kept with the patient's chart. The **chart** is a record that contains physician's notes, medication orders, nurses' notes, medication administration records, and lab results.

There are several different types of medication orders:

- Admitting orders—An **admitting order**, also called an admission order, is an order that is written by the physician when the patient is admitted to the hospital.

- Stat orders—A **stat order** is an emergency order that must be processed quickly and delivered to the patient for immediate administration.

- Continuation orders—A **continuation order** is similar to a refill; it indicates that the medication previously ordered should be continued.

Hospitals have policies on standard care orders and the number of times the physician must review and approve the orders. These policies may vary from one hospital to another.

The nurse, unit secretary, or unit clerk periodically checks all patients' charts for new orders that need to be sent to various departments in the hospital. The hospital pharmacy receives all medication orders that need to be filled for each patient in the hospital. The orders may contain oral, parenteral, and as-needed medications. The orders must also contain all necessary information from the patient's record such as the full name, medical-record number, room number, diagnosis, date of birth, other medications, drug allergies, and vital statistics such as weight. These orders may be received via fax, electronically, or via a pneumatic tube system.

When an order is received by the pharmacy, a pharmacy technician or pharmacist enters the order into the computer. The pharmacist then verifies the accuracy of the transcription by checking the original order against what is entered into the patient's medical record. As the orders are signed off, labels are printed. Then, the technician fills the order; the pharmacist verifies that the pharmacy technician has placed the correct drug, dose, and route into the package (which is labeled for the patient); and the pharmacist

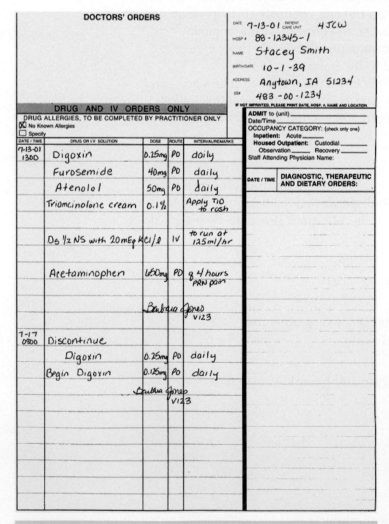

FIGURE 15.1 A hospital medication order.

signs off on the order, indicating that it has been filled correctly. When the medication reaches the floor, the nurse will administer the medication according to the instructions on the medical record. The nurse will document that the medication was given to the right patient at the right time and with the correct drug, dose, route, and frequency according to the order on the medication administration record.

Unit Dose

Most hospitals dispense medications for patient use as a unit dose. A **unit dose** is an individually prepackaged medication for a specific patient for a single administration.

A unit-dose drug-distribution system allows for individual doses to be prepared and dispensed, and for a 24-hour supply of many medications to be sent to the floor. This type of drug-distribution system reduces errors because the drug is ready to be administered as is. The label of a unit-dose medication, which must adhere to federal and state regulations, includes the brand and generic name (if the brand is dispensed) of the drug, the strength, the manufacturer, a bar code, the lot number, and the expiration date. If the generic drug is dispensed, it has only the generic name and not the brand name on the label.

The pharmacy technician fills unit-dose orders for each individual patient from a computer list. Each order is then placed in a unit-dose cart that is bound for a particular floor or area of the hospital. Each cart has individually labeled drawers for each patient. The unit-dose cart is then delivered to the floor. Some unit-dose carts contain two drawers for each patient—one that contains the unit doses of medication for administration for that day and another that is used to fill medication orders for the next day.

Although unit doses are more expensive because they have higher packaging costs than a single dose of the same drug from a retail pharmacy, a unit-dose system has many advantages. This system reduces nursing time because the dose is ready for a single administration, reduces medication errors, prevents tampering with medications, and makes charging and crediting easier. Unopened unit doses can be returned to drug stock, which minimizes waste.

> A unit-dose system reduces nursing time and medication errors, prevents tampering with medications, makes charging and crediting easier, and minimizes waste.

Unit-dose medication orders can be filled by a pharmacy technician with a final check by the pharmacist or filled directly by the pharmacist. These orders can also be filled by an automated robotic system. The automated robotic system uses bar-code scanning technology to recognize the medications. Each unit dose has an identifying bar code that is specific for that medication. A robotic arm uses suction to collect the unit doses and transfer them to a collection area. The patient's medications are then placed in a bag or tray for delivery to the nursing unit.

Automated robotic systems improve efficiency, minimize dispensing errors, and make it easier to manage inventory. These systems also free up the pharmacist to spend more time examining adverse effects and consulting on

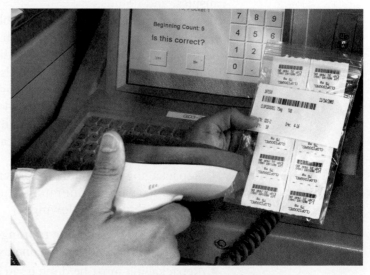

A unit-dose medication is a drug that is packaged for a single administration. A unit-dose label should include the name, strength, dosage form, lot number, and expiration date.

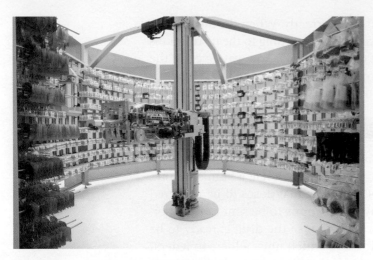

An automatic robotic system fills prescriptions using bar-code technology.

effective drug therapy for each patient. One such system is the Pyxis MedStation. It uses bar-code scanning to ensure accurate medication dispensing and to ensure that the right medication is sent to the nursing unit. The pharmacy technician can easily pick the medication and deliver the medication to the correct MedStation system.

A final check must be performed for all orders that are not filled directly by the pharmacist. For those orders that are filled by an automated robotic system, the pharmacist must also perform a final check. Each state has different guidelines on the percentage of filled unit doses that must be checked by the pharmacist. The medications' bar codes are scanned at the pharmacy and are scanned again by nurses before administration to the patient to make sure the patient is receiving the correct medication.

The pharmacy technician plays an important role in filling unit-dose medication orders. The pharmacy technician often prints the medication administration record and fills unit-dose orders for each individual patient from this record. The pharmacy technician also stocks and maintains inventory, checks for expired drugs, and delivers the unit doses to patient-care areas.

Repackaging Medications

Medications may need to be repackaged by pharmacy personnel. For example, this might occur because the medication is not available from the manufacturer in a unit dose, the order calls for a dose that is not available as a unit dose, the unit dose is not stocked by the pharmacy, or for easy return to stock if not used. Alternatively, the hospital pharmacy might prefer to make its own unit-dose packaging because doing so can be less expensive than purchasing them from a manufacturer. Common dosage forms of drugs that are normally repackaged include oral medications such as tablets, capsules, and liquids.

Technicians are usually responsible for determining which medications should be prepared in unit doses based on utilization. Bulk medications are pulled from stock and made into unit doses. The type of unit-dosing equipment used will vary depending on the amount of drug that needs to be repackaged. Packaging machines, counting trays, heat-sealed zipper-lock bags, glass or plastic bottles, blister packs, amber blister packs, bubble packs, heat-sealed trays, plastic or glass liquid cups, heat-sealed aluminum cups, and syringes can all be used for repackaging. Whatever packaging is used, it should ensure the physical stability of the drug and be labeled per state requirements for repackaging.

Repackaging requirements can vary from state to state. The U.S. Pharmacopeia (USP) has developed minimum requirements for repackaging medications. These guidelines include the following:

- Personnel must have the training, education, and experience to ensure the original drug properties are retained when repackaged.
- Repackaging must be done in an area suitable for repackaging.
- Equipment must be clean, maintained, and sanitized to prevent malfunction and contamination.

- The label must include the product name and strength, lot number, manufacturer, and beyond-use date.
- Records showing the name of the manufacturer, lot number, expiration date, date of repackaging, and initials of repackager must be maintained.
- The medication must be repackaged in a container that ensures the stability and integrity of the drug.

Proper procedures must be followed when repackaging medications. These include maintaining accuracy, using proper technique, and maintaining documentation. **Good manufacturing practices (GMPs)** are FDA guidelines designed to guarantee the delivery of safe and effective products to the patient. When preparing unit-dose medications, these guidelines should be followed. GMP guidelines include the following:

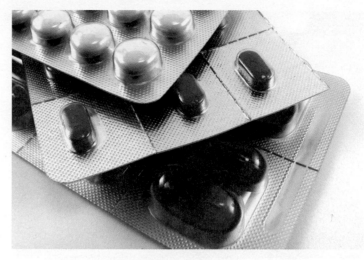

Common drug dosage forms that are repackaged include oral medications such as tablets and capsules.

- Medications must be checked by a pharmacist.
- Equipment must be clean
- Packaging must be appropriate for the drug
- Records must be maintained
- The expiration date given is generally one year from the date of filling unless the manufacturer's expiration date is less than one year from the date of filling. In that case, the earlier date is given as the expiration date.

The pharmacy must document all drugs that have been repackaged using a repackaging control log **TABLE 15.1**. This information is usually kept in a binder near the repackaging area. The pharmacist must check the stock bottle from which the unit doses were made, the unit-dose label, the repackaging log, and the final unit-dose package before it is used to fill unit orders. Information that must be recorded in this log includes the following:

- The date on which the drug was repackaged (including month, day, and year)

Date	Generic Name	Brand Name	Strength	Dosage form	Quantity	MFG	MFG lot number	Pharmacy log number	Expiration date	Tech	Pharmacist

Table 15.1   An Example of a Repackaging Control Log

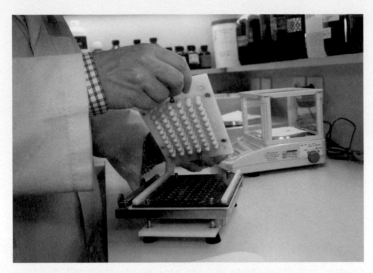

A pharmacy technician prepares unit-dose medications.

- The drug's name (generic and brand) and strength
- The dosage form
- The manufacturer's name
- The manufacturer's expiration date
- The quantity repackaged
- The pharmacy lot number
- The pharmacy beyond-use date
- The initials of the technician
- The initials of the pharmacist

The information on the label of the unit dose should include the drug's generic name and brand name, strength, dosage form, pharmacy lot number, and pharmacy beyond-use date.

When repackaging medications, non-sterile technique can be used. Technicians should wear a lab coat, pull hair back, wash hands thoroughly, wear gloves, and wear a face mask if needed. All equipment should be clean. Repackaging should take place in a designated low-traffic repackaging area. If pill trays are used, the trays should be washed after each use. Only one item should be repackaged at a time because having multiple drugs on the countertop can lead to errors or contamination.

Medication Dispensing and Filling

Medication orders are received by the hospital pharmacy, entered into the computer, and filled on a continual basis until the patient is discharged from the hospital. These medication orders make up a patient's medication profile. A **medication profile** is a list of all the medications a patient receives. After orders are entered into the system, a **unit-dose profile**, or medication profile, is generated. This profile includes the name, strength, formulation, and route and time of administration for each medication. Unit-dose profiles for multiple patients are generated to create a **cart-fill list**, which includes all the aforementioned information for each medication that the patient receives. The cart-fill list is generated at the same time each day by the pharmacy technician. If a medication is ordered after the cart has been filled and sent to the floor, the order is filled and sent to the floor with enough medication to cover the patient until the next fill.

The pharmacy uses the medications remaining in the cart as a quality-assurance mechanism to figure out why the doses were not administered. The pharmacy technician should notify the pharmacist when unit doses of certain drugs remain in the unit-dose carts.

What Would You Do?

Question: You are repackaging amoxicillin from a bulk container into unit doses. You used a counting tray to count 100 capsules and are ready to put them into a blister pack. You repackage all 100 capsules and clean the repackaging area, but forget to clean the counting tray. You receive an emergency order for another medication and repackage it into unit doses. You realize that the patient is allergic to penicillin and that you forgot to clean the counting tray. What would you do?

Answer: It is possible that the new medication may have been contaminated with amoxicillin because the counting tray was not washed. You should clean the tray and get a new supply of the medication and repackage it. To minimize the chance of contamination, it is important to start and finish with a clean work surface.

Schedule II, Schedule III, and Schedule IV controlled substances are not kept in unit-dose carts. They must be kept in a narcotic cabinet or a locked automated floor stock system.

Floor Stock

In some areas of a hospital, the pharmacy must maintain preauthorized levels of medications. The medications and supplies kept on hand and stored on the floors are referred to as **floor stock**. Although most hospitals store an adequate supply of medications and supplies on the floor, the Joint Commision discourages the use of floor stock. These medications may vary from one patient unit to another, depending on the type of services it provides. Ointments and creams are examples of bulk items that are kept as floor stock. The pharmacy normally receives daily supply orders from specialty areas with requests to replace floor stock. The technician should also check the floor stock for expired or outdated drugs and make sure the supplies are sufficient in quantity and are stored properly. Automated delivery systems for floor stock store frequently used medications. This frees up nursing time, records all charges for medications taken out of the system, tracks inventory, stores medication safely, and tracks all medications dispensed. Each dose taken from the automated delivery system is matched with a medication order, thereby ensuring that the right patient receives the right drug. The nurse who retrieves the medication from floor stock must record his or her initials.

Controlled Substances

All Schedule II controlled substances must be kept in a locked cabinet. Narcotics are commonly kept in certain areas of the hospital in floor stock inventory. To prevent diversion, documentation of use for each dose must be recorded. The name of the medication, date and time administered, quantity (administered and wasted), and patient name must be recorded on a controlled drug administration record. It must also be verified with the medication order and nursing notes.

In a manual system, at the end of each nursing shift, the controlled drug administration record must be reconciled. The name of the medication, the amount given, the name of the doctor prescribing the medication, and the nurse administering the medication must be recorded. It must also be initialed by another health professional who witnessed the recording.

With an automated delivery system, the floor stock is replenished by the pharmacy technician. The names of the pharmacy technician and the receiving nurse are recorded for each dose of narcotic that is added to floor stock. In an automated system, the recordkeeping, inventory, and date of removal from floor stock is tracked by the system. All discrepancies must be resolved immediately and with a witness. Narcotic inventory records may need to be reconciled by a pharmacist. The Drug Enforcement Administration (DEA) is a federal regulatory body that has published regulations for enforcing the acquisition, storage, dispensing, and documentation of all controlled substances. The DEA works with local and state agencies to ensure compliance with these regulations. Often, state laws regarding the acquisition, dis-

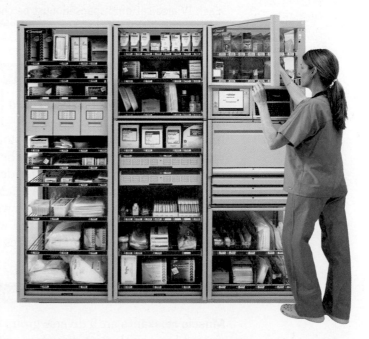

An automated delivery system is used to keep floor stock of certain medications.

pensing, and documentation of controlled substances are more stringent than DEA regulations.

Intravenous Admixture Service

Most hospital pharmacies provide sterile parenteral preparations such as antibiotics, IV fluids, and nutrition. An **IV admixture service** prepares parenteral medications in a sterile environment. These medications are administered to the patient intravenously, intramuscularly, intradermally, or subcutaneously. The IV admixture service is staffed by pharmacists and pharmacy technicians who have expertise in and knowledge in preparation and dispensing of IV preparations. These medications are prepared in a clean-room environment under a laminar-flow hood to prevent contamination and maintain sterility.

Many hospital pharmacies also have a **total parenteral nutrition (TPN) service** within the IV admixture service. The TPN service may consist of a dietician, physician, pharmacist, and nurse. The TPN service specializes in the preparation of **total parenteral nutrition (TPN)**. TPN is used for patients who cannot or should not get their nutrition through eating. It may include a combination of sugar and carbohydrates (for energy), proteins (for muscle strength), lipids (fat), electrolytes, and trace elements. The solution may contain all or some of these substances, depending on the patient's condition. A TPN is administered directly into a large vein, usually over 24 hours. Special training is required for a pharmacy technician to prepare intravenous admixtures.

A TPN provides all the nutritional needs for a patient who is unable to eat.

The pharmacy technician must physically inspect each IV medication for particulate matter and precipitate. The product is often checked under special lighting by the technician and pharmacist.

Each IV medication dispensed must be checked for particulate matter and precipitate.

Medication Administration Record

A **medication administration record (MAR)** is a manual or electronic patient-specific record that includes the names of all drugs the patient receives, doses, routes and times of administration, start and stop dates, and any special instructions. The nurse records his or her initials next to the exact time each medication was administered. Drugs that are administered as needed (prn) are listed separately on the MAR. With the advent of the electronic MAR (eMAR), bar-code technology is used each time a drug is administered to a patient. A wristband with a bar code on the patient is linked to his or her eMAR and is matched with the bar code of the drug. A nurse scans the bar code on the patient and matches it with the bar code on the medication.

Drug Insights: Muscle and Joint Disease and Pain

Muscle relaxants are a diverse group of drugs approved by the FDA to treat spasticity caused by neurological disorders or for musculoskeletal conditions. Muscle spasms can be caused by musculoskeletal conditions such as back and neck injury or neurological conditions such as multiple sclerosis. Nonsteroidal anti-inflammatory drugs are also used to treat other disorders that involve the muscles and joints.

Muscles and Joints

The skeletal system consists of bones and the tissues that connect them, such as tendons, ligaments, and cartilage. The skeletal system provides support for the human body.

Bones are connected to each other at joints. A **joint** is the place where two or more bones meet **FIGURE 15.2**. Joints allow the body to move in many ways and make the skeleton flexible. Joints can be classified according to structure, function, or region. Joints classified by their structure can be divided into the following types:

- **Fibrous joints** connect bones without allowing any movement. The bones of your skull and pelvis are held together by fibrous joints. The union of the spinous processes and vertebrae are fibrous joints.

- **Cartilaginous joints** are joints in which the bones are attached by cartilage. These joints allow for only a little movement, such as in the spine or ribs.

- **Synovial joints** allow for much more movement than cartilaginous joints. Cavities between bones in synovial joints are filled with synovial fluid. This fluid helps lubricate and protect the bones. Bursa sacks contain the synovial fluid.

Muscles and joints work together to move body parts by working in pairs of flexors and extensors. The flexor muscle contracts to bend a limb at a joint. When the movement is completed, the extensor muscle contracts to straighten the limb at the same joint. Muscles are connected to bones by cordlike tissues called tendons. Muscles can be grouped into the following three types **FIGURE 15.3**:

- Skeletal—Skeletal muscles hold the skeleton together, give the body its shape, and allow voluntary movements. These muscles are also called striated muscles because they are made up of fibers that have horizontal stripes.

- Smooth—Smooth muscles are controlled by the nervous system. The contraction of these muscles is involuntary. Smooth muscles are found in the walls of the stomach and intestines and in the walls of blood vessels.

- Cardiac—Cardiac muscles are involuntary muscles found in the heart.

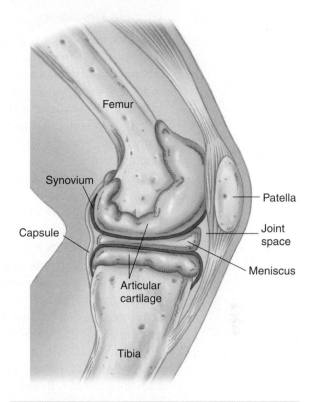

FIGURE 15.2 Anatomy of a joint.

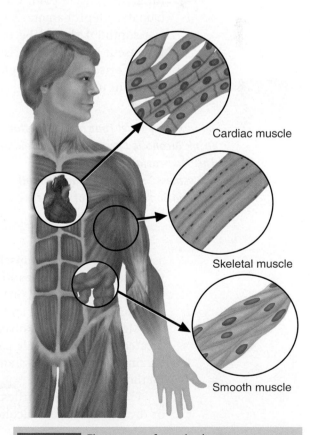

FIGURE 15.3 Three types of muscle tissue.

Muscle Relaxants

The somatic system is a network of nerves that relay messages to the central nervous system (CNS) from the external environment and return messages back to the body. This system regulates the nerves that control voluntary movements of the skeletal muscles and impulses from sensory receptors. The neurotransmitter acetylcholine binds with nicotinic receptors on the muscle cell membrane, causing a release of calcium. When calcium is released, it causes contraction in the muscle fibers. The enzyme acetylcholinesterase breaks down acetylcholine, causing relaxation. Acetylcholine is a neurotransmitter that plays an important role in learning and memory and in sending messages from nerves to muscles. Parasympathetic receptors that respond to acetylcholine are located on smooth muscle cells and cardiac muscle cells. Anticholinergics, or cholinergic blockers, prevent acetylcholine from combining with the receptor, causing nerve impulses to stop.

Many disorders involve inappropriate or excessive muscle contractions, and some involve atrophy, or wasting away of muscles from lack of use. A muscle relaxant is used to reduce muscle contractions or tension by blocking the release of acetylcholine or by preventing acetylcholine from reaching nicotinic receptors. Muscle relaxants are used to reduce spasticity caused by musculoskeletal conditions such as back and neck pain or neurological conditions such as multiple sclerosis. Side effects that are common to all muscle relaxants include sedation, dizziness, drowsiness, and GI upset.

Baclofen (Lioresal) is a centrally acting skeletal muscle relaxant. It inhibits the transmission of reflexes at the spinal cord. It is indicated for spasticity associated with multiple sclerosis or spinal cord injury. Baclofen should be taken with food or milk to minimize GI upset. Baclofen may cause dizziness or drowsiness.

Carisoprodol (Soma) is a centrally acting skeletal muscle relaxant. It is indicated for acute muscle pain. Carisoprodol is metabolized to its active metabolite, meprobamate. Meprobamate (Equanil, Miltown) is a Schedule IV controlled substance. Carisoprodol should be taken with food. Alcohol consumption should be avoided because it increases the risk of toxicity. Carisoprodol may cause dizziness or drowsiness. Carisoprodol, though not scheduled according to the DEA, is a controlled substance in many states.

An auxiliary label that reads "Do Not Drink Alcoholic Beverages When Taking This Medication" and "May Cause Drowsiness" should be placed on all prescription containers of chlorzoxazone.

Chlorzoxazone (Parafon Forte DSC) is a centrally acting skeletal muscle relaxant. It is indicated for acute muscle pain. Its mechanism of action is similar to baclofen in that it inhibits the transmission of reflexes at the spinal cord. It may cause dizziness or drowsiness. Avoid alcohol while taking chlorzoxazone.

Cyclobenzaprine (Flexeril) is a centrally acting skeletal muscle relaxant. It is indicated for spasms associated with acute muscle pain. It may cause dizziness or drowsiness. Avoid alcohol while taking cyclobenzaprine.

Metaxalone (Skelaxin) is indicated for muscle spasms. It may cause dizziness or drowsiness, headache, and upset stomach.

Methocarbamol (Robaxin) is a centrally acting skeletal muscle relaxant. It is indicated for acute muscle pain and muscle pain associated with tetanus. It may cause dizziness or drowsiness and change the color of urine. Avoid alcohol while taking methocarbamol.

Orphenadrine (Norflex) is indicted for acute muscle pain. It may cause dizziness or drowsiness. Avoid alcohol use.

Dantrolene (Dantrium) is a direct-acting agent that works directly on the muscles by inhibiting calcium release. It may cause fatigue, dizziness, drowsiness, diarrhea, and photosensitivity. Avoid alcohol use.

Diazepam (Valium) is a benzodiazepine that acts by enhancing the effects of the neurotransmitter gamma-aminobutyric acid (GABA) in the brain. It may be used to treat muscle spasms in some neurologic diseases. Common side effects include drowsiness, fatigue, and loss of balance. Alcohol or other medicines causing sedation may add to the sedative effects of diazepam.

Muscle relaxants are not classified as controlled substances. Even so, they are often abused, and patients should be monitored for signs of abuse.

Inflammation and Swelling

An analgesic is any drug used to relieve pain. Analgesics are classified as either narcotic (containing opiods) or non-narcotic (not containing opioids). A non-narcotic analgesic can be used to treat mild to moderate pain, inflammation, or fever. Acetaminophen, aspirin, and nonsteroidal anti-inflammatory drugs are non-narcotic analgesics used to treat acute mild to moderate pain. Except for acetaminophen, these drugs prevent the formation of prostaglandins by inhibiting the enzyme cyclooxygenase, thereby decreasing the number of pain impulses received by the CNS. The body does not store prostaglandins; they are synthesized and released during inflammation. The inhibition of cyclooxygenase reduces the synthesis of prostaglandins, which reduces their influence at the site of inflammation.

A decrease in the synthesis of prostaglandins can also reduce a fever. Endogenous **pyrogens** are produced in response to bacterial or viral infections. These pyrogens stimulate the release of prostaglandins, which cause the body to produce a fever.

Non-narcotic analgesics can cause gastrointestinal irritation. Prostaglandins protect the lining of the stomach by promoting mucosal production; preventing the production of prostaglandins can result in ulceration.

Salicylates

Salicylates are analgesics because they help reduce or relieve pain. In addition, they are **antipyretics**, because they help reduce fever. An antipyretic is any drug that reduces a fever. They also exhibit anti-inflammatory activity. Acetylsalicylic acid (ASA) is known more commonly by the generic name aspirin. It also decreases the clotting ability of platelets, and is used to decrease the risk of blood clotting in patients with stroke or cardiovascular disease. Salicylates are indicated for treatment of arthritis, inflammation of arthritis, menstrual cramps, muscle aches and pains, fever, and headache.

Salicylates should not be taken after surgery, by patients with bleeding disorders, by hemophiliac patients, or by patients with bleeding ulcers. Salicylates should not be used during pregnancy; if they are used, it should be only under direct supervision of a physician. Salicylates should also not be taken with methotrexate because this can lead to methotrexate toxicity. Salicylates can increase bleeding times in patients also taking warfarin. Side effects of salicylates include GI upset, tinnitus (ringing in the ears), and loss of platelet function.

Aspirin toxicity can occur in doses greater than 4g/day, although patients with arthritis frequently take doses greater than 4g/day. Mild intoxication is characterized by ringing in the ears, headache, and mental confusion. Severe intoxication can cause delirium, convulsions, nausea, and abnormal breathing.

Aspirin should not be given to individuals under the age of 19 because of the risk of Reye's syndrome. If a person takes aspirin while suffering from a viral infection such as chicken pox, the person may develop Reye's syndrome. Symptoms of Reye's syndrome include vomiting, listlessness, drowsiness, disorientation, confusion, delirium, convulsions, and coma.

Aspirin toxicity can occur in patients taking doses greater than 4g/day.

Children should not take aspirin because they can develop Reye's syndrome.

Choline magnesium trisalicylate is used to reduce fever and relieve pain, inflammation, and stiffness caused by arthritis. It should be taken with food to minimize GI upset. The brand-name version of this drug is no longer available.

Acetaminophen

Acetaminophen (Tylenol) helps reduce or relieve pain and fever, but exhibits no anti-inflammatory activity. Unlike aspirin, acetaminophen can be used with caution and as directed by a healthcare professional during pregnancy. It should be used cautiously in patients with liver disease or who are alcoholics. Acetaminophen can be used by patients with peptic ulcers, those taking medications for gout, those taking anticoagulants such as warfarin, those with clotting disorders such as hemophilia, those at risk for Reye's syndrome, and those with post-surgical pain. Acetaminophen has minimal side effects. It does not cause GI upset, bleeding, or platelet changes.

Acetaminophen exhibits no anti-inflammatory activity.

Although this drug is readily available in many OTC products, it is a very toxic substance and overdose is serious threat. Many consumers believe that because a product is over-the-counter that it is safer than prescription drugs. Consumers should be made aware of acetaminophen toxicity. No more than 4g of acetaminophen should be taken in one day. Doses of more than 4g/day can cause severe liver damage or liver failure. Damage caused by acetaminophen can be irreversible and deadly. If an acute overdose is suspected, the administration of acetylcysteine acts as an antidote. It is only effective when given within hours of acute overdose. There is no treatment for liver damage caused by chronic overuse of acetaminophen.

The risk of acetaminophen overdose had prompted the FDA to issue the following:

On January 13, 2011, FDA announced that it is asking manufacturers of prescription acetaminophen combination products to limit the maximum amount of acetaminophen in these products to 325 mg per tablet, capsule, or other dosage unit. FDA believes that limiting the amount of acetaminophen per tablet, capsule, or other dosage unit in prescription products will reduce the risk of severe liver injury from acetaminophen overdosing, an adverse event that can lead to liver failure, liver transplant, and death.

Patients should not take more than 4g of acetaminophen in one day.

Mixed Analgesics

Mixed analgesics are combinations of two or more analgesic drugs in a single dosage unit such as a tablet or capsule. These combination products contain analgesics with different modes of action and provide more effective pain relief than that which could be achieved if a single analgesic was used alone. These drugs typically include an opioid such as hydrocone or oxycodone combined with a non-narcotic analgesic such as acetaminophen or ibuprofen. Most of these drugs are classified as controlled substances by the DEA, but some mixed analgesics such as Ultracet (tramadol/acetaminophen) are not scheduled drugs.

The most common mixed analgesic, and the most commonly dispensed medicine overall in community pharmacies, is the combination of hydrocodone and acetaminophen. This combination is available in a variety of strengths and under numerous brand names including Vicodin, Norco, and Lortab, among others.

These drugs are very popular because they work well. However, they are also heavily abused and their use should be monitored closely. One common risk is acetaminophen toxicity, which can occur with overuse. This is of extra concern with those known to abuse alcohol, as both alcohol and acetaminophen are very taxing on a patient's liver.

Arthritis and Related Diseases

Arthritis is inflammation of one or more joints FIGURE 15.4 . It can result in pain, stiffness, and limited movement. **Osteoarthritis** is a degenerative joint disease that results in loss of cartilage. In osteoarthritis, the top layer of cartilage breaks down and wears away, which causes the bones under the cartilage to rub together, resulting in pain, swelling, and loss of motion of the joint. Osteoarthritis develops over time. Risk factors include being overweight, increasing age, and joint injury. It can occur in any joint, but usually affects joints of the hands, knees, hips, and spine.

Bursitis is an inflammation of a bursa, a small, fluid-filled sac that acts as a cushion between a bone and muscles, tendons, or skin. Bursitis is commonly caused by overuse or direct trauma to a joint. Infection, arthritis, gout, thyroid disease, and diabetes can also cause bursitis.

Rheumatoid arthritis is an autoimmune disease that causes inflammation of the joints. An **autoimmune disease** occurs when the body's tissues are attacked by their own immune system. The antibodies in the blood target the body's own tissues. There is no known cure for rheumatoid arthritis. The goal of treatment is to reduce inflammation and pain, maximize joint function, and prevent joint destruction.

Some drugs used to treat rheumatoid arthritis modify the immune system. As a result, they often make the body more susceptible to infections, cancer, and other illnesses. The symptoms of rheumatoid arthritis include fatigue, decreased appetite, low-grade fever, stiffness, and muscle and joint pain. Inflammation occurs in multiple joints and is usually symmetrical, meaning that it occurs in the same joints on either side of the body. Chronic inflammation can cause body-tissue damage that can lead

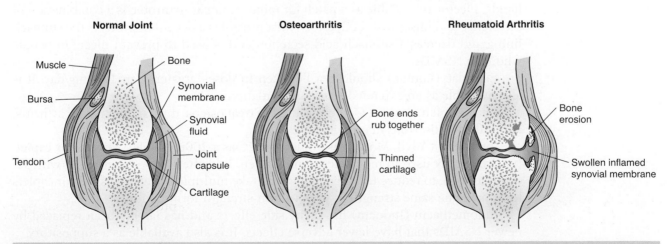

FIGURE 15.4 Normal and arthritic joints.

to loss of cartilage and erosion and weakness of the bones, resulting in deformity, destruction, and loss of function. Rheumatoid arthritis is a systemic disease. Inflammation can affect organs. There is no singular test for diagnosis of rheumatoid arthritis. The diagnosis is based on the presentation of the joints involved, joint stiffness in the morning, presence of blood rheumatoid factor, X-ray changes, rheumatoid nodules, and turbid synovial fluid.

Nonsteroidal Anti-inflammatory Drugs

Nonsteroidal anti-inflammatory drugs (NSAIDs) are first-line drugs used to reduce inflammation, pain, and swelling associated with arthritis. They do not reduce joint destruction. NSAIDs are also used for headaches, menstrual cramps, aches, and fever. NSAIDs prevent the formation of prostaglandins in the tissues by inhibiting the enzyme cyclooxygenase, thereby decreasing the number of pain impulses received by the CNS.

The most common side effect of NSAIDs is GI upset. Prostaglandins protect the lining of the stomach by promoting mucosal production and mucosal blood flow; preventing the production of prostaglandins can result in ulceration and inhibit its protective effects. To minimize GI upset, NSAIDs should always be taken with food and in the lowest possible dose for a short period. Proton pump inhibitors, antacids, and sucralfate (Carafate) are sometimes administered to protect the stomach and minimize the GI effects associated with NSAID use. NSAIDs can also cause kidney damage. Other side effects include liver dysfunction, tinnitus, dizziness, drowsiness, dry mouth, and clotting abnormalities.

NSAIDs can interact with other NSAIDs, beta-blockers, digoxin, methotrexate, and warfarin.

Traditional NSAIDs

Traditional NSAIDs block the action of cyclooxygenase I and II. These NSAIDS are used to ease pain and inflammation, but they may also cause bleeding and stomach upset.

Diclofenac (Voltaren, Arthrotec, Cataflam, Solaraze, Flector) is an NSAID that is marketed in several dosage forms to treat a variety of inflammatory conditions. Diclofenac can cause hepatotoxicity and frequent monitoring of liver function should be performed. It is comparable to aspirin, with a longer duration of action. Cataflam has a rapid onset of action because it is absorbed in the stomach. Voltaren is available as a topical gel formulation for relief of pain of osteoarthritis in the knees and hands. Flector is available as a patch for minor trauma. Arthrotec is a combination of diclofenac and misoprostol (Cytotec). Misoprostol is a drug that protects the stomach lining and decreases stomach-acid secretion and is used to prevent ulcers in people who take NSAIDs.

Etodolac (Lodine) should not be taken in doses greater than 1200mg/day. It is also available as an extended-release formulation.

Flurbiprofen (Ansaid, Ocufen) is used to treat osteoarthritis, rheumatoid arthritis, and inflammation and itching in the eye.

Ibuprofen (Advil, Motrin) is available OTC as a 200mg tablet, capsule, or caplet. It is frequently used to reduce fever in children. It is often taken, alternating with acetaminophen, to reduce fever. Patients often take multiple tablets, capsules, or caplets to achieve the same strength as prescription-strength formulations.

Indomethacin (Indocin) has many side effects and has largely been replaced by newer NSAIDs that have fewer adverse effects. It is also available as a suppository.

Ketorolac (Toradol) is used to treat moderate to severe pain. It was the first NSAID to become available in an injectable formulation in the U.S. It is marketed for short-term use (up to five days) because of GI toxicity. Intramuscular or intravenous ketorolac is comparable in analgesic efficacy to moderate doses of morphine. This drug is also available as a tablet.

Mefenamic acid (Ponstel) should not be used for more than one week or two to three days for dysmenorrhea. It is more effective than aspirin for dysmenorrhea.

Meloxicam (Mobic) is approved for osteoarthritis and rheumatoid arthritis. It may cause less GI toxicity than other NSAIDs.

Nabumetone (Relafen) should be taken in the morning with breakfast to minimize the risk of stomach upset.

Naproxen sodium is available OTC as Aleve. It is frequently prescribed for patients who have cardiovascular disease. Naproxen is also available by prescription in combination with sumatriptan (Treximet) and esomeprazole (Vimovo).

Piroxicam (Feldene) can be taken once daily to achieve therapeutic effects.

Sulindac (Clinoril) is metabolized in the liver. It must be metabolized to its active metabolite to exert its therapeutic effect.

Cox-2 Inhibitors

Cyclooxygenase I (COX-1) and **cyclooxygenase II (COX-2)** are enzymes that convert arachadonic acid to prostaglandin, resulting in pain and inflammation. COX-1 enzymes maintain the normal lining of the stomach and are involved in kidney and platelet function. COX-2 enzymes are present at the sites of inflammation. Traditional NSAIDs are nonselective because they inhibit both COX-1 and COX-2 enzymes. Inhibition of COX-1 is responsible for GI- and kidney-adverse effects, while inhibition of COX-2 is responsible for anti-inflammatory effects. As a result, a new class of NSAIDs called COX-2 inhibitors has been developed to selectively block only the COX-2 enzyme; it has anti-inflammatory effects with minimal GI effects.

Celecoxib (Celebrex) is the only COX-2 inhibitor available on the market. Patients who are allergic to sulfonamides may also be allergic to celecoxib. It should be taken with food to minimize GI upset.

Disease-Modifying Antirheumatic Drugs

Disease-modifying antirheumatic drugs (DMARDs) are now used early in the treatment of rheumatoid arthritis to prevent irreversible damage to joints and minimize toxicities associated with NSAIDs. They have no immediate analgesic effects, but over time can control symptoms and have been shown to delay and possibly stop progression of the disease.

Most non-biologic DMARDs have a slow onset of action and require frequent monitoring for adverse effects. Biologic DMARDs bind to **tumor necrosis factor (TNF)**, a pro-inflammatory cytokine, present in the synovium of patients with rheumatoid arthritis.

Abatacept (Orencia) is a genetically engineered fusion protein that interferes with T-cell activation, which plays a role in the inflammatory process. It can be used in patients who have not responded to non-biologic or biologic DMARDs. It should not be given with biologic DMARDs. Abatacept can increase the risk of serious infections and malignancies.

Adalimumab (Humira) is a biologic anti-TNF antibody. It can increase the risk of serious infections and malignancies.

Anakinra (Kineret) is a genetically engineered interleukin-1 receptor antagonist that inhibits the effects of interleukin-1. Injection-site reactions including pain, redness, and itching are common.

Azathioprine (Imuran) is an immunosuppressive purine analogue that is used to treat rheumatoid arthritis, which does not respond to other treatments. It can cause hepatitis and bone-marrow suppression.

Cyclophosphamide (Cytoxan) is a cytotoxic drug that is a nitrogen mustard alkylating agent generally used for severe cases of rheumatoid arthritis. It can increase the risk of infection and malignancies. It can also cause bone-marrow suppression, GI upset, hair loss, and liver toxicity. The drug can also cause irreversible damage to the bladder if the patient is not hydrated.

Etanercept (Enbrel) is a fusion protein that inhibits TNF. It is indicated for treatment of patients with moderate to severe rheumatoid arthritis that does not respond to other treatments. Injection-site reactions are the most common side effect. Etanercept can increase the risk of serious infections and malignancies.

Hydroxychloroquine (Plaquenil) is an antimalarial used to treat mild rheumatoid arthritis. Blurred vision and difficulty seeing at night are common side effects.

Infliximab (Remicade) is a TNF inhibitor used to treat rheumatoid arthritis, Crohn's disease, and ulcerative colitis. It can increase the risk of serious infections and malignancies.

Leflunomide (Arava) is an oral inhibitor of pyrimidine synthesis used to treat rheumatoid arthritis. It can be used as initial therapy instead of methotrexate or in addition to methotrexate. It can reduce symptoms, limit damage to joints, and improve function. Diarrhea, rash, and hair loss are common side effects. Liver function should be monitored while taking leflunomide.

Methotrexate (Trexall) is used to treat mild, moderate, and severe rheumatoid arthritis. It can reduce symptoms, limit damage to joints, and improve function. It is an antifolate that is toxic to rapidly dividing cells. Side effects include hair loss, nausea, and bone-marrow suppression. Liver function should be monitored while taking methotrexate.

Drugs for Gouty Arthritis

Gouty arthritis is more commonly referred to as gout. Gout is a disease that results from a buildup of uric acid, which leads to the formation of tiny crystals of urate (**tophi**) that deposit in tissues, especially joints. This leads to joint inflammation. The most common site of buildup is in the small joint at the base of the big toe. Other joints that are commonly affected include the ankles, knees, wrists, fingers, and elbows. Symptoms of acute attacks of gout include pain, swelling, reddish discoloration, and tenderness. In chronic gout, tophi are commonly found around the fingers, at the tips of the elbows, in the ears, and around the big toe. Gout is the result of overproduction of uric acid or improper excretion of uric acid. Drugs such as thiazide diuretics, aspirin, niacin, cyclosporine, pyrazinamide, and ethambutol can cause elevated levels of uric acid and lead to gout.

Allopurinol (Zyloprim) is a xanthine oxidase inhibitor that lowers uric-acid levels by inhibiting xanthine oxidase, the enzyme that converts xanthine into uric acid. It is effective in preventing recurrences of acute gout arthritis and reducing the size of tophi. It can cause rash and hepatotoxicity.

Colchicine (Colcrys) is the drug of choice for treatment of acute gout attacks. It is a xanthine oxidase inhibitor. It lowers uric-acid levels by inhibiting xanthine oxidase, the enzyme that converts xanthine into uric acid. Adverse effects include abdominal pain, diarrhea, nausea, and vomiting.

Febuxostat (Uloric) is also a xanthine oxidase inhibitor that lowers uric-acid levels by inhibiting xanthine oxidase, the enzyme that converts xanthine into uric acid. It is effective in preventing recurrences of acute gout arthritis and reducing the size of tophi. Adverse effects include liver function abnormalities, nausea, arthralgia (pain in joints), and rash.

NSAIDs are used to treat acute exacerbations of gout. Indomethacin is the most common NSAID used for this indication.

Probenecid-colchicine (Col-Probenecid) is a combination of a xanthine oxidase inhibitor (colchicine) and a uricosuric agent (probenecid), which increases urinary acid excretion. It can increase the risk of kidney stones.

Sulfinpyrazone (Anturane) prevents reabsorption of uric acid in the kidney.

Tech Math Practice

Question 1: Calculate the volume of medication that must be prepared to provide 12.5mg to a patient using the following information:

Name of drug: Imuran 5mg/mL

Answer: Use the ratio-proportion method: $\frac{12.5mg}{xmL} = \frac{5mg}{1mL}$. Then cross-multiply: $xmL = (12.5mg) \times \frac{1mL}{5mg} = 2.5mL$.

Question: How many milliliters of meperidine 50mg/mL must be prepared to provide 30mg of meperidine to the patient?

Answer: Use the ratio-proportion method: $\frac{xmL}{30mg} = \frac{1mL}{50mg}$. Then cross-multiply: $xmL = (30mg) \times \frac{1mL}{50mg} = 0.6mL$.

Question: How many milligrams of Imuran are in 5mL of a 5mg/1mL solution?

Answer: Use the ratio-proportion method: $\frac{xmg}{5mL} = \frac{5mg}{1mL}$. Then cross-multiply: $xmg = (5mL) \times \frac{5mg}{1mL} = 25mg$.

Question: How many grams of drug A are present in a 500mL of a 1:500 solution?

Answer: Use the ratio-proportion method: $\frac{xg}{500mL} = \frac{1g}{500mL}$. Then cross-multiply: $xg = (500mL) \times \frac{1g}{500mL} = 1g$.

Question: A patient needs to take a solution of potassium chloride to supplement potassium due to chronically low potassium levels. Potassium chloride is available in solution as 20mEq/15mL. The physician has ordered 12mEq of potassium chloride. How many milliliters will be prepared?

Answer: Use the ratio-proportion method: $\frac{xmL}{12mEq} = \frac{15mL}{20mEq}$. Then cross multiply: $xmL = (12mEq) \times \frac{15mL}{20mEq} = 9mL$.

Question: A physician has ordered that 15mL of sodium chloride be added to a patient's TPN. If the sodium chloride in stock is 4mEq/mL, how many milliequivalents of sodium chloride will be in 15mL of solution?

Answer: Use the ratio-proportion method: $\frac{xmEq}{15mL} = \frac{4mEq}{1mL}$. Then cross-multiply: $xmEq = (4mEq) \times \frac{15mL}{1mL} = 60mEq$.

Question: Ketorolac tromethamine is supplied as a 2mL single-dose vial at a concentration of 60mg/2mL. How many milligrams of ketorolac are contained in 1.7mL?

Answer: Use the ratio-proportion method: $\frac{xmg}{1.7mL} = \frac{60mg}{2mL}$. Then cross-multiply: $xmg = (60mg) \times \frac{1.7mL}{2mL} = 51mg$

Question: **A physician has ordered potassium chloride 24mEq to be added to a TPN. Potassium chloride is available at a concentration of 2mEq/mL. What volume of potassium chloride should be added to the TPN?**

Answer: Use the ratio-proportion method: $\frac{24mEq}{xmL} = \frac{2mEq}{1mL}$. Then cross-multiply: $xmL = (24mEq) \times \frac{1mL}{2mEq} = 12mL$.

Question: **Express the components of a 1 percent steroid cream as a weight-in-weight solution.**

Answer: A 1 percent cream is a compound that contains 1g of steroid in a total of 100g of cream.

Question: **Express the components of a 5% dextrose in water solution in the form of a weight-in-volume solution.**

Answer: A 5% dextrose solution contains 5g of dextrose in 100mL of D_5W.

Question: **How many grams of dextrose are in 1.5L of D_5W?**

Answer: D_5W means 5% dextrose in water, or a concentration of 5g/100mL. Use the ratio-proportion method: $\frac{xg}{1,500mL} = \frac{5g}{100mL}$. Then cross-multiply: $xg = (1,500\ mL) \times \frac{5g}{100mL} = 75g$.

Question: **If there are 40g of dextrose in a 2L IV solution, what is the percentage strength of the solution?**

Answer: Convert 2L to milliliters using the ratio-proportion method: $xg/100mL = 40g/2,000mL$. Then cross-multiply: $xg = (100mL) \times \frac{40g}{2,000mL} = 2$, or 2 percent.

Question: **A medication order calls for furosemide 20mg tid. You are filling a 24-hour unit-dose supply for this patient. How many tablets will be needed for this patient?**

Answer: tid means three times a day. A 24-hour supply would mean that you would need to dispense three tablets for this patient.

Question: **A medication order calls for furosemide 20mg qid. You are filling a 24-hour unit-dose supply for this patient. How many tablets will be needed for this patient?**

Answer: qid means four times a day. A 24-hour supply would mean that you would need to dispense four tablets for this patient.

Question: **A 24-hour supply unit-dose cart has already been sent to the floor. An emergency prescription is called to the pharmacy for ibuprofen 800mg qid at 1400. The medication is to be dispensed at 0800,1200,1600, and 2200. If the next cart is delivered the next day at 0900, how many doses of ibuprofen should be dispensed?**

Answer: Three doses for 1600 and 2200 for day one and 0800 for the next day are needed to get the patient through to the next delivery at 0900.

WRAP UP

Chapter Summary

- The hospital is a complex organization with many departments, all working together to provide emergency, medical, trauma, and surgical care to the community.

- Hospitals serve many functions that include providing treatment, diagnosis and testing, education and support programs, training of health professionals, and research to advance medical knowledge.

- The director of pharmacy is the pharmacist responsible for all of the hospital's pharmacy services.

- The services provided by a hospital pharmacy are similar to those provided by a community pharmacy, but hospital pharmacies also dispense oral medications, parenteral medications, biologics, and chemotherapy that are often not provided by a typical community pharmacy.

- In a hospital, when the doctor writes a prescription for a patient, it is in the form of a medication order.

- Most hospitals dispense medications for patient use as a unit dose. This can save money and reduce the chance of medication errors.

- Medications may need to be repackaged by pharmacy personnel because they are not available from the manufacturer in a unit dose or stocked by the pharmacy, or so that the dose can be returned to stock if it is not used. An order may also call for a dose that is not available as a unit dose. The hospital may also prefer to make its own unit-dose packaging because doing so can be less expensive than purchasing from a manufacturer.

- An intravenous admixture service can reduce the chance of medication errors.

- A medication administration record is used by the nurse to document when medications are given to a patient.

- Muscle relaxants are a diverse group of drugs approved by the FDA to treat spasticity caused by neurological disorders or for musculoskeletal conditions.

- A muscle relaxant is used to reduce muscle contractions or tension by blocking the release of acetylcholine, by preventing destruction of acetylcholine at nicotinic receptors, or by preventing acetylcholine from reaching nicotinic receptors. Muscle relaxants are used to reduce spasticity caused by musculoskeletal conditions such as back and neck pain or neurological conditions such as multiple sclerosis.

- Analgesics are used to treat mild to moderate pain, inflammation, and fever.

- An analgesic is any drug used to relieve pain.

- A non-narcotic analgesic is used to treat mild to moderate pain, inflammation, and fever. Acetaminophen, acetylsalicylic acid (aspirin), and non-steroidal anti-inflammatory drugs are non-narcotic analgesics used to treat acute mild to moderate pain.

- Salicylates help reduce or relieve pain (analgesic) and fever (antipyretic). They also exhibit anti-inflammatory activity.

- Acetaminophen (Tylenol) helps reduce or relieve pain and fever, but exhibits no anti-inflammatory activity.

- Mixed analgesics are drugs that contain both an NSAID, aspirin, or acetaminophen, and a narcotic.

- Arthritis is inflammation of one or more joints. It can result in pain, stiffness, and limited movement.

- Nonsteroidal anti-inflammatory drugs are first-line drugs used to reduce inflammation, pain, and swelling associated with arthritis. They do not reduce joint destruction.

- Cyclooxygenase I (COX-1) and cyclooxygenase II (COX-2) are enzymes that convert arachadonic acid to prostaglandin, resulting in pain and inflammation.

- Disease-modifying antirheumatic drugs (DMARDs) are used early in the treatment of rheumatoid arthritis to prevent irreversible damage to the joints and minimize toxicities associated with NSAIDs. They have no immediate analgesic effects, but over time can control symptoms and have been shown to delay and possibly stop progression of the disease.

- Colchicine is the drug of choice used to treat gout.

WRAP UP

Learning Assessment Questions

1. A prescription written in the hospital is referred to as which of the following?
   A. Prescription order
   B. Medication administration record
   C. Medication order
   D. Formulary

2. The director of pharmacy is responsible for which of the following?
   A. Staffing the pharmacy
   B. Managing the budget
   C. Complying with hospital policies
   D. All of the above

3. Which of the following is a non-narcotic drug that is used to treat pain, inflammation, and fever?
   A. Muscle relaxant
   B. Analgesic
   C. Disease-modifying antirheumatic drug
   D. Skeletal muscle relaxant

4. The most commonly dispensed mixed analgesic is a combination of which of the following two drugs?
   A. Hydrocodone and acetaminophen
   B. Oxycodone and acetaminophen
   C. Hydrocodone and ibuprofen
   D. Hydrocodone and naproxen

5. Which of the following is a disorder in which the body's own immune system attacks and destroys tissues in the body?
   A. Autoimmune disease
   B. Psoriasis
   C. Osteoarthritis
   D. Gout

6. Which of the following is a disease that results from a buildup of uric acid, which leads to the formation of tiny crystals of urate (tophi) that deposit in tissues (especially joints)?
   A. Rheumatoid arthritis
   B. Muscle spasticity
   C. Gout
   D. Arthritis

7. Hospital pharmacy services include which of the following?
   A. Filling a 24- to 72-hour supply of medication orders
   B. Dispensing unit-dose packaging
   C. Delivering medications to the floor for routine or emergency use
   D. All of the above

8. A unit dose system does which of the following?
   A. Reduces medication errors
   B. Makes charging and crediting easier
   C. Minimizes waste
   D. All of the above

9. An IV admixture service prepares which of the following?
   A. Parenteral medications in a sterile environment
   B. Capsules using the punch method
   C. Nonsterile preparations
   D. All of the above

10. Which of the following is a degenerative joint disease that results in loss of cartilage?
    A. Muscle spasticity
    B. Arthritis
    C. Gouty arthritis
    D. All of the above

11. Which of the following is the drug of choice for treatment of gout?
    A. Relafen
    B. Colchicine
    C. Indomethacin
    D. Ketorolac

WRAP UP

12. Which NSAID is frequently prescribed for patients with cardiovascular disease?

    A. Naproxen sodium

    B. Indomethacin

    C. Piroxicam

    D. Ketorolac

13. A muscle relaxant reduces muscle contractions or tension by blocking the release or preventing the destruction of which of the following?

    A. Histamine

    B. Dopamine

    C. Acetylcholine

    D. Norepinephrine

14. Side effects that are common to all muscle relaxants include all but which of the following?

    A. Sedation

    B. Dizziness

    C. Seizures

    D. GI upset.

15. All prescription containers of chlorzoxazone should contain which of the following auxiliary labels?

    A. "Do Not Drink Alcoholic Beverages When Taking This Medication"

    B. "May Cause Drowsiness"

    C. All of the above

    D. None of the above

16. Which of the following is the active metabolite of carisoprodol?

    A. Meprobamate

    B. Baclofen

    C. Chlorzoxazone

    D. Acetaminophen

17. Taking aspirin can cause children who have been exposed to viral infections such as chicken pox to develop which of the following?

    A. Rash

    B. Liver disease

    C. Hepatitis

    D. Reye's syndrome

18. Aspirin toxicity can occur in patients taking doses greater than which of the following?

    A. 3g/day

    B. 1g/day

    C. 2g/day

    D. 4g/day

19. Which of the following is the only COX-2 inhibitor currently available on the market?

    A. Celecoxib

    B. Rofecoxib

    C. Advil

    D. Tylenol

20. Acetaminophen displays all but which of the following?

    A. Antipyretic activity

    B. Analgesic activity

    C. Anti-inflammatory activity

    D. All of the above

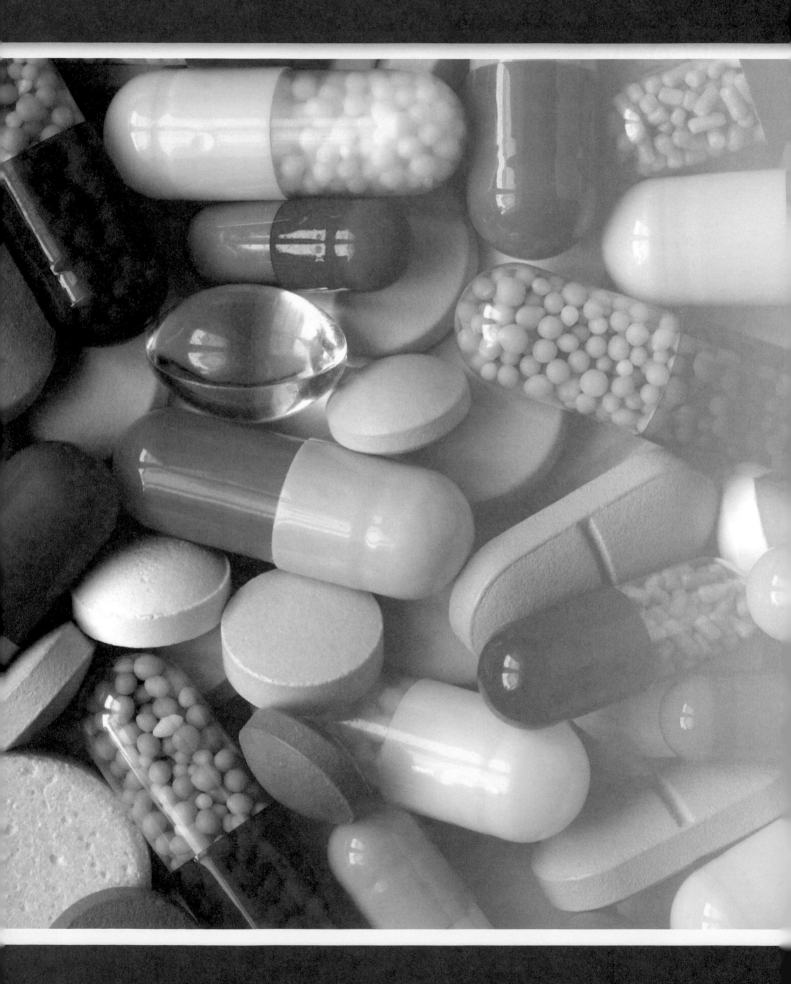

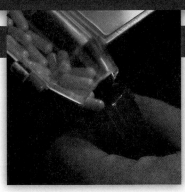

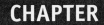
Labs for Institutional Pharmacy

OBJECTIVES

After reading this chapter, you will be able to:

- Fill a 24-hour medication cart.
- Prepare unit dose medications with tablets and capsules.
- Fill and record narcotic floor stock.
- Prepare oral syringes.
- Use an automated drug dispensing system
- Identify common hormonal disorders and explain the drugs used to treat them.

KEY TERMS

Acne
Addison's disease
Adrenal gland
Adrenocorticotropic
     hormone (ACTH)
Androgens
Calcitonin
Chlamydia
Condoms
Cortex
Corticosteroid
Corticotropin releasing
     factor (CRF)
Cortisol
Crash carts
Cretinism
Crushing
Cushing disease
Diabetes mellitus
Dwarfism

Endocrine system
Epididymitis
Epiphyseal fusion
Erectile dysfunction
Estrogen
Exophthalmos
Genital herpes
Gluconeogenesis
Glucocorticoids
Glycosuria
Goiter
Gonorrhea
Graves' disease
Growth hormone (GH)
Growth hormone
     releasing factor
     (GHRF)
Gynecomastia
Hormones
Hyperglycemia

Hyperthyroidism
Hypoglycemia
Hypothalamus
Hypothyroidism
Impotence
Inhibitors
Insulin
Ketoacidosis
Libido
Medulla
Menopause
Menstrual cycle
Mineralocorticoids
Myxedema
Negative feedback
     mechanism
Ovaries
Pancreas
Parathyroid gland
Pelvic inflammatory

disease (PID)	Progestin	Testosterone
Perpetual log book	Resorption	Thyroglobulin
Pineal body	Retinopathy	Thyroid gland
Pituitary gland	Sexually transmitted	Thyroid-stimulating
Polydypsia	disease (STD)	hormone (TSH)
Polyuria	Syphilis	Thyroxine (T$_4$)
Priapism	Target	Triiodothyronine (T$_3$)
Progesterone	Testes	Virilization

Chapter Overview

Filling a 24-hour medication cart, filling and checking floor stock, filling and recording narcotic floor stock, and preparing oral syringes are important basic functions that a pharmacy technician performs in an institutional setting. Common hormonal disorders and hormone-replacement therapy, as well as proper documentation of hormone-replacement products, will also be discussed.

Lab: Filling a 24-Hour Medication Cart

A 24-hour medication cart fill is a basic function that a pharmacy technician working in an institutional setting performs. It may also be referred to as medication fill or medication pick. Although specific cart-fill procedures may vary from one institution to another, the basic functions are the same. In larger hospitals, the fill may be performed by automated machines or robots instead of by the pharmacy technician. However, the pharmacy technician still plays a vital role in stocking the medications in the automated filling machine, documenting the medication information, checking expiration dates, and ensuring the cart-fill process is running smoothly. Additionally, the pharmacy technician is responsible for manual picks for those medications not stocked in the robot or machine.

Filling the medication cart that is sent up to the floor and patient-care areas involves referring to a cart-fill list **FIGURE 16.1** or pick list. The cart-fill list is a list of unit-dose profiles for multiple patients. It includes the following information for each medication that the patient receives:

- Name
- Strength
- Formulation
- Directions (sig)
- Route and time of administration

It can contain a prescription number for each medication and does require the quantity of medication that should be dispensed for each cart fill. The quantity placed in each patient drawer is calculated based on the sig and the frequency of cart fill. The cart-fill list is usually generated each morning by the pharmacy technician.

Always check the expiration date of every dose before putting it into the medication cart.

Although the frequency of cart fills can vary from one institution to another, for this lab, the technician will perform a 24-hour cart fill.

Patient Name:	
Drug name	
Strength	
Formulation	
Directions (sig)	
Route and time of administration	

FIGURE 16.1 A cart-fill list.

Supplies Needed

- Cart-fill list
- Individual patient drawer, bin, or bag
- Pharmacy lab with unit-dose medications
- Pharmacy reference books or online access to reputable pharmacy references

Steps

Addition means that you are adding or increasing the quantity by a given number.

1. Gather the necessary supplies and place them at a clean workstation.

2. Put your initials or name (as is required by the practice site or individual state law) and the date on the cart-fill list.

3. Familiarize yourself with the different areas where unit-dose medications are stored in the pharmacy lab. Keep yourself aware of changes in location of products and generic substitutions to ensure the correct drug is pulled for use in the fill. (Knowing what each medication is used for may help you locate where medications are stored.)

4. Looking at the cart-fill list, obtain the drugs you need from the appropriate bins. Match each drug, dose, and dosage form to the cart-fill list to make sure that what you have picked is exactly the same as what is needed. (Refer to Table 4.1 in Chapter 4 for a review of prescription sigs to assist in calculating the number of medication units needed for each dose.)

5. Double-check the expiration date on each unit dose of medication.

6. Examine the packaging for each medication to ensure it contains medication that is viable for use—that it is not open, it is not broken, it is not missing components, and it does not contain the wrong number of units.

7. Place the appropriate amount of medication in each patient's drawer, bin, or bag. Make sure the quantity placed in each drawer matches that required on the cart-fill list.

Some cart-fill lists are already generated by the pharmacy with the "quantity to dispense" of each medication already calculated.

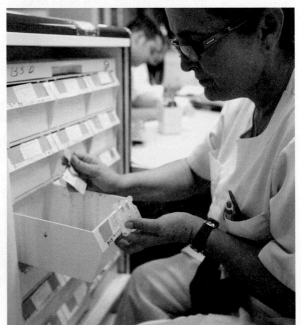

A pharmacy technician fills a medication cart drawer.

Rx Number	Drug Name	Strength	Sig	Quantity to Dispense	Primary Use
101	Hydrochlorothiazide	25mg	Give 1 tablet po tid		
102	Ranitidine	150mg	Give 1 tablet po bid		
103	Coumadin	1mg	Give 1 tablet po daily		
104	Amoxicillin	250mg	Give 1 tablet po tid		
105	Ibuprofen	200mg	Give 2 tablets po q8h prn		
106	Levothyroxine sodium	0.025mg	Give 1 tablet po bid		
107	Docusate sodium	100mg	Give 1 capsule po tid prn		

FIGURE 16.2 Cart-fill list form (Example 1).

Rx Number	Drug Name	Strength	Sig	Quantity to Dispense	Primary Use
1101	Atorvastatin	40mg	Give 1 tablet po bid		
1102	Bromocriptine	0.8mg	Give 4 tablets po daily		
1103	Coumadin	1mg	Give 1 tablet po daily		
1104	Torsemide	10mg	Give 1 tablet po bid		
1105	Ibuprofen	800mg	Give 1 tablet po q8h prn		
1106	Levothyroxine sodium	0.100mg	Give 1 tablet po daily		
1107	Paroxetine	10mg	Give 2 tablets po daily		
1108	Valsartan	40mg	Give 2 tablets po bid		

FIGURE 16.3 Cart-fill list form (Example 2).

When performing a cart fill, watch out for abbreviations such as SR or CR. Drugs whose names are followed by these abbreviations are not the same as those without these abbreviations.

8. The cart is now ready for the pharmacist to check. Place the cart-fill list in the patient's drawer for the instructor to check or sign off.

FIGURE 16.2 and **FIGURE 16.3** show two examples of a cart-fill list form.

Lab: Filling and Checking Stock Medications

In many hospitals, the pharmacy maintains preauthorized levels of certain medications on each floor. The medications and supplies kept on hand and stored on the floors are referred to as stock medications. The medications stocked may vary from one patient unit to another, depending on the type of services the unit provides. Medications kept as stock medication generally include those drugs that need to be administered immediately.

The pharmacy normally receives daily supply orders from specialty areas with requests to replace stock medications. The technician should also check the floor stock for expired or outdated drugs, and make sure the supplies are sufficient in quantity and are stored properly. Accurate filling of the stock medication request form and checking of the stock medications ensures that the nursing staff will have the necessary medications available for prompt administration to the patient.

The preferred method for stocking medications on floors is in automated drug dispensing systems. However, some hospitals still maintain stock medications and supplies on hand and commonly refer to them as floor stock. Stock medication generally does not include critical-care medications that require compounding by the pharmacy or narcotics. Critical-care medications are kept in emergency carts commonly known as **crash carts**, which are brought to the patient's bedside for immediate administration. Narcotics are kept in a locked cabinet, locked dispensing device, or other secure area as designated by specific state and federal guidelines. To prevent diversion, documentation of use for each dose of narcotic must be recorded when stocking the narcotic cabinet and when the nurse removes it from the cabinet and dispenses it to the patient.

Narcotics are kept in a secure, locked area that is not part of the regular floor stock items.

Supplies Needed

- Completed stock medication request form
- Pharmacy lab with stock medication items

Steps

This lab is divided into three parts.

- The first part is filling stock medication requests.
- The second part is double-checking stock medication fills, which is important for ensuring that the stock medication items you filled were correct. (In some states, pharmacy technicians are allowed to perform the double check. In other states, the double check must be performed by the pharmacist.)
- The third part is a final check. The final check ensures that the right drug, strength, and dose reach the patient-care area.

Part 1: Filling Floor Stock

1. Prepare a clean workstation.
2. Put your initials or name (as is required by the practice site or individual state law) and the date on the stock medication request form.
3. Filling and checking each stock medication or dose requires knowledge of your state's expiration-date requirements. To ensure that the stock medication is acceptable, you must first ask your instructor for the state regulations regarding expiration dates.
4. Looking at the stock medication request form, find the first item that needs to be filled. The number in the fill column will indicate the quantity requested for that item. Only medications with an amount indicated in the fill column should be replaced. If there is no amount indicated in the fill column, you do not need to fill that medication.

Carefully match the name of the drug, formulation, strength, and quantity that you pull to the stock medication request form. The drug pulled must match what is ordered on the stock medication request form.

5. Looking at the stock medication request form, pull the quantity needed to fill the first item on the list.

6. Check the expiration date of the item pulled to make sure it meets state requirements.

7. Place the item on the countertop away from other medications to ensure that item is not mixed with other medications and thus placed in an incorrect bin, causing a medication error.

8. Looking at the stock medication request form, move to the next item on the list, paying careful attention to match the drug, dose, and quantity to that requested on the stock medication request form. Also check the expiration date.

9. Continue pulling all the items on the stock medication request form.

10. After all the items on the stock medication request form have been pulled, arrange them on your workspace in the order the items appear on the floor-stock request form. This will enable your instructor to check the items easily and prevent medication errors.

11. At the bottom of the stock medication request form, fill in the blanks for the following: Filled By and Today's Date.

Part 2: Checking Stock Medication Fills

12. Find another student to check your stock medication request form.

13. Looking at the completed stock medication request form, verify that the name strength, formulation, and quantity of the first medication, match exactly what is requested on the form.

14. Check the expiration date of each dose to make sure it meets state requirements as part of the double-check process.

15. Repeat steps 13 and 14 for each medication on the stock medication request form, going down the form one line at a time, until all the medications are checked. Mark on the form any errors that you find while checking.

These forms often have a place for errors. That way, errors that are made can be addressed and solutions can be created to prevent these errors from recurring.

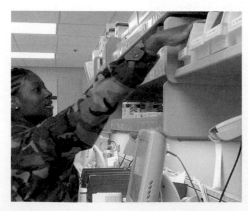

A pharmacy technician performs a double check.

16. Write the total number of errors on the blank at the bottom of the form.

17. Enter your name in the Checked By blank.

Part 3: Final Check

18. Exchange your stock medication request form with the other student's.

19. Show the other student any errors that were made on his or her form.

20. Correct the errors identified by the student who checked your stock medication request form, and then double-check these corrections.

STOCK MEDICATION REQUEST FORM		
Unit: Obstetrics/Gynecology		
Fill #	**Medication Requested**	**Par Level**
4	Acetaminophen 325mg tablets	8
5	Acetaminophen 500mg caplets	8
	Amoxicillin 250mg capsules	6
	Azithromycin 250mg tablets	6
	Ciprofloxacin 500mg tablets	6
2	Dexamethasone 8mg/2mL injectable vial	4
	Diphenhydramine 25mg capsules	10
	D_5W 1000mL IV bag	6
	$D_5\frac{1}{2}NS$ 1000mL IV bag	6
4	Dulcolax soft gel capsules	10
	Erythromycin 250mg tablets	6
2	Furosemide 20mg tablets	10
	Ibuprofen 200mg tablets	10
3	Ibuprofen 800mg tablets	10
1	Maalox 30mL unit-dose cups	4
2	Metoclopramide 10mg tablets	6
1	Mylanta 30mL unit-dose cups	4
	NS 1,000mL IV bag	6
	$\frac{1}{2}NS$ 1,000mL IV bag	6
	Tucks medicated pads 1 jar	1
Filled By:		
Date:		
Checked By:		
Final Check by Instructor:		
Number of Errors:		

FIGURE 16.4 Stock medication request form.

21. Ask for a final check from your instructor. Your instructor will look at both the form you filled out and the one you checked.

   FIGURE 16.4 shows an example of a stock medication request form.

Lab: Unit Dose Preparation of Tablets or Capsules

Unit doses are used in hospitals to increase efficiency by making drug formulations ready to administer. Because manufacturers do not prepare all drugs in a unit-dose form, and individual orders may require nonstandard doses, the pharmacy technician may need to repackage medications.

Supplies Needed

- Medi-Cup blisters
- Fil-form 25 template
- Lid-label cover sheet

- Roll-E-ZY press piece
- Pharmacy lab with bulk bottles of medications
- Pharmacy reference books, including a brand/generic drug handbook or Internet access
- Repackaging documentation log

Steps

1. Prepare a clean workstation.
2. Preparing unit doses of a medication requires knowledge of your state's expiration-date requirements. To ensure that the unit dose is acceptable, you must ask your instructor for the state regulations regarding expiration dates.
3. Place a sheet of Medi-Cup blisters in the Fil-form 25 template.
4. Fill each Medi-Cup blister with the desired medication.
5. Peel away the protective liner from the lid-label cover sheet.
6. Place the lid-label cover sheet over the filled Medi-Cup blisters.
7. Using the Roll-E-ZY press-piece, seal the cover sheet to the Medi-Cup blisters.
8. Labeled Medi-Cup blisters are separated at the perforations before use. The label should contain the following information: drug name and strength, date of repackaging, lot number, and expiration date.
9. Fill the repackaging control log with the correct information.
10. Ask for a final check from your instructor.

Lab: Filling and Recording Narcotic Floor Stock

In institutional settings, all controlled substances (Schedules II–V) must be kept in a locked cabinet. Narcotics are commonly kept in certain patient areas as floor-stock inventory. To prevent diversion, documentation of use for each dose must be recorded. Narcotics should not be left unattended. The name of the medication, date and time administered, quantity (administered and wasted), and patient name must be recorded on a controlled drug administration record. It must also be verified with the medication order and nursing notes.

In some hospitals, the pharmacy technician is responsible for ordering, filling, maintaining, and replenishing the narcotic floor stock. Schedule II substances for floor stock can be ordered from wholesalers using the DEA 222 form. The pharmacist must sign all DEA 222 forms.

A pharmacy technician can maintain the **perpetual log book** or perpetual inventory record to record all narcotics that are withdrawn and added to the narcotic floor stock. This is the official record for all Schedule II substances kept in the narcotic cabinet. A separate log book is also kept for Schedule III–V controlled substances. It is extremely important to accurately and correctly document all entries into the perpetual log book. **FIGURE 16.6** contains an example of a perpetual log book.

Following proper procedures when recording entries in the perpetual log book can minimize the risk of making an error. Proper procedures for recording include the following:

- All entries into the log book should be clearly and legibly written in black ink. If there is an error in the entry, simply cross it out by making a single line through the entire entry. Initial the entry and circle the initials. Errors should never be erased, whited out, or blacked out.

See Reverse of PURCHASER'S Copy for Instructions		No order form may be issued for Schedule I and II substances unless a completed application form has been received (21 CFR 1305.01).		OMB APPROVAL No. 1117-0010

TO: (Name of Supplier)
PHARMA, INC.

STREET ADDRESS
3131 Grand Ave., Suite B

CITY and STATE
CITY, ST 12345

DATE
09/09/11

TO BE FILLED IN BY SUPPLIER
SUPPLIER'S DEA REGISTRATION No.

TO BE FILLED IN BY PURCHASER

LINE No.	No. of Packages	Size of Packages	Name of Item	National Drug Code	Packages Shipped	Date Shipped
1	12	50mL	Fentanyl CIT, 15mg/mL			
2	5	20mL	Demerol HCL, 100mg/mL			
3						
4						
5						
6						
7						
8						
9						
10						

2 ◄ No. OF LINES COMPLETED

SIGNATURE OF PURCHASER OR HIS ATTORNEY OR AGENT

BE SURE TO SIGN FORM

Date Issued
06-01-11

DEA Registration No.
BL9876543

Name and Address of Registrant
DOE, JOHN EDWARDS MD
ABC CLINIC
1234 MAIN STREET
ANYWHERE, USA   **11223**

Schedules
2, 2N, 3, 3N, 4, 5

Registration as a
PRACTITIONER

No. of this Order From
123456789

DEA Form 222
(Aug. 1990)

U.S. OFFICIAL ORDER FORMS — SCHEDULES I & II
DRUG ENFORCEMENT ADMINISTRATION
SUPPLIER'S Copy 1

45579700

FIGURE 16.5 A DEA 222 form. This form is used to order narcotics. All pharmacies that order narcotics must use the DEA 222 form.

PERPETUAL LOG BOOK

Drug Name, Strength, Dosage Form: _____

NDC: _____

Manufacturer: _____

Date	Invoice #	Department/ Floor	Quantity +/– Quantity Dispensed	Remaining Balance	Initials	Checked/ Verified By

FIGURE 16.6 Perpetual log book.

> All entries into the perpetual log book must be clearly and legibly written using black ink. All errors must be crossed out with a single line and initialed.

- Withdrawals from inventory should be clearly written in ink.
- Each entry should be recorded on the next available line. If there are no more available lines, start a new sheet. In order to prevent tampering of records or recorded entries, never leave any blank lines between entries.

> Never leave blank lines between entries in a perpetual log book.

- All entries should be in order of date.
- When starting a new sheet, transfer the last entry and balance onto the first line of the new sheet. Clearly and legibly fill out the information at the top of the record, including the name, strength, formulation, and manufacturer of the controlled substance.

Federal law requires that all narcotic records be kept in a secure area in the pharmacy for at least two years. The state board of pharmacy, the DEA, and other regulatory agencies may ask to review all records pertaining to controlled substances.

> All narcotic inventory records must be kept in the pharmacy for a minimum of two years.

Supplies Needed

- Narcotic floor-stock request form
- Perpetual log book (there are separate ones for CII and CIII–CV)
- Pharmacy lab with a locked narcotic cabinet or room with narcotic floor stock items
- Counting tray
- Spatula
- Calculator
- Black pen
- Pharmacy reference books, including a brand/generic drug handbook, or Internet access

Steps

1. Prepare a clean workstation.
2. Write your name and date on the narcotic floor-stock request form.
3. Filling and checking each narcotic floor-stock medication or dose requires knowledge of your state's expiration-date requirements. To ensure that the floor stock is acceptable, you must first ask your instructor for the state regulations regarding expiration dates.
4. Locate the relevant perpetual log book (there are separate ones for CII and CIII–CV substances) and find the first medication on the narcotic floor-stock request form **FIGURE 16.7**. Double-check to make sure that what is requested on the narcotic floor-stock request form is exactly the same as that listed on the perpetual log book.
5. On the first available line, record today's date and your initials in the appropriate fields. In the Department/Floor field, record the words "actual count."

NARCOTIC FLOOR-STOCK REQUEST FORM		
Unit: Obstetrics/Gynecology		
Percocet 5/325 × 25 Starting Balance:____ Quantity Dispensed:_____ Remaining Balance:_____		
MS Contin 30mg × 25 Starting Balance:____ Quantity Dispensed:_____ Remaining Balance:_____		
Vicodin ES 7.5mg/750mg × 10 Starting Balance:____ Quantity Dispensed:_____ Remaining Balance:_____		
Instructor's Initials:_____ Grade:_____		

FIGURE 16.7 Narcotic floor-stock request form.

6. Unlock the narcotic cabinet or room and locate the first item ordered on the narcotic floor-stock request form.

7. Pull the medication. Double-check to make sure it is exactly the same as what is requested on the request form. Check the expiration date to make sure it is acceptable and follows state regulations for expiration dates.

8. Count all tablets or capsules for the specified medication.

9. Using black pen, record the total number of capsules or tablets counted and your initials in the Remaining Balance field in the perpetual log book. This is the actual count.

10. Pull the requested number of unit-dose capsules or tablets necessary to complete the order request. If you do not have enough unit-doses of the medication needed to complete the order, notify your instructor.

11. On the next line, record the date, the department, floor, or unit number and your initials in the appropriate fields.

12. Using black pen, record in the Quantity +/– Quantity Dispensed field the quantity of drug that was pulled to complete the order request.

13. Subtract the quantity pulled from the original balance and, using a black pen, enter the result in the Remaining Balance field. This amount should equal the quantity left in the bin.

14. Report any discrepancies in the actual count and balance to your instructor.

15. Referring to the perpetual log book, fill in the Balance, Quantity Dispensed, and Remaining Balance fields on the narcotic floor-stock refill form for the medication you just pulled from the bin.

16. Going down the narcotic floor-stock refill form, pull the next medication requested by following the same procedures.

17. After all the information has been recorded in the perpetual log book and the narcotic floor-stock refill form, and all the drugs have been pulled, ask for a final check from your instructor.

Figure 16.7 contains an example of a narcotic floor-stock request form.

Lab: Preparing Oral Syringes

Some oral liquid medications are available as unit-dose cups, but many are supplied to the hospital in bulk bottles. The pharmacy technician must then prepare individual oral syringes by withdrawing individual doses from a bulk bottle. This requires the

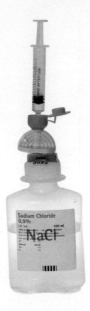

An adapter is placed on the mouth of the bulk bottle to aid in the withdrawal of the medication into each syringe.

use of a special adapter that fits on the mouth of the bulk bottle. The syringes are then labeled for dispensing.

Preparing oral syringes requires calculating the amount of liquid to withdraw from the bulk bottle into each syringe. The calculation is based on the concentration of the medication and the dose of medication needed. In this lab, you will prepare three different doses of ibuprofen. The doses that will be drawn up from the bulk bottle are ibuprofen 200mg, 100mg, and 50mg.

Supplies Needed

- Bulk bottle of ibuprofen oral suspension (100mg/5mL)
- One 10mL oral syringe
- One 5mL oral syringe
- One 3mL oral syringe
- Three oral syringe caps
- Oral syringe bottle adapter
- Calculator

Steps

1. Wash hands thoroughly.
2. Prepare a clean workstation.
3. Gather all the supplies needed to perform the lab.
4. Verify that the medication you have is the correct name, strength, and formulation.
5. On a separate sheet of paper, perform the calculations needed to determine how many milliliters will need to be withdrawn from the bulk bottle to prepare each dose. Make sure to write your name and date on your paper. (Your instructor will check your calculations sheet at the end of this lab.)
6. Remove the cap from the bulk bottle of ibuprofen.
7. Attach the bottle adapter to the mouth of the bulk bottle. Make sure the bottle adapter is firmly and securely placed so that only the top one or two rings of the adapter are visible.
8. Select the appropriate syringe for the dose you are preparing and the appropriate syringe cap for the size of syringe. Use the smallest size syringe that will fit the entire dose.
9. Insert the tip of the syringe into the hole of the bottle adapter. Invert the bottle so that the bottle is on top of the syringe.
10. Pull the plunger of the syringe down so the ibuprofen liquid flows into the syringe. When the syringe is one-third full, expel the fluid and air bubbles in the syringe by pushing the plunger so the liquid goes back into the bulk bottle.
11. Pull down on the plunger a second time so the ibuprofen liquid again flows into the sy-

In a hospital or long-term care setting in which healthcare professionals administer medications, oral syringes are for one-time use. They should be discarded after the dose is administered to the patient. Oral syringes may be used multiple times to administer medication when accompanying a prescription provided by a patient or caregiver outside of a healthcare setting. The oral syringe should be rinsed in warm water and left to dry after each dose is administered.

ringe. Repeat this process, called **crushing**, several times to expel the fluid and air bubbles.

12. Pull down on the plunger until the desired volume of ibuprofen is in the syringe. Make sure the volume in the syringe matches the calculation you performed.

13. Invert the bottle again so the syringe is on top of the bottle. Holding the barrel of the syringe, detach the syringe from the adapter by twisting the syringe.

14. Place a syringe cap on the tip of the syringe.

15. Label the syringe and the plastic container that will store the syringe.

16. Place the labeled syringe in the plastic container that has just been labeled.

17. Place the completed syringe aside for your instructor to check.

18. Repeat steps 7 through 14 for the remaining two doses of ibuprofen.

19. Ask your instructor to check all three filled syringes, the bulk medication bottle, and your math calculations.

To determine the amount of liquid to draw up in each syringe, use the ratio-proportion method. Look at the label of the bulk bottle from which you will be drawing up the doses and find the concentration of the medication. The concentration of ibuprofen is 100 mg/mL.

So, for example, to determine how many milliliters need to be withdrawn from the bulk bottle to obtain the desired 200mg dose of ibuprofen, use the ratio-proportion method like so: $\frac{100mg}{5mL} = \frac{200mg}{xmL}$]. Then cross-multiply: $xmL = (200mg \times 5mL) \div 100mg = 10mL$. The amount you need to withdraw from the bulk bottle is 10mL.

To determine how many milliliters need to be withdrawn from the bulk bottle to obtain the desired dose of ibuprofen 100mg, you again use the ratio-proportion method: $\frac{100mg}{5mL} = \frac{100mg}{xmL}$. Then cross-multiply: $xmL = (100mg \times 5mL) \div 100mg = 5mL$. The amount you need to withdraw from the bulk bottle is 5mL.

Finally, to determine how many milliliters need to be withdrawn from the bulk bottle to obtain the desired dose of ibuprofen 50mg, you again use the ratio-proportion method: $\frac{100mg}{5mL} = \frac{50mg}{xmL}$. Then cross-multiply: $xmL = (50mg \times 5mL) \div 100mg = 2.5mL$. The amount you need to withdraw from the bulk bottle is 2.5mL.

Lab: Charging and Refilling a Crash Cart

Crash carts are kept on hand to ensure that needed equipment, medication, and supplies are within reach when a patient experiences a potentially life-threatening condition or emergency. Crash carts may also be called code carts or crash trays.

Crash carts or code carts are kept on hand to deliver medications to a patient during a potentially life-threatening emergency.

The arrangement of the crash cart and the contents within the cart will vary depending on the institution. The crash cart contains medications that are used in emergency situations, such as epinephrine and atropine. The cart may also contain supplies and medications needed for parenteral administration, because a patient who is experiencing a respiratory or cardiac emergency will need prompt administration of medication.

When a patient has a respiratory or cardiac emergency, a code (a life-threatening situation) is called by the staff. A code team (a group of doctors and nurses) uses the medications and supplies from the crash cart to treat the patient. The crash cart is kept locked at all times and unlocked only when needed by the code team.

After a crash cart has been unlocked and the code has ended, a new cart is brought to the floor and the used crash cart is returned to the pharmacy so that the items used can be charged to the patient and the cart can be refilled. The pharmacy is usually the lead department on the cart fill, but it may be coordinated by a central supply or other department. The pharmacy technician often performs both the filling/refilling the cart and the billing for the pharmacy stock used when the crash cart is needed for a patient. These tasks generally need to be done quickly to ensure the carts are always ready for use. The pharmacy technician should also check the expiration dates on all the medications in the cart and replace those items that do not meet state requirements for expiration dates. The final step in preparing a code cart for use is to cover the tray of medications with a plastic seal or to lock the cart so that the ready-for-use medications cannot be tampered with or borrowed when there is not an actual emergency. The pharmacy tray usually has different identification than the supply trays, which are filled by another department. The trays are marked with color-coded stickers, labels, or tray colors to differentiate which is the medication or pharmacy tray and which are from the other departments. The supply tray in the cart is filled in departments other than the pharmacy. Once the cart is completely restocked, it is ready to be re-issued. Often, a "Code Blue" cart will also be used in a healthcare setting. This cart is the first one to be used when an emergency or "Code Blue" is called. This cart needs to be refilled, checked, and exchanged immediately so that one is always ready for use. The pharmacy technician usually delivers the cart and signs it out to the floor.

Supplies Needed

- Crash cart or tray
- Crash-cart charge form
- Crash-cart refill form

Steps

This lab is divided into two parts: charging the patient and refilling the crash cart. You use your crash-cart charge form to charge the patient for the items used during the code. Then, using the crash-cart refill form, you will refill the crash cart so that it can be ready to use for the next code. A sample crash-cart charge form appears in **FIGURE 16.8**; **FIGURE 16.9** contains a sample crash-cart refill form.

Special delivery systems are often used to deliver medications needed during an emergency situation. These device systems are often found in crash carts. Such systems include devices like the Abboject or Bristoject, which contain the medication in ready to use or pre-filled syringes.

Part 1: Charging the Patient

1. Prepare a clean workstation.
2. Write your name and today's date on the crash-cart charge form.
3. Look up the brand/generic names of any of the items on the crash-cart charge form with which you are unfamiliar.
4. Know the state's requirements for medication expiration dates. Check the expiration dates of each medication in the crash cart.

Medication/Supply	Par Level	Quantity to Charge Patient
Alcohol pads	20	
8.4% sodium bicarbonate injection USP 50mEq pre-filled syringe	3	
2g lidocaine (8mg/mL) vial	5	
Atropine sulfate injection USP 1mg pre-filled syringe	4	
2% lidocaine HCl injection USP 100mg/5mL pre-filled syringe	4	
1:10,000 epinephrine injection, 0.1mg/mL ampule	4	
Vented IV tubing	2	
Bacteriostatic normal saline 30mL vial	4	
Dextrose 50%, 25g syringe	4	
Heparin 5,000u/mL syringe	4	
Naloxone 0.4mg/mL syringe	2	
Furosemide 100mg/10mL vial	2	
Potassium chloride 2mEq/mL 20mL vial	2	
Calcium chloride 10% pre-filled syringe	2	
Potassium chloride 2mEq/mL 20mL vial	2	
Dopamine 1,600mcg/250mL IV bag	2	
0.9%NS 1L bag	4	
D_5W 1L bag	4	

FIGURE 16.8 Crash-cart charge form.

Medication/Supply	Par Level	Expiration Date
Alcohol pads	20	
8.4% sodium bicarbonate injection USP 50mEq pre-filled syringe	3	
2g lidocaine (8mg/mL) pre-filled syringe	5	
Atropine sulfate injection USP 1mg pre-filled syringe	4	
2% lidocaine HCl injection USP 100mg/5mL pre-filled syringe	4	
1:10,000 epinephrine injection, 0.1mg/mL ampule	4	
Vented IV tubing	2	
Bacteriostatic normal saline 30mL vial	4	
Dextrose 50%, 25g syringe	4	
Heparin 5,000u/mL syringe	4	
Naloxone 0.4mg/mL syringe	2	
Furosemide 100mg/10mL vial	2	
Potassium chloride 2mEq/mL 20mL vial	2	
Calcium chloride 10% pre-filled syringe	2	
Potassium chloride 2mEq/mL 20mL vial	2	
Dopamine 1,600mcg/250mL IV bag	2	
0.9%NS 1L IV bag	4	
D_5W 1L bag	4	

FIGURE 16.9 Crash-cart refill form.

5. Find the first item on the crash-cart charge form. Then open the top drawer or tray of the crash cart and attempt to find the first item on the form. You may have to look in multiple drawers to find the item. Make sure the item you pull from the cart is the same as the one on the crash-cart charge form.

> The technician should be careful when removing items from a crash cart that has been opened. Often, it will contain open vials or ampules or used syringes.

6. Count the quantity remaining of that item in the crash cart. This quantity should match the quantity on the crash-cart charge form. If it does not, the difference between what is in the crash cart and the quantity on the form represents the quantity used to treat the patient. This is also the quantity that needs to be replaced in the crash cart.

7. On the crash-cart charge form, write down the number of items that were used by the patient and need to be replaced.

8. Going down the crash-cart charge form, repeat steps 5 through 7 until all the missing items have been noted.

9. After all the information has been recorded on the crash-cart charge form, ask the pharmacist to check or verify your work.

Part 2: Refilling the Crash Cart

1. Write your name and today's date on the crash-cart refill form.

2. Using the crash-cart refill form, locate the first item to be refilled. Verify that the expiration date of the medication already in the crash cart meets the state requirements for expiration dates.

3. Refill the quantity needed to bring the item up to par level.

> All medications in the crash cart should meet state requirements for expiration dates.

4. On the crash-cart refill form, record the earliest expiration date of the medication. For example, if there are two ampules of the same medication, but they have different expiration dates, use the earliest expiration date.

5. Place these items in the appropriate section or drawer of the crash cart.

6. Going down the crash-cart refill form, repeat these steps until all items on the refill form have been checked and refilled.

For Further Practice

A central supply worker brings a used crash cart to the pharmacy. As the pharmacy technician, you receive this cart. Central supply has replenished their trays and now needs the pharmacy to refill the medications in the pharmacy tray in the crash cart. You must count each item that is returned in the cart and compare this to the items that were used and written on the crash-cart charge form during or immediately following the use of the cart for a patient emergency. (Sometimes these numbers do not match, which means that during the emergency situation, some of the medications used were not accurately documented.) You must also make sure that everything used is documented for billing to the patient on the crash-cart charge form. You must then refill the cart off of this list.

To begin, look at the returned crash-cart charge form **FIGURE 16.10** and write in the quantity of each item to be charged to the patient.

Patient Name: Jane Doe				
Date: August 22, 2011				
Time: 5:02 p.m.				
Nurse Signature:				
Medication/Supply	Par Level	Quantity Used	Quantity Returned to PY	Quantity to Charge Patient
Alcohol pads	20	8	10	
8.4% sodium bicarbonate injection USP 50mEq	3	1	1	
2g lidocaine (8mg/mL) vial	5	0	5	
Atropine sulfate injection USP 1mg	4	0	4	
2% lidocaine HCl injection USP 100mg/5mL	4	0	4	
1:10,000 epinephrine injection, 0.1mg/mL	4	0	4	
Vented IV tubing	2	2	0	
Bacteriostatic normal saline 30mL vial	4	2	0	
Dextrose 50%, 25g syringe	4	0	4	
Heparin 5,000u/mL syringe	4	0	4	
Naloxone 0.4mg/mL syringe	2	0	2	
Furosemide 100mg/10mL vial	2	0	2	
Potassium chloride 2mEq/mL 20mL vial	2	0	2	
Calcium chloride 10% pre-filled syringe	2	0	2	
Potassium chloride 2mEq/mL 20mL vial	2	0	2	
Dopamine 1,600mcg/250mL IV	2	0	2	
0.9%NS 1L	4	2	2	
D_5W 1L	4	1	2	

FIGURE 16.10 The returned crash-cart charge form.

Using the crash-cart refill form **FIGURE 16.11**, fill in the quantity of each medication/supply that is needed to refill the items used to the par level. Check the expiration date and record it for each item in the cart, including the items that are *not* being refilled. For the purposes of this lab, use the last day of the month for the expiration dates. Sign and date the cart in the appropriate space and return it to the instructor.

Lab: Filling or Refilling an Automated Drug Storage and Dispensing System

Large hospitals often use automated drug storage and dispensing systems to help with the storing, dispensing, record keeping, and charging of medications. This type of system consists of a cabinet that is linked to a computer or laptop. The computer or laptop is in turn linked to the pharmacy department. There are several brands and manufacturers of these types of systems, but they are all similar in the way they work.

The advantages of using an automated drug storage and dispensing system include the following:

- Immediate access for nursing staff
- Convenience for stocking and dispensing medications
- Accurate inventory verification

Medication/Supply	Par Level	Quantity Refilled	Expiration Date
Alcohol pads	20		
8.4% sodium bicarbonate injection USP 50mEq	3		
2g lidocaine (8mg/mL) pre-filled syringe	5		
Atropine sulfate injection USP 1mg	4		
2% lidocaine HCl injection USP 100mg/5mL	4		
1:10,000 epinephrine injection, 0.1mg/mL	4		
Vented IV tubing	2		
Bacteriostatic normal saline 30mL vial	4		
Dextrose 50%, 25g syringe	4		
Heparin 5,000u/mL syringe	4		
Naloxone 0.4mg/mL syringe	2		
Furosemide 100mg/10mL vial	2		
Potassium chloride 2mEq/mL 20mL vial	2		
Calcium chloride 10% pre-filled syringe	2		
Potassium chloride 2mEq/mL 20mL vial	2		
Dopamine 1,600mcg/250mL IV	2		
0.9%NS 1L IV bag	4		
D_5W 1L	4		
Date:			
Pharmacy Technician Signature:			
Pharmacist Signature:			

FIGURE 16.11 Sample crash-cart refill form.

- Decreased labor cost
- Reduced errors
- Patients are charged automatically
- Prevention of drug diversion or theft

What Would You Do?

Question: The nurse calls the pharmacy and asks that you please send up two more of every item on the automated drug storage and dispensing system refill request form. What do you do?

Answer: You should gently remind the nurse that an automated drug storage and dispensing system refill request form must be filled out completely to requisition items for refilling the system.

The pharmacy technician is usually responsible for refilling and maintaining the inventory of an automated drug storage and dispensing system. This exercise involves learning how to refill medication needed for an automated drug storage and dispensing system. (Note that in most classroom settings, an automatic drug storage system will not be available; for this reason, this lab takes a more theoretical approach than others in this book.)

Supplies Needed

- Automated drug storage and dispensing system refill request form
- Pharmacy lab with sample stock items found in an automated drug storage and dispensing system
- Automated drug storage and dispensing system

Steps

1. Find a clean workstation.

2. Write your name and today's date on the automated drug storage and dispensing system refill request form.

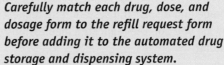

Carefully match each drug, dose, and dosage form to the refill request form before adding it to the automated drug storage and dispensing system.

3. Filling and checking an automated drug storage and dispensing system requires knowledge of your state's expiration-date requirements. To ensure that the medication is acceptable, you must know the state regulations regarding expiration dates. For this exercise, use the last day of the month in which you complete this work.

4. Looking at the automated drug storage and dispensing system refill request form, find the first item that needs to be replaced. Make sure the item you pull from stock is the same as the one on the refill request form. The drug name, strength, dosage form, and quantity must match that requested on the refill request form.

5. Pull out the quantity required from stock and place it on your workstation. Check the expiration date of each unit dose or item that needs to be refilled and make sure it meets your state's requirements.

6. Going down the automated drug storage and dispensing refill request form, repeat these steps until all items on the refill form have been pulled.

7. After you have pulled all the items on the refill request form, arrange them in the order in which they appear on the refill request form. In a real-world setting, the pharmacist would then verify your work, although in some pharmacies, the pharmacist completes the check after the items are places in a zipper lock bag.

8. Place the medications pulled in a zipper lock bag with a label for delivery to each floor.

In a real pharmacy setting, the pharmacy technician would then take the completed refill request form and all the medications to the automated drug storage and dispensing system. The technician would then enter a login and password assigned to him or her for access to the system and for completing the fill or refill. The name of each medication to be refilled would be entered into the computer, after which the drawer or cell that contains this medication would open up. After the drawer or cell is opened, the computer would ask for the exact number of items in the drawer. This is a double-check. If the actual count matches what is shown in the computer, the pharmacy technician would select Yes. If it does not, the pharmacy technician would select No, and enter the correct quantity into the computer. The quantity of the item that is going to be added would then be entered into the system. The computer would ask for verification of the new count. The drawer should be closed when the fill is completed. The technician would double-check that the drawer indeed is closed. This process would then be repeated until all the medications on the refill request form have been placed in the automated drug storage and dispensing system. After all the

What Would You Do?

Question: The completed automated drug storage and dispensing system refill request form above is given to you, the pharmacy technician, to fill. How would you do this?

Answer: You would locate the items on the automated drug storage and dispensing system refill request form. Most pharmacies will have them located in one specific area for quick and accurate refilling of the system. You would then count out the number of items needed for each request and double-check that the correct medication and quantity are pulled and this matches the request form. You will also check the expiration date. Each medication requested should be set aside for checking by the pharmacist. Once the pharmacist has verified the medication requests, you can then add the medications to the system.

What Would You Do?

Question: You've received an automated drug storage and dispensing system refill request form. How do you add the requested medications to the system?

Answer: You enter the refill information into the system and double-check that the drawer or tray that opens up to be filled is indeed for the medication that has been requested and filled. This can be done by double-checking the labeling or identification numbers on the tray. Additionally, you should always double-check to ensure no other medications other than those that are assigned to that specific drawer are actually in the drawer.

medications have been placed in the system, the refilling pharmacy technician would log out of the computer. The system would generate a printout that shows the inventory of the medications. It would also highlight any discrepancies noted during the refilling process. This would need to be rectified upon return to the pharmacy. The printout would be placed in a designated file or storage site in the pharmacy.

FIGURE 16.12 shows an automated drug-storage and dispensing system refill request form. The automated request form may be generated from the computer system and printed out or it may be completed by hand from a nurse on the floor where the system is located.

For Further Practice

Review this sample automated drug storage and dispensing system refill request form **FIGURE 16.13** and fill in the quantity to refill section. Sign the form in the filled

Medication	Quantity Used	Par Level	Quantity to Refill
Acetaminophen 325mg tablets	10	20	
Acetaminophen 500mg caplets	8	20	
Ampicillin 125mg vials	5	5	
Ampicillin 500mg vials	4	5	
Ampicillin 1g vials	10	10	
Bacteriostatic NS 30mL vials	4	10	
Cimetidine 150mg tablets	2	10	
Diphenhydramine 25mg tablets	8	10	
Heparin lock flush 100 units/5mL	6	20	
Furosemide 20mg tablets	4	10	
Metoclopramide 5mg/5mL vial	3	5	
Furosemide 100mg/10mL vial	2	5	
Milk of magnesia 30mL unit dose cup	2	10	
Calcium chloride 10% vial	2	2	
Potassium chloride 2mEq/mL 20mL vial	2	5	
Promethazine 25mg/mL ampule	2	5	
0.9%NS 1L IV bag	4	10	
D_5W 1L IV bag	4	10	
Filled By:			
Pharmacy Technician Signature:			
Verified By:			
Pharmacist Signature:			
Date:			

FIGURE 16.12 Automated drug storage and dispensing system refill request form.

Medication	Quantity Used	Par Level	Quantity to Refill
Acetaminophen 325mg tablets	10	20	
Acetaminophen 500mg caplets	8	20	
Ampicillin 125mg vials	5	5	
Ampicillin 500mg vials	4	5	
Ampicillin 1g vials	10	10	
Bacteriostatic NS 30mL vials	4	10	
Cimetidine 150mg tablets	2	10	
Diphenhydramine 25mg tablets	8	10	
Heparin lock flush 100 units/5mL	6	20	
Furosemide 20mg tablets	4	10	
Metoclopramide 5mg/5mL vial	3	5	
Furosemide 100mg/10mL vial	2	5	
Milk of magnesia 30mL unit dose cup	2	10	
Calcium chloride 10% vial	2	2	
Potassium chloride 2mEq/mL 20mL vial	2	5	
Promethazine 25mg/mL ampule	2	5	
0.9%NS 1L IV bag	4	10	
D_5W 1L IV bag	4	10	
Filled By:			
Pharmacy Technician Signature:			
Verified By:			
Pharmacist Signature:			
Date:			
Instructor Sign Off			

FIGURE 16.13 Sample automated drug storage and dispensing system refill request form for practical exercise.

by section. Have a fellow student verify your form and sign in the pharmacist section. Turn your completed automated drug storage and dispensing system refill request form in to the instructor.

Drug Insights: Hormonal Disorders

The **endocrine system** is a system of glands that produce and secrete hormones **FIGURE 16.14**. These **hormones**, or chemical messengers, are released directly into the bloodstream. They regulate mood, growth and development, tissue function, metabolism, sexual function, and reproduction. The hormones that regulate these activities are also used to treat hormonal disorders.

The Endocrine System

The endocrine system is composed of the following:

- Thyroid gland—The **thyroid gland** is a gland that secretes hormones that stimulate metabolic activity, growth, and the activity of the nervous system

- Hypothalamus—The **hypothalamus** is an area of the brain that produces hormones that control body temperature, moods, sex drive, and the release of hormones.
- Pituitary gland—The **pituitary gland** is a gland that produces hormones that affect the activity of other endocrine glands and specific organs of the body.
- Parathyroid gland—The **parathyroid gland** is the gland that produces parathyroid hormone.
- Adrenal glands—The **adrenal glands** are located directly above the kidneys. They are composed of two layers of tissue: the medulla and the cortex.
- Pineal body—The **pineal body** is a gland that produces and secretes melatonin, a hormone that regulates the circadian cycle.
- Ovaries—**Ovaries** are female organs responsible for hormones that regulate the menstrual cycle and pregnancy.
- Testes—**Testes** are male sex glands that produce testosterone.
- Pancreas—The **pancreas** aids in hormone production and digestion.

The endocrine system glands secrete hormones that maintain homeostasis by regulating physiological processes. The tissue or organ that these hormones affect is called its **target**. As mentioned, the pituitary gland produces hormones that affect the activity of other endocrine glands and specific organs of the body.

The endocrine system is regulated by an intricate **negative feedback mechanism** that involves a particular gland, the hypothalamic-pituitary axis, and autoregulation. This feedback mechanism is the primary regulatory mechanism used to maintain homeostasis. The hormone levels in the endocrine system are regulated by a negative feedback mechanism in almost the same way that a thermostat regulates the temperature in a room. In negative feedback, the stimulus results in actions that reduce the stimulus. If a gland stops producing a hormone or secretes too much or too little hormone, various conditions of the endocrine system may result.

Thyroid Disorders

The thyroid gland is located at the base of the neck. It produces and secretes three hormones, **thyroxine (T4)**, **triiodothyronine (T_3)**, and **calcitonin**, that stimulate metabolic activity, growth, and the activity of the nervous system. The thyroid gland needs iodine to synthesize T_3 and T_4; each hormone is named according to the number of iodine atoms in its structure. T_3 and T_4 are stored as **thyroglobulin**; the body breaks down thyroglobulin before it can be released into the bloodstream. T_3 is more potent than T_4. These hormones are transported via the bloodstream, where they bind to a specific protein. This reaction helps trigger the metabolism of proteins, fats, and carbohydrates. The hypothalamic-pituitary axis produces **thyroid-stimulating hormone (TSH)**, which stimulates the thyroid to produce T_3 and T_4. When the levels of these hormones rise, the pituitary produces and releases less TSH. Calcitonin is involved in the regulation of calcium levels. Calcitonin inhibits the **resorption** of calcium from the bone and kidney.

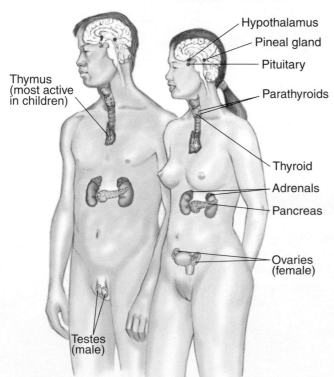

Thymus (most active in children)

Testes (male)

Hypothalamus
Pineal gland
Pituitary
Parathyroids
Thyroid
Adrenals
Pancreas
Ovaries (female)

FIGURE 16.14 The endocrine system.

Hypothyroidism

Hypothyroidism is a condition that occurs when the thyroid gland is not able to produce and secrete sufficient levels of T_3 and T_4. This can be caused by a lack of iodine in the diet, inflammation of the thyroid gland, tumors that affect the thyroid gland, surgical removal of the thyroid, radioactive iodine therapy, or the absence of a thyroid gland. Some children who are born without a thyroid gland or whose thyroid gland does not function properly may develop cretinism or dwarfism. **Cretinism** can cause severe mental retardation. **Dwarfism** can cause a child's growth to be stunted. A lack of iodine in the diet can cause a decrease in the production of T_3 and T_4 because iodine is necessary for the synthesis of T_3 and T_4.

The signs and symptoms of hypothyroidism may vary depending on the severity of hormone deficiency. Symptoms may include the following:

- Fatigue
- Sluggishness
- Constipation
- Dry skin
- Puffy face
- Hoarse voice
- Unexplained weight gain
- Brittle fingernails
- Cold intolerance

Hypothyroidism may cause **myxedema**. Symptoms of myxedema include low blood pressure, decreased breathing, unresponsiveness, and in rare cases, coma.

Patients with hypothyroidism manage their condition with hormone-replacement therapy. In patients with hypothyroidism due to tumors, surgery is indicated to remove all or part of the thyroid gland. Thyroid hormone-replacement drugs need to be taken for a patient's whole life.

The drug of choice for thyroid hormone replacement is levothyroxine sodium. Levothyroxine sodium may cause cardiotoxicity, or injury to the heart. The patient should be advised to report any signs of chest pain, palpitations, or heat intolerance to his or her physician. It can also alter the protein binding of other drugs. Although all FDA-approved levothyroxine products are considered to be therapeutically equivalent, small compositional variabilities may affect the blood levels of these drugs. The Approved Drug Products with Therapeutic Equivalence Evaluations (*Orange Book*) provides ratings for the equivalence of levothyroxine products.

> The technician should verify that all prescription refills for levothyroxine are filled with *Orange Book*–rated equivalent products.

TABLE 16.1 shows drugs used for thyroid hormone-replacement therapy.

Hyperthyroidism

Hyperthyroidism is a condition caused by oversecretion of hormones from the thyroid gland. It is primarily caused by Graves' disease, **goiter** (an enlargement or swelling of the thyroid gland), a tumor in the pituitary that causes overproduction of TSH, or postpartum thyroiditis. **Graves' disease** is an autoimmune disorder in which the body makes antibodies to TSH receptors. Graves' disease may cause **exophthalmos**, or bulging of the eye.

Table 16.1   Drugs Used for Thyroid Hormone-Replacement Therapy

Class	Generic Name	Brand Name	Dosage Forms Available
T₃	Liothyronine sodium	Cytomel, Triostat	Tablet, injection
T₄	Levothyroxine sodium	Levothroid, Levoxyl, Synthroid, Tirosint, Unithyroid	Tablet
Combined T₃ and T₄	Thyroid, pork	Armour Thyroid	Tablet
	Liotrix	Thyrolar	Tablet

The signs and symptoms of hyperthyroidism may vary depending on the severity of hormone deficiency. Symptoms may include the following:

- Sudden weight loss
- Goiter
- Rapid heartbeat
- Increased appetite
- Sweating
- Heat intolerance
- Nervousness
- Fatigue
- Difficulty sleeping

If hyperthyroidism is the result of a tumor, treatment could include surgery to remove the tumor (thyroidectomy) or radiation to destroy or shrink part or all of the tumor. **TABLE 16.2** lists drugs used to treat hyperthyroidism. Removal of the thyroid gland can cause hypothyroidism, which would require thyroid hormone replacement therapy.

Both propylthiouracil (PTU) and methimazole (Tapazole) inhibit the synthesis of thyroid hormone, reducing the risk of surgical complications during a thyroidectomy. PTU also blocks the conversion of T₄ to T₃. Radioactive iodine is absorbed in the thyroid tissue, where it destroys the thyroid cells.

Male Sex Hormones

As mentioned, the adrenal glands are located directly above the kidneys. Each adrenal gland is composed of two layers of tissue: the medulla and the cortex. Along with other hormones, the cortex produces androgens and estrogens, which are the sex hormones. The androgens and estrogens are controlled by follicle-stimulating hormone (FSH), and luteinizing hormone (LH), which are the pituitary hormones. **Androgens** are male hormones produced by the testes. The testes also produce the male hormone

Table 16.2   Drugs Used for Hyperthyroidism

Generic Name	Brand Name	Dosage Forms Available
Propylthiouracil	N/A	Tablet
Methimazole	Tapazole	Tablet
Radioactive iodine	N/A	Capsule, oral solution

testosterone. **Testosterone** is responsible for male characteristics and sperm production, red blood cell production, **libido** (sex drive), and fat distribution.

When there is an insufficient amount of male sex hormone production and secretion (hypogonadism), androgens must be replaced. Insufficient production of male sex hormone can be caused by underdevelopment of the genitals during fetal development, injury, or infection. Androgen-replacement therapy may be used to treat hypogonadism in men. It may also be used to treat testosterone deficiencies in women. Androgen-replacement therapy may cause the following conditions:

- Virilization—**Virilization** describes the development of male characteristics in a female.
- Hirsutism—Hirsutism describes excess facial and body hair growth in women.
- Priapism—**Priapism** involves a persistent erection that is usually painful.
- Gynecomastia—**Gynecomastia** refers to the enlargement of the gland tissue of the male breast.
- Acne—**Acne** describes the inflammation of the skin due to overactivity of hormones on the skin's oil glands.

Testosterone undergoes extensive first-pass metabolism in the GI tract and liver. Various testosterone products have been developed to counteract this. Testosterone can be delivered through a variety of dosage forms. Because it is not as painful as an injection, many men prefer transdermal patches or gels. Some testosterone gels can be applied to the back, abdomen, or thigh. A buccal tablet is also available for testosterone-replacement therapy.

All testosterone products are classified as Schedule III controlled substances.

A deficiency of testosterone may also cause male **impotence**, also known as **erectile dysfunction**. Impotence can also be caused by alcoholism, cigarette smoking, and some drugs. Alprostadil (Caverject) is available as a penile injection or a urethral suppository (Muse) to treat erectile dysfunction. Caverject vials and Muse suppositories should be refrigerated until dispensed. They may be stored at room temperature for up to three months. Common side effects of alprostadil include local irritation and burning.

The patient should be instructed to wash his hands with soap and water after applying a product containing testosterone.

Phosphodiesterase **inhibitors** such as sildenafil (Viagra), vardenafil (Levitra), and tadalafil (Cialis) are now the drugs of choice for first-line therapy for erectile dysfunction. They increase blood flow to the penis by causing the penile arteries and corpus cavernosal smooth muscle to relax. These drugs are contraindicated in patients also taking nitrates. Patients taking these drugs should be advised to avoid alcohol. Sildenafil may also cause blurred vision. Vardenafil is often used in patients who do not respond to sildenafil (Viagra) treatment. Tadalafil has a longer duration of action than sildenafil and vardenafil. Tadalafil is effective for 36 hours, and can be taken daily in a more maintenance fashion. **TABLE 16.3** lists drugs commonly used to treat erectile dysfunction.

Female Sex Hormones

The cortex of the adrenal gland produces the sex hormone estrogen. The follicle-stimulating hormone (FSH) and luteinizing hormone (LH) are pituitary hormones that control the sex hormones. The ovaries secrete the hormones estrogen and progesterone. **Estrogen** stimulates the development of breasts and genitals, produces endometrial

Table 16.3   Common Drugs Used for Erectile Dysfunction

Class	Generic Name	Brand Name	Dosage Forms Available
Testosterone-containing products	Testosterone	Androderm, AndroGel, Striant, Testoderm, Fortesta	Gel, injection, buccal tablet, transdermal patch
	Methyltestosterone	Android, Testred	Capsule, tablet
Phosphodiesterase inhibitors	Sildenafil	Viagra	Tablet
	Tadalafil	Cialis	Tablet
	Vardenafil	Levitra	Tablet
Prostaglandin	Alprostadil	Muse, Edex, Caverject	Injection, urethral suppository

Phosphodiesterase inhibitors are contraindicated in patients taking nitrates.

growth, increases production of cervical mucus, and regulates the **menstrual cycle**. **Progesterone** prepares the uterus for implantation of the fertilized ovum. It also stimulates the development of ducts and glands of the breasts to prepare for lactation. FSH triggers estrogen levels to rise, which causes LH to be secreted. Administration of these hormones can prevent pregnancy, relieve the symptoms of menopause, and help prevent osteoporosis. They can also be used to control menstrual cycles and their symptoms by regulating the levels of estrogen and progestin in the body.

Estrogen

Estrogen is a female hormone formed in the ovaries. The hypothalamic-pituitary axis releases FSH, which stimulates estrogen production for the first 14 days of the menstrual cycle and progesterone for days 14 through 28 of the menstrual cycle. As the levels of both estrogen and progesterone rise, the hypothalamus does not produce or release gonadotropin-releasing hormone.

Symptoms of estrogen deficiency include irregular bleeding, irregular menstrual cycles, hot flashes, vaginal dryness, dysparenuia, and urethral and bladder atrophy. The amount of estrogen production declines at the start of menopause. Loss of ovarian function can lead to **menopause** and tissue atrophy. Hormone-replacement therapy can help relieve the symptoms of estrogen deficiency associated with menopause. Side effects of estrogen include swollen breasts, dizziness, acne, skin-color changes, and breakthrough bleeding. All estrogens are contraindicated for use during pregnancy.

Progestins

Progesterone is the female hormone secreted during the second half the menstrual cycle, which typically runs 28 days. Progesterone blocks ovulation by inhibiting the secretion of LH. **Progestin** is a synthetic form of progesterone. Progestin is used to prevent pregnancy, prevent uterine cancer in woman who take hormone-replacement therapy, regulate menstrual cycles, and treat menstrual dysfunction. When a progestin is combined with estrogen, the dosage of progestin is measured in milligrams and the

What Would You Do?

Question: A patient in the pharmacy asks for a refill of an estrogen-containing product. You notice that she is pregnant. What should you do?

Answer: Ask the patient to wait; then ask the pharmacist to speak to the patient.

Table 16.4 Common Drugs Used as Estrogen- and Progestin-Replacement Therapy

Class	Generic Name	Brand Name	Available Formulations
Progestin-only	Progesterone	Crinone	Vaginal gel
	Medroxyprogesterone	Provera, Depo-Provera, Depo-SubQ Provera 104	Tablet, injection
	Norethindrone	Aygestin	Tablet
Estrogen-only	Estropipate	Ogen	Tablet
	Conjugated estrogens	Premarin, Cenestin, Enjuvia	Tablet, cream
	Esterified estrogen	Menest	Tablet
	Estradiol	Estrace, Estraderm, Divigel, Elestrin, Femring, Vivelle Dot, Estring, Estrasorb	Vaginal cream, tablet, transdermal patch, gel

estrogen component in micrograms. Side effects of progestins include weight gain, stomach pain, headaches, mood swings, anxiety, acne, and insomnia.

Hormone-Replacement Therapy

Hormone-replacement therapy is used to treat symptoms of menopause. Patients who take estrogen supplements should be advised not to smoke cigarettes because it can increase the risk of blood clots. Hormone-replacement therapy may increase the risk of breast cancer. The decision to use hormone-replacement therapy and whether the benefits in reducing menopausal symptoms outweigh the risks of breast cancer are up to the individual patient and her physician. TABLE 16.4 outlines common drugs used for hormone-replacement therapy.

Patients on estrogen-replacement therapy should be advised to not smoke cigarettes.

Combination therapy with an estrogen and progestin is used for women with an intact uterus. Estrogen-replacement therapy, like naturally occurring estrogen, can cause a thickening of the uterine lining, which can lead to uterine cancer. A progestin prevents this thickening and is therefore given in combination with an estrogen. TABLE 16.5 lists combination drugs used in hormone-replacement therapy.

Table 16.5 Combination Drugs Used as Estrogen- and Progestin-Replacement Therapy

Generic Name	Brand Name	Available Formulations
Conjugated estrogen-medroxyprogesterone	Premphase, PremPro	Tablet
Estradiol-levonorgestrel	Climara Pro	Patch
Estradiol-norethindrone	Activella, CombiPatch	Tablet, patch
Estradiol-norgestimate	Prefest	Tablet
Ethinyl estradiol-norethindrone	Femhrt	Tablet

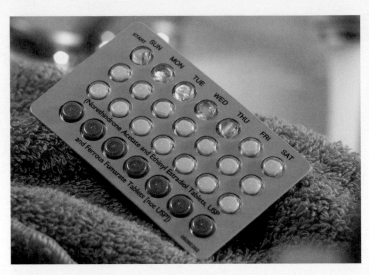

Birth control pills are the most commonly used contraceptive.

Oral Contraceptives

Oral contraceptives, also known as "the pill," are used as a form of birth control to prevent fertilization of an ovum and subsequent pregnancy. Oral contraceptives are available as progestin-only contraceptives (known as mini-pills) or as combinations of estrogen and progestin. These pills interfere with hormones that regulate the menstrual cycle. The estrogen content of the pill suppresses production of LH and FSH, which prevents the egg from being released and maturing. Progestin suppresses the production of LH and alters the composition of the cervical mucus of the endometrium, making it unsuitable for sperm to penetrate and for the fertilized ovum to implant.

Combination oral contraceptives are available in the following formulations. These formulations are designed to mimic the natural hormonal cycle:

- Monophasic—In monophasic formulations, the estrogen and progestin content of each pill remains constant throughout the cycle.
- Biphasic—In biphasic formulations, the estrogen content of each pill is the same, but the progestin dose is increased during the second half of the cycle.
- Triphasic—In triphasic formulations, the amount of progestin varies in all three phases.

Most traditional combination oral contraceptives are packaged as a 21/7 cycle (21 days of active tablet and seven days of placebo, or an iron supplement in some cases), resulting in 13 bleeding episodes per year. Newer regimens include fewer hormone-free days per 28 day cycle (2–4 placebo tablets) or extended-cycles with fewer withdrawal bleeds per year. One low-dose combination oral contraceptive (Lybrel-levonorgestrel/ethinyl estradiol) is taken once daily while contraception is desired, without any placebo or pill-free interval. Progestin-only contraceptives are usually taken once a day, without a pill-free interval.

All oral contraceptives should be taken at the same time each day. If a dose is missed, it should be taken as soon as the patient remembers, and the next dose should be taken according to the regular schedule. If two doses are missed, two tablets should be taken for the next two days, and alternative forms of contraception should be used for the next seven days. If three doses are missed, the patient should use another form of contraception and start a new cycle of medication seven days after the last pill was taken. If a patient misses a dose of a progestin-only contraceptive, advise the patient to consult her physician.

Oral contraceptives have other benefits as well, such as regular menstrual cycles, improvement in acne, and reduced menstrual flow. They may also reduce the risk of endometrial and ovarian cancer. Side effects of oral contraceptives include nausea, weight gain, vomiting, mood swings, headache, and breast tenderness. More serious side effects include blood clots, stroke, or other cardiovascular complications. Smoking increases the risk of developing blood clots and stroke.

Many drugs taken concurrently with oral contraceptives, including rifampin (Rifadin), several anti-HIV agents, and anticonvulsants, can induce the metabolism of oral contraceptives, thus decreasing their effectiveness.

The majority of oral contraceptives in the U.S. contain ethinyl estradiol estrogen and levonorgestrel or norethindrone progestin. Ethinyl estradiol-drosperinone (found in Yasmin and Yaz) may reduce bloating because it contains drospirenone, a spironolactone analogue that has diuretic activity. Yasmin has a 28-day cycle, while Yaz is taken as 24 active tablets and a placebo for four days. Yaz is also approved for treatment of acne.

Ethinyl estradiol-levonorgestrel (Seasonale, Introvale, Quasense, Seasonique, LoSeasonique, Lybrel) is available in many combinations. Seasonale, Introvale, and Quasense are taken on a 91-day cycle (84 days of active pills and seven days of placebo). Seasonique and LoSeasonique are taken on a 91-day cycle, but instead of a placebo, the patient takes 10mcg of ethinyl estradiol for seven days. Women taking these pills have only four periods per year.

Some combination oral contraceptives that contain ethinyl estradiol-norethindrone such as Estrostep, Loestrin, and Loestrin 24 Fe are also approved for the treatment of acne. Estrostep Fe and Loestrin 24 Fe also contain an iron supplement to replace iron lost during menses. **TABLE 16.6** contains commonly used oral contraceptives.

Emergency contraceptives may prevent pregnancy if used within 72 hours of unprotected sex. Levonorgestrel (Plan B One-Step and Next Choice) are available for emergency contraception without a prescription to anyone 17 years of age and older, and with a prescription for younger women. Ulipristal acetate (Ella) can be used up to five days after unprotected intercourse.

Drugs Used During Childbirth

Drugs can be used during childbirth to alleviate or control pain or induce labor. They can also be used to promote cervical ripening or prevent hemorrhage following delivery.

Table 16.6 Commonly Used Oral Contraceptives

Class	Generic Name (Progestin/Estrogen)	Brand Name	Available Formulations
Combination oral contraceptives	Ethynodiol diacetate/ethinyl estradiol	Zovia, Kelnor	Tablet
	Norethindrone/ethinyl estradiol	Ovcon, Necon, Norinyl, Ortho-Novum 1/35, Ortho-Novum 7/7/7, Tri-Norinyl	Tablet
	Norgestrel/ethinyl estradiol	Ogestrel, Low-Ogestrel	Tablet
	Norgestimate/ethinyl estradiol	MonoNessa, Ortho-Cyclen, TriNessa, Ortho Tri-Cyclen	Tablet
	Desogestrel/ethinyl estradiol	Ortho-Cept, Cyclessa, Mircette	Tablet
	Drospirenone/ethinyl estradiol	Yasmin, Yaz, Beyaz	Tablet
	Norethindrone acetate/ethinyl estradiol	Loestrin Fe, Loestrin 24 Fe, Estrostep Fe	Tablet
	Levonorgestrel, ethinyl estradiol	Aviane, Lutera, Introvale, Quasense, Seasonale, Lybrel, Seasonique, LoSeasonique	Tablet
	Mestranol/norethindrone	Necon, Norinyl	Tablet
	Dienogest/estradiol valerate	Natazia	Tablet
Progestin-only	Norethindrone	Camila, Micronor	Tablet

Dinoprostone (Cervidil, Prepidil, Prostin E2) promotes cervical ripening, meaning the cervix prepares for delivery. Cervidil is available as a vaginal insert, Prepidil as a gel, and Prostin E2 as a suppository.

Methylergonovine (Methergine) is available as a tablet or injection. It causes constriction of the blood vessels in the uterus, preventing bleeding or hemorrhage when the uterine fails to contract after delivery.

Oxytocin (Pitocin) stimulates contraction of the uterine smooth muscle and is used to induce labor.

Drugs used to control pain during labor and delivery must balance the benefits of alleviating pain for the mother and the risks of toxicity for the baby. Butorphanol, fentanyl, and morphine are used to control pain during labor and delivery. An epidural can also be given to control pain.

Sexually Transmitted Diseases (STDs)

A **sexually transmitted disease (STD)** is a disease that can be transmitted by sexual intercourse. Symptoms may appear on the genitalia of males or females **FIGURE 16.15**.

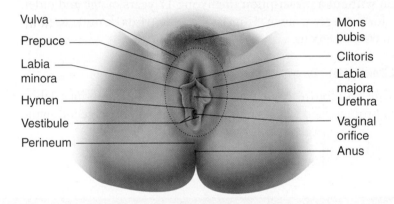

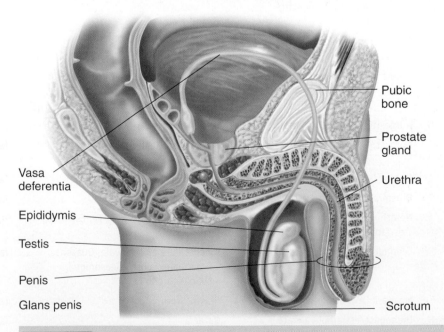

FIGURE 16.15 The anatomy of the male and female genitals.

Sometimes, diseases that are referred to as STDs are actually not transmitted sexually. These diseases can be transmitted by nonsexual modes such as through childbirth, close contact with an infected individual, or from shared use of needles. STDs are caused by bacterial, viral, fungal, and protozoan infections. The symptoms of STDs can vary according to the severity and type of infection. Some STDs such as chlamydia, gonorrhea, hepatitis, and HIV are on a list of nationally notifiable infectious conditions. If a patient is diagnosed with one of the diseases on this list, the physician must notify the local health department. This list is updated annually by the Centers for Disease Control and Prevention (CDC).

The CDC publishes a list of nationally notifiable infectious conditions, which is updated yearly. This list can be found at http://www.cdc.gov/osels/ph_surveillance/nndss/phs/infdis2011.htm.

Symptoms for many STDs are not noticeable in the early stages of infection, which results in more transference of infection between partners. Because infection is spread by sexual contact, education and protection are important measures to prevent the spread of STDs. Abstaining from sexual contact or having a monogamous relationship with a partner who is not infected are the most effective ways to avoid getting an STD. Latex **condoms** are also effective because they create a barrier against infection. Oral contraceptives or contraceptive gels do not protect against the transmission of STDs. Some vaccines such as Gardasil (human papillomavirus quadrivalent types 6, 11, 16, and 18) have been developed to protect against human papillomavirus (HPV) infections. Acquired immunodeficiency syndrome (AIDS), an STD that is caused by the human immunodeficiency virus (HIV), is discussed in Chapter 7.

Abstaining from sexual contact or being in a monogamous relationship with a partner who is not infected are the best ways to avoid getting an STD.

Chlamydia

Chlamydia is caused by an infection from the bacterium *Chlamydia trachomatis*. Chlamydia can be transmitted during vaginal, oral, or anal sex. It can also be transmitted from an infected mother to a child during vaginal delivery in childbirth. Chlamydia is known as the "silent disease" because most women have no symptoms. If left untreated, it can permanently damage a woman's reproductive organs, leading to infertility. Infection can result in urethritis and **pelvic inflammatory disease (PID)** (an infection of the uterus, fallopian tubes, or other reproductive organs that causes symptoms such as lower abdominal pain) in women and **epididymitis** (a painful condition of the ducts attached to the testicles that may lead to infertility if left untreated) in men. Chlamydial infection can also be found in the rectum of receivers of anal intercourse and in the throats of those having oral sex with an infected partner.

Gonorrhea

Gonorrhea is caused by an infection from the bacterium *Neisseria gonorrhoeae*. It can affect the anus, eyes, mouth, genitals, or throat. Gonorrhea is spread through sexual contact with the penis, vagina, mouth, or anus. It can also be transmitted from an infected mother to a child during delivery. Some men have no symptoms, while others have symptoms including burning when urinating or penile discharge that appear between one and 14 days after infection. Most women infected with gonorrhea have no symptoms. If they do have symptoms, the cause is often mistaken for a bladder or

Table 16.7   Drugs Commonly Used to Treat Sexually Transmitted Diseases

Class	Generic Name	Brand Name	Available Formulations
Antibiotics	Azithromycin	Zithromax	Tablet, suspension, injectable
	Ceftriaxone	Rocephin	Injectable
	Cefotetan	Cefotan	Injectable
	Doxycycline	Vibramycin, Doryx	Capsule, suspension
	Erythromycin	E-mycin, Ery-tab	Capsule, tablet, suspension
	Penicillin G benzathine	Bicillin L-A	Injectable
	Metronidazole	Flagyl	Capsule, tablet, injectable
Antifungals	Fluconazole	Diflucan	Tablet, suspension, injectable
Antivirals	Acyclovir	Zovirax	Tablet, capsule, suspension, injectable, ointment
	Famciclovir	Famvir	Tablet
	Valacyclovir	Valtrex	Tablet

vaginal infection. Infection can result in pelvic inflammatory disease (PID) in women and epididymitis in men.

Syphilis

Syphilis is caused by an infection from the bacterium *Treponema pallidum*. Syphilis is transmitted through direct contact with a syphilis sore. Sores occur on the genitals, vagina, anus, lips, or mouth, or in the rectum. Syphilis is spread through vaginal, anal, or oral sex. It can also be transmitted from an infected mother to a child during pregnancy. Transmission may occur from persons who are unaware they are infected because many people who are infected do not have any symptoms for years.

Genital Herpes

Genital herpes is caused by the herpes simplex virus type 1 (HSV-1) or type 2 (HSV-2). HSV-2 infection is transmitted during oral or genital sexual contact with someone who has a genital HSV-2 infection. HSV-1 commonly causes "fever blisters" or infections of the mouth and lips. A person with HSV-1 can transmit the virus through oral sex to another person's genitals.

Most people with herpes aren't aware they are infected. An outbreak usually occurs within two weeks after the virus is transmitted, and the sores usually heal within two to four weeks. To prevent transmission of herpes to a baby during childbirth, a Caesarean delivery is performed if the mother has active genital herpes at delivery. **TABLE 16.7** lists drugs commonly used to treat sexually transmitted diseases.

Adrenal Gland Disorders

The adrenal glands are located directly above the kidneys. The adrenal gland is composed of two layers of tissue: the medulla and the cortex. The **medulla** synthesizes and secretes the catecholamines, epinephrine and norepinephrine. These hormones are activated by the sympathetic nervous system. When activated, they stimulate the "fight or flight" reaction. That is, when the body is presented with a stressful situation, the body prepares itself for fight or flight. The **cortex** synthesizes three hormones: **corticosteroids** (glucocorticoids and mineralocorticoids), androgens, and estrogens.

Glucocorticoids are involved in the metabolism of lipids, carbohydrates, and proteins. **Mineralocorticoids** regulate the secretion of water and sodium by the kidney. **Cortisol** is the primary steroid hormone secreted by the adrenal gland. Cortisol is involved in the conversion of fatty acids and protein to glucose (**gluconeogenesis**), regulation of blood pressure, inflammatory response, insulin release, and immune function.

The production of cortisol is regulated by the hypothalamic-pituitary axis. The hypothalamus produces **corticotropin releasing factor (CRF)**. CRF stimulates the pituitary to produce **adrenocorticotropic hormone (ACTH)**, which stimulates the release of cortisol from the adrenal cortex. The production of cortisol follows a circadian rhythm cycle.

Addison's disease results from a deficiency of corticosteroids caused by damage to the adrenal cortex. Treatment includes replacement with corticosteroids administered daily. Symptoms of Addison's disease include the following:

- Low blood pressure
- Chronic diarrhea
- Darkening of the skin
- Fatigue
- Extreme weakness
- Weight loss
- Hyperkalemia
- Salt craving

Cushing disease results from the release of too much ACTH from the pituitary. ACTH stimulates the production and release of cortisol, meaning that people with Cushing disease have too much cortisol. It is usually caused by a tumor or excess growth of the pituitary. Treatment may involve surgery or radiation to remove the pituitary tumor or it may involve removal of the adrenal glands. Symptoms include the following:

- Round, red full face (moon face)
- Fat deposits above the waist
- Acne
- Purple marks on the skin of the abdomen, thighs, and breasts

Corticosteroids are synthetic drugs that mimic the natural effects of cortisol. The effects of corticosteroids, mainly anti-inflammatory effects, are attributed to their glucocorticoid activity, while the side effects are due to their mineralocorticoid properties. Corticosteroids are used to treat a variety of skin disorders and asthma. Corticosteroids are usually administered in the morning to mimic the natural circadian rhythm of the body. These drugs should be used cautiously in patients with cardiovascular disease, diabetes, immunosuppressed patients, and those with GI disease. Corticosteroids can also cause suppression of the hypothalamic-pituitary axis. When they are discontinued, the dosage should be tapered to minimize withdrawal symptoms because the normal production of steroids by the body has been turned off. **TABLE 16.8** lists some common corticosteroids.

Diabetes

Diabetes mellitus is a chronic disease that results from a deficiency in the production of insulin (type 1) or a resistance to insulin (type 2). If diabetes is not treated, it can result in serious complications and death.

Table 16.8	Some Common Corticosteroids	
Generic Name	**Brand Name**	**Available Formulations**
Cortisone acetate	N/A	Tablet
Hydrocortisone (various salts)	Solu-Cortef, many others	Injectable, lotion, cream, tablet
Prednisone	Deltasone	Tablet, solution
Prednisolone (various salts)	Pediapred, Pred Forte	Ophthalmic suspension, ointment, syrup
Methylprednisolone	Medrol, Solu-Medrol	Tablet, injectable
Triamcinolone	Many	Inhaler, cream, ointment, spray
Betamethasone (various salts)	Celestone Soluspan, Beta-Val, Diprolene,	Cream, lotion, ointment, injectable
Dexamethasone	Decadron	Ophthalmic ointment and suspension, tablet, elixir, injectable
Mometasone	Elocon, Asmanex Twisthaler, Nasonex	Powder for inhalation, cream, ointment, lotion, nasal spray

The pancreas produces and releases insulin. **Insulin** is involved in the transportation of glucose into the cells, stimulates protein synthesis, releases fatty acids from fat deposits, and increases ion transport into the tissues. Insulin plays an important role in maintaining blood glucose levels.

People with diabetes have high blood glucose levels, either because they do not produce enough insulin or because they don't utilize insulin properly. When this happens, the kidneys are not able to reabsorb the excess amount of glucose and the glucose spills out into the urine. When blood glucose levels are high, it is referred to as **hyperglycemia**.

Type 1 Diabetes

Type 1 diabetes is most commonly identified in children and young adults. This type of diabetes is not outgrown as patients mature into adulthood and can also be diagnosed in adults. Type I diabetes is caused by destruction of the beta cells in the pancreas, which results in the inability to produce insulin. Some patients also produce antibodies to these beta cells, which also results in the inability to produce insulin.

Type 2 Diabetes

Type 2 diabetes is more common in obese patients and adults. Insulin is released from the beta cells in the pancreas, but the receptors are resistant to insulin. As a result, glucose is not absorbed because the cells do not respond to insulin.

Gestational Diabetes

Gestational diabetes occurs in women during pregnancy. Blood glucose levels usually return to pre-pregnancy levels after childbirth. Gestational diabetes can be treated through diet, exercise, and sometimes, insulin injections.

Symptoms and Complications of Diabetes

Patients with diabetes are at risk for secondary complications if their diabetes is not well controlled or managed. Symptoms include the following:

- Infections
- **Glycosuria** (glucose spilling into the urine)
- Increased appetite
- **Polyuria** (increased urination)
- Nocturia (excessive urination at night)
- Numbness
- Taking a long time for a wound to heal
- **Polydypsia** (excessive thirst)
- Visual changes
- Weight loss
- **Ketoacidosis** (the body cannot utilize glucose because there isn't enough—or any—insulin)

Complications include the following:

- Retinopathy—**Retinopathy** describes a condition in which the blood vessels in the retina become damaged. It can lead to blindness.
- Peripheral neuropathy—Peripheral neuropathy describes a condition in which the nerves don't get enough blood supply, which can lead to numbness and tingling.
- Atherosclerosis—Atherosclerosis refers to plaque buildup in the arteries.
- Nephropathy—Nephropathy refers to kidney disease.
- Infections—Specifically, complications include infections of the feet, urinary tract, and vagina.

Treatment

For patients with type 1 diabetes, treatment consists of insulin injections and proper diet and exercise. For patients with type 2 diabetes, treatment consists of lifestyle modifications (diet and exercise) and medications. Patients should also be advised to maintain proper hygiene, take good care of their feet, and check their feet for numbness, swelling, and redness because they are more susceptible to infections. Monitoring blood glucose levels is important to prevent short-term and long-term complications.

Insulin

There are two types of insulin used for type 1 diabetes:

- Human insulin, which is made in a laboratory and is chemically identical to human insulin
- Natural insulin, taken from pigs (porcine) or cows (bovine)

Most patients are treated with human insulin. Insulin is available either in prefilled syringes or pens or in vials. Regular insulin is a clear liquid, while mixtures of insulin are suspensions. Unopened insulin vials should be stored in the refrigerator and administered at room temperature. Insulin is classified as

Regular insulin does not need to be mixed before administration. Mixtures of insulin need to be mixed before administration by rolling the vial between the hands several times to mix the suspension. The vials should not be shaken because it will make the insulin unstable.

Table 16.9   Some Common Insulin Preparations

Duration of Action	Generic Name	Brand Name
Short-acting	Regular insulin	Humulin-R, Novolin R
Rapid-acting	Insulin lispro	Humalog
	Insulin aspart	Novolog
	Insulin glulisine	Apidra
Intermediate-acting	NPH	Novolin N, Humulin N
	Insulin zinc	Humulin L
Long-acting	Insulin glargine	Lantus
	Insulin detemir	Levemir
Mixed long- and short-acting	Isophane and regular insulin	Humulin 50/50, Humulin 70/30, Novolin 70/30
	Lispro and lispro protamine	Humalog mix 50/50, Humalog mix 75/25

The majority of insulin preparations are offered in similar packages and in vials containing the same amount of volume. They all also have similar labeling. Pay attention to the package labeling to ensure that the right insulin is dispensed.

short-acting, rapid-acting, intermediate-acting, or long-acting, based on its duration of action. Most diabetics require a combination of a short-acting insulin and a long-acting insulin. **TABLE 16.9** lists common insulin preparations.

Depending on the type of insulin, it can be injected subcutaneously or intramuscularly. Only regular insulin can be administered intravenously. When given subcutaneously, the sites of injection should be rotated. Insulin is best absorbed from the abdomen, then the arms and legs, and then the buttocks.

Sometimes, blood sugar levels drop below normal, resulting in **hypoglycemia**, or a deficiency of glucose in the bloodstream. Hypoglycemia can be caused by skipping meals, too much exercise, certain medications, and improper doses of diabetic medications. Hypoglycemia can be treated by giving the patient more sugar, such as peanut butter, soft drinks, or fruit juice. Glucose tablets and gels can also be used to treat hypoglycemia. A glucagon emergency kit can be used to counteract hypoglycemia and can be used when sugar cannot be given. Glucagon is a hormone that raises the level of glucose in the blood. Symptoms of hypoglycemia include the following:

- Confusion
- Double vision or visual disturbances
- Sweating
- Thirst
- Numbness or tingling
- Palpitations

Noninsulin Injections

Some patients with type 2 diabetes mellitus may also use noninsulin medications such as exanatide (Byetta). It stimulates the beta cells in the pancreas to produce insulin and slows the rate of gastric emptying. Pramlintide (Symlin) also works by slowing gastric emptying. It is approved for use in patients with type 1 or type 2 diabetes.

Oral Hypoglycemic Drugs

Oral hypoglycemic drugs are used to treat patients with type 2 diabetes mellitus. They are not effective for patients with type 1 diabetes mellitus because they work by stimulating the pancreas to release insulin. In type 1 diabetes mellitus, there is no insulin for the body to release.

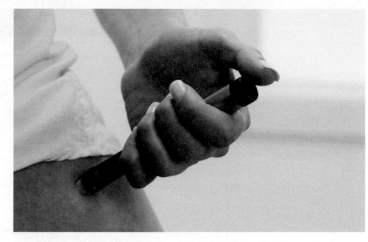

A patient injecting insulin.

First-generation sulfonylureas increase insulin release. Newer drugs with fewer side effects have been developed; as a result, these older drugs are rarely used. Second-generation sulfonylureas also work by stimulating the release of insulin.

Alpha-glucosidase inhibitors inhibit the enzyme alpha-glucosidase, interfering with hydrolysis of carbohydrates and delaying the absorption of glucose. They lower postprandial (after a meal) hyperglycemia.

Biguanides increase peripheral glucose utilization and decrease intestinal absorption of glucose.

Thiazolidinediones lower blood glucose by increasing insulin sensitivity of fat tissue, skeletal muscles, and the liver.

Non-sulfonylurea secretagogues stimulate the beta cells of the pancreas to release insulin. Like sulfonylureas, they are only effective for treatment of type 2 diabetes mellitus.

Gliptins enhance the effects of incretin, a hormone that stimulates the beta cells of the pancreas to release insulin. It also inhibits glucagon production. **TABLE 16.10** outlines some common oral hypoglycemic drugs.

Growth Disorders

Growth hormone (GH) is a mixture of amino acids that is secreted by the pituitary gland in response to **growth hormone releasing factor (GHRF)**. GHRF is secreted by the hypothalamus. Growth hormone plays an important role on carbohydrate, protein, and fat metabolism and in the growth of skeletal muscles. Children diagnosed with GH deficiency may have growth failure or serious problems relating to heart strength, lung capacity, bone density, or immune-system function. For many children with GH deficiency and growth failure, this problem can be corrected by replacement growth-hormone therapy.

Growth rates vary from child to child. Age, sex, genetic disorders, malnutrition, chronic illness, and stress are all factors that affect the growth of a child. Endocrine system and non-endocrine–related disorders such as chromosomal defects or abnormal growth of bone can also cause a delay in growth. Some children have constitutional growth delay. These children grow at a normal rate when they are younger, but then go through puberty much later than their peers. On X-ray, their bones tend to look younger than those of other normal children their age. These children will generally have a late growth spurt. Some children may be shorter than their peers because of genetics.

Human growth hormone is made by recombinant DNA technology. The younger a patient is started on growth hormone–replacement therapy and before epiphyseal fusion, the more likely he or she will be to catch up on growth. Usually, the maximum increase in height is noted within the first year of therapy. Once **epiphyseal fusion**

Table 16.10 Some Common Oral Hypoglycemic Drugs

Generic Name	Brand Name	Available Formulations
Biguanides		
Metformin	Glucophage, Glucophage XR	Tablets
	Fortamet	Tablets
	Riomet	Solution
Second-Generation Sulfonylureas		
Glimepiride	Amaryl	Tablets
Glipizide	Glucotrol, Glucotrol XL	Tablets
Glyburide	Diabeta	Tablets
	Micronase	Tablets
	Glynase Prestab	Micronized tablets
Non-sulfonylurea Secretagogues		
Nateglinide	Starlix	Tablets
Repaglinide	Prandin	Tablets
Thiazolidinediones		
Pioglitazone	Actos	Tablets
Rosiglitazone	Avandia	Tablets
Alpha-Glucosidase Inhibitors		
Acarbose	Precose	Tablets
Miglitol	Glyset	Tablets
Gliptins		
Sitagliptin	Januvia	Tablets
Other		
Exanatide	Byetta	Prefilled pen
Pramlintide	Symlin	Prefilled pen, vial

Table 16.11 Commonly Used Synthetic Human Growth Hormones

Generic Name	Brand Name	Available Formulations
Somatropin recombinant	Humatrope	Injectable

has occurred (that is, the epiphyseal plates at the end of the long bones are fused), there is little, if any, increase in growth. Treatment should be continued throughout adolescence to avoid slowing of the rate of growth. Growth hormone is not effective for some patients such as those who have a genetic predisposition to being short, Down syndrome, bone disorders, or cardiac disease. **TABLE 16.11** lists commonly used synthetic growth hormones.

Tech Math Practice

Question: **You are asked to prepare 6mL of hydrocortisone stock solution with a concentration of 5mg/mL from a 100mg/2mL hydrocortisone vial. How many milliliters of hydrocortisone are needed?**

Answer: The stock solution concentration is 100 mg/2mL. It can be further reduced by dividing both the numerator and denominator by 2, which is the common factor to yield 50mg/mL. First use the ratio proportion method: $\frac{50mg}{mL} = \frac{5mg}{xmL}$. Then cross-multiply: $xmL = 5mg \div 50mg \times 1mL = 0.1mL$. 0.1mL of hydrocortisone stock solution is needed.

Question: **How many milliliters of diluent are needed in the preceding question?**

Answer: Subtract the amount of hydrocortisone needed from the amount in the stock solution: 6mL − 0.1mL = 5.9mL of diluent.

Question: **How many milliliters of methylprednisolone 40mg/mL must be prepared to provide 30mg of methylprednisolone to the patient?**

Answer: Use the ratio-proportion method: $\frac{xmL}{30mg} = \frac{1mL}{40mg}$. Then cross-multiply: $xmL = (30mg) \times 1mL \div 40mg = 0.75mL$.

Question: **How many milligrams of diflucan are in 100mL of a 2mg/1mL solution?**

Answer: Use the ratio-proportion method: $\frac{xmg}{100mL} = \frac{2mg}{1mL}$. Then cross-multiply: $xmg = (100mL) \times 2mg \div 1mL = 200mg$.

Question: **How many grams of cortisone are present in a 500mL of a 1:500 solution?**

Answer: Use the ratio-proportion method: $\frac{xg}{500mL} = \frac{1g}{500mL}$. Then cross multiply: $xg = (500mL) \times 1g \div 500mL = 1g$ of cortisone.

Question: **A medication order calls for fluconazole 50mg tid. You are filling a 24-hour unit-dose supply for this patient. How many tablets will be needed for this patient?**

Answer: tid means three times a day. A 24-hour supply would require you to dispense three tablets for this patient.

Question: **Humatrope is supplied as a 6mg/mL injectable syringe. How many milligrams of drug are contained in 0.6mL?**

Answer: Use the ratio-proportion method: $\frac{6mg}{1mL} = \frac{xmg}{0.6mL}$. Then cross-multiply: $xmg = (6mg \times 0.6mL) \div 1mL = 3.6mg$.

WRAP UP

Chapter Summary

- The endocrine system is responsible for maintaining homeostasis.

- A negative feedback mechanism involving the hypothalamic-pituitary axis and gland helps maintain homeostasis.

- The thyroid gland produces hormones that stimulate various body tissues to increase metabolic activity.

- Hypothyroidism and hyperthyroidism are disorders of the thyroid gland. Hypothyroidism is treated with thyroid hormone-replacement therapy. Hyperthyroidism is treated with propylthiouracil or methimazole.

- Male impotence can be treated with testosterone products.

- All testosterone substances are classified as Schedule III controlled substances.

- Testosterone is responsible for male characteristics and sperm production, red blood cell production, libido, and fat distribution.

- Estrogen stimulates the development of breasts and genitals, produces endometrial growth, increases cervical mucus, and regulates the menstrual cycle.

- Progesterone prepares the uterus for implantation of the fertilized ovum. It also stimulates the development of ducts and glands of the breasts to prepare for lactation.

- Contraceptives are available in a variety of dosage forms including pills, creams, patches, implants, and rings.

- Most oral contraceptives available are a combination of an estrogen and a progestin.

- Most STDs are transmitted via sexual activity. Corticosteroids are used as anti-inflammatory and immunosuppressant drugs.

- Addison's disease and Cushing disease are disorders of the adrenal gland.

- Type 1 diabetics are treated with insulin and are usually children or young adults.

- Type 2 diabetics are usually treated with lifestyle modifications and drugs.

- A deficiency in growth hormone can cause growth failure. Replacing growth hormone before epiphyseal fusion can help a child grow to his or her natural height.

Learning Assessment Questions

1. Which of the following is the corticosteroid involved in carbohydrate, lipid, and protein metabolism?

   A. Mineralocorticoid

   B. Glucocorticoid

   C. Testosterone

   D. Estrogen

2. A deficiency of corticosteroids caused by damage to the adrenal cortex can lead to which of the following?

   A. Addison's disease

   B. Cushing disease

   C. Gluconeogenesis

   D. Hyperthyroidism

3. Growth hormone plays an important role in which of the following?

   A. Carbohydrate metabolism

   B. Growth of skeletal muscles

   C. Fat metabolism

   D. All of the above

4. Which sexually transmitted disease is also known as the "silent disease"?

   A. Chlamydia

   B. Syphilis

   C. Genital herpes

   D. HIV

5. Corticosteroids are used mainly for which of the following effects?

   A. Anti-metabolic effects

   B. Anti-inflammatory effects

   C. Renal effects

   D. Cardiac effects

6. All entries into the perpetual log book must be clearly and legibly written using which of the following?

   A. Red pen

   B. Blue pen

   C. Black pen

   D. Pencil

7. Which of the following forms is used to order Schedule II controlled substances?

   A. DEA 222 form

   B. DEA 121 form

   C. DEA 111 form

   D. DEA 150c form

8. The endocrine system is composed of which of the following glands?

   A. Thyroid

   B. Hypothalamus

   C. Pituitary

   D. All of the above

9. The thyroid gland produces and secretes which of the following?

   A. Estrogen

   B. Calcitonin

   C. Testosterone

   D. Serotonin

10. Which of the following is a condition caused by oversecretion of hormones from the thyroid gland?

    A. Hypothyroidism

    B. Hypogonadism

    C. Hyperthyroidism

    D. Diabetes mellitus

11. Symptoms of hypothyroidism include which of the following?

    A. Hoarse voice

    B. Unexplained weight gain

    C. Brittle fingernails

    D. All of the above

12. Which of the following is the hormone responsible for male sex characteristics and sperm production?

    A. Estrogen

    B. Testosterone

    C. Progestin

    D. Progesterone

13. The ovaries secrete which of the following hormones?

    A. Estrogen

    B. Progestin

    C. Progesterone

    D. Both A and B

14. Estrogen does which of the following?

    A. Stimulates the development of breasts and genitals

    B. Produces endometrial growth

    C. Regulates the menstrual cycle

    D. All of the above

15. A patient on estrogen-replacement therapy should be advised to do which of the following?

    A. Avoid smoking cigarettes

    B. Drink lots of water

    C. Take the medicine with alcohol

    D. Take the medicine only when symptomatic

16. The estrogen content of an oral contraceptive does which of the following?

    A. Suppresses production of LH

    B. Suppresses production FSH

    C. Increases production of LH

    D. Both a and b

17. Which of the following is a low-dose combination oral contraceptive that is taken for 365 days a year, without any placebo or pill-free interval?

    A. Seasonale

    B. Seasonique

    C. Lybrel

    D. Yasmin

18. Which of the following stimulates contraction of the uterine smooth muscle?

    A. Oxytocin

    B. Hydrocortisone

    C. Estrogen

    D. Progestin

19. Which of the following is the drug of choice for the treatment of type 1 diabetes?

    A. Metformin

    B. Byetta

    C. Symlin

    D. Insulin

20. Complications of diabetes include which of the following?

    A. Polyuria

    B. Polydypsia

    C. Visual changes

    D. All of the above

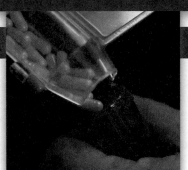

Infection Control

OBJECTIVES

After reading this chapter, you will be able to:

- Discuss the types of disease-causing pathogens.
- Understand sterilization procedures.
- Identify sources of and prevent contamination.
- Use guidelines for controlling infections.
- Recognize the importance of vaccinations for healthcare workers.
- List the guidelines for standard precautions.
- Prepare compounded sterile products.
- Summarize topical, ophthalmic, and otic medications and their uses.

KEY TERMS

Acne vulgaris
Actinic keratosis
Antiseptic
Apocrine sweat glands
Asepsis
Autoclave
Basal cell carcinoma
Candidiasis
Carbuncle
Catheter-associated
    urinary tract
    infection (CAUTI)
Cellulitis
Central line-associated
    bloodstream
    infection (CLABSI)
Cerumen
Clostridium difficile

(*C. diff*) infection
Compounded sterile
    product (CSP)
Conjunctivitis
Contamination
Dermatitis
Dermis
Disinfectant
Eccrine sweat glands
Eczema
Emollients
Epidermis
Erythema
Folliculitis
Furuncle
Germ theory of disease
Glaucoma
Hand hygiene

Handwashing
Healthcare-associated
    infection (HAI)
Hypodermis
Immunomodulatory
    agent
Impetigo
Keratoacanthoma
Keratococonjunctivitis
Melanoma
Mold
Nosocomial infection
Otalgia
Pathogens
Pediculosis
Percutaneous
    absorption
Photosensitivity

Protist	Sterilization	USP 797
Pruritis	Stratum corneum	Ventilator-associated
Ringworm	Subcutaneous tissue	pneumonia (VAP)
Sebaceous glands	Surgical site infections	Vertigo
Sebum	(SSIs)	Yeast

Chapter Overview

Sterile procedures and practices are frequently used in hospital, institutional, home health care, and community settings to reduce the risk of infection. The dangers associated with inadequate or incomplete sterilization are plenty. An understanding of the nature of infection-causing organisms is critical to applying safe sterilization procedures and implementing infection-control practices. Also, knowledge of the published guidelines will aid in adhering to proper practices that limit the risk of infection. Pharmacy technicians are integral to maintaining infection-control practices in all pharmacy settings by adhering to published guidelines and institution-specific infection-control policies. Pharmacy technicians must also uphold rigorous standards of personal and environmental cleanliness and hygiene.

The Burden of Healthcare-Associated Infections

A **healthcare-associated infection (HAI)**, also known as a **nosocomial infection**, may occur during the course of medical care. An HAI is considered to be associated with a medical intervention if it occurs at least 48 hours after hospital admission, or up to one month after surgery. (This window is extended to one year for hip-replacement surgery.) An HAI can lead to debilitating or deadly consequences for patients. Eliminating these infections is essential in healthcare today. HAIs are recognized as a critical public-health issue that demands attention.

HAIs impose a significant burden on healthcare resources. Worldwide, at least 7 million HAIs occur each year. Nearly 2 million HAIs occur each year in the United States; approximately 100,000 of these result in death. HAIs affect nearly 10 percent of hospitalized patients in developed countries. In intensive-care units, this prevalence increases to 40 percent. In developing countries, the proportion of hospitalized patients who experience HAIs is at least 25 percent.

Estimates of the direct economic costs associated with HAIs range from roughly $30 billion to $45 billion annually in the United States. Direct costs include medications, treatments, procedures, and equipment and supplies associated with the infection. Additionally, there are indirect and intangible costs, including lost wages, decreased productivity, psychological stress, and pain and suffering.

HAIs affect all patient populations, including newborns, children, and adults. Patients with compromised immune systems are particularly vulnerable to HAIs. In a hospital setting, organisms are exposed to a plethora of antibiotics, allowing them ample opportunity to develop resistance to medications. This makes

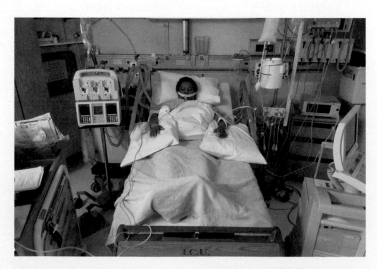

Healthcare-associated infections cause substantial morbidity, mortality, and excess healthcare costs.

HAIs even more dangerous and contributes to the public health crisis of antimicrobial resistance.

Fortunately, many HAIs are preventable. Healthcare workers can take action to prevent the spread of infectious diseases in all healthcare settings. Adherence to infection-prevention guidelines ensures safe healthcare for all patients.

Infections and Organisms

Only relatively recently have scientists completely understood the role that microorganisms play in infectious diseases. Microorganisms were recognized in the late 17th century, although their role in infection was not discovered until nearly 200 years later.

The Germ Theory of Disease

The idea that microorganisms can cause disease is called the **germ theory of disease**. In the late 19th century, Louis Pasteur originated and proved the germ theory after conducting experiments with beverage contamination. He, along with several of his contemporary scientists, also believed that microorganisms caused physical and chemical changes in the organic material they infected. Based on this belief, Pasteur proposed the idea of eliminating infections by preventing the entry of microorganisms into the human body. Pasteurization, the process of heating and cooling food and liquid to slow microbial growth, was named after Pasteur.

Joseph Lister, a surgeon in Pasteur's time, applied Pasteur's work to human medicine. He began by soaking surgical dressings in a mild phenol solution known to kill bacteria, and later developed other techniques for preventing surgical infections. Although updated, Lister's washing and gowning methods are still practiced in medicine and pharmacy today. Listerine, one of the most common brands of mouthwash in the United States, is named after Lister.

Microorganisms

Thousands of microorganisms have been identified, but not all cause disease. In fact, some are essential to healthy functioning in the human body, as in the case of bacteria in the human gastrointestinal tract that help digest food. Bacteria that do not cause harm to humans are also present in yogurt. Yeast are microorganisms used to ferment wine. However, some microorganisms are **pathogens**, or disease-causing organisms.

Bacteria

Bacteria are small, single-celled living microorganisms. They possess no nuclear membrane, mitochondria, Golgi bodies, or endoplasmic reticulum, which are all structures of the cell. Bacteria reproduce by cell division.

Bacteria are classified according to their characteristics and spatial arrangement. Bacterium exist in one of three shapes: sphere (cocci), rod (bacilli), and spiral (spirochetes). They may live as single cells or in pairs, chains, or clusters. Bacteria are sometimes identified by Gram-staining as either Gram-positive or Gram-negative,

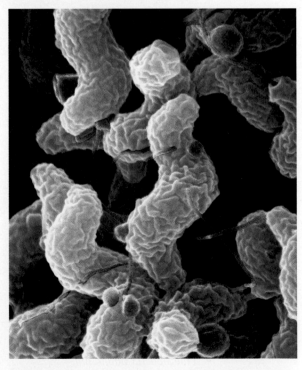

Some bacteria, such as *C. jejuni*, have a spiral or corkscrew structure.

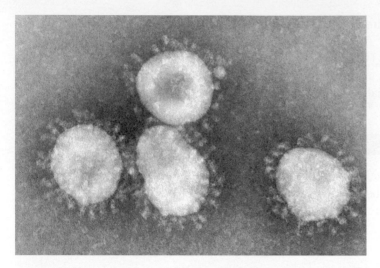

Coronaviruses have a halo or crown-like appearance when viewed under an electron microscope.

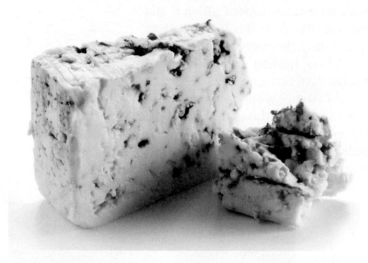

Penicillium roqueforti and *Penicillium glaucum* contribute to the flavor and texture of blue cheese.

Ten pathogens account for 84 percent of HAIs:
- Coagulase-negative *Staphylococci*
- *Staphylococcus aureus*
- *Enterococcus spp.*
- *Candida spp.*
- *Escherichia coli*
- *Pseudomonas aeruginosa*
- *Klebsiella* pneumonia
- *Enterobacter spp.*
- *Cinetobacter baumannii*
- *Klebsiella oxytoca*

distinguishable by their color under a microscope. The different colors apparent after staining are a result of structural differences in the bacterial cell wall and plasma membrane. Gram-positive cells present as a purple-blue color, while Gram-negative cells appear as a pinkish-red color.

Common infection-causing bacteria include the following:

- *Acinetobacter*
- *Burkholderia cepacia*
- *Clostridium difficile (C. diff)*
- *Clostridium sordellii*
- *Enterobacter*
- *Klebsiella*
- Methicillin-resistant *Staphylococcus aureus* (MRSA)
- *Mycobacterium abscessus*
- *Mycobacterium tuberculosis*
- *Pseudomonas aeruginosa*
- Vancomycin-resistant *Enterococci* (VRE)

Viruses

A virus is the smallest of all infectious microorganisms. It cannot be viewed except with an electron microscope. Some microbiologists (scientists who study microbes) classify viruses as microorganisms, or living things. Others do not classify viruses as living organisms, because they cannot reproduce on their own. A virus requires a host body in which to reproduce.

A virus contains either DNA or RNA (but not both) enclosed in a protein shell. Diseases caused by viruses range from simple, common illnesses to deadly infections. Viruses are discussed in full detail in the "Drug Insights" section of Chapter 7.

Common infection-causing viruses include the following:

- Herpes simplex virus
- Human immunodeficiency virus (HIV)
- Human papillomavirus (HPV)
- Influenza virus
- Measles virus
- Mumps virus
- Norovirus
- Rabies virus
- Rhinovirus

- Rotavirus
- Varicella zoster virus

Fungi

Fungi are parasitic microorganisms, living on or in other organisms. Fungi feed on dead and decaying organic material. They reproduce by producing spores that can travel through the air.

One common group of fungi is molds. Some molds are not harmful and do not cause disease. In fact, some molds are the source of antibiotics that fight disease. Others facilitate the aging of cheese and wine.

Fungi have a more complex structure than other microorganisms, and possess a well-defined nucleus, mitochondria, Golgi bodies, and endoplasmic reticulum, which are structures of the cell. As unicellular forms, fungi are called **yeast**. When they exist in a filamentous arrangement, they are called **mold**. Some fungi can exist in either form. Fungal infections are discussed in detail in Chapter 7.

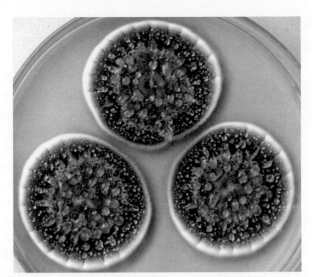

Penicillium chrysogenum is the source of penicillin-related antibiotics.

Most fungi do not cause disease. Those that do are usually opportunistic in nature, affecting primarily immunocompromised hosts. Common infection-causing fungi include the following:

- *Blastomycoses*
- *Candida*
- *Coccidioides*
- *Cryptococcus*
- *Histoplasma*

Protozoa

Protozoa are single-celled parasites, also classified as **protists** because they belong to the kingdom Protista. They are animal cells and contain a nucleus, an endoplasmic reticulum, digestive vacuoles, and organs of motility, including cilia, flagella, or pseudopods. Protozoa require a moisture-rich environment.

Common infection-causing protozoa include the following:

- *Amoeba*
- *Plasmodium*
- *Trypanosoma*

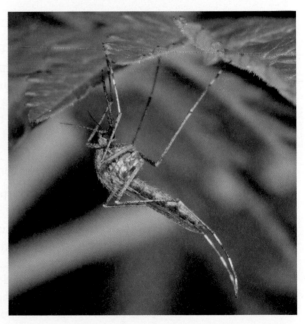

Mosquitoes transmit the malaria-causing protist *Plasmodium* to humans.

Types of Infections

HAIs are associated with a variety of procedures, instruments, and devices used in medicine. Some of the most common infections include **surgical site infections (SSIs)**, **central line-associated bloodstream infections (CLABSIs)**, **ventilator-associated pneumonia (VAP)**, **catheter-associated urinary tract infections (CAUTIs)**, and *Clostridium difficile* **(*C. diff*)** infections. These infections may result from contaminated equipment or surfaces or the unclean hands of a healthcare worker transferring microorganisms

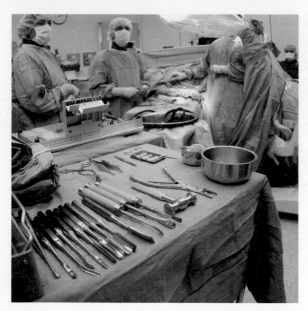

Proper sterilization of surgical instruments helps prevent SSIs.

to a patient. CLABSIs, CAUTIs, and VAP account for nearly two-thirds of all HAIs.

Surgical Site Infections (SSIs)

An SSI occurs after surgery in the part of the body where the surgery took place. Sometimes, these infections are superficial and only involve the skin. Other times, the infection involves organs, tissues, implanted material, or the bloodstream.

Surgeon technique and sterilization procedures influence the incidence of SSIs. Antibiotic prophylaxis to prevent SSIs is routine practice for many surgical procedures.

Central Line-Associated Bloodstream Infections (CLABSIs)

A central line is a tube placed in a large vein in the neck, chest, or arm to administer fluids, blood, or medications. A CLABSI occurs when infection-causing agents enter the bloodstream through a central line. The placement of a central line disrupts the integrity of the skin, making it easier for bacteria and fungi to enter the body.

Preventing CLABSIs involves proper hand hygiene, proper infection-control practices, and prompt removal of the central line when it is no longer necessary.

Ventilator-Associated Pneumonia (VAP)

A ventilator is a machine that helps a patient breathe by providing air for inflation of the lungs under positive pressure, through a tube directly into the patient's nose or mouth or through a hole in the front of the neck. VAP is an infection of the lung that develops while a patient is on a ventilator. An infection occurs when microorganisms enter the tube and travel to the patient's lungs. Poor infection control and contaminated equipment are cited as causative factors for VAP.

Catheter-Associated Urinary Tract Infection (CAUTI)

A catheter is a tube inserted into the bladder to drain urine. A CAUTI occurs when microorganisms enter the urinary tract, including the bladder and kidneys, through the catheter. The prevention of CAUTIs relies on proper technique, sterilization, and removal of catheters when they are no longer necessary.

The Centers for Medicare and Medicaid Services will not reimburse hospitals for some health-care-associated infections that are considered preventable. This forces healthcare organizations to strengthen their efforts to prevent transmission of disease and to control infections.

Clostridium Difficile (C. diff) Infections

C. difficile or C. diff is a bacterium that often grows after prolonged antibiotic use. *C. diff* infections of the gastrointestinal tract cause diarrhea and colitis. Exposure to *C. diff* often occurs from contaminated surfaces or improper hand hygiene. *C. diff* may be little more than nuisance gastrointestinal upset, but *C. diff* infections can result in death. HAIs associated with *C. diff* are increasing, and hygiene and sterilization techniques that prevent other types of HAIs may not be effective against *C. diff*.

Preventing Healthcare-Associated Infections

HAIs endanger patient health and safety. As a result, federal, state, local, and institutional programs that focus on HAI prevention are on the rise. Strategies to prevent the transmission of infectious microorganisms in a healthcare setting improve practice and increase the quality of care provided.

Harmful microorganisms are everywhere, from the air we breathe to the surfaces we touch to the food we eat and the water we drink. Controlling the presence of infection-causing agents is essential to preventing HAIs. Understanding how these microorganisms contaminate our surroundings is critical to applying proper sterile preparation techniques and following institutional policies and procedures to ensure patient safety. By making infection control a multidisciplinary priority, the spread of HAIs can be controlled through the practice of effective hygiene measures, the identification of risk factors, and responsible antibiotic use.

Contamination

Contamination is the presence of microorganisms or chemicals on or near a structure, area, person, or object. Touch is the most common means of contamination. Millions of potentially harmful microorganisms live on normal skin and under fingernails. When they exist on healthy skin, they generally do not cause harm. When introduced into the body through a catheter, a central line, a needle, or an open wound, however, these microorganisms can cause serious infections.

Hand washing is the easiest way to prevent the spread of disease and to prevent contamination of sterile surfaces by touch. Wearing gloves and hair coverings also reduces the risk of contamination by touch.

Tell patients that handwashing is the simplest way to reduce the spread of disease.

Microorganisms are found in the air, on particles of dust, and in droplets of moisture. When sterile equipment or objects are prepared, special equipment should be used to decrease the flow of air around the objects, preventing contamination as much as possible.

Water is also a source of contamination. Moisture, whether from tap water or from a body fluid, contains microorganisms that may develop into bacteria. Sterile objects and surfaces should not come in contact with potentially contaminated moisture.

If you have a respiratory tract infection, such as a cold, or are sneezing or coughing, you will likely contaminate objects, surfaces, and persons around you. Thus, you should not conduct compounding or other practices requiring sterile conditions. For the safety of your co-workers and patients, it is safest to work only when you are healthy.

Sterilization

Asepsis is the absence of infection-causing microorganisms. **Sterilization** is any process that destroys infection-causing microorganisms and brings about asepsis. Proper sterilization destroys all types of microorganisms present on an object or a surface; it is not necessary to identify the specific type of organism that may be present. Several methods of sterilization are used in hospitals, including moist-heat, dry-heat, mechanical, gas, and chemical sterilization.

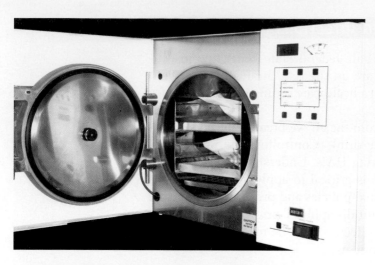

An autoclave can be used to sterilize medical equipment.

Moist-Heat Sterilization

Moist-heat sterilization is a common practice, not only in hospital settings, but in home kitchens. Submerging objects or food in boiling water for 10 minutes kills most infection-causing organisms.

An **autoclave**, a machine that generates both heat and pressure, is often used for moist-heat sterilization in hospital and institutional settings. The autoclave generates moist heat of 121°C (270°F) under pressure of 15 pounds per square inch (psi). Under these conditions, most microorganisms are destroyed in about 15 minutes. An autoclave occupies quite a large amount of space, however, and the equipment is expensive. New means of sterilization are increasing in popularity owing to these disadvantages.

Dry-Heat Sterilization

Dry-heat sterilization, such as flaming (holding a small object in the flame of a burner), destroys microorganisms. To sterilize objects with dry heat, a temperature of 170°C must be maintained for at least two hours, making the process impractical and potentially expensive. Dry heat, in the form of incineration, is used for disposing of contaminated objects.

A higher temperature is needed to sterilize with dry heat than with moist heat because liquid more easily transfers heat than dry air.

Mechanical Sterilization

Mechanical sterilization is a process that removes microorganisms from a liquid or gas by trapping them in a screen- or sieve-like device when the liquid or gas is passed through the device. Mechanical sterilization is used for heat-sensitive solutions, including culture media, enzymes, vaccines, and antibiotics. Filters are often used to prepare pharmaceutical products, both by manufacturers and when compounding individual prescriptions or medication orders.

Filters are commercially produced with a variety of pore sizes. The choice of filter depends on the microbe that needs to be removed. In pharmacy practice, 0.22 and 0.5 micron filters are used to sterilize IV solutions and ophthalmic preparations.

Gas Sterilization

Gas sterilization uses ethylene oxide to sterilize objects that are sensitive to or destroyed by heat. This process requires special equipment, techniques, and handling procedures. The gas is highly flammable and, therefore, poses a danger to operators of the equipment. Prepackaged fluids and bandages are often sterilized by this method in large manufacturing facilities.

Chemical Sterilization

Chemical sterilization destroys microorganisms on objects or surfaces using a disinfectant. Iodine, isopropyl alcohol, and chlorinated bleach are common disinfectants.

Personal Practices

Healthcare workers are instrumental in the prevention of contamination and disease transmission. Failure to adhere to guidelines, policies, and procedures directing personal practices regarding hygiene and infection control leads to higher rates of HAIs.

In a healthcare setting, all employees must follow standard precautions. In addition, each healthcare organization must have an infection-control policy for its staff in order to receive accreditation from the Joint Commission.

Standard precautions are practices employed to prevent the transmission of infection and contamination. They are based on the principle that all blood, body fluids, secretions, excretions (except sweat), non-intact skin, and mucous membranes may contain infectious

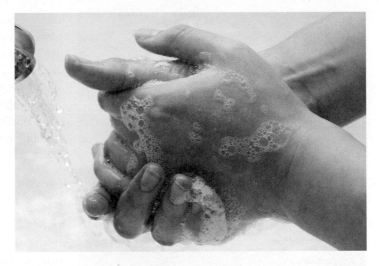

Handwashing and hand hygiene are important practices to control the spread of infection.

agents. Pharmacy workers must participate in training sessions regarding blood-borne pathogens so they not only understand various aspects of contamination, but are also aware of ways to prevent exposure and transmission of infections. For example, training includes the interpretation of room signs that indicate patient isolation (such as droplet or contact isolation) and the precautions and procedures that should be followed if access to these rooms is necessary.

Hand Hygiene

Hand hygiene is the easiest and most important method of infection control. It involves the use of alcohol-based sanitizers or washes that do not need water. These products are preferred to **handwashing** when the hands are not visibly dirty because of the superior antimicrobial action of alcohol-based products compared to soap. They are also quick, inexpensive, and easy to use. To use alcohol-based sanitizers, apply a small amount to your palm and rub your hands together, covering all surfaces of your hands and fingers with the product. Continue until hands are dry. Alcohol-based sanitizers are readily available in most hospitals, as well as in many public settings.

Jewelry and artificial nails decrease the value of hand hygiene in preventing contamination and disease transmission. Many institutions have policies advising against these types of embellishments as part of their infection-control practices. Some institutions have expanded such policies, banning white coats, ties, and even long sleeves for healthcare workers in an effort to promote infection control.

Simple handwashing prevents contamination by touch and reduces the transmission of infection-causing microorganisms. Proper hand-washing technique requires wetting the hands with warm water; scrubbing with soap to cover the hands, nails, and wrists for at least 30 seconds;

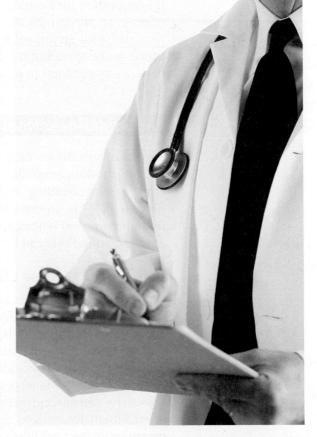

White coats have been banned in some hospitals because they are often infrequently laundered and have been found to carry disease-causing organisms.

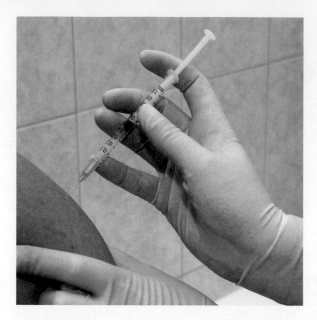

Healthcare workers are encouraged to stay up to date on vaccinations and receive an annual flu shot.

rinsing with warm water; and drying with a clean paper towel. Use a towel to turn off the faucet after your hands are clean and dry.

> To ensure an adequate length of time for handwashing, many school-aged children are taught to sing a simple song such as "Old MacDonald Had a Farm" or the alphabet song while scrubbing their hands with soap and water.

Gloves

Gloves are recommended as part of an infection-control policy because they prevent the transmission of bacteria living on the skin of healthcare workers to patients or objects. Handwashing and hand-hygiene practices may not eliminate all microorganisms, so gloves are necessary for any healthcare worker with direct patient contact or those preparing products for administration to patients. Proper hand hygiene and handwashing is still required, even if gloves are worn routinely. Gloves are often made of latex or vinyl, and both offer equal levels of protection. Gloves should be worn only once and then discarded into a designated container.

Vaccination

It is important for healthcare workers to remain up to date on their own vaccinations in order to prevent disease transmission to patients. Most hospital staff members are provided with an annual flu shot, which decreases the risk of workers getting sick, prevents the spread of the flu from healthcare workers (many of whom may not experience symptoms) to hospitalized patients, and maintains productivity.

Guidelines, Monitoring, and Research for Infection Control

Several organizations have established guidelines and requirements for sterile product preparation, surveillance procedures for monitoring infections, and prevention strategies for avoiding disease transmission. Existing prevention strategies cannot prevent all HAIs, so investment in research is critical for improving infection control. By improving surveillance, research, and communication, the infection-control goal of eliminating HAIs can be met.

Centers for Disease Control and Prevention

The Centers for Disease Control and Prevention (CDC) is a federal agency that protects public health and safety by evaluating disease prevention and control practices, promoting occupational health and safety, endorsing injury prevention, and supporting educational activities. One function of the CDC is to monitor HAI data from several sources and provide recommendations and strategies for effective infection control. The CDC is responsible for preparing and publishing reports on antibiotic sensitivity and susceptibility, drug-of-choice guidelines, dosage intervals, and lengths of treatment for various conditions. The CDC also focuses on preventing disease transmission in healthcare settings to protect both patients and healthcare workers. Guidelines regarding hand hygiene, protective clothing, and vaccinations are provided by the CDC. Although not legally binding, adherence to these guidelines and recommendations are required for accreditation and approval by evaluating agencies and government bodies.

Active Bacterial Core Surveillance

The CDC's Active Bacterial Core surveillance (ABCs) is a laboratory- and population-based monitoring system for bacterial pathogens that are potential public-health concerns. ABCs provides the infrastructure needed for identifying risk factors for bacterial disease, reviewing vaccine effectiveness, evaluating bacteria implicated in disease, and monitoring the effectiveness of prevention programs. Currently, ABCs provides surveillance for six bacteria: group A and group B *Streptococcus* (GAS, GBS), *Haemophilus influenza*, *Neisseria meningitides*, *Streptococcus pneumonia*, and MRSA.

Emerging Infections Program

The CDC partners with states and local communities to track specific pathogens and concentrate on HAI issues through the Emerging Infections Program's (EIP's) Healthcare-Associated Infection-Community (HAIC) interface. This collaborative program of 10 state health departments and academic medical centers focuses on innovation of HAI surveillance, changes in HAI epidemiology, and new clinical practices that reduce HAIs. The EIP program concentrates on coordinating reporting of HAIs, improving data collection regarding HAIs, evaluating antibiotic use and the emergence of antimicrobial resistance, and assessing the characteristics of disease-causing pathogens.

National Healthcare Safety Network

The National Healthcare Safety Network (NHSN) is a public health-surveillance system operating in all 50 states, Washington, D.C., and Puerto Rico. All types of healthcare facilities are invited to participate in NHSN: acute care hospitals, long-term–care facilities, rehabilitation centers, ambulatory surgery centers, outpatient dialysis centers, and psychiatric hospitals. NHSN facilitates the sharing of information between healthcare facilities. Under this network, data collected can be used in a timely manner to improve patient safety at local and national levels.

Surveillance for Emerging Antimicrobial Resistance Connected to Healthcare

Surveillance for Emerging Antimicrobial Resistance Connected to Healthcare (S.E.A.R.C.H.) is a voluntary surveillance network for hospitals, health departments, professional organizations, and laboratories. S.E.A.R.C.H. collects data on the occurrence of *Staphylococcus aureus* that has intermediate or complete resistance to vancomycin, known as vancomycin-intermediate *S. aureus* (VISA) or vancomycin-resistant *S. aureus* (VRSA), respectively. VISA and VRSA are emerging healthcare pathogens and growing public-health concerns.

Prevention Epicenters Program

The CDC's Prevention Epicenters Program conducts infection-control research. It coordinates investigators and innovative research across a wide spectrum of topics relevant to HAI prevention. Through this research, the CDC has made possible the validation of numerous bacterial-detection tests, exploration of emerging pathogens, confirmation of protocols for isolating and preventing contamination by healthcare pathogens, and the development of models for testing the effectiveness of disinfectants.

USP Chapter 797 Standards

Compounding of sterile products requires clean facilities and equipment, specialized training of personnel, air-quality control, and knowledge of stability and sterilization procedures. In 2004, the United States Pharmacopeia (USP) established the first enforceable requirements for the preparation of compounded sterile products. A **compounded sterile product (CSP)** is a sterile product that is prepared outside of a manufacturing facility.

CSPs include small- and large-volume injectable preparations, irrigation fluids, dialysis solutions, total parenteral nutrition, vaccines, and antitoxins.

The USP's requirements—published in Chapter 797 of the National Formulary, commonly known as **USP 797**—focus on sterility and stability of CSPs. USP 797 is designed to help protect patients from infections transmitted by pharmaceutical products and to protect staff working with CSPs. State boards of pharmacy, the Food and Drug Administration, the Joint Commission, the Pharmacy Compounding Accreditation Board, and other regulatory and accreditation bodies may support and enforce USP 797 requirements.

All pharmacy staff, including pharmacy technicians, must understand and adhere to USP 797 guidelines when compounding sterile products. Each state board of pharmacy has specific guidelines for following the minimum standards recommended in USP 797. These guidelines ensure that preparations are free of microbial contamination and patient harm is prevented. USP 797 requirements are numerous and stringent. The brief discussion provided here is only an overview; each facility or institution participating in the preparation of CSPs will have a formal training program to ensure understanding of and compliance with USP 797.

Sterility and stability are important considerations for CSPs. That is because these products are often placed in direct contact with internal body fluids and tissues where infections and complications can easily occur.

Responsibilities of Healthcare Facilities

USP 797 provides guidelines, procedures, and compliance requirements for all facilities that compound CSPs. USP 797 applies to all persons, places, and disciplines that conduct sterile compounding. The risk of contamination of CSPs is high, and the consequences could be deadly for a patient. Therefore, USP 797 requirements are quite stringent compared to requirements for compounding nonsterile products.

To meet USP 797 standards, healthcare facilities must determine the risk level of compounding completed in their facilities, perform a gap analysis to determine what compliance requirements are not being met, and develop an action plan to implement compliant compounding practices. Action plans might include things as simple as handwashing, proper gowning, or wearing gloves. They will include quality-assurance procedures, protocols for sampling sterility and stability of CSPs, procedures for cleaning spills, training requirements for personnel, or maintenance of cleaning logs.

Environmental Quality and Control

USP 797 has stringent environmental standards to control airborne contamination of CSPs. A sterile compounding room must include separate areas for gowning and washing hands, collecting supplies and drugs, and preparing CSPs. The levels of contamination allowed in each of the three sections are progressively lower.

An important piece of equipment for maintaining air quality in the clean room where CSPs are prepared is a laminar airflow workbench (LAFW). A horizontal positive-pressure LAFW is used to compound nonhazardous CSPs; a vertical negative-pressure LAFW is used to compound hazardous CSPs. The different patterns of airflow offer different levels of protection for the person compounding potentially hazardous products. A horizontal LAFW and a vertical LAFW cannot be located in the same room. LAFWs cannot be located near high-traffic areas, doorways, air vents, or any other area that could produce an air current and lead to CSP contamination.

Personal Cleansing and Gowning

To meet USP 797 standards, personnel who are compounding CSPs must remove all outerwear prior to entering the area for washing and gowning. After handwashing, personnel must don protective booties, a head covering, a gown, and a facial mask. These products must be disposable, non-shedding, and fit snuggly to the body. Hands are washed again with an alcohol-based product or chlorhexidine gluconate. Once hands are dry, sterile gloves are donned.

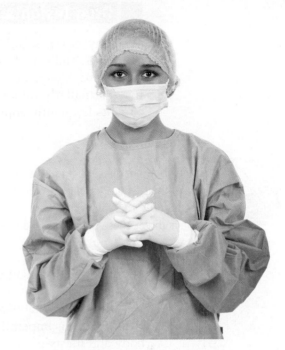

A gown, gloves, head covering, mask, and shoe covers are required for personnel preparing CSPs.

Storage and Beyond-Use Dates

USP 797 standards direct the use of a beyond-use date for CSPs. A beyond-use date identifies the time by which the preparation must be used to avoid chemical degradation, instability, or contamination. It is an estimate of the risk level of contamination of a specific product. In contrast, an expiration date provided by a manufacturer is the manufacturer's estimate of a product's shelf life. Beyond-use dates are based on the stability, sterility, risk level, and storage conditions of a CSP. Each institution or facility can set its own beyond-use dates based on reliable testing, but most facilities use the USP recommendations for establishing beyond-use dates. The USP recommendations are presented in **TABLE 17.1**.

Low-risk preparations are CSPs prepared entirely under sterile conditions using proper aseptic technique; preparations that involve only the transfer, measuring, or mixing of closed or sealed packages; single sterile product transfers; or manually mixing and measuring no more than three ingredients for an admixture. A single, sterile ingredient placed into a delivery system is a low-risk preparation. Medium-risk preparations are CSPs involving multiple small doses of sterile ingredients, complex manipulations, or an unusually long duration of compounding. TPN is a medium-risk preparation. High-risk preparations are CSPs that involve nonsterile ingredients, sterile ingredients exposed to air contaminants, or nonsterile products that are stored more than six hours before sterilization. An epidural is a high-risk preparation.

Table 17.1 USP Beyond-Use Date Recommendations Based on Risk Level of Contamination and Storage Conditions

	Low-Risk Preparations	Medium-Risk Preparations	High-Risk Preparations
Controlled room temperature (< 25°C/ < 77°F)	48 hours	30 hours	24 hours
Refrigerator (2–8°C/36–46°F)	14 days	7 days	3 days
Freezer (< –20°C/< –4°F)	45 days	45 days	45 days

Drug Insights: Topical, Ophthalmic, and Otic Medications

A variety of types and formulations of drugs are available to treat disorders of the skin, eyes, and ears. Disorders range from acute pain to seasonal allergies to chronic conditions. Many of these products are available as over-the-counter (OTC) products. It is particularly important for pharmacy technicians to be familiar with these, as patients frequently approach community pharmacies for help in choosing a self-care product.

Remember, pharmacy technicians may not counsel patients. Pharmacy technicians may not discuss drug therapy or health-related questions. Always direct these questions to a pharmacist.

Anatomy and Physiology of Skin

The skin is the largest organ in the human body, accounting for more than 10 percent of body weight. The skin acts as a barrier, protecting the body from chemical, physical, and microbial injury. The skin also acts as the body's main source of sensory input and is the primary organ for temperature regulation.

Skin is remarkably resilient and is the human body's primary defense mechanism. Healthy skin is imperative, not only for aesthetic value, but for maintaining a healthy body and lifestyle.

Skin Regions

The skin is divided into three regions **FIGURE 17.1** that have distinct components and functions:

- Epidermis—The **epidermis** is the outermost layer of skin. It contains compact, stratified squamous epithelial cells. The epidermis lacks blood supply. The epidermis is continually shedding dead, dry cells and producing new, healthy cells. The epidermis produces glands, nails, and hair. The **stratum corneum** is the outermost layer of the epidermis, and is the layer of cells exposed to the environment. The stratum corneum is composed of between 10 and 20 percent water by weight, and its water content affects its flexibility. Water content is influenced by humidity, temperature, or physical or chemical trauma. When water content falls below 10 percent, the stratum corneum becomes chapped, or dry and brittle, and cracks easily. Any such loss of integrity of the outer layer of skin exposes the body to infection from pathogens or contamination from other irritants.
- Dermis—The **dermis** is the second layer of skin. It is 40 times thicker than the epidermis. The dermis supports the epidermis and separates it from the lower layers of skin. The dermis is composed of elastic and connective tissue, and contains blood vessels and nerves. The dermis is responsible for sensory input.
- Hypodermis—The **hypodermis**, also known as **subcutaneous tissue**, is the innermost layer of the skin. It contains loose connective tissue and fatty tissue firmly anchored to the dermis. The fatty component of the hypodermis facilitates temperature control, maintains food reserves, and provides cushioning for the body.

Skin Functions

The most important function of the skin is to serve as a barrier between the body and the external environment. The skin's ability to protect the body depends on the condition and integrity of the skin, which is influenced by factors such as age, im-

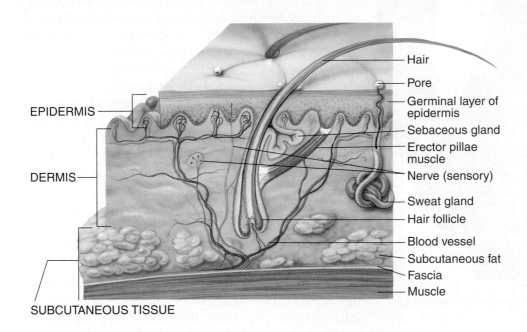

EPIDERMIS

DERMIS

SUBCUTANEOUS TISSUE

Hair
Pore
Germinal layer of epidermis
Sebaceous gland
Erector pillae muscle
Nerve (sensory)
Sweat gland
Hair follicle
Blood vessel
Subcutaneous fat
Fascia
Muscle

FIGURE 17.1 The structure of human skin.

munologic status, other diseases or medical conditions, medications, and any other disorders that affect the structure of the stratum corneum.

The skin contributes to sensory input, temperature control, pigment development, emotional expression, and vitamin D synthesis. The skin also controls the loss of moisture from the body and moisture penetration into the body.

The skin contains **sebaceous glands** and **sweat glands**. Sebaceous glands secrete an oily substance (**sebum**) that prevents the skin and hair from becoming too dry. Sebum is also toxic to some bacteria, offering an additional layer of protection from infection. Two types of sweat glands are located in the skin. **Eccrine sweat glands** produce sweat containing water and salts. **Apocrine sweat glands** are located deeper in the skin than eccrine glands and produce sweat that contains organic material. Sweat produced by apocrine glands generates an odor when it is broken down by bacteria on the skin. Apocrine glands located in the skin of the external ear canal produce **cerumen**, a wax-like substance that plays host to antibacterial and antifungal activity.

Hair and nails are appendages of the skin. They protect the skin from damage and are important in the healthy functioning of skin.

Absorption of Drugs

The health and integrity of the skin influence the absorption and onset of action of topical medications. All topical formulations of drugs require release of the drug, and absorption and distribution to the site of action. Drugs may be intended for treatment of disorders of the layers of skin itself, or for distribution to systemic circulation. Absorption through the stratum corneum is often the rate-limiting step in the absorption of drugs through the skin, since it acts as a barrier to **percutaneous absorption** (absorption through the skin). Because it does not contain blood vessels, absorption through the stratum corneum takes place by passive diffusion (the movement of biochemicals and substances across the cell membrane). Once through this outermost protective

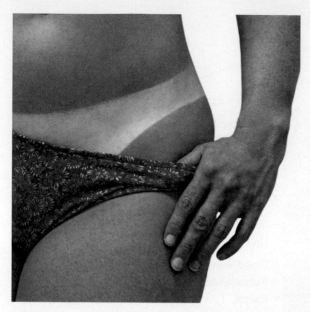

Exposure to the UV radiation from the sun can lead to sunburn on unprotected skin.

layer of skin, the blood supply in the dermis and subcutaneous tissue facilitate drug absorption and distribution.

Hydration aids in diffusion through the stratum corneum. Inflammation also increases diffusion through the stratum corneum, so caution should be advised in applying topical preparations to inflamed or irritated skin. Particularly if large surface areas are involved, an increase in drug absorption could lead to unwanted or hazardous side effects.

Common Skin Disorders and Treatments

An estimated 5 percent of Americans suffer from chronic skin, hair, or nail conditions that require treatment. Countless more suffer from infrequent acute or seasonal conditions. A majority of people aged 65 years or older have two or more skin conditions.

Dermatitis is a nonspecific term describing any condition of the skin characterized by redness, or **erythema**, and inflammation. The terms "dermatitis" and "**eczema**" are used interchangeably. Dermatitis is often used to describe inflammatory conditions of the skin of unknown origin. However, if the cause of the inflammation or irritation is known, the type of dermatitis will be indicated.

Sun-Induced Disorders

Ultraviolet (UV) radiation is produced by the sun. Both UV-A and UV-B radiation damage the epidermis. Repeated exposure to UV radiation causes cumulative damage to the skin and may lead to premature aging of the skin and skin cancer. The most effective way to reduce the risks of UV radiation is to avoid excessive sun and UV radiation exposure. Sunscreens are available to protect the skin from the effects of UV-A and UV-B rays when sun exposure is necessary.

The most common sun-related skin disorder is sunburn. It is most often a first-degree or superficial burn and is accompanied by redness, pain, tenderness, and edema. Avobenzone, titanium dioxide, and zinc oxide are topical preparations that prevent UV radiation from damaging the skin. Applying these products to the skin prior to sun exposure will reduce the incidence of sunburn.

The sun protection factor (SPF) is an indicator of the effectiveness of sunscreens. The SPF is determined by comparing the amount of radiation that causes erythema on skin protected with sunscreen to the amount of radiation that causes the same amount of erythema on unprotected skin. If the dose of radiation required to induce redness is 10 times higher with the sunscreen than without, the product will be designated with an SPF of 10. The higher the SPF, the more protection the product offers and the more effective the product is at preventing sunburn.

Photosensitivity is an abnormal sensitivity to light, and can include an increased sensitivity of the skin to sunlight. Many drugs cause photosensitivity, so patients should be advised to use caution when taking these medications because the risk of sun-induced skin disorders is high. Other medical conditions, soaps, plants, and cosmetics may also induce photosensitivity.

A list of common photo-sensitivity-inducing drugs follows:

- Antidepressants—These include amitriptyline, clomipramine, doxepin, imipramine, nortriptyline, and trazodone.
- Antihistamines—These include brompheniramine, chlorpheniramine, clemastine, cyproheptadine, dimenhydrinate, diphenhydramine, doxylamine, hydroxyzine, meclizine, and promethazine.
- Antihypertensives—These include captopril, diltiazem, enalapril, hydralazine, labetalol, lisinopril, minoxidil, and nifedipine.
- Antipsychotics—These include chlorpromazine, fluphenazine, haloperidol, perphenazine, thioridazine, and thiothixene.

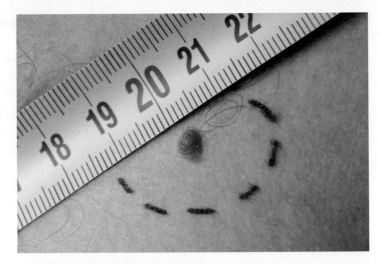

Melanoma may appear as a small lesion on the skin.

- Diuretics—These include acetazolamide, chlorothiazide, chlorthalidone, furosemide, hydrochlorothiazide, metolazone, and triamterene.
- Estrogens/progestins—These include estradiol, ethinyl estradiol, medroxyprogesterone, norethindrone, and norgestrol, which is available in combination forms.
- Fluroquinolones—These include ciprofloxacin, levofloxacin, norfloxacin, and ofloxacin.
- Hypoglycemics—These include acetohexamide, chlorpropamide, glipizide, lyburide, and tolbutamide.
- NSAIDs—These include diclofenac, fenoprofen, ibuprofen, indomethacin, ketoprofen, naproxen, piroxicam, sulindac, and tolmetin.
- Sulfonamides—These include sulfadiazine, sulfmethoxazole, sulfasalazine, and sulfisoxazole.
- Tetracyclines—These include demeclocycline, doxycycline, minocycline, and tetracycline.

Skin cancer can occur after prolonged exposure to damaging UV radiation. Several types of skin cancer are recognized. **Actinic keratosis** is a precancerous condition that results from overexposure to the sun. It is characterized by scaly lesions on the skin. **Basal cell carcinoma** is a slow-growing tumor that rarely metastasizes. **Keratoacanthoma** is an epithelial tumor that exhibits initially rapid growth, but then regresses and heals. **Melanoma** is a highly malignant cancer; sunburn significantly increases the risk of developing melanoma. Preventing unnecessary exposure to UV radiation is the best way to prevent skin cancer. Frequent self-checks of the skin is an important early-detection tool for all types of skin cancer. Once skin cancer is diagnosed, it must be treated by a dermatologist or an oncologist.

Take care to place warning labels on medications that may cause photosensitivity: "Avoid Prolonged Exposure to the Sun." Advise patients to use sunscreen regularly while taking these drugs.

Treating sun-damaged skin improves the skin's condition by restoring hydration and skin integrity and decreasing pain and inflammation associated with sunburn. The most common topical drugs used to treat sun-damaged skin include aloe gel, hydrocortisone, benzocaine, and lidocaine. Aloe gel has soothing, cooling properties, and also promotes wound healing. In addition, it has antibacterial and antifungal properties. Hydrocortisone is a topical corticosteroid that decreases inflammation and aids in pain relief. Benzocaine and lidocaine are topical anesthetics that provide temporary pain relief.

ABCs of Skin-Cancer Detection

An easy-to-use mnemonic device helps patients remember how to complete self-checks for skin cancer detection:

- A is for "asymmetry"—A skin-cancer lesion will have varied size, shape, or color. A benign mole or discoloration on the skin will appear symmetrical and uniform in size, shape, and color.
- B is for "border"—The edges of a skin-cancer lesion will be uneven or blurry.
- C is for "color"—Skin-cancer lesions will not have a uniform or consistent color throughout the lesion.
- D is for "diameter"—Most melanomas are at least ¼ of an inch in diameter, approximately the size of a pencil eraser.
- E is for "evolving"—Skin-cancer lesions will change over time. Patients should be advised to note changes in their skin, including changes in size, color, shape, or elevation of skin lesions, or the appearance of new symptoms such as bleeding, crusting, or itching.

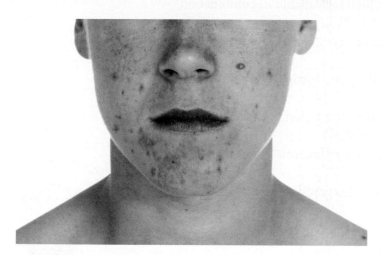

Acne lesions most commonly appear on the face.

Acne

Acne vulgaris results from increased secretions from the sebaceous glands. This gives the skin an oily appearance. Its severity fluctuates as a result of stress. Due to the increased activity of the glands in puberty, acne is most often linked to this age group. However, acne can affect people of any age. Acne is not a direct threat to physical health, but it can have devastating effects on mental and psychosocial health.

Papular lesions associated with acne are most common on the head, face, and neck, but can affect other parts of the body. A blackhead forms when the duct of a sebaceous gland becomes blocked due to excess sebum production. The gland and the hair follicle then become enlarged with sebum, forming a papule. If the papule becomes infected with *P. acnes*, a pustule will form, surrounded by redness and inflammation.

The goal of acne treatment is to prevent the ducts of the sebaceous glands from becoming blocked with sebum. Cleansing skin with mild soap and water can help maintain skin that is free of lesions. In cases of moderate to severe acne that do not respond to simple cleansing regimens, topical or systemic antibiotics may be initiated to control the growth of *P. acnes*. Several antibiotics may be used, including several of the tetracyclines, erythromycin, and sulfamethoxazole/trimethoprim. Oral contraceptives are also frequently prescribed to female patients as part of a regimen to control hormone fluctuations that exacerbate acne.

Common acne medications are presented in **TABLE 17.2**. All the products presented are only available by prescription, with the exception of benzoyl peroxide, which is available OTC.

Table 17.2 Common Acne Treatments		
Generic name	**Brand name**	**Dosage Forms Available**
Adapalene	Differin	Cream, gel, topical solution
Azelaic acid	Azelex	Cream
Azithromycin	Zithromax	Injection, oral liquid, tablet
Benzoyl peroxide	Brevoxyl, Zoderm	Cream, lotion, soap
Clindamycin-benzoyl peroxide	BenzaClin	Gel
Tetracycline	Sumycin	Capsule, suspension, tablet
Tretinoin	Retin-A	Capsule, cream, gel, topical solution

Atopic Dermatitis and Dry Skin

Atopic dermatitis is most commonly seen in infants, children, and young adults. It is the most common skin condition that occurs in children. In adults, atopic dermatitis usually occurs with other skin conditions, such as dry skin, hand dermatitis, and contact dermatitis.

Atopic dermatitis is often a manifestation of an allergy. Many patients with atopic dermatitis experience seasonal allergies, asthma, or chronic allergic rhinitis. Soaps, detergents, chemicals, temperature changes, mold, dust, pollen, or emotional stress can worsen atopic dermatitis. Patients with atopic dermatitis are often very sensitive to irritants and allergens.

Atopic is a term used to describe any condition with a hereditary or genetic component.

Atopic dermatitis often appears as redness and chapping of the cheeks, but may also affect the face, neck, and torso. Classically, infants experience atopic dermatitis beginning at age two to three months, and the condition usually resolves between two and four years of age. When atopic dermatitis occurs later in life, the redness and dryness appears on flexor surfaces (knees, elbows, or the collar area of the neck). Lesions are usually symmetrical. Atopic dermatitis is accompanied by intense **pruritus** (itching). The constant itching and scratching is associated with discomfort, and can damage the skin to the point of causing inflammation, open wounds, and infection.

Dry skin can be caused by numerous factors, including occupational and environmental exposures. Patients may not consume enough water, or may bathe too frequently or bathe with water that is too hot or with soaps that remove too much oil from the body, all of which decrease skin hydration. Dry skin is more common in older people because as the skin ages, the epidermis becomes thinner and rougher, unable to retain moisture. Also, hormonal changes decrease the amount of sebum produced by the body, decreasing natural lubrication of the skin. Arid, windy, or cold environments also increase the occurrence of dry skin.

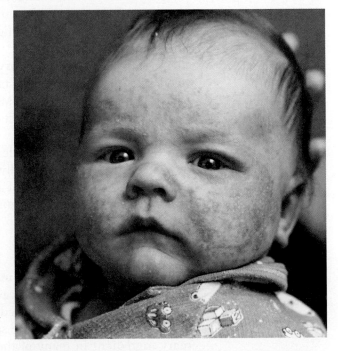

Atopic dermatitis often appears during infancy or childhood.

Dry skin may cause a mild itch, or it may progress to roughness, scaling, loss of flexibility, inflammation, or severe pruritus. As with atopic dermatitis, this decrease in skin health can lead to open wounds or infections. The goals of atopic-dermatitis and dry-skin treatments are to maintain skin hydration, relieve or minimize symptoms of itching, and avoid factors that aggravate these conditions.

Numerous OTC products are available to restore skin's hydration. Bath oils, oatmeal soaks, and gentle cleansers containing myriad ingredients are commonly used. The effectiveness of one type of product over another has not been proved; patient preference is important in selecting such a product. **Emollients**, most of which contain mineral oil or petrolatum, should be applied frequently to maintain skin hydration and flexibility.

Excessive bathing with soap and water may increase skin dryness and aggravate atopic dermatitis or dry skin.

Topical hydrocortisone is available without a prescription to treat dermatitis and dry skin. It is a corticosteroid that reduces redness, swelling, heat, pain, and itch associated with several skin disorders. Hydrocortisone is available in cream and ointment preparations. It is available without a prescription concentrations of 0.5 percent and 1 percent. (Higher concentrations are available by prescription.) It should be applied sparingly to the affected area three to four times daily. Hydrocortisone can mask the symptoms of a dermatologic infection, so confirm that the area intended for application is not infected before use. If the skin does not improve after seven days of hydrocortisone treatment, the patient should seek medical advice.

Other topical corticosteroids are available to treat the redness, swelling, and itching associated with dermatitis, dry skin, and various other skin conditions. All corticosteroids should be used sparingly and applied to the affected area as a thin film. Systemic absorption of corticosteroids can lead to suppression of the hypothalamic-pituitary axis (HPA). HPA is a set of interactions in the endocrine system that respond to stress and regulate body functions like digestion, immune function, and metabolism. So, the lowest-potency formulations that are effective should be used, and products should not be used for more than two weeks. HPA suppression leads to decreased levels of cortisol; symptoms include fatigue, depression, weight loss, immune system dysfunction, and sleep disturbances.

Topical corticosteroids vary greatly in their potency, delivery system, and effectiveness. Low-potency products are used to treat areas where the skin is thin, such as the face, armpits, or genitals. Medium-potency products are used on the trunk, arms, or legs. High-potency products should be reserved for skin conditions that do not respond to other treatments.

Most products are available as a cream and an ointment, and some are available as gels or foams. Creams generally have a lower potency than ointments; the potency of gels is usually between that of a cream and an ointment. Other than hydrocortisone, all topical corticosteroids require a prescription. Common topical corticosteroids are listed in **TABLE 17.3**.

Viral Infections

Warts and cold sores are the most common skin disorders caused by viruses. Warts are a tumor of the epidermis caused by a virus. Genital warts are a sexually transmitted disease. Warts are removed surgically or by freezing with liquid nitrogen. OTC products are available for the self-treatment of small warts. Salicylic acid is the primary ingredient in many of these products. However, newer products are available for removal by freezing.

Table 17.3 Common Topical Corticosteroids

Generic Name	Brand Name	Dosage Forms Available
Aclometasone	Aclovate	Cream, ointment
Amcinonide	Cyclocort	Cream, lotion, ointment
Betamethasone	Beta-Val, Diprolene, Diprosone, Luxiq	Cream, foam, lotion, ointment
Clobetasol	Clobex, Temovate, Olux	Cream, ointment, foam
Diflorasone	Florone, Psorcon	Cream, ointment
Fluocinolone	Capex, Synalar	Cream, ointment
Fluticasone	Cutivate	Cream, lotion, spray, ointment
Halcinonide	Halog	Cream, ointment
Mometasone furoate	Elocon	Cream, ointment
Triamcinolone	Kenalog	Cream, lotion, ointment

A combination of dimethyl ether and propane (Wartner) is also available to remove warts. It is available as an aerosol device that contains propane and is a form of cryotherapy. If used correctly, this product is as effective as the cryotherapy completed in physician's offices.

Imiquimod (Aldara) is a prescription-only product that is approved to remove external perianal and genital warts. Imiquimod is an immunomodulator.

Cold sores are caused by the herpes simplex 1 virus (HSV1). HSV1 and another member of the herpes simplex family, HSV2, also cause genital warts, commonly transmitted by sexual contact. Most cases of genital herpes are caused by HSV2. Most people are infected with HSV1, but it usually remains dormant in the body. An outbreak of the virus, evidenced by cold sores on the face, may be triggered by stress, hormonal changes, environmental factors, or sun exposure. The herpes simplex virus is highly contagious and can be spread by sharing personal items or from close contact with the infected area during an outbreak. Cold sores may be mild and cause little pain, or they may appear in severe, recurrent outbreaks accompanied by pain and fever.

Untreated, cold sores will resolve in one to two weeks. Oral antiviral medications, including acyclovir, famciclovir, and valacyclovir, are available for the systemic treatment of herpes simplex virus. Docosanol (Abreva) is a topical OTC product that treats cold sores. If applied at the first signs of a sore, it blocks the virus from invading other cells. Docosanol must be applied five times daily.

Fungal Infections

Fungal skin infections are among the most common skin disorders. **Candidiasis** is a common fungal infection caused by *Candida albicans* that usually occurs in the mouth, where it is known as thrush, or in the vagina. Clotrimazole and miconazole are effective for treating candidiasis. Nystatin, frequently prescribed as a mouth rinse, can also be used for thrush. It may be swallowed or spit out of the mouth, depending on the prescriber's instructions and the indication for use.

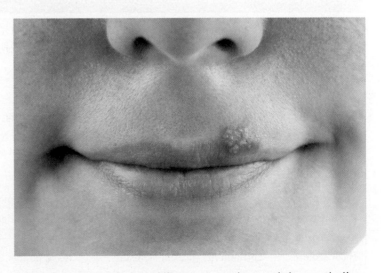

Cold sores appear as lesions, blisters, or a rash around the mouth, lips, and gums.

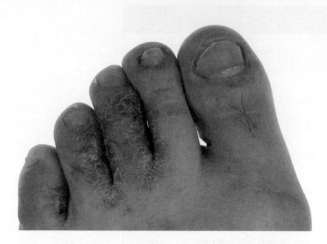

Tinea pedis, also known as athlete's foot, causes red, scaly patches of skin.

Ringworm (tinea) is a common infection that produces a characteristic ring structure on the skin, although the infection may also produce large, scaly, dry patches of skin. There may also be blistering, oozing discharge, or encrustations of the damaged skin. Ringworm infections are usually superficial and affect the hair, nails, and skin. Tinea infections are named for the areas of the body they affect: tinea capitis (scalp), tinea cruris (groin), tinea corporis (body), tinea pedis (feet), and tinea unguium (nails). Tinea infections are usually caused by one of three fungi: *Trichophyton*, *Microsporum*, or *Epidermophyton*. The term *ringworm* is a misnomer, as the infectious organism is not a worm, but a fungus. The name is derived from the characteristic red rings that look like worms underneath the surface of the skin.

Tinea infections affect nearly one-quarter of the United States population at any one time. Simple, brief exposure to a fungal pathogen can lead to an infection, and broken, damaged, or unhealthy skin significantly increases the risk of infection.

The goals of treatment of tinea infections are to provide symptom relief, cure the existing infection, and prevent future infections. Tinea pedis, tinea corporis, and tinea cruris can usually be resolved with OTC self-treatment. Tinea unguium and tinea capitis should be evaluated by a physician. Common treatments for tinea infections, as well as the conditions they treat, are presented in **TABLE 17.4** .

Most antifungals stop the growth of the infecting fungus, but terbinafine and butenafine kill the fungus.

Table 17.4 Common Treatments for Tinea Infections

Generic Name	Brand Name	Dosage Form	Conditions
Griseofulvin	Fulvicin-U, Fulvicin-F, Grifulvin V	Oral suspension, tablet	Tinea capitis, tinea corporis, tinea unguium
Butenafine	Lotrimin Ultra, Mentax	Cream	Tinea corporis, tinea cruris, tinea pedia
Terbinafine	Lamisil	Cream, gel, oral granules, topical spray, tablet	Tinea corporis, tinea cruris, tinea pedia
Clotrimazole	Lotrimin AF	Cream, topical solution	Tinea cruris, tinea pedis, candidiasis
Ciclopirox	Penlac, Loprox	Cream, gel, shampoo, topical solution, topical suspension	Tinea unguium
Itraconazole	Sporanox	Capsule, oral liquid, IV injection	Tinea unguium
Ketoconazole	Nizoral	Shampoo	Tinea capitis
Miconazole	Lotrimin AF, Micatin, Monistat	Cream, powder, spray	Tinea cruris, tinea pedis, candidiasis
Tolnaftate	Tinactin Antifungal, Lamisil AF	Cream, powder, spray	Tinea cruris

Bacterial Infections

Bacterial infections affecting the skin occur as a result of improper wound healing or as a primary infectious disease. Some minor infections can be self-treated with OTC products, but many require systemic antibiotics to cure the infection.

Impetigo is a superficial skin infection. It is highly contagious and common among children. It is especially prevalent in warm, humid climates, and among populations with poor hygiene. Elderly and immunocompromised patients may also be affected. Impetigo causes redness, blisters, and encrustations of the skin. It is often caused by *Staphylococcus* or *Streptococcus* bacteria. Small lesions can be treated

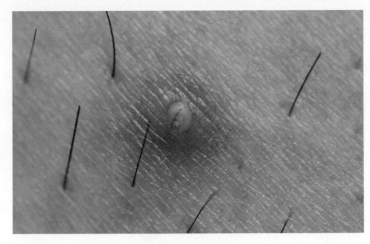

Folliculitis is the inflammation of a hair follicle.

with topical antibiotics, but large or widespread lesions require systemic antibiotics. Mupirocin (Bactroban) is a topical cream or ointment that is effective for impetigo.

Cellulitis is a bacterial skin infection that produces redness, warmth, swelling, and pain. The infection can spread rapidly, and can lead to serious systemic infections if left untreated. Systemic antibiotics are required for cellulitis. It is often caused by *Staphylococcus* or *Streptococcus* bacteria, and antibiotic selection is based on local sensitivity data and patient factors. (Antibiotic selection is described in detail in the "Drug Insights" section of Chapter 6.)

Folliculitis is the inflammation of a hair follicle. It produces a red nodule, but is not usually associated with pain. In healthy individuals, mild folliculitis resolves on its own or with mild topical treatment. A **furuncle**, more commonly known as a boil, is an infection of the sebaceous gland and hair follicle, usually caused by *Staphylococcus* bacteria. It is a deeper, more widespread infection than folliculitis. Furuncles are associated with itching, redness, and swelling. Local pain and pus formation accompany a furuncle. A **carbuncle** is a group of infected hair follicles. Carbuncles signify a deeper and more widespread infection than furuncles. Pain, redness, swelling, drainage, fever, and systemic toxicity are possible. Treatment of moderate to severe folliculitis, furuncles, and carbuncles requires systemic antibiotic therapy.

External Parasites

Pediculosis is an infestation of lice. Lice are wingless parasites with well-developed legs. Lice use the human body as a host and receive nourishment from human blood. Different species of lice infect the body (*Pediculosis humanus corporis*), the head (*Pediculosis humanus capitus*), or the pubic area (*Phthirus pubis*). Lice are spread by direct contact with an infested person's head, body, or personal items. Lice generally do not spread disease, but do cause intense itching and discomfort.

Head lice are the most common type of pediculosis and occur most frequently in school-aged children. Body lice are larger than head lice and infest people who do not change their clothes frequently, such as homeless people or soldiers on extended military campaigns. Public lice are also known as crab lice, and infest people from all geographic and demographic regions, as well as all levels of hygiene. In addition to the pubic area, these lice may infest armpits, eyelashes, mustaches, beards, and eyebrows. Pubic lice may be transmitted during sexual contact.

The goal of treatment of a pediculosis infection is to rid the host of lice and their eggs. A pediculicide, several of which are available as OTC products, is applied to the

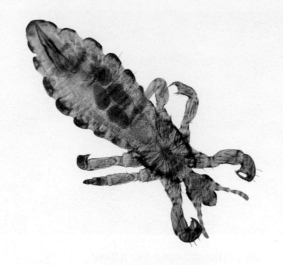

A photomicrograph of *Pediculosis humanus capitus*.

affected area of the body and left in place for a specified amount of time. The hair or body is then combed or cleaned to remove the dead or dying lice and eggs. The treatment should be repeated after seven to 10 days to rid the body of any newly hatched lice. Avoiding future infestations requires cleaning all clothing, bedding, and objects that came in contact with the infested person and not sharing personal items with other people.

A combination of pyrethrum and piperonyl butoxide (Pronto, Rid) is an OTC pediculicide, available as a shampoo, gel, and spray. Pyrethrum is an extract from the chrysanthemum seed and a natural insecticide. Although pyrethrum is extremely non-toxic, patients with allergies to ragweed may be sensitive to pyrethrum. Permethrin (Nix) is an alternative OTC pediculicide available as a cream or lotion. Permethrin (Elimite) is a stronger formulation and is prescription only. Permethrin kills lice for up to 14 days after its initial application.

Lindane is a shampoo or lotion used to treat all varieties of pediculosis. This drug is only available as a prescription and should be reserved for infestations that do not respond to OTC products.

Antiseptics and Disinfectants

An **antiseptic** is a substance that inhibits the growth of infection-causing microorganisms. It does not necessarily kill them. A **disinfectant** is a chemical applied to an object or surface to remove microorganisms. The goal of antiseptics and disinfectants is to prevent the spread of infectious agents. These agents may be applied to instruments, work surfaces, or body areas.

Following are several examples of antiseptics and disinfectants:

- Isopropyl alcohol is available in many strengths, but the 90-percent solution is the only one effective as an antiseptic and disinfectant. It can be used safely on a variety of surfaces, including the body. Isopropyl alcohol removes most bacteria, but also kills some bacteria. It is effective at cleaning minor wounds, although it produces a stinging sensation when applied to broken skin.

- Sodium hypochlorite (Clorox bleach) is commonly used in household cleaning to kill microorganisms, deodorize surfaces, and remove stains. It can also be used to clean surfaces and floors in the pharmacy.

- Hexachlorophene (pHisoHex) is a surgical scrub that inhibits the growth of bacteria on the skin. It is particularly effective against gram-positive bacteria.

- Povidone-iodine (Betadine) is a wound-cleaning solution with rapid antimicrobial activity. It is the most effective disinfectant available and does not cause stinging or burning when applied to wounds. It is effective against a wide variety of pathogens, including bacteria, fungi, viruses, and protozoa.

- Zinc oxide is a topical mild astringent that also has weak antiseptic properties. It is used to treat minor skin irritations, including those caused by diaper rash.

- Hydrogen peroxide is an inexpensive, effective disinfectant. It is used to clean open wounds and is often used to cleanse oral cavities prior to dental procedures. When hydrogen peroxide is applied to a surface, oxygen is released, which produces the antiseptic activity. Hydrogen peroxide is the most commonly used first-aid antiseptic.

- Chlorhexidine gluconate (Hibiclens) is a topical antimicrobial agent used as a surgical scrub, hand cleanser, wound irrigant, and oral dental rinse called Perio-Guard, which is used to treat gingivitis and periodontitis. It is effective against both gram-negative and gram-positive bacteria, as well as yeast.

- Carbamide peroxide, like hydrogen peroxide, releases oxygen on contact with tissues. It is used as an antiseptic agent in dental procedures, and to treat oral ulcers and dental sores. It can also be used to treat topical sores and to cleanse wound areas.

Common Eye Conditions and Treatments

The location and exposure of the eye make it susceptible to contamination and infection. However, the eye has protective mechanisms to prevent the entry of foreign bodies into the eye and to maintain the health and comfort of the eye. See **FIGURE 17.2** for an illustration of the structure of the human eye.

Many otic products available to treat conditions or disorders of the eye must be instilled directly into the eye, either as a drop of solution or suspension or as an ointment. Proper procedures for instilling eye drops and ointments into the eye must be followed for maximum effectiveness. Patients must be aware that the tip of the dropper or tube must remain clean. As always, direct the pharmacist to counsel patients more if they do not understand the directions on the label or package. To prevent the spread of infection, the bottle or dropper should never come in direct contact with the eye. Also, eye preparations should never be shared. Contact lenses should be removed before placing eye drops or ointments in the eye.

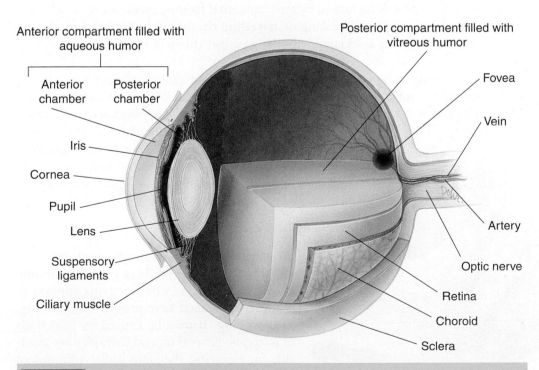

FIGURE 17.2 A cross-section of the human eye.

Steps for Instilling Eye Drops

1. Wash hands thoroughly.
2. Tilt head back and gently pull down on the lower eyelid.
3. Place dropper directly over the eye. Be careful not to touch the surface of the eye with the dropper.
4. Instill a drop into the pocket of the eyelid.
5. Slowly release the lower eyelid and close the eye. Minimize blinking or squeezing the eyelid for several minutes.
6. If more than one drop is required, wait five minutes in between drops to ensure that the first drop is not washed away by subsequent drops.

Steps for Applying Ointment to the Eye

1. Wash hands thoroughly.
2. Tilt head back and gently pull down on the lower eyelid.
3. Place tube of ointment directly over the eye. Be careful not to touch the surface of the eye with the tube.
4. Squeeze a ribbon of ointment from the tube and let it fall into the pocket of the eyelid.
5. Slowly release the lower eyelid and close the eye. Gently roll the eye around to distribute the ointment.

Chronic Dry Eye

Chronic dry eye (**keratococonjunctivitis**) is one of the most common disorders affecting the eye. It affects more than 4,000,000 people in America. With this condition, the eye is not able to produce enough tears to lubricate and nourish the eye. It is characterized by a sandy or gritty sensation in the eye, and may be accompanied by redness.

Chronic dry eye may be caused by environmental factors, medications, or chronic medical conditions. OTC lubricating or rewetting drops can be instilled in the eye to relieve the symptoms associated with dry eye, but this will not correct the condition.

Recent evidence has proved the role of an immune-mediated inflammatory process in chronic dry eye, and it can be successfully treated with an **immunomodulatory agent**, which is a drug that alters the response of the immune system. Cyclosporine (Restasis), an immunomodulatory agent, increases tear production and decreases inflammation. While cyclosporine is not absorbed systemically from the eye, it may cause decreased immune function in the eye.

A man instilling eye drops into his eye.

Conjunctivitis

Conjunctivitis is an inflammation of the outer membrane of the eye. It is more commonly known as pink eye. Conjunctivitis appears as redness, increased tear production, itching, and swelling. It may be caused by infections or allergies. Several topical therapies are available for reducing the signs and symptoms of conjunctivitis, including vasoconstrictors, mast

Table 17.5 Common Otic Preparations for Conjunctivitis

Class	Generic Name	Brand Name	Dosage Forms Available
Corticosteroids	Loteprednol	Alrex, Lotemax	Ophthalmic suspension
Mast cell stabilizers	Pemirolast	Alamast	Ophthalmic solution
Antihistamines	Ketotifen	Zaditor	Ophthalmic solution
	Epinastine	Elestat	Ophthalmic solution
	Olopatadine	Patanol	Ophthalmic solution
Antibiotics	Gatifloxacin	Zymar	Ophthalmic solution
	Moxifloxacin	Vigamox	Ophthalmic solution

cell stabilizers, antihistamines, corticosteroids, antibiotics, and antiviral agents. Some common agents for treating conjunctivitis are presented in TABLE 17.5 .

Glaucoma

Glaucoma is a common disorder of the eye characterized by increased ocular pressure. The increased pressure is a result of an imbalance of the production and drainage of fluid within the eye. The pressure damages the optic nerve and causes partial vision loss. Glaucoma may occur as a result of a genetic predisposition or eye injury or disease.

The goals of glaucoma treatment are to correct the pressure in the eye and to prevent further damage to the optic nerve. In certain cases, corrective surgery may be appropriate treatment for glaucoma. Several classes of drugs are used to treat glaucoma, including alpha-adrenergic agonists, prostaglandins and prostaglandin analogs, and carbonic anhydrase inhibitors. These products are available as solutions or suspensions for instillation directly into the eye. Systemic effects from most of these agents are uncommon. Acetazolamide (Diamox) is an oral agent for the systemic treatment of glaucoma. Common glaucoma treatments are presented in TABLE 17.6 .

Common Ear Conditions and Treatments

Disorders of the ear are common, and range from pain (otalgia), to excess wax in the ear canal, to complicated infections. In contrast to other medical conditions, 87 percent of patients with ear complaints seek medical care. The structures of the human ear are detailed in FIGURE 17.3 .

What Would You Do?

Question: A mother enters your community pharmacy with prescriptions for both of her children. Both children, a two-year-old boy and a four-year-old girl, were just diagnosed with bacterial conjunctivitis by their pediatrician. They both received prescriptions for Vigamox, one drop into both eyes, three times daily for seven days. Vigamox is very expensive and the mother cannot afford two bottles. She requests that you only fill one of the prescriptions so that her children can share one bottle. What should you tell her?

Answer: The pharmacy technician should ask the pharmacist to consult with the mother. The pharmacist will explain to the mother that these are two separate prescriptions intended for two separate patients. To only fill one prescription and use it in both children has the potential to spread infection from one sibling's eye to the other sibling's eye and is thus not a sterile process, as well as not a legal use of the prescription. In some pharmacies, a payment plan may be worked out. If this is still not an option for the parent, the pharmacist should contact the prescriber to identify a less expensive prescription option if available.

Patients with glaucoma should be cautioned to avoid cold remedies, appetite suppressants, drugs for motion sickness, and sleep aids. These products may increase intraocular pressure.

Table 17.6 Common Drugs for the Treatment of Glaucoma			
Class	**Generic Name**	**Brand Name**	**Dosage Forms Available**
Alpha-adrenergic agonists	Brimonidine	Alphagan P	Ophthalmic solution
	Apraclonidine	Iopidine	Ophthalmic solution
Prostaglandin-related agents	Latanoprost	Xalatan	Ophthalmic solution
	Bimatoprost	Lumigan	Ophthalmic solution
Carbonic anhydrase inhibitors	Brinzolamide	Azopt	Ophthalmic suspension
	Dorzolamide	Trusopt	Ophthalmic solution
	Travoprost	Travatan	Ophthalmic solution

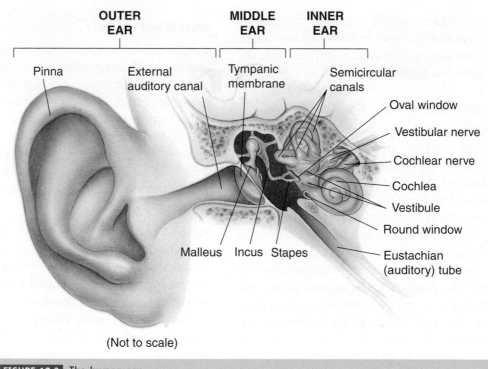

(Not to scale)

FIGURE 17.3 The human ear.

Ear Pain

Otalgia caused by otitis media requires a prescription analgesic solution, antipyrine-benzocaine (A/B Otic), to be administered directly into the ear. Additionally, cipro-floxacin-dexamethasone suspension (Ciprodex) is a combination of an antibiotic and a steroid that fights bacteria that cause ear infections and reduces inflammation associated with infections.

Solutions should not be administered to individuals with tubes in their ears or a ruptured eardrum. Suspensions, however, may be safely used in these patients.

Earwax Solvents

Excess cerumen in the ear canal is one of the most common ear complaints seen in general practice. Excess or impacted cerumen can lead to pain, ringing in the ears, **vertigo** (a type of dizziness in which an individual feels a sense of motion even when still), hearing loss, and damage to the ear canal.

OTC and prescription products are available to remove excess wax from the ear. The products soften, loosen, and remove excess wax that builds up in the ear canal. Carbamide peroxide solution (Debrox) is available as an OTC preparation.

Sometimes, physicians prescribe eye drops for use in the ear. This practice is safe and can be effective, depending on the condition. However, eardrops should never be used in the eye. When in doubt, clarify the route of administration of an otic or ophthalmic preparation.

Earwax protects the ear from dust, infectious agents, irritants, foreign particles, and water. Attempts to remove normal earwax can lead to impacted cerumen and damage the ear canal.

Tech Math Practice

Question: How many milligrams of lidocaine are contained in 2mL of a 1.5% lidocaine solution for injection?

Answer: 1.5% solution = 1.5g lidocaine/100mL.

1.5g lidocaine/100mL = xg lidocaine/2 mL.

Cross-multiply and solve for x. $x = 0.03$g.

0.03g × 1,000mg/1g = 30mg.

Question: How many grams of travoprost are contained in 5mL of a 0.004% travoprost ophthalmic solution?

Answer: 0.004% solution = 0.004g travoprost/100mL.

0.004g travoprost/100mL = xg travoprost/5mL.

Cross-multiply and solve for x. $x = 0.0002$g.

Question: How many grams of isoproterenol are contained in 5mL of a 1:5,000 isoproterenol solution for injection?

Answer: 1:5,000 solution = 1g isoproterenol/5,000mL.

1g isoproterenol/5,000mL = xg isoproterenol/5mL.

Cross-multiply and solve for x. $x = 0.001$g.

Question: How many micrograms of epinephrine are contained in 3mL of a 1:1,000 epinephrine solution for injection?

Answer: 1:1,000 = 1g epinephrine/1,000mL.

1g epinephrine/1,000mL = xg epinephrine/3mL.

Cross-multiply, and solve for x. $x = 0.003$g.

0.003g × 1,000mg/1g × 1,000mcg/1mg = 3,000 micrograms.

Question: **Normal saline contains 0.9% sodium chloride. How many grams of sodium chloride were administered to a patient if he received 500mL of normal saline?**

Answer: 0.9% solution = 0.9g sodium chloride/100mL.

0.9g sodium chloride/100mL = xg sodium chloride/500mL.

Cross-multiply and solve for x. x = 4.5g.

Question: **Itraconazole (Sporanox) is available in 25mL vials with a concentration of 10mg/mL. An adult patient needs a dose of 200mg twice daily. What volume of solution for injection is required?**

Answer: Dose = 200mg × 2 doses/day = 400mg/day.

400mg × 1mL/10mg = 40mL.

Question: **A multidose vial of flu vaccine has a total volume of 5mL. The recommended adult dose is 0.5mL. How many doses are available in each vial?**

Answer: 0.5mL/1 dose = 5mL/x doses.

Cross-multiply and solve for x. x = 10 doses.

WRAP UP

Chapter Summary

- Healthcare-associated infections cause substantial morbidity and mortality worldwide. As many as 100,000 people die each year in the United States due to healthcare-associated infection.

- The germ theory of disease was developed in the late 19th century and offered the idea that microorganisms caused disease. Early research led to the development of infection-control practices that are still used today.

- Common pathogens include several types of bacteria, viruses, fungi, and protozoa.

- The most common healthcare-associated infections include central line-associated bloodstream infections, catheter-associated urinary tract infections, ventilator-associated pneumonia, *C. difficile* infections, and surgical site infections.

- Contamination includes the presence of disease-causing organisms on surfaces, objects, or people. Contamination occurs through touch, air, and water. Decreasing contamination is essential to infection control.

- Sterilization procedures destroy pathogens. Several methods of sterilization are used in healthcare, including moist-heat sterilization, dry-heat sterilization, mechanical sterilization, gas sterilization, and chemical sterilization.

- Hand hygiene, handwashing, wearing gloves, and obtaining vaccinations are important personal strategies for preventing disease transmission.

- The Centers for Disease Control and Prevention have established several monitoring and research programs that facilitate compliance with sterility guidelines, communication, and surveillance. These efforts improve current infection-control practices and will help eliminate future healthcare-associated infections.

- The USP published enforceable guidelines concerning the preparation of compounded sterile products in Chapter 797 of the National Formulary. The guidelines include requirements for monitoring, environmental quality and control, personal practices, and standards for storage and beyond-use dates.

- The skin is the largest organ in the body. It functions as a protective barrier and prevents the entry of pathogens and foreign objects into the human body.

- Sun-induced skin disorders are caused by overexposure to the UV radiation from the sun. Sun-induced damage can range from premature aging to skin cancer. Prevention is the most effective strategy against sun-induced skin damage, and a variety of sunscreens are available to protect the skin.

- Acne vulgaris is a skin disorder that results from the overproduction of sebum. Lesions form when the sebaceous glands become blocked and infected by *P. acnes*. Cleansing regimens may effectively treat acne, but systemic antibiotics might be necessary in severe cases.

- Atopic dermatitis and dry skin are common skin disorders. Both conditions can result from a number of causes, including occupational or environmental exposures, seasonal allergies, or stress. Emollients are the most effective treatment and serve to hydrate the skin and maintain its flexibility. Topical hydrocortisone may be used to decrease the redness and inflammation associated with dry skin.

- Various topical corticosteroids are available in a range of potencies and dosage forms to treat the redness, swelling, heat, pain, and itching associated with many skin disorders.

- Warts and cold sores are caused by viral infections of the skin. OTC products are available for the self-treatment of these conditions.

- Candidiasis and ringworm are common fungal infections of the skin. OTC products are available for the self-treatment of these infections.

- Impetigo, cellulitis, folliculitis, furuncles, and carbuncles are bacterial infections of the skin. They are usually caused by *Streptococcus* or *Staphylococcus* bacteria. The treatment of these conditions usually requires systemic antibiotic therapy.

- Pediculosis is the infestation of lice. Pyrethrin and permethrin are available as OTC products for the self-treatment of a lice infestation. Lindane is available with a prescription for lice infestations that do not respond to other treatment.

- Antiseptics and disinfectants can be used topically and on mucus membranes to cleanse wounds or the skin. Many of these agents are highly effective and inexpensive, including isopropyl alcohol and hydrogen peroxide.

- Chronic dry eye is a condition in which the eye is not able to produce enough tears to lubricate and nourish the eye. Lubricating or rewetting drops may be instilled to decrease the symptoms associated with dry eye. Cyclosporine can be used to increase tear production.

- Conjunctivitis is the inflammation of the outer layer of the eye. It is characterized by redness, itching, increased tear production, and swelling. Conjunctivitis may be caused by allergies or an infection. Corticosteroids, mast cell stabilizers, antihistamines, and antibiotics are available for treating the underlying cause of conjunctivitis.

- Glaucoma is an eye disorder characterized by increased pressure within the eye. The pressure damages the optic nerve and causes vision loss. Topical and systemic preparations are available that decrease the ocular pressure. Topical preparations include alpha-adrenergic agonists, prostaglandin-related agents, and carbonic anhydrase inhibitors.

- Ear pain is a common disorder of the ear and may result from an infection of the ear. Prescription analgesics for the ear are available, as are topical antibiotics to treat the cause of the infection.

- Patients who have tubes in their ears may not use solutions of otic products; otic suspensions may be safely used.

- Excess ear wax can cause pain, discomfort, and hearing loss. OTC and prescription products are available to help remove excess wax.

Learning Assessment Questions

1. A healthcare-associated infection can occur up to how long after surgery?
   A. Six months
   B. One month
   C. 48 hours
   D. Two years

2. How many healthcare-associated infections occur in the United States each year?
   A. 7,000,000
   B. 100,000
   C. 2,000,000
   D. 300,000

3. Which of the following is not a direct cost of healthcare-associated infections?
   A. Lost wages
   B. Testing supplies
   C. Additional medical procedures
   D. Medications needed to treat the infection

4. Which pathogen is not a living organism?
   A. Fungi
   B. Protozoa
   C. Bacteria
   D. Virus

5. Which of the following is a common cause of healthcare-associated infections?
   A. *Staphylococcus aureus*
   B. *Cryptococcus*
   C. *Trypanosoma*
   D. *Mycobacterium tuberculosis*

6. Which infections account for nearly two-thirds of health care-associated infections?
   A. MRSA, VRE, and *C. diff*
   B. *Enterococcus*, *Pseudomonas*, and *Candida*
   C. VRSA, SSIs, and rotavirus
   D. CLABSIs, CAUTIs, and VAP

7. What is the most common source of contamination?

   A. Air

   B. Touch

   C. Water

   D. Food

8. Which of the following is true regarding sterilization techniques?

   A. Isopropyl alcohol can be used to disinfect contaminated surfaces.

   B. An autoclave requires temperatures of 121°C for two hours in order to achieve sterilization.

   C. Dry-heat sterilization is economical and inexpensive.

   D. Gas sterilization uses carbon dioxide to sterilize prepackaged equipment and supplies.

9. Which of the following is not an important personal practice in infection control?

   A. Wearing gloves

   B. Removing excess jewelry and artificial nails in patient-care settings

   C. Receiving a flu shot

   D. Wiping hands with iodine-based disinfectants

10. What is the purpose of USP Chapter 797?

    A. To establish practice guidelines to prevent microbial contamination of pharmaceutical products and maintain patient safety

    B. To assess the characteristics of disease-causing pathogens

    C. To provide training programs for pharmacists regarding aseptic technique

    D. To provide a framework for antibiotic drug selection for select infections

11. Which of the following is the correct beyond-use date for an admixture of one sterile preparation placed into a large-volume sterile fluid, if stored at room temperature?

    A. 48 hours

    B. 12 hours

    C. 14 days

    D. Three days

12. Which of the following is an important piece of equipment for maintaining air quality when preparing CSPs?

    A. Beyond-use date

    B. Laminar airflow workbench

    C. Alcohol-based sanitizers

    D. Controlled room temperature

13. Which of the following does not affect the absorption of drugs through the skin?

    A. The amount of blood vessels present in the skin

    B. Water content of the skin

    C. Thickness of the skin

    D. Pigment of the skin

14. Which class of drugs is not likely to cause photosensitivity?

    A. Antidepressants

    B. Fluoroquinolones

    C. Penicillin-based antibiotics

    D. Diuretics

15. Which topical corticosteroid is available over the counter, without a prescription?

    A. Betamethasone

    B. Hydrocortisone

    C. Clobetasol

    D. Terbinafine

WRAP UP

16. A furuncle is most commonly caused by which microorganism?

    A. *Pediculosis*

    B. *Streptococcus*

    C. *Candida albicans*

    D. *Staphylococcus*

17. Pyrethrin is a derivative of what?

    A. Chrysanthemum seed

    B. Vitamin D

    C. *Epidermophyton*

    D. Herpes simplex 1 virus

18. The antiseptic activity of hydrogen peroxide is related to what property?

    A. Increased hydration

    B. The stinging sensation when it is applied to open wounds

    C. The release of oxygen

    D. Its effectiveness against yeast

19. Which drug can be used to treat chronic dry eye?

    A. Cyclosporine

    B. Acetazolamide

    C. Olopatadine

    D. Ciprodex

20. Which agents are available to treat otalgia?

    A. Povidone-iodine

    B. Carbamide peroxide

    C. Antipyrine-benzocaine

    D. Ciprofloxacin-dexamethasone

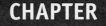
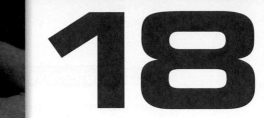

Sterile Compounding

OBJECTIVES

After reading this chapter, you will be able to:

- Describe the characteristics of sterile preparations for parenteral administration.
- Explain the common types of small- and large-volume parenteral preparations.
- Use techniques and equipment to prepare sterile products.
- Perform calculations used in the preparation of sterile products.
- Safely prepare and work with hazardous agents.
- Compare and contrast recombinant drugs and chemotherapeutic agents.
- Discuss the preparation of TPN.

KEY TERMS

Acidic solution
Active immunity
Adaptive immune system
Alkaline solution
Ampule
Anemia
Antecubital area
Aseptic technique
B-cell
Benign tumor
Biologic response
    modifier
Cancer
Carcinogen
Cell-mediated immunity
Cloning
Closed-system transfer
    device
Continuous infusion

Cytopenia
Cytotoxic drug
Deltoid
Dialysis
Electrolyte
First-pass metabolism
Gluteus maximus
Hematocrit
Hemoglobin
Humoral immunity
Hyperosmotic
Hypertonic
Hypo-osmotic
Hypotonic
Innate immune system
Intermittent infusion
Iso-osmotic
Isotonic
IV piggyback (IVPB)

IV push
IV set
Large-volume parenteral
    (LVP)
Lymphatic system
Lymphocyte
Malignant tumor
Metastasis
Mitotic spindle fibers
Monoclonal antibody
Mutagen
Needle
Needle gauge
Needle length
Neoplasm
Neoplastic disease
Neutropenia
Osmolarity
Osmotic pressure

Parenteral product	Rescue drug	Teratogen
Passive immunity	Small-volume parenteral	Transcription
Prime	(SVP)	Translation
Replication	T-cell	Vastus lateralis

Chapter Overview

In a pharmacy setting, the preparation of sterile medications for individual use is called sterile compounding. Sterile compounding requires specialized training and technique, and factors such as pH, tonicity, buffers, and preservatives must be considered. USP-797 defines a sterile product as one that is prepared according to the manufacturer's instructions, one that contains non-sterile ingredients that must be sterilized before patient administration, or any biologic, diagnostic, drug, nutrient, or radiopharmaceutical product that possesses either of the first two characteristics, including baths and soaks for live tissues and organs, implants, inhalations, injections, powder for injection, irrigations, metered sprays, ophthalmic preparations, or otic preparations.

Sterile Products for Parenteral Administration

Parenteral products are preparations that are intended for administration by injection, either through the skin or through other external tissue such as mucous membranes or connective tissue, rather than through the gastrointestinal tract. Parenteral administration allows the active drug to be delivered directly to an organ, a lesion, a muscle, a nerve, or other body tissue. Parenteral administration is preferred over oral administration when a patient is unable to take medications orally, such as when a patient is noncompliant, potentially causing harm to himself or herself or others; unconscious; or vomiting. Parenteral administration is appropriate when drug action is required immediately and when a drug is not therapeutically active after oral administration, such as when it is inactivated by the gastrointestinal tract or first-pass metabolism by the liver. **First-pass metabolism** is the phenomenon by which a large fraction of active drug is lost through metabolism by the liver, so that only a small fraction of active drug reaches systemic circulation. First-pass metabolism significantly reduces the bioavailability of a drug. Bioavailability refers to the degree to which a drug is absorbed and becomes available at the intended site of action. Products for intravenous administration are defined as having a bioavailability of 1 or 100 percent. When a drug has a bioavailability of 100 percent, the entire quantity of drug is delivered directly to systemic circulation and is available for the body to use. Most drugs administered by any route other than intravenous (orally, topically, subcutaneously) have a bioavailability of less than 1.

Fluids, electrolytes, and nutrients may be administered parenterally for patients unable to take nutrition by mouth, such as patients who are vomiting repeatedly, patients with physical obstructions in the gastrointestinal tract, or patients who are unconscious.

Drugs that experience high rates of first-pass metabolism include buprenorphine, cimetidine, diazepam, imipramine, lidocaine, midazolam, meperidine, morphine, propranolol, and verapamil.

Characteristics of Parenteral Products

One of the most important features of parenteral products is the requirement that they be sterile—that is, free from particulate matter, contaminants, and microorganisms. In hospital and home health care settings, pharmacy technicians are responsible for preparing parenteral products for administration. Pharmacy technicians must pay special attention to policies and procedures that ensure compliance with USP 797 guidelines for compounding sterile products. USP 797 guidelines are discussed in Chapter 17. The product itself must be sterile, as must the equipment used for administration.

Parenteral products must be free of pyrogens, or organic substances capable of inducing fever. Pyrogens usually arise from microbial contamination of sterile products and are responsible for many febrile reactions (reactions that induce a fever) that patients experience following intravenous injections.

The parenteral route of administration is needed in certain situations. However, it is typically more expensive than other routes, requires a specially trained staff to prepare and administer, and can pose increased risk to the patient. Once administered, a parenteral product cannot be removed. Any problems with dose or adverse effects are difficult, if not impossible, to reverse. Because the products are administered directly into the body, there may be pain or tissue damage associated with administration.

The physical and chemical properties of parenteral solutions must not damage or alter the properties of blood, blood vessels, or body tissues. Specifically, intravenous products must be iso-osmotic and isotonic compared to the blood **FIGURE 18.1**. An **iso-osmotic** solution has the same number of particles dissolved in solution, or **osmolarity**, as the blood. **Osmotic pressure** is related to osmolarity and is defined as the pressure required to maintain equilibrium between solutions. An **isotonic** solution for parenteral administration has the same osmotic pressure as the blood. A solution that is less concentrated, or has lower osmolarity or osmotic pressure, than another solution is said to be **hypo-osmotic** or **hypotonic**, respectively. A solution that has a higher osmolarity or osmotic pressure than another is said to be **hyperosmotic** or **hypertonic**, respectively.

Normally, blood has an osmolarity of 285mOsm/L. Normal saline (0.9 percent sodium chloride) is an example of an isotonic solution. Isotonic solutions have an osmolarity between 280 and 310mOsm/L. If a solution is hypertonic or hypotonic compared to blood, it will cause red blood cells in the body to lose water or take in water, respectively, damaging the blood cells.

pH is a measurement of the number of hydronium ions in a solution and is an indicator of how acidic or alkaline a solution is. The pH scale ranges from 0 to 14, and 7 indicates a neutral compound. Pure water has a pH of 7. An **alkaline solution** is any solution with a pH greater than 7. An **acidic solution** has a pH of less than 7.

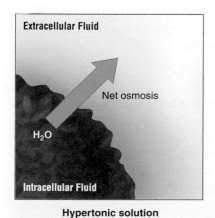
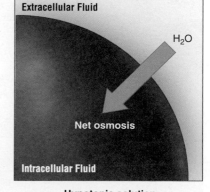

FIGURE 18.1 Hypertonic, isotonic, and hypotonic solutions compared to blood.

The pH of blood is 7.4. This denotes that blood is slightly alkaline. Products for parenteral administration should have a neutral pH close to 7. Blood pH must remain as close as possible to 7.4 at all times to maintain health.

Chemical and physical properties of parenteral products are important for patient administration and for compounding the product. If two products have markedly different pH values or concentrations, they may be incompatible in solution. A telltale sign of incompatibility is the formation of a precipitate (a solid substance that separates from the solution) in a pharmaceutical preparation. If it is large enough, the precipitate can prevent the flow of solution out of a syringe or bag of fluid. Small precipitates may enter the bloodstream and damage a blood vessel or cause a blood clot to form. A visual inspection of the final parenteral product is necessary to check for precipitate formation. Administering multiple drugs may require the use of separate IV bags if two or more incompatible drugs must be delivered.

> The premier reference for evaluating the compatibility and stability of drugs is *Trissel's Stability of Compounded Formulations*, frequently consulted in hospital pharmacies and home infusion pharmacies.

Storage conditions are an important consideration when evaluating the physical and chemical properties of drug solutions. For example, some drugs must remain refrigerated to maintain drug stability, while others cannot be refrigerated. And, many drugs are stable when exposed to light, while other drugs must be stored in specialized containers or in amber-colored bags to protect from exposure to light. Pharmacy technicians involved in compounding parenteral products must be aware of storage and compounding requirements. Failure to adhere to such guidelines can render a drug ineffective, which is an expensive and unsafe outcome.

"Subcutaneous" should not be abbreviated using "SQ" or "SC," as these abbreviations can easily be misinterpreted. Instead, "subQ," "sub-Q," or "subcutaneous" should be used. Verify all abbreviations that are unclear or unapproved.

Routes of Administration for Parenteral Products

Drugs can be injected into almost any area of the body, including into a vein (intravenous, abbreviated IV), into a muscle (intramuscular, abbreviated IM), into the skin (intradermal, abbreviated ID), or under the skin (subcutaneously, abbreviated sub-Q/subQ.) Less commonly, drugs are injected directly into joints (intra-articular), the fluid surrounding a joint (intrasynovial), the spinal column (intraspinal), spinal fluid (intrathecal), an artery (intra-arterial), or the heart (intracardiac).

Intravenous

Drugs administered by the IV route offer a rapid onset of action. Most superficial veins are suitable for IV administration, but the veins in front of the elbow (the **antecubital area**) are routinely chosen for administration. These veins are large, easy to see, and easy to reach with a needle.

Both small and large volumes of drugs can be administered via IV. Drugs, nutrients, elec-

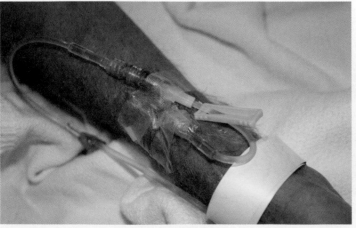

The veins on the front of the arm are often used for IV administration.

trolytes, amino acids, and other therapeutic products can be administered by IV. The IV route is preferred for drugs that require close monitoring of blood levels.

The primary disadvantage of IV administration is the possibility of a blood-clot formation induced by touching the vein wall with a needle or catheter. A blood clot is more likely to form when the drug solution is irritating to the body's tissues. When blood clots break loose and flow through the blood, they can lead to serious, life-threatening blockages in the lungs, brain, or other major blood vessels.

IV administration can be in the following forms:

- Continuous infusion—With a **continuous infusion**, the drug is placed into a large volume of base solution and slowly and continuously dripped into a vein. In this case, the drug and fluid are administered simultaneously. Continuous drug levels are obtained in the blood. Vein irritation is minimized because the concentration of drug is greatly reduced when placed in a dilute solution. A continuous infusion requires constant monitoring by pharmacy and nursing staff because the drug is administered without interruption. If the infusion is stopped early for any reason, part of the drug will not be administered.

> *Potassium products are never administered by healthcare providers via IV push because of the risk of cardiotoxicity. Potassium products should be diluted in large volumes and administered via a slow infusion. Pharmacy technicians prepare the ingredients and compound IV admixtures, which contain potassium products. Pharmacy technicians may also play a role in preventing medication errors that involve the administration of potassium.*

- Intermittent infusion—With an **intermittent infusion**, a drug is placed in an intermediate volume of base solution (usually 25mL to 100mL) and infused over a specified period (for example, 15 to 60 minutes) at regularly spaced intervals (for example, every six hours.) This route of administration requires monitoring during the infusion to assess for adverse reactions, but does not require continuous monitoring like a continuous infusion. The complete drug dose is given in a relatively short period, and the blood levels of drug do not remain constant as in a continuous infusion. Intermittent infusions cannot be used to administer fluids or some electrolytes, or for administration directly to an organ or tissue.

- Bolus dose or IV push—A bolus dose or **IV push** is the administration of a drug using a syringe over a short period (usually minutes or less). The drug is placed directly into the vein. Bolus administration may be used for a one-time dose or repeated at scheduled intervals. This form of administration requires less monitoring than infusions and can be used in emergencies, when rapid action is needed. Bolus doses can cause irritation to the veins because the drug solutions are more concentrated than doses given by infusion. Drug levels are less consistent when administered as boluses compared to infusions. Drug toxicity is more likely with a bolus dose because a high concentration of drug is administered over a short period.

Intramuscular

IM injections are administered deep into a skeletal muscle, usually the **deltoid** (upper arm), **gluteus maximus** (buttocks), or **vastus lateralis** (top of the leg). Proper administration of IM injections requires insertion of the needle at a 90-degree angle to the muscle. IM injection is appropriate for non-irritating drugs. IM injections do not result in a rapid onset of

> *The healthcare professional who administers the IV medication should remain with the patient to assess adverse reactions or side effects from the medication. Monitoring patients who receive medication by IV administration is for the safety of the patient.*

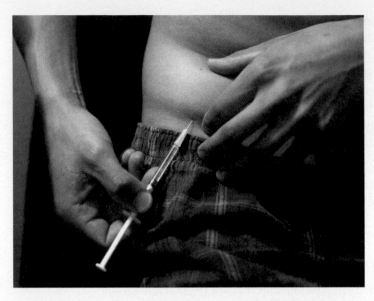

Insulin doses are often administered by subcutaneous injection.

action, but do lead to a prolonged duration of effect. Injuries relating to IM injections usually result from the point of entry of the needle or the deposition of drug solution. Fluid or pus accumulation, blood clots, bruising, and scars can occur, but these events are rare.

The volume of drug administered is limited by the size of the muscle. In adults, up to 2mL can be administered into the deltoid, and 5mL can be administered into the gluteus maximus. However, these upper limits of injection volumes may cause pain and discomfort. IM injections are usually limited to half of the maximum volume, usually 1mL for the deltoid and 2 to 2.5mL for the gluteus maximus.

The vastus lateralis is the preferred site for IM injection in children because it is the largest muscle in children's bodies and has no major nerves or blood vessels. Children under three years old may not receive injections of more than 1mL into the vastus lateralis.

If a large volume of solution is required for IM injection, the dose may be divided into two syringes and injected into separate sites.

Subcutaneous

The subQ route of IV administration is used for small volumes of medication. Drug solutions are administered into the subcutaneous layer of fat beneath the surface of the skin, between the dermis and the muscle, usually on the outer surface of the upper arm, the anterior surface of the thigh, or the lower portion of the abdomen. Proper administration of a subcutaneous injection requires needle insertion at a 45-degree angle to the surface of the skin. The site of injection should be rotated when frequent injections are administered, such as daily insulin injections. The maximum volume of drug administered by the subQ route is 2mL. Volumes greater than approximately 1.3mL cause painful pressure at the site of administration, so subQ doses are often limited to 1mL if possible. Thick suspensions are not appropriate for subQ administration.

Intradermal

ID injections are administered between the vascular layer of skin between the dermis and the epidermis. Usually, the anterior portion of the forearm is used for ID administration. This route is frequently used for diagnostic skin tests, such as tuberculosis testing or allergy desensitization, in which systemic absorption would be dangerous. ID injections are limited to very small volumes, often less than 0.1mL, but can range from 0.02mL to 0.5mL.

Types of Parenterals

Countless products are available for parenteral administration. These are often divided into **small-volume parenterals (SVPs)**, which are preparations that contain 100mL or less, and **large-volume parenterals (LVPs)**, which contain more than 100mL. TABLE 18.1 presents common SVPs and LVPs used in pharmacy practice.

Table 18.1   Commonly Used Products for Parenteral Administration

Component/Product	Contents	Abbreviation	Category
Commonly Used Additives in Small-Volume Parenterals			
Cimetidine injection	150mg/mL	N/A	Histamine 2 antagonist
Dexamethasone injection	4 or 10mg/mL	N/A	Glucocorticoid
Digoxin injection	100 or 250mcg/mL	N/A	Cardiac glycoside
Furosemide injection	10mg/mL	N/A	Diuretic
Heparin sodium injection	1 unit/mL, 2 units/mL, 10 units/mL, 100 units/mL, 1,000 units/mL, 5,000 units/mL, 10,000 units/mL, 20,000 units/mL	N/A	Anticoagulant
Insulin injection	100 or 500 units/mL	Various	Antidiabetic agent, hormone
Magnesium sulfate injection	500mg/mL	$MgSO_4$	Electrolyte
Potassium acetate	2 or 4mEq/mL	K acetate	Electrolyte
Potassium chloride	2mEq/mL	KCl	Electrolyte
Potassium phosphate	4.4mEq potassium and 3mmol phosphorous per mL	K Phos or KPO_4	Electrolyte
Sodium bicarbonate	4.2% (5mEq/10mL), 7.5% (8.92mEq/10mL), 8.4% (10mEq/10mL)	NaBicarb; $NaHCO_3$	Electrolyte
Sodium chloride injection	0.45%, 0.9%, 3%, 5%, 14.6%, or 23.4% sodium chloride (normal saline)	NS	Electrolyte
Selenium	40mcg/mL	Se	Trace element
Zinc	1mg/mL	Zn	Trace element
Large-Volume Parenterals			
Dextrose injection	2.5% dextrose in water	$D_{2.5}W$	Fluid and nutrient replacement
	5% dextrose in water	D_5W	Fluid and nutrient replacement
	10% dextrose in water	$D_{10}W$	Fluid and nutrient replacement
	20% dextrose in water	$D_{20}W$	Fluid and nutrient replacement
Dextrose and lactated Ringer's solution	5% dextrose in lactated Ringer's solution	D_5LR	Fluid, nutrient, and electrolyte replacement
Dextrose and sodium chloride injection	5% dextrose and 0.9% sodium chloride (normal saline)	D_5NS	Fluid, nutrient, and electrolyte replacement
	5% dextrose and 0.45% sodium chloride (normal saline)	$D_5\frac{1}{2}NS$	Fluid, nutrient, and electrolyte replacement
	2.5% dextrose and 0.45% sodium chloride (normal saline)	$D_{2.5}\frac{1}{2}NS$	Fluid, nutrient, and electrolyte replacement

(continues)

Table 18.1 **Commonly Used Products for Parenteral Administration** *(Continued)*			
Component/Product	**Contents**	**Abbreviation**	**Category**
Lactated Ringer's solution	2.7mEq calcium, 4mEq potassium, 130mEq sodium, and 28mEq lactate per liter of sterile water (equivalent to 0.2g calcium chloride, 0.3g potassium chloride, 6g sodium chloride, and 3.1g sodium lactate, per liter)	LR	Fluid and electrolyte replacement; systemic alkalinizer
Ringer's solution for injection	147mEq sodium, 4mEq potassium, 4.5mEq calcium, and 156mEq chloride per liter of sterile water (equivalent to 8.6g sodium chloride, 0.3g potassium chloride, and 0.33g calcium chloride per liter)	N/A	Fluid and electrolyte replacement
Sodium chloride injection	0.9% sodium chloride in sterile water	NS	Fluid and electrolyte replacement; isotonic vehicle

Concentrations of solutions for parenteral administration are presented by a variety of different measurements: percentage, mmol/L, mg/mL, mEq/L, etc. Verify accurate conversions, calculations, and manipulations when handling multiple parenteral solutions.

Small-Volume Parenterals

An SVP is usually used for delivering a medication at a controlled rate. SVPs may be either single or multi-dose products. When an SVP is prepared to be added to a running IV, it is known as an **IV piggyback (IVPB)**. An IVPB may contain as few as 25mL or as many as 100mL in a mini bag. The IVPB is infused into the IV line for a short time in order to administer all of the medication.

The chemical abbreviation for magnesium sulfate is MgSO₄ and a commonly seen abbreviation is MagSO₄. Although commonly used by prescribers, these two abbreviations should not be used in writing prescription orders as they lead to medication errors. These abbreviations are often confused with MSO₄ which is another abbreviation (also not recommended) to prescribe morphine sulfate.

Frozen Products

Many SVPs are available in prepackaged, frozen mini bags. These types of products decrease labor-intensive preparation of individual SVPs and increase convenience. Products remain frozen until a patient-specific order is received; at that point, a mini bag is thawed at room temperature or in a microwave, depending on the manufacturer's instructions. A product-specific expiration date is placed on the thawed mini bag. After it has been thawed, a product cannot be refrozen. Most hospitals purchase frozen mini bags containing commonly used antibiotics.

Closed-System Transfer Device

A recent innovation in the administration of SVPs is a packaging system known as a **closed-system transfer device** (a.k.a., piggyback). Such systems minimize preparation time and workload, decrease costs and drug wastage, and reduce the possibility of contamination. Only a few products are available in a closed-system device, most of which are antibiotics. Each system varies by manufacturer, but the concept is uniform: The drug, which has not been reconstituted, is paired with an IV solution for reconstitution. The system is opened and the drug is reconstituted immediately prior to administration. The products do not need to be thawed, frozen, or refrigerated. In a hos-

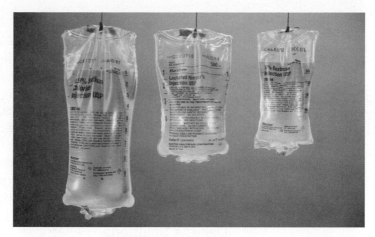

Solutions for parenteral administration are commercially available in a variety of volumes.

pital or institutional setting, a closed system that is not used may be returned to the pharmacy and dispensed to another patient in most states; there is no drug wastage or contamination. Safety is maximized because no measuring or manipulation of the ingredients is required.

Large-Volume Parenterals

LVPs are used to replace fluids, provide electrolytes or nutrients, and deliver medications. LVPs are administered by slow continuous IV infusion. LVPs are commonly available in 250mL, 500mL, and 1,000mL sizes. The base solution may contain varying concentrations of sodium chloride, dextrose, or electrolytes to which drugs or other additives are incorporated.

Total Parenteral Nutrition

When patients cannot tolerate oral feedings or they have experienced a significant loss of water or electrolytes, then solutions of water, dextrose, trace elements, and electrolytes can be administered through LVPs. In patients unable to take in oral nutrition for more than a few days, total parenteral nutrition (TPN) containing carbohydrates, fat, amino acids (FreAmine), multivitamins (MVI), electrolytes, and trace elements are administered to maintain calorie requirements. TPN is useful for patients with physical barriers to gastrointestinal intake of nutrition, patients with anorexia, or patients undergoing chemotherapy. TPN additives are patient-specific. Many hospitals have specialized teams of physicians, nurses, pharmacists, and dieticians who formulate and direct the care of patients who need TPN.

A TPN may contain several dozen additives. Therefore, it must be compounded carefully, with attention paid to the order in which ingredients are added to the base, how to filter the compounded product, and how to store the finished product. Some institutions employ an automated compounding device that facilitates the preparation of multiple TPNs. The programmable device aids in calculating the amount of additives needed and coordinates the manipulation of additives. Such a system helps to prevent errors, reduces the possibility of contamination, and increases accuracy and precision in compounding TPNs.

A TPN must be administered through a central venous catheter, also called a central line, which is inserted into the subclavian vein in the neck. A large vein is required for administration because a TPN is hypertonic compared to blood and the large volume (up to 2L per day) requires dilution in the blood.

Irrigation

Solutions for the irrigation of body wounds or tissues are also subject to rigorous standards of sterile product preparation. These solutions are not injected directly into veins, but are employed outside the circulatory system. Irrigation solutions are used to bathe or wash wounds, surgical incisions, or body tissues. Solutions for irrigation are commonly manufactured and available in large-volume bottles that facilitate the rapid pouring of solutions into areas of the body where cleansing and irrigation is needed.

Although many irrigation solutions have the same composition as injectable solutions, the two dosage forms are packaged and handled differently. Solutions for irrigation must always be prominently labeled "Not for Injection."

Dialysis Solutions

Normally, the kidneys act as a filter for the blood, removing waste products and excreting them from the body. **Dialysis** is a process that filters the blood of waste products when the kidneys are not able to do so, such as in the case of acute poisoning, chronic kidney disease, or renal failure. Dialysis uses the principles of osmosis to remove waste products from the body. Dialysis solutions are prepared to contain dextrose, vitamins, minerals, electrolytes, and amino acids. The solutions are hypertonic, which prevents their absorption into the circulatory system. The concentration of ingredients in the dialysis solution encourages the diffusion of water, toxic substances, and metabolites from the body into the dialysis solution, where it is removed by a specialized pump. Dialysis solutions are commercially available, but pharmacy technicians may have to adjust their composition or prepare them from scratch, based on individual patient needs.

Specialized Systems of Delivery

In addition to solutions for parenteral administration, other sterile products may need to be administered to patients. Pellets and implants are available for subcutaneous administration and provide for a continuous release of medication over an extended period—up to several years. Pellets and implants are often used for hormone therapy, which is designed to treat cancers or provide contraception. The pellets or implants may contain up to 100 times the dose of a drug given by another route of administration. This necessitates less-frequent administration and provides a prolonged therapeutic effect.

Preparing Sterile Products

Most parenteral products are manufactured by pharmaceutical companies in large-scale facilities. However, when individualized products are required, manipulations of admixtures and injections are needed. Individualization like this is performed in hospital, home-health, and institutional pharmacy settings. Specialized training is required to ensure compliance with safety standards when compounding or preparing sterile products for administration to patients.

Aseptic Technique

In a pharmacy-compounding setting, **aseptic technique** is the procedure by which sterile products are prepared and equipment and facilities are cleaned to avoid contamination. The goal of aseptic technique is to maintain asepsis in the clinical setting. The room where pharmacy products are compounded using aseptic technique should be cleaned routinely to maintain an aseptic environment. Aseptic technique may be used when preparing doses from single- or multiple-dose vials, opening ampules or other containers to make an IV solution, or preparing small- or large-volume parenteral products for patient administration. The guidelines of aseptic technique when working in a laminar flow hood are as follows:

- Remove all outerwear.
- Remove all jewelry and other restricted items, such as nail polish or artificial nails.
- Abstain from eating or drinking during preparation of sterile products.
- Wear protective attire, including a non-shedding laboratory coat or gown, head and facial hair covers, facemask, and shoe covers.
- Wash hands with antimicrobial soap according to proper hand-washing guidelines.
- Wipe down supplies and workspace with 70 percent isopropyl alcohol.
- Wash hands again and don gloves.
- Do not take any unnecessary supplies into the laminar workbench, such as pens, paper, calculators, or labels.
- Avoid touching the hair or face while in the sterile workspace.
- Avoid talking, sneezing, or coughing while in the sterile workspace.
- Place materials at least 6 inches inside the outer edges of the workbench. Do not place items anywhere in which they might obstruct airflow.
- Use separate needles or instruments for each manipulation.

Vials

Before an additive can be placed into a larger-volume parenteral product for administration, it must be withdrawn from a vial or an ampule using aseptic technique. Vials are available in single- and multiple-dose varieties. The hard rubber stopper on top of a vial can harbor contaminants, so it must be cleaned with isopropyl alcohol before the solution is withdrawn.

Vials are closed systems. Therefore, fluid cannot be withdrawn unless an equal volume of air is added to the vial. The needle and syringe are used to introduce air into the vial and to withdraw the needed amount of fluid. The plunger of the syringe is drawn back, filling the barrel with air, to the volume that needs to be withdrawn. The tip of the needle is inserted at an angle, and then straightened to enter the vial at 90 degrees. Using this technique, the bevel heel of the needle enters the rubber stopper at the same location as the bevel tip. This prevents coring, or the breaking of a small piece of rubber into the solution.

Depress the plunger and dispense all the air in the syringe. Invert the vial with the syringe still inserted. Pull back the plunger to the desired volume of solution. Withdraw the needle from the syringe. The rubber stopper will close and seal the remaining contents of the vial.

For multiple-dose vials, note a beyond-use date on the outside of the vial. In most cases, a single-dose vial must be used within one hour or discarded. A multiple-dose vial can usually be used for 28 days when stored under appropriate conditions.

Ampules

An **ampule** is a glass container with a single dose of active ingredient. An ampule contains no preservatives. Ampules can be challenging because the glass neck of the ampule must be broken in order to withdraw the solution.

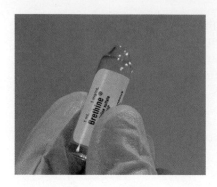

The neck of an ampule must be broken in order for the solution to be withdrawn.

First, tap the top of the ampule or gently invert the ampule and swirl it back upright to remove any solution from the top of the container. Next, clean the neck of the ampule with an alcohol swab. Cover the top of the ampule with the alcohol swab and grasp the top of the ampule between the thumb and index finger. Quickly snap the neck of the ampule away from your body. The neck of the ampule is scored to facilitate opening.

After the ampule is opened, tilt the ampule, place the needle bevel near the opening, and withdraw the desired volume of solution. Use a needle with a filter to remove any fragments of glass, paint chips, or other particles that may have fallen in to the ampule. Remove this needle and replace with a new needle before injecting the contents from the ampule into a larger-volume solution or admixture.

Syringes and Needles

Syringes are used for the preparation and administration of sterile pharmaceutical products. Syringes are also used in non-sterile environments for oral use and irrigation. The term syringe refers to the calibrated reservoir and the plunger of a device intended to deliver medication to a body or introduce it to another delivery sys-

Filter needles should be used only for moving liquids one direction.

tem. **FIGURE 18.2** shows the components of a syringe and needle. Most syringes are made of plastic, but some are made of glass. Glass syringes are expensive and are used only for medications that are absorbed by plastic. Plastic syringes are available from manufacturers as sterile products, individually wrapped for convenience and storage. Plastic syringes are inexpensive and disposable.

The plunger and the tip of the syringe must remain sterile to ensure asepsis. These components must not be touched. Only the flange and the barrel may be touched.

Syringes are available in a variety of sizes for medical use, ranging from 0.25mL to 60mL. When manipulating solutions with a syringe, choose the smallest size syringe that will measure the desired volume.

A **needle** is attached to a syringe and is the component that actually enters the medication vial, the container to hold medication for dispensing, or the body. Needles are made of aluminum or stainless steel. Needles vary in gauge and length. **Needle gauge** refers to the diameter of the needle. The larger the diameter, the smaller the gauge. For example, a 28-gauge needle has a smaller diameter than a 25-gauge needle. Needles for medical use are available in gauges ranging from 33 to 13. Commonly used **needle lengths** range from ⅜ inches to 2 inches. Needle gauge and length are important considerations for patient administration, mostly because of patient comfort and site of administration. Syringes and needles needed for compounding must be the appropriate size and length to accurately and precisely measure the appropriate additives under sterile conditions.

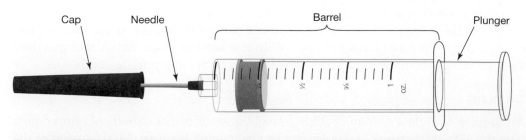

FIGURE 18.2 The components of a syringe and needle.

A smaller needle gauge indicates a larger diameter and a larger needle gauge indicates a smaller diameter.

IV Sets

An **IV set** is a sterile, disposable device used to administer IV medications or fluids from an IV container or reservoir. The IV tubing is usually made of polyvinyl chloride (PVC), although IV sets made from other materials are available for cases of incompatibilities or instabilities.

The IV set consists of several basic components: a spike to connect to the IV container, a drip chamber for trapping air, a clamp for controlling the flow rate of the solution, and flexible tubing to deliver the infusion to the injection site. The tubes attached to the IV set range in length from 6 inches to 120 inches. Technicians must **prime** the tube before administering medication to a patient via an IV set to remove all the air and particulate matter from inside the tube. Priming the IV tube removes all particles and air from the tube and allows a small amount of solution to flow into the tubing. This decreases the chance of injecting air or foreign particles into a patient's body.

> *Nitroglycerin and fat emulsions cannot be administered using a PVC IV set. Nitroglycerin adheres to the plastic in the bag and tubing. Fat emulsions dissolve a plasticizer that is added to PVC, which may be harmful to patients.*

Nurses are traditionally responsible for maintaining and using IV sets, but pharmacy personnel may sometimes be involved in the selection and use of IV sets for training purposes, for priming tubes for chemotherapeutic agents, or for transferring fluid from one container to another.

Calculations for Sterile Products

Basic math skills are involved in the safe and efficient compounding and administration of sterile products. Due to the sensitive nature of parenteral administration, technicians should always double-check calculations and measurements when preparing sterile products.

IV Flow Rates

IV flow rates are usually expressed in milliliters per hour (mL/hr) and may be as slow as 42mL/hr or as fast as 150mL/hr, depending on the clinical needs of the patient. Lower rates are used to maintain patency in the IV line.

Pharmacy staff usually denote IV flow rates in milliliters per hour, but nurses often prefer to calculate drops per minute. Help other hospital staff members convert between flow rates if needed. To calculate drops per minute of an IV infusion, use the following equation:

$$x \text{ Drops/Min} = \frac{\text{Volume of Fluid}}{\text{Delivery Time in Hours}} \times \frac{\text{Drops of IV Set}}{\text{mL of IV Set}} \times \frac{1\text{hr}}{60 \text{ min}}$$

Electrolyte Requirements

An **electrolyte** is a fluid containing a dissolved mineral salt. Electrolyte solutions are often measured in milliequivalents (mEq), which are related to molecular weight. Electrolytes are available in concentrations of mEq/mL. When compounding electrolyte solutions or TPNs, it may be necessary to calculate the volume that contains an ordered amount of electrolyte. Use a simple ratio to calculate the volumes needed for compounding.

Hazardous Agents

Special attention is required in the preparation and handling of cytotoxic drugs and hazardous agents. A **cytotoxic drug** is any drug that has a toxic effect on cells. Cytotoxic drugs are frequently used in cancer chemotherapy, nuclear pharmacy, antiretroviral therapy, biologic hormones, and bioengineered drugs. Common cytotoxic drugs are listed in TABLE 18.2.

In the case of specific treatments, the risks to the patient are outweighed by the benefits of the drugs. However, a risk of exposure exists for the pharmacist, technician, or other healthcare provider handling and preparing the drugs for administration. Healthcare providers need to be aware of the risks, as well as how to mitigate the dangers of exposure. Exposure of healthcare personnel to cytotoxic drugs should be minimized, while maintaining requirements for safety and asepsis. If handled properly, the exposure risk is minimal, but pharmacy personnel should be aware of the risks of working with hazardous chemicals.

Risks of Working with Hazardous Materials

Cytotoxic drugs target rapidly dividing cells in the body, including those in the immune system, blood cells, hair cells, gonadal cells, embryonic and fetal cells, and cancer cells. Therefore, these drugs have carcinogenic, mutagenic, and teratogenic potential. A **carcinogen** is a cancer-causing substance. A **mutagen** is substance that can cause a genetic mutation. A **teratogen** is a substance that interferes with normal fetal development.

Long-term exposure to cytotoxic drugs can cause cancers, birth defects, miscarriages, and chromosomal damage. Pregnant women should never handle or come in contact with cytotoxic agents. Short-term exposure to cytotoxic drugs may cause lightheadedness, dizziness, nausea, vomiting, and allergic reactions. Direct contact with cytotoxic drugs can cause irritation or injury to the skin, eyes, and mucus membranes.

Handling and Preparing Sterile Products Using Hazardous Agents

Gloves are worn whenever cytotoxic drugs are handled for stocking, inventory, disposal, or preparation of parenteral products. When receiving a shipment of cytotoxic drugs, the products should be immediately taken to the storage area and inspected. Broken containers of cytotoxic drugs are considered hazardous spills and must be contained and cleaned accordingly. Procedures for cleaning spills are discussed later in this section. Cytotoxic drugs are stored separate from other non-hazardous drugs in order to prevent contamination, possible exposure, and errors in taking the wrong drug off the shelf.

Exposure to cytotoxic drugs usually occurs through inhalation of droplets or absorption through the skin. Exposure to cytotoxic agents may occur during any step

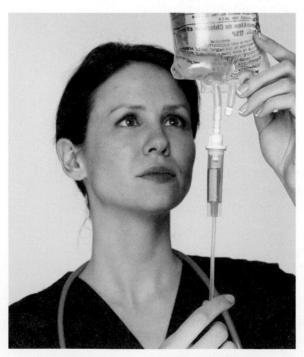

Nurses often calculate the rate of IV administration as the number of drops per minute.

Table 18.2 Common Cytotoxic Drugs

Class	Generic Name	Brand Name
Antiviral agents	Ganciclovir	Cytovene, Vitrasert
Chemotherapeutic/ antineoplastic agents	Aldesleukin	Proleukin
	Anastrozole	Arimidex
	Asparaginase	Elspar
	Bleomycin	N/A
	Busulfan	Busulfex, Myerlan
	Carboplatin	Paraplatin-AQ
	Carmustine	BiCNU, Gliadel
	Cisplatin	Platinol
	Cyclophosphamide	Cytoxan
	Cytarabine	Cytosar
	Dactinomycin	Cosmegen
	Daunorubicin	Cerubidine
	Doxorubicin	Adriamycin
	Estramustine	Emcyt
	Etoposide	Toposar
	Exemestane	Aromasin
	Hydroxyurea	Droxia, Hydrea
	Idarubicin	Idamycin PFS
	Ifosfamide	Ifex
	Irinotecan	Camptosar
	Letrozole	Femara
	Mercaptopurine	Purinethol
	Methotrexate	Rheumatrex, Trexall
	Oxaliplatin	Eloxatin
	Temozolomide	Temodar
	Topotecan	Hycamtin
	Vinblastine	Velban
	Vincristine	Vincasar
Hypnotic	Chlorambucil	Leukeran
Immunosuppressant	Azathioprine	Imuran

involved in the preparation of pharmaceutical products: withdrawing needles from vials, using needles or syringes for drug transfer, opening ampules, or removing air from a syringe. Personnel should wear protective clothing to minimize the chance of exposure to cytotoxic drugs. The same personal protective clothing is required for handling cytotoxic drugs as for compounding sterile products, with the addition of a requirement for wearing a lint-free, nonabsorbent, cuff-sleeved gown, wearing two pairs of gloves (double-gloving), and wearing eye protection. The first pair of gloves should be worn under the cuff of the gown, and the second pair should be worn over the cuff. Gloves should be changed every 20 to 30 minutes with continuous use, or removed immediately after a puncture or contamination. Nitrile gloves are thicker than latex gloves and may be used as an alternative to double-gloving.

If protective clothing or equipment is visibly contaminated, immediately remove and replace it. If a cytotoxic drug comes in contact with the skin, immediately wash the affected area with soap and water. If a cytotoxic drug comes in contact with the eyes, flush the eyes with copious amounts of water for at least 15 minutes; then seek medical attention. Exposure from a needle stick should be presented for medical attention immediately.

Syringes and containers containing cytotoxic drugs should always be adequately labeled. Syringes, needles, tubing, bottles, vials, gloves, gowns, and any other equipment used in preparing or handling cytotoxic drugs should be disposed of in a puncture-resistant container that is labeled to warn of its cytotoxic contents. Cytotoxic drugs are considered regulated waste, and, as such, must be disposed of in accordance with local, state, and federal laws.

Preparation of cytotoxic drugs should take place in a vertical laminar flow biological safety cabinet or bacteriological glove box. A biological safety cabinet is an enclosed, ventilated workspace that prevents exposure to cytotoxic drugs. A bacteriological glove box is a sealed container that allows workers to manipulate objects or drugs inside the container through gloves installed in the side of the box without breaching the contained space. Drug administration sets for hazardous agents should be attached and primed inside a safety cabinet.

When working with vials of cytotoxic drugs, the procedure for withdrawing fluids differs slightly from that used in the preparation of nonhazardous products. Namely, when inserting air into the vial, the volume of air introduced into the vial must be slightly smaller than the volume of fluid that will be withdrawn. This produces a vacuum inside the vial and prevents solution from being expelled from the vial when the needle is withdrawn.

Cytotoxic oral drugs may be handled in hospital or community pharmacies. Personnel handling or dispensing these agents should wear gloves, a gown, and a respirator. Contaminated equipment should be cleaned with detergent and water immediately after use. Patients should be informed and counseled of the risks of handling cytotoxic drugs and requirements for storage.

Spills of Hazardous Materials

Spills of hazardous materials should be immediately contained and cleaned to prevent exposure to other individuals. Spill kits are necessary to properly clean hazardous spills. As such, spill kits should be readily available in every pharmacy that handles or prepares hazardous chemicals. A spill kit should contain all the necessary equipment to safely manage a cytotoxic drug spill: a nonabsorbent, lint-free gown; two pairs of gloves; a respirator mask; one pair of goggles; absorbent towels or spill cloths; hazard labels; spill-control pillows; a scoop and brush; plastic disposal bags; and a "CAUTION: Chemo Spill" sign.

Small spills (5mL or less) of cytotoxic drugs outside of a safety cabinet should be wiped up with absorbent gauze. The area should then be cleaned three times with detergent and clean water. Large spills should be covered with absorbent sheets. Respirators should be worn if there is a danger of aerosol generation of the cytotoxic drug. Chemical inactivators should not be applied to a spill, due to the risk of producing hazardous by-products. Contaminated surfaces should be cleaned with detergent and water.

Quality Assurance for the Preparation of Sterile Products

Each pharmacy must develop and enforce a quality-assurance program to ensure that sterile preparations are compounded safely and accurately. A quality-assurance program is a systematic method used to identify areas for improvement in patient care and to address and correct them with clerical, administrative, or educational actions. Such actions might include changes to policies and procedures, personnel training, process validation, equipment evaluation, or improved labeling or documentation. In implementing a quality-assurance program, pharmacies improve quality of care, manage risk, and control infection transmission. Pharmacy personnel should remain up to date on training, continually refine and perfect skills necessary for sterile compounding, and follow institutional and federal guidelines for the handling of sterile products. These actions ensure the safety of the patient, as well as the safety of the healthcare worker.

Drug Insights: The Immune System, Recombinant Drugs, and Chemotherapy

Innovative technology is changing the shape of healthcare administration. New discoveries enable clinicians to use modified genetic material and specialized agents that target rapidly dividing cells in the body to treat serious diseases, including immune system dysfunctions and many types of cancer. Many of these drugs are expensive and require specialized training for handling, preparation, and administration.

The Immune System

The immune system protects the body by attacking and destroying invading pathogens. It adapts to its environment and evolves based on previous exposures. The immune system exhibits several remarkable characteristics:

- Specificity—Specificity is the ability to distinguish between different pathogens
- Memory—Memory is the ability to mount a quick response to pathogens that are similar to previous pathogens
- Mobility—Mobility is the ability of local immune reactions to produce systemic effects
- Replication—**Replication** is the ability to reproduce cellular components of the immune system to amplify its response
- Redundancy—Redundancy is the ability to produce components with the same effect from multiple origins

These highly complex characteristics make the immune system a powerful defense against invading organisms. The immune system is difficult to control with drug therapy. To manipulate an immune response with drugs, the structure and components of the immune system must be understood.

Structure and Function of the Immune System

The body's first lines of defense against invading pathogens are exterior defenses: skin, mucus, saliva, normal bacterial flora, the acidic environment of the stomach, and the flushing effect of tears, urination, diarrhea, vomiting, coughing, and sneezing. A disruption in the normal defenses of the body can allow penetration by a pathogen.

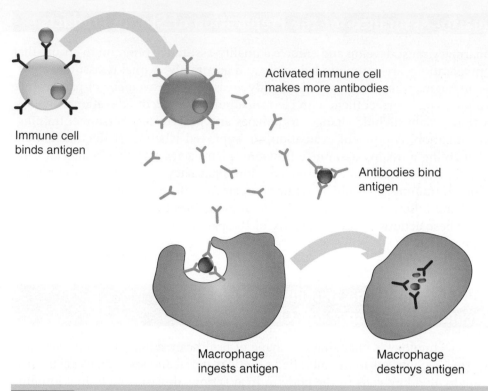

Immune cell
binds antigen

Activated immune cell
makes more antibodies

Antibodies bind
antigen

Macrophage
ingests antigen

Macrophage
destroys antigen

FIGURE 18.3 An antibody response to a bacterial antigen.

If pathogens penetrate the body's exterior defenses, the **innate immune system** will halt the progression of an infection. Innate immunity is present at birth and uses a limited number of cells to mount an immune response.

An antigen is any substance or pathogen that causes the immune system to produce an antibody. An antibody, also called an immunoglobulin, is a Y-shaped protein that identifies and neutralizes pathogens **FIGURE 18.3**. The human body can respond to an antigen in many different ways through the adaptive immune system. The **adaptive immune system** is the division of the immune system that exhibits specificity and memory. The adaptive immune response is divided into two components: cell-mediated immunity and humoral immunity. The two main cell types that participate in the adaptive immune response are the T-cells and B-cells. These cells contain antigen-specific receptors capable of recognizing a specific antigen and coordinating an immune response against it.

A **T-cell** is a type of **lymphocyte**, or white blood cell. In **cell-mediated immunity**, T-cells bind to the surface of cells that display antigens and trigger a response. The response may include other lymphocytes or cytotoxic cells, such as killer T-cells. T-cells defend against intracellular infections, including viral infections.

A **B-cell** is also a lymphocyte. B-cells are responsible for **humoral immunity**. In response to a pathogen, B-cells secrete pathogen-specific antibodies. B-cells neutralize pathogens before they enter host cells.

An immunoglobulin, or antibody, is a protein with an attached sugar molecule that reacts to a specific antigen. Five types of immunoglobulins have been identified:

- IgG—IgG is the most common type of immunoglobulin. It is also the smallest immunoglobulin. After the first exposure to an antigen, small amounts of IgG are produced. After subsequent exposures, large amounts of IgG are produced.

- IgM—IgM is produced after the first exposure to an antigen. IgM is sensitive to antigens on the surface of red blood cells and is responsible for the effects of blood-type mismatches.

- IgA—IgA is produced by cells of the mucus membranes of the respiratory and gastrointestinal tract. It is also found in tears, saliva, and nasal fluids. IgA prevents pathogens from adhering to epithelial cells. IgA is also present in breast milk, which transfers immunity to infants. (IgG and IgM are also present in breast milk, but in low concentrations.)

- IgE—IgE is the least common type of antibody. Most of the IgE in the body is attached to mast cells, where it causes the release of histamine and other inflammatory substances. IgE is responsible for allergic and hypersensitivity reactions.

- IgD—IgD is located on the surface of B-cells and is involved in B-cell differentiation. IgD might play a role in autoimmune diseases, but its exact role in the immune system has not been clearly defined.

After an immune response is initiated (either from exposure to an invading pathogen or to a vaccine designed to stimulate the immune system), **active immunity** is developed. Active immunity gives the immune system a memory, enabling it to fight the same pathogen quickly on the next exposure. In contrast, **passive immunity** is the acquisition of antibodies without the immune system mounting a response. The most common example of passive immunity is the transfer of antibodies from a mother to a developing fetus during pregnancy or to an infant during breastfeeding. In the case of passive immunity, a host possesses antibodies to specific pathogens, but the host's own immune system did not produce them. Passive immunity does not confer lifelong protection, but provides defense until the host's own immune system is able to produce its own antibodies.

Lymphatic System

The **lymphatic system** is part of the immune system **FIGURE 18.4**. It includes a network of vessels that carry lymph (which is interstitial fluid that has entered the lymphatic system), the lymph nodes, and the lymphoid organs. Lymphatic vessels are made of a single layer of epithelial cells. Lymph capillaries, the smallest of the vessels, have one-way valves to direct the unidirectional flow of lymph around the body. Lymph capillaries flow into larger lymph vessels, which ultimately empty into subclavian veins. The lymphatic system carries proteins and fluid that have leaked out of the circulatory system back to the blood. The lymphatic system also carries fat and fat-soluble vitamins absorbed from the gastrointestinal tract to the circulating blood.

Lymph nodes are bell-shaped organs distributed throughout the body. Lymph nodes contain lymphocytes and phagocytes. As lymph flows through the lymphatic vessels, it passes through lymph nodes. Foreign materials in the lymph are removed by phagocytosis.

The thymus and bone marrow produce and store early lymphocytes, and are considered primary lymphoid organs. Secondary lymphoid organs include the spleen, the adenoids, and the tonsils. Secondary lymphoid organs contain lymphocytes that are activated in response to an antigen. These lymphocytes are responsible for initiating the adaptive immune response.

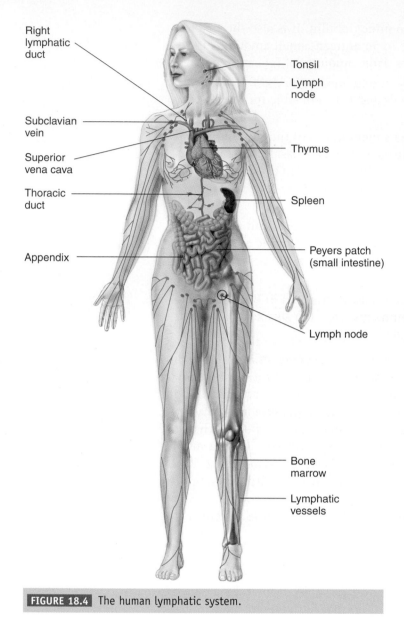

Right lymphatic duct

Subclavian vein

Superior vena cava

Thoracic duct

Appendix

Tonsil

Lymph node

Thymus

Spleen

Peyers patch (small intestine)

Lymph node

Bone marrow

Lymphatic vessels

FIGURE 18.4 The human lymphatic system.

Immunosuppressants

The immune system is excellent at recognizing and attacking anything that is foreign to the body. This includes transplanted organs. The concept of immunosuppression was developed to facilitate organ transplants by inhibiting the body's natural immune response. Drugs used specifically for organ transplants are called anti-rejection drugs.

Because immunosuppressants inhibit critical steps in fighting infections, patients receiving immunosuppression therapy are at increased risk for infections. Continuous monitoring of immunosuppression therapy for effectiveness and adverse reactions is necessary. Common immunosupression drugs are presented in **TABLE 18.3** .

Azathioprine is used to prevent rejection in solid organ transplants. It is also used to treat rheumatoid arthritis, because this disease has an autoimmune component.

Cyclosporine inhibits the production of interleukin-2. Cyclosporine is administered with azathioprine and/or corticosteroids to prolong survival in kidney, liver, heart, and bone-marrow transplants.

Mycophenolate inhibits the production of T- and B-cells. It is used to prevent rejection in kidney transplants.

Tacrolimus inhibits T-cell activation. It is used to prevent rejection in liver, kidney, heart, lung, or small-bowel transplants. Sirolimus also inhibits T-cell activation. It is used to prevent rejection in kidney transplants.

Monoclonal Antibodies

Monoclonal antibodies have been developed to protect against various diseases and infections, as well as to treat certain cancers. A **monoclonal antibody** (MAb or mAb) is produced in a laboratory from clones of B-cells that are targeted to specific anti-

Table 18.3 Common Immunosuppressants		
Generic Name	**Brand Name**	**Dosage Forms Available**
Azathioprine	Imuran	IV, tablet
Cyclosporine	Sandimmune, Neoral	Capsule, IV, oral liquid
Mycophenolate	CellCept	Capsule, IV, oral liquid, tablet
Sirolimus	Rapamune	Oral liquid, tablet
Tacrolimus	Prograf	Capsule, IV

gens, including those present in cancer cells. MAbs are structurally related to naturally occurring antibodies: IgG, IgM, IgA, IgE, and IgD. IgG and IgM are most commonly used therapeutically.

MAbs stimulate the body's natural immune defenses to target specific cells. MAbs function is several distinct ways. First, they can make the target cell easier to identify for the immune system. Second, MAbs can block receptors and prevent cell signaling, which, in turn, impairs the growth of target cells.

Cyclosporine oral suspension may be dispensed to patients in a community setting. Advise patients to review the instructions on mixing this drug with a beverage. Sandimmune may be mixed with milk, chocolate milk, or orange juice. Neoral may be mixed with apple juice or orange juice. Only glass containers and a glass syringe should be used when measuring and administering cyclosporine. Plastic or Styrofoam utensils or instruments should never be used. Ask a pharmacist to counsel the patient.

Last, MAbs can be combined with radioactive elements to target radiation delivery to specific cells, either for treatment or diagnostic tests. MAbs may likewise be combined with other drugs for targeted delivery, which prevents injury to healthy cells.

Cytopenias—specifically, low red blood cells, low white blood cells, and low platelets—are the primary side effects of therapy with MAbs. The immune system becomes hyperactive at the target cells and the rest of the body is left with an underactive immune system, which increases the risk for infection in patients receiving therapy with MAbs. MAbs may cause injection site pain and reactions, including burning, numbness, or tingling; nausea and vomiting; changes in blood pressure; allergic reactions; fever; and a rapid heartbeat. Pre-medications are usually administered prior to MAb administration to help prevent side effects associated with the infusion, including an antihistamine such as diphenhydramine, acetaminophen, and/or a corticosteroid.

MAbs are rarely considered first-line therapy. They are prescribed when other therapies have failed. MAbs are considered high-alert medications because of the danger associated with inappropriate or accidental use.

MAbs are named according to their origin and their site of action. The first part of the name signifies the distinctive name of the product. Next, the target of the antibody is noted:

- bac—Bacteria
- ci—Cardiovascular
- col—Colon
- got—Testis
- gov—ovary
- li(m)—Immune system
- les—Infections
- mel—Melanoma
- mar—Mammary
- mul—Musculoskeletal system
- n(e)(ur)—Nervous system
- pr(o)—Prostate
- vi(r)—Virus
- tu—Miscellaneous or multiple targets

The origin of the antibody is then conveyed:

- a—Rat
- axo—Rat/mouse hybrid
- e—Hamster

- i—Primate
- o—Murine/mouse
- u or zu—Human
- xi—A combination of sources
- xizu—A combination of human and other sources

Finally, the suffix mab indicates that an agent is a monoclonal antibody.

For example, the name infliximab signifies that the product is a MAb from a combination of sources (xi) that targets the immune system (li). (In fact, infliximab is indicated for the treated of autoimmune diseases.) Likewise, palivizumab identifies that the MAb is from a human origin (zu) and treats viral infections (vi). (Palivizumab is used to treat infections from respiratory syncytial virus.)

Common MAbs and the diseases or conditions they treat are listed in **TABLE 18.4**.

Confirm that appropriate pre-medications are ordered for a patient when dispensing monoclonal antibodies. If no antihistamine or acetaminophen is ordered, check with the pharmacist to see if these drugs are indicated.

Recombinant DNA Drugs

Recombinant DNA technology is used to manufacture therapeutic agents. DNA is the hereditary information contained in humans and many other living organisms. In this case, sequences of DNA that contain the genetic code of the target protein are inserted into a bacterium's DNA. The bacterium rapidly divides and produces the protein of interest. After large-scale **cloning**, or duplication, and growth of the bacteria, the protein is harvested, purified, and packaged for administration.

Table 18.4   Common Monoclonal Antibodies

Generic Name	Brand Name	Indication
Abciximab	ReoPro	Cardiovascular disease
Adalimumab	Humira	Autoimmune inflammatory disease
Alemtuzumab	Campath	Chronic lymphocytic leukemia
Basiliximab	Simulect	Transplant rejection
Bevacizumab	Avastin	Colorectal cancer, small-cell lung cancer
Cetuximab	Erbitux	Colorectal cancer
Daclizumab	Zenapax	Transplant rejection
Efalizumab	Raptiva	Psoriasis
Gemtuzumab	Mylotarg	Acute myeloid leukemia
Infliximab	Remicade	Autoimmune inflammatory disease
Natalizumab	Tysarbi	Multiple sclerosis
Omalizumab	Xolair	Allergy-related inflammatory disease
Palivizumab	Synagis	Respiratory syncytial virus
Panitumumab	Vectibix	Colorectal cancer
Ranibizumab	Lucenetis	Macular degeneration
Rituximab	Rituxan, Mabthera	Non-Hodgkin's lymphoma
Tositumomab	Bexxar	Non-Hodgkin's lymphoma
Trastuzumab	Herceptin	Breast cancer

Many diseases arise from protein dysfunction, and protein-based therapeutic agents that are highly specific are increasing in availability as recombinant technology improves and drug development intensifies. Insulin is a common example of a therapeutic agent that uses recombinant technology. Continued growth in the field of recombinant DNA drugs is expected.

Colony-Stimulating Factors

Blood contains many distinct cell types **FIGURE 18.5**. A colony-stimulating factor (CSF) stimulates blood-cell production in the bone marrow. Colony-stimulating factors are used to treat **anemia** (a decrease in the number of red blood cells), **neutropenia** (a decrease in the number of white blood cells), and **cytopenia** (a decrease in any type of blood cell).

CSFs treat cytopenias relating to chemotherapy, bone-marrow dysfunction, chronic kidney disease, hematological disorders, and infectious diseases. The availability of CSFs has decreased the use of blood transfusions, which has decreased the risks that can occur with chronic exposure to blood components. CSFs also help optimize chemotherapy regimens because CSFs can correct cytopenias related to chemotherapy, meaning that chemotherapy does not need to be delayed or discontinued. CSFs are expensive and require specialized storage, preparation, and administration. All CSFs are available only by prescription, and all must be administered via injection. Common CSFs are presented in **TABLE 18.5**.

Epoetin alfa is a synthetic form of erythropoietin, which is naturally produced by the kidneys. Epoetin alfa is used to treat anemia associated with end-stage renal disease as well as anemias that do not respond to other treatment. Frequent blood tests are required to assess the effectiveness and safety of epoetin alfa. If the patient's

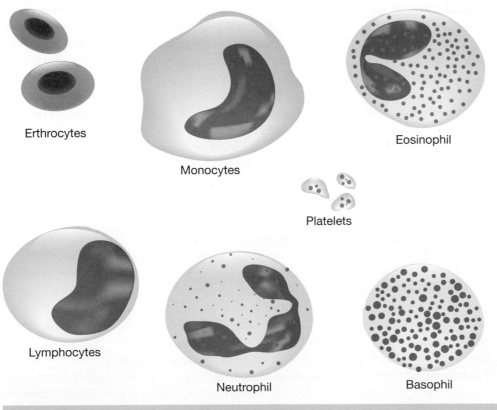

Erthrocytes

Monocytes

Eosinophil

Platelets

Lymphocytes

Neutrophil

Basophil

FIGURE 18.5 Blood contains many distinct cell types.

Table 18.5 Common Colony-Stimulating Factors	
Generic Name	**Brand Name**
Epoetin alfa	Procrit, Epogen
Filgrastim	Neupogen
Pegfilgrastim	Neulasta
Sargramostim	Leukine

What Would You Do?

Question: You work in a hospital pharmacy where pharmacy technicians are responsible for confirming laboratory results prior to administration of colony-stimulating factors. You receive an order for Procrit for a 55-year-old male receiving chemotherapy. The patient's hemoglobin is 12g/dL. Would you dispense the Procrit?

Answer: Do not initiate therapy with epoetin alfa if the hemoglobin is greater than 10g/dL. Reassess the laboratory results routinely and initiate treatment when the hemoglobin falls below 10g/dL, if still indicated as ordered by the physician. Colony-stimulating factors should be used at the lowest possible dose and for the shortest length of time needed to avoid a blood transfusion.

hematocrit, or portion of red blood cells in the blood, exceeds 36 percent, or the **hemoglobin**, the concentration of iron-containing protein, exceeds 10g/dL, epoetin alfa should not be administered. In some hospital settings, the pharmacy technician is responsible for ensuring that the appropriate lab work has been completed prior to administration of epoetin alfa.

Filgrastim increases the production of white blood cells and granulocytes. Filgrastim should not be administered within 24 hours before or 24 hours after chemotherapy. Filgrastim is not compatible with normal saline and must be mixed with 5 percent dextrose. Dextrose flushes should be dispensed with filgrastim so nurses can clean saline out of the IV tubing before administering filgrastim.

Pegfilgrastim is a long-acting form of filgrastim. It has a polyethylene glycol component that increases the duration of action and, therefore, requires less frequent dosing than filgrastim. Pegfilgrastim is used to prevent infections in patients receiving chemotherapy; one dose of pegfilgrastim is administered after each chemotherapy cycle. Pegfilgrastim is dispensed in a prefilled syringe.

Sargramostim increases the growth of white blood cells after bone-marrow or stem-cell transplantation, which decreases the length of antibiotic treatment, reduces infections, and shortens hospital stays. Sargramostim may be administered daily for up to 30 days, and frequent monitoring of blood cell counts is recommended. Sargramostim cannot be mixed with dextrose; it should be reconstituted in sterile water, and normal saline should be used for infusion of this product.

Immune System Therapies

A **biologic response modifier** enhances immune activity so the body can effectively attack and kill pathogens. An intact immune system is critical to controlling the growth of disease, and biologic response modifiers are used to treat cancers, rheumatoid arthritis, acute coronary syndrome, immunologic disorders, and a host of other conditions. These agents can cause adverse effects, ranging from nausea and vomiting to flu-like symptoms, a skin rash, bleeding disorders, or cardiotoxicity. Common biologic response modifiers are presented in TABLE 18.6 .

Interferons are small proteins that are naturally produced by the immune system in response to viral infections or tumor proliferation. As a therapeutic family, interferons possess antiviral, antiproliferative, and immune-modulating properties. Interferons increase the activity of cytotoxic cells within the immune system. They also prolong the cell cycle and increase cell size. Interferons inhibit the growth of blood vessels in

Table 18.6	**Common Biologic Response Modifiers**	
Generic Name	**Brand Name**	**Clinical Use/Indication**
Aldesleukin (interleukin-2)	Proleukin	Treatment of metastatic renal-cell cancer and metastatic melanoma
Denileukin diftitox	Ontak	Treatment of recurrent cutaneous T-cell lymphoma
Interferon alfa-2b	Intron A	Treatment of chronic hepatitis B, chronic hepatitis C, hairy-cell leukemia, malignancy melanoma, AIDS-related Kaposi's sarcoma, non-Hodgkin's lymphoma
Interferon beta-1a	Avonex, Rebif	Treatment of relapsing forms of multiple sclerosis
Interferon beta-1b	Betaseron	Treatment of relapsing forms of multiple sclerosis
Interferon gamma-1b	Actimmune	Reduce infections associated with chronic granulomatous disease; treatment of severe, malignant osteopetrosis
Oprelvekin (interleukin-11)	Neumega	Prevention of severe thrombocytopenia

tumors and block cancer-regulating genes that direct the uncontrolled growth rate of tumors. Because of their widespread activities, interferons can alter gene expression in healthy cells or activate proteins that control normal cell growth and function.

Interleukins are proteins that function as signaling molecules. They are naturally produced as part of the immune system. Interleukin-2 promotes B- and T-cell growth and differentiation. It also increases the activity of cytotoxic immune cells. Interleukin-2 can differentiate between tumor cells and healthy cells, leaving healthy cells undamaged. Interleukin-11 increases the production of platelets. Administration of interleukin-based therapies should be completed under the supervision of trained personnel. Serious adverse reactions have occurred related to aldesleukin and oprelvekin therapy, including vascular leak syndrome, impaired neutrophil production, and severe lethargy, somnolence, or coma with interleukin-2, and anaphylactic reactions with interleukin-11. In general, the effects are manageable with supportive care after the therapy is discontinued.

Denileukin diftitox is a fusion protein containing both interleukin-2 and diphtheria toxin. This formulation allows the toxic effects of the diphtheria toxin to be delivered only to cells with a high affinity for interleukin-2, such as cancer cells. The diphtheria toxin inhibits protein synthesis within the cancer cells and leads to cell death. Denileukin diftitox can produce acute hypersensitivity reactions and vascular leak syndrome.

Cancer and Chemotherapy

Cancer is a large group of diseases characterized by uncontrolled cellular growth, local tissue invasion, and distant metastases. Cancer incidence is increasing. It is the leading cause of death among Americans aged 85 years or younger, claiming more than half a million lives every year.

Types of Tumors

Cancer is defined by the presence of a tumor, or **neoplasm**—an abnormal growth of cells that originates in a single cell with altered or damaged DNA. Therefore, cancer is also called a **neoplastic disease**. Usually, cells grow and multiply when the body needs them, and then die when the body does not need them. Healthy cells also stop growing when they come in contact with other cells, so as to not become overcrowded. In cancer, cells do not respond to signals to stop growing or to die.

Tumors can arise from any of the basic tissues of the body: epithelial tissue, connective tissue (which includes muscle, bone, and cartilage), lymphoid tissue, and nerve tissue. As tumors grow and cancerous cells spread, they lose some of their original characteristics, although most cancer cells retain enough of the original cell's traits that it is possible to identify their precise origin. **Benign tumors**—those that are not harmful, progressive, or recurrent—are named by adding the suffix oma to the end of the cell or organ of origin. Hence, a fibroma is a benign tumor of fibrous connective tissue. Benign tumors are not considered cancerous. Benign tumors are most often localized masses, and the tumor cells resemble the originator cells. These tumors do not spread to other tissues and rarely recur once removed surgically.

The suffixes carcinoma and sarcoma describe **malignant tumors**—that is, invasive or progressive tumors arising from epithelial tissue and connective tissue, respectively. Therefore, a fibrosarcoma is a malignant tumor of fibrous connective tissue. Lymphoma and leukemia designate cancers found in blood-forming tissues, and blastomas are cancers arising from embryonic tissues. Blastomas are most often seen in children. Unlike benign tumors, malignant tumors are invasive and spread to surrounding tissues and organs. **Metastasis** is the spread of cancerous cells from the primary site to distant sites to form new tumors. As the cells grow and metastasize, they lose the characteristics of the original cell and lose their ability to carry out normal cellular functions. Recurrence of malignant tumors is common, even after removal of the primary tumor.

Chemotherapy Agents

The treatment of cancer depends on the type of cancer and the amount of growth or spread of the original tumor. If the cancer is confined to one location in the body, surgery may be used to remove the tumor. If the tumor has only spread to the lymph nodes, these may also be successfully removed with surgery. If surgery cannot remove the presence of all cancerous tumors, radiation therapy, biological agents, or chemotherapy can be used instead of or in addition to surgery.

Several classes of chemotherapy agents are available to treat a multitude of cancers. Chemotherapy agents may be used alone or in combination with other drugs or treatments. Chemotherapy agents are usually classified by their mechanism of action. Some agents fall into more than one class. Common chemotherapy agents are presented in **TABLE 18.7**, according to their most well-defined mechanism of action.

Chemotherapy regimens are developed and implemented based on the type of cancer being treated and the presence of metastases, as well as patient-specific factors including body weight, body surface area, age, kidney function, and complete blood counts. Each of these parameters is assessed regularly, prior to administering chemotherapy. Incorrect doses or time intervals could have detrimental consequences to the patient and result in ineffective or unsafe treatment.

The goals of chemotherapy are to cure cancer and remove all traces of the disease. If this is not possible, chemotherapy is used to prolong survival and decrease symptoms associated with cancer.

Antimetabolites resemble naturally occurring metabolites, including nucleotides, and are incorporated into the cell's own DNA. However, antimetabolites cannot be used by cells in the same productive manner as the actual metabolite, so normal cellular functions

When methotrexate is dispensed in a community setting, the Institute for Safe Medication Practices (ISMP) encourages providing patients with written information regarding the dosing schedule and the risks associated with incorrect dosing. If possible, dispense methotrexate in prepackaged dose packs to decrease confusion or errors in dosing. Confirm that the patient understands the dosing schedule and instruct him or her to speak with the physician or pharmacist if he or she has any questions.

Table 18.7 Common Chemotherapy Agents

Class	Generic Name	Brand Name	Dosage Forms Available
Antimetabolites	Azacytidine	Vidaza	Injection, IV
	Capecitabine	Xeloda	Tablet
	Cladribine	Leustatin	IV
	Cytarabine	Cytosar	Injection, IV
	Decitabine	Dacogen	IV
	Fludarabine	Fludara	IV
	Fluorouracil	Adrucil, Carac, Efudex, Fluoroplex, Fluorouracil	Injection, IV, topical preparation
	Gemcitabine	Gemzar	IV
	Mercaptopurine	Purinethol	Tablet
	Methotrexate	Rheumatrex, Trexall	Injection, tablet
	Pentostatin	Nipent	Injection
	Thioguanine	Tabloid	Tablet
Plant alkaloids	Docitaxel	Taxotere	IV
	Paclitaxel	Onxol, Taxol, Abraxane	IV
	Vinblastine	Velban	IV
	Vincristine	Vincasar PFS	IV
	Vinorelbine	Navelbine	IV
Topoisomerase inhibitors	Daunorubicin (daunomycin)	Cerubidine	IV
	Doxorubicin	Adriamycin PFS	IV
	Epirubicin	Ellence	IV
	Etoposide	VePesid	Capsule, IV
	Idrarubicin	Idamycin	IV
	Mitoxantrone	Novantrone	IV
	Teniposide	Vumon	IV
Alkylating agents	Carmustine	BiCNU	IV
	Cyclophosphamide	Cytoxan	IV, tablet
	Dacarbazine	N/A	IV
	Ifosfamide	Ifex	IV
	Lomustine	CeeNU	Capsule
	Temozolomide	Temodar	Capsule
Heavy metal compounds	Cisplatin	Platinol	IV
	Carboplatin	Paraplatin	IV
	Oxaliplatin	Eloxatin	IV
Nitrogen mustards	Chlorambucil	Leukeran	Tablet
	Melphalan	Alkeran	IV, tablet
	Thiotepa	N/A	IV

(continues)

Table 18.7   Common Chemotherapy Agents *(Continued)*

Class	Generic Name	Brand Name	Dosage Forms Available
Tyrokinase inhibitors	Dasatinib	Sprycel	Tablet
	Erlotinib	Tarceva	Tablet
	Imatinib	Gleevec	Tablet
	Nilotinib	Tasigna	Capsule, tablet
Modified steroid hormones	Aminoglutethimide	Cytadren	Tablet
	Bicalutamide	Casodex	Tablet
	Flutamide	Eulexin	Capsule
	Goserelin	Zoladex	Implant
	Leuprolide	Eligard, Lupron Depot, Viadur	Implant, injection
	Megestrol	N/A	Oral suspension, tablet
	Mitotane	Lysodren	Tablet
	Triptorelin	Trelstar	Injection
Estrogen-receptor antagonists	Fulvestrant	Faslodex	Injection
	Tamoxifen	Nolvadex	Tablet
Aromatase inhibitors	Anastrozole	Arimidex	Tablet
	Exemestane	Aromasin	Tablet
	Letrozole	Femara	Tablet

cease. Antimetabolites often resemble purines, pyrimidine, or folate. Antimetabolites used in chemotherapy prevent the replication of DNA, RNA, and proteins.

Chemotherapy Roadmaps

Roadmaps are error-prevention tools used in cancer chemotherapy. As the name implies, a roadmap is analogous to a map that you would use when you travel. Much like the packet you pick up from a travel agent before you leave on a long trip, the roadmap is a step-by-step itinerary for cancer treatment. It is based on protocols that help ensure that the correct drugs, doses, and monitoring are completed while patients are on the road from point A, cancer, to point B, a hoped-for remission or cure. The roadmap, which is usually several pages long, includes important patient data, a schedule of when drugs are to be given, and laboratory and other therapeutic or diagnostic procedures to be completed. The roadmap stays with the patient chart and is updated constantly so that all team members know where they are at all times. A copy of the protocol or plan for the future treatment is a part of the permanent record. Chemotherapy is sometimes based on body surface area, a measurement derived from height and weight. This and other crucial patient information is updated on the roadmap each time a patient comes in for treatment.

Plant alkaloids are derived from the periwinkle (vinca) plant. Also called vinca alkaloids, this class of drugs inhibits cell division by inhibiting the formation of **mitotic spindle fibers**, the fibers that separate the strands of DNA during replication.

Topoisomerase is an enzyme responsible for maintaining DNA structure during replication and transcription. (**Transcription** is the process by which a strand of RNA is made that corresponds to a strand of DNA.) When DNA unwinds itself, strain is placed on the helical structure; topoisomerase cleaves the DNA strand and forms temporary bonds to prevent DNA damage during replication and transcription. Topoisomerase inhibitors prevent this action, which causes DNA strands to break, leading to cell death.

Alkylating agents exert their antineoplastic activity by inhibiting DNA and protein synthesis. These agents bind to DNA and prevent the unwinding of the DNA double helix that must take place prior to replication and transcription. Alkylating agents are the oldest and arguably most useful class of chemotherapy drugs. Alkylating agents are cytotoxic, mutagenic, teratogenic, and carcinogenic. Resistance to these agents can develop after prolonged use because of increased DNA repair capabilities of cancer cells.

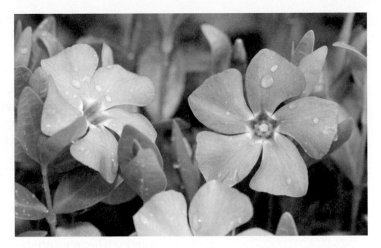

Some chemotherapy agents are derived from plant-based compounds, such as those found in the periwinkle (*Vinca spp.*) plant.

Heavy metal compounds are also classified as alkylating agents. They are platinum derivatives that bind to DNA and form bonds between pairs of guanines. The bonds cause the DNA to bend and break, producing cellular damage and cell death. Heavy metal compounds can cause severe hypersensitivity reactions, including anaphylaxis.

Nitrogen mustards are chemically related to mustard gas, a chemical weapon used in World War I. Nitrogen mustards irreversibly bind to DNA and RNA, inhibiting the reproduction of the cell. Nitrogen mustards are most effective against cells that are in a resting phase, not actively growing and dividing cells.

Tyrokinase (or tyrosine kinase) is an enzyme that promotes cell growth and proliferation among many types of cells. By blocking the action of this enzyme, tyrokinase inhibitors decrease cell growth and proliferation. In general, these agents present fewer side effects than other chemotherapy agents.

Hormone-based therapies target cancer cells that originate from cells under steroid hormone control such as breast, prostate, and endometrial cancers. Tumors often regress when the hormone controlling the tumor growth is inhibited. Some agents are modified hormones that can act as hormone antagonists or suppress normal hormone production. Estrogen receptor antagonists and aromatase inhibitors inhibit the normal production and function of steroid hormones. These estrogen-based therapies can cause hot flashes, nausea, and weight gain. They are generally used to prevent the recurrence of breast cancer.

Complications of Chemotherapy

Many of the drugs used to treat chemotherapy cannot be specifically targeted to cancer cells. Therefore, any cells in the body that are rapidly growing or dividing, such as cells of the skin, mucus membranes, or immune system, are vulnerable to these drugs' cytotoxic effects. Common side effects of chemotherapy include pain, nausea and vomiting, oral toxicity and tissue injury, hair loss, blood-related disorders, and decreased immune function. Many of these side effects are manageable with additional drug therapy.

Comfort and quality of life are important considerations in comprehensive cancer treatment. Therefore, pain management and control of gastrointestinal complications are essential to treating the patient's entire well-being, rather than just the cancer.

Pain, nausea, and vomiting related to cancer and chemotherapy are managed according to general principles of analgesia and antiemesis, described in Chapters 8 and 12, respectively.

Oral complications are common among patients receiving chemotherapy. Because the cells of the oral mucosa are rapidly dividing, they suffer from the effects of chemotherapy. Oral ulcerations and irritations can impair a patient's ability to eat and can pose a risk for infection, both of which can interfere with the effectiveness of chemotherapy regimens. Oral complications cannot be prevented during chemotherapy, but they can be managed to promote healing and decrease pain. Cevimeline (Evoxac), chlorhexidine gluconate (Peridex), hydrogen peroxide (Peroxyl), phenol solutions, and several other solutions are available that offer cleansing of the oral cavity coupled with pain relief and local antimicrobial activity.

Rescue drugs can be administered after chemotherapy to decrease the risk of side effects associated with chemotherapy. Once the chemotherapeutic agent has been in the body long enough to exert its effects on the cancer cells, the rescue drug is administered to act as an antidote to the chemotherapy and prevent its cytotoxic effects on healthy cells. Amifostine (Ethyol) is a rescue drug administered after cisplatin to reduce kidney toxicity. It is also administered after radiation therapy to treat head and neck cancer or rectal cancer. Dexrazoxane (Zinecard) reduces cardiotoxicity associated with doxorubicin administration in postmenopausal women with metastatic breast cancer. Leucovorin, also known as folinic acid, is administered after methotrexate and decreases toxicity associated with impaired folic-acid synthesis.

Tech Math Practice

Question: **A physician orders 500mL of D$_5$W to be administered over four hours. The IV set delivers 10 drops/mL. How many drops should be administered to the patient each minute?**

Answer: x drops/min = $\frac{\text{Volume of Fluid}}{\text{Delivery Time in Hours}} \times \frac{\text{Drops of IV Set}}{\text{mL of IV Set}} \times \frac{\text{1hr}}{\text{60min}}$

x drops/min = $\frac{\text{500mL}}{\text{4hr}} \times \frac{\text{10 drops of IV Set}}{\text{mL of IV Set}} \times \frac{\text{1hr}}{\text{60min}}$ = 20.83 drops/min, or rounded up to 21 drops/min.

Question: **If a 1-L continuous IV infusion is running at 125mL/hr, how often will a new infusion be needed?**

Answer: How long an IV lasts depends on the volume and the flow rate. This can be expressed by the following equation:

Time of IV = $\frac{\text{Volume of Solution (mL)}}{\text{Flow Rate (}^{mL}/_{hr}\text{)}}$.

In this case, the time of IV = $\frac{\text{1,000mL}}{\text{125mL/hr}}$ = 8 hours, so the infusion will need to be replaced every 8 hours.

Question: **You prepared a 75mL IV infusion to be administered over 60 minutes. It will be administered using an IV set with a flow rate of 15 drops/mL. The nurse wants to know the administration rate in drops/minute.**

Answer: x drops/min = $\frac{\text{Volume of Fluid}}{\text{Delivery Time in Hours}} \times \frac{\text{Drops of IV Set}}{\text{mL of IV Set}} \times \frac{\text{1hr}}{\text{60min}}$

x drops/min = $\frac{\text{75mL}}{\text{1hr}} \times \frac{\text{15 Drops of IV Set}}{\text{mL of IV Set}} \times \frac{\text{1hr}}{\text{60min}}$ = 18.75 drops/min, or rounded to 19 drops/min.

Question: **A physician orders a volume of 500mL to be administered over 12 hours using a microdrip IV set that delivers 60 drops/mL. What is the flow rate of this infusion in drops/min?**

Answer: x drops/min = $^{\text{Volume of Fluid}}/_{\text{Delivery Time in Hours}} \times {}^{\text{Drops of IV Set}}/_{\text{mL of IV Set}} \times {}^{\text{1hr}}/_{\text{60min}}$

x drops/min = $^{\text{500mL}}/_{\text{12hr}} \times {}^{\text{60 Drops of IV Set}}/_{\text{mL of IV Set}} \times {}^{\text{1hr}}/_{\text{60min}}$ = 41.67 drops/min, or rounded to 42 drops/min.

Question: **A nurse is using an IV set with a drip rate of 20 drops/mL to administer 42 drops per minute. If 500mL needs to be administered to the patient, how long will the infusion last? What will the flow rate be in mL/hr?**

Answer: x drops/min = $^{\text{Volume of Fluid}}/_{\text{Delivery Time in Hours}} \times {}^{\text{Drops of IV Set}}/_{\text{mL of IV Set}} \times {}^{\text{1hr}}/_{\text{60min}}$

42 drops/min = $^{\text{500mL}}/_{\text{xhr}} \times {}^{\text{20 Drops of IV Set}}/_{\text{mL of IV Set}} \times {}^{\text{1hr}}/_{\text{60min}}$

Cross-multiply and solve for x: $x$hr = $^{\text{500mL}}/_{\text{42 drops/min}} \times {}^{\text{20 drops of IV Set}}/_{\text{mL of IV Set}} \times {}^{\text{1hr}}/_{\text{60min}}$ = 4hr

Flow rate = 500mL ÷ 4hr = 125mL/hr.

Question: **A physician orders sodium chloride 2mEq/kg/day for a patient weighing 135lbs. Sodium chloride is available in a solution containing 4mEq/mL. How many milliliters will be needed to prepare this product for 24 hours?**

Answer: Dose = 135lbs $\times {}^{\text{1kg}}/_{\text{2.2lbs}} \times {}^{\text{2mEq}}/_{\text{1kg}}$ = 122.7mEq, or rounded to 123mEq.

Volume: $^{\text{4mEq}}/_{\text{1mL}} = {}^{\text{123mEq}}/_{\text{xml}}$

Cross-multiply and solve for x: x = 30.75mL.

WRAP UP

Chapter Summary

- Parenteral products are administered via injection. They allow drug delivery directly to an organ, lesion, muscle, nerve, body tissue, or systemic circulation. Parenteral products are preferred when patients are unable to take medications by mouth, when immediate drug action is required, or when drugs are inactivated after oral administration.

- Parenteral products must be sterile. Because of stringent requirements for aseptic preparation of compounded sterile products, parenteral products are expensive and time-consuming to prepare.

- Parenteral products must be isotonic to the blood to prevent damage to blood cells. Sodium chloride is an isotonic vehicle that is often used as a base solution for parenteral administration.

- Parenteral products may be administered via several routes of administration: intravenous, intramuscular, intradermal, subcutaneous, intra-articular, intrasynovial, intraspinal, intrathecal, intra-arterial, and intracardiac.

- Small-volume parenterals contain less than 100mL. They may be administered alone or as an IV piggyback. Large-volume parenterals contain more than 100mL and include solutions for nutrition, fluid replacement, dialysis, and irrigation.

- Preparation of parenteral products requires knowledge of and adherence to safety precautions and aseptic technique practices, as well as the use of specialized equipment, including syringes and needles and IV sets.

- Calculations are necessary for preparing and administering IV solutions. Pharmacy personnel report flow rates in mL/hr, but nurses often prefer to calculate drops/min.

- Cytotoxic drugs have a toxic effect on cells. When used therapeutically in specific disease states, cytotoxic drugs are beneficial. When exposure to hazardous agents occurs during the preparation or handling of pharmaceutical products, healthcare workers can suffer from carcinogenic, mutagenic, or teratogenic consequences.

- Personal protective clothing and equipment should be worn when handling cytotoxic drugs for stocking, inventory, disposal, or compounding. Exposure to cytotoxic drugs can occur during any of these processes. To minimize exposure, cytotoxic drugs should always be compounded in a vertical laminar flow biological safety cabinet or a bacteriological glove box. Any drugs, materials, or equipment used in preparing or handling cytotoxic agents should be disposed of in appropriate containers, in accordance with local, state, and federal regulations. Patients receiving cytotoxic agents on an outpatient basis should be informed of the risks associated with handling and administering hazardous agents.

- Spill kits are required for any pharmacy that works with cytotoxic drugs. A quality-assurance program guarantees that any lapses in patient or worker safety due to the handling or preparation of cytotoxic drugs are addressed and corrected.

- The immune system is the body's defense against invading pathogens. The immune system adapts and evolves in response to its environment and pathogen exposure.

- Exterior defenses are the body's first line of defense. Innate immunity is a non-specific defense mounted to destroy pathogens by phagocytosis; innate immunity includes monocytes, macrophages, neutrophils, basophils, mast cells, eosinophils, and natural killer cells. The adaptive immune system mounts a pathogen-specific defense against invading organisms.

- The adaptive immune system includes cell-mediated immunity, orchestrated by T-cells, and humoral immunity, directed by B-cells. B-cells produce antibodies in response to antigens.

- The lymphatic system is a component of the immune system that carries interstitial fluid through a network of lymph nodes that act as filters. The lymph system removes invading pathogens from the body, returns proteins and fluid to the circulatory system, and carries fat and fat-soluble vitamins to blood.

- Immunosuppressants decrease the functionality of the immune system. This concept is important in organ transplant to prevent the body from attacking the new organ, which it sees as a foreign pathogen. Patients receiving immunosuppression therapy are at increased risk for infection.

- Monoclonal antibodies are laboratory-produced targeted antibodies. They can be used to treat a variety of autoimmune and cardiovascular diseases, infections, and cancers. Monoclonal antibodies are high-alert medications because of the risk of serious side effects. Pre-medications should be administered with monoclonal antibodies to decrease the risk of infusion-related reactions.

- DNA is the genetic material present in all living organisms. DNA can replicate itself, and directs the production of proteins through the processes of transcription and translation. (**Translation** is the process by which ribosomes read the nucleotide sequence from RNA and assemble proteins.) Recombinant DNA technology is used to produce therapeutic agents by inserting specific DNA sequences into a bacterium. The bacterium grows and multiplies, and produces the protein specified by the DNA sequence.

- Colony-stimulating factors (CSFs) are therapeutic compounds produced by recombinant DNA technology. CSFs treat cytopenia related to chemotherapy and other disease states. CSFs require routine monitoring, as well as specialized storage, handling, and administration techniques.

- Biologic response modifiers are agents produced through recombinant DNA technology that enhance the body's own immune defenses. They are modifications of naturally occurring immune system proteins. Biologic response modifiers are used to treat cancer, autoimmune disease, and acute coronary syndrome.

- Cancer is a group of diseases defined by uncontrolled cellular growth, local tissue invasion, and distant metastases. A tumor, or neoplasm, is a hallmark sign of cancer. Benign tumors are isolated and not progressive or recurrent. Malignant tumors are invasive and progressive tumors.

- Several classes of chemotherapeutic agents are available to treat cancer. Most classes of drugs interrupt the normal processes of DNA replication or cell growth and proliferation. If a complete cure of cancer is not possible, the goals of chemotherapy are to prolong survival and decrease the symptoms associated with cancer.

- Chemotherapy targets rapidly dividing cells. Therefore, even healthy cells are vulnerable to the effects of chemotherapy, particularly the skin, oral mucosa, and immune system. Adverse effects of chemotherapy cannot be prevented, but they can be managed with supportive care. Rescue drugs can serve as antidotes to chemotherapy to prevent damage to healthy cells.

Learning Assessment Questions

1. Parenteral administration of fluid, electrolyte, or nutritional products is preferred in all but which of the following situations?

   A. When a patient is unconscious

   B. When a patient is vomiting repeatedly

   C. When a drug is inactivated by oral administration

   D. Parenteral administration is preferred in all of the above situations

2. Which of the following is not true of parenteral administration?

   A. Dosage errors cannot always be easily corrected.

   B. They are inexpensive to prepare.

   C. Parenteral products result in a rapid onset of action.

   D. Chemical incompatibilities may render the drug ineffective.

3. Which of the following solutions is considered isotonic when compared to blood?

   A. Acetic acid solution

   B. 5% dextrose in water

   C. Lactated Ringer's solution

   D. 0.9% sodium chloride

4. Which of the following is not considered a parenteral route of administration?

    A. Intramuscular

    B. Sublingual

    C. Intrasynovial

    D. Intrathecal

5. Which of the following is not a type of IV administration?

    A. Continuous infusion

    B. Intermittent infusion

    C. IV push

    D. Irrigation

6. Which of the following pairs correctly matches the injection site and the maximum volume for an intramuscular injection for an adult?

    A. Vastus lateralis, 1mL

    B. Gluteus maximus, 5mL

    C. Deltoid, 1mL

    D. Gluteus maximus, 2mL

7. Which of the following is a not benefit of a closed-system transfer device?

    A. Preparation time is decreased.

    B. Costs are decreased.

    C. Consistency is increased.

    D. Patient comfort is increased.

8. How must total parenteral nutrition be administered?

    A. Via subcutaneous injections to the abdomen

    B. Via a central venous catheter

    C. Through a nasogastric tube

    D. To a vein in the antecubital area

9. Which of the following is not used as an irrigation solution?

    A. Acetic acid solution

    B. 10% dextrose in water

    C. Lactated Ringer's solution

    D. Sodium chloride

10. Which of the following is a not principle of aseptic technique?

    A. All outerwear and jewelry should be removed.

    B. Protective clothing should be worn, including a non-shedding laboratory coat, hair covers, a facemask, shoe covers, and gloves.

    C. A calculator, a pen, and a label should be brought to the work area to minimize the need to leave and re-enter the sterile workspace.

    D. One should avoid touching the face or hair while in the sterile workspace.

11. What is a teratogen?

    A. A substance that causes cancer

    B. A substance that activates an immune response

    C. A substance that acts as an antidote to a chemotherapeutic agent

    D. A substance that interferes with normal fetal development

12. Which of the following does not need to be part of a hazardous-spill cleanup kit?

    A. A cell phone or other communication device

    B. Two pairs of gloves

    C. A respirator mask

    D. A "Caution" sign

13. Which of the following is not a benefit of colony-stimulating factors?

    A. They prolong survival in kidney transplant recipients.

    B. They decrease the need for blood transfusions.

    C. They manage the side effects of chemotherapy.

    D. They can be used to treat anemia related to several disease states.

14. Filgrastim must be administered with what solution?

    A. Normal saline

    B. Dextrose

    C. Water

    D. Lactated Ringer's

15. Interferons possess which of the following sets of properties?

    A. Carcinogenic, mutagenic, and teratogenic

    B. Antiviral, antiproliferative, and immune-modulating

    C. Specificity, mobility, and redundancy

    D. Cardiotoxicity and nephrotoxicity

16. Which of the following is part of the body's first line of defense against invading pathogens?

    A. Saliva

    B. Cell-mediated immunity

    C. Natural killer cells

    D. The innate immune system

17. Which type of immunity is conferred by vaccines?

    A. Innate immunity

    B. Redundant immunity

    C. Passive immunity

    D. Adaptive immunity

18. What is the most common subtype of immunoglobulin?

    A. IgG

    B. IgA

    C. IgD

    D. IgE

19. Which of the following is a primary lymphoid organ?

    A. Adenoids

    B. Spleen

    C. Bone marrow

    D. Tonsils

20. What is the source of the monoclonal antibody called bevacizumab?

    A. Mouse

    B. Human

    C. Hamster

    D. Primate

21. What is the target of the monoclonal antibody called natalizumab?

    A. Immune system

    B. Cardiovascular system

    C. Viral infections

    D. Nervous system

22. Nitrogen mustards are most effective against which type of cells?

    A. Cells that are undergoing the process of transcription

    B. Cells in a resting phase

    C. Cells that are larger than normal size

    D. Cells that are rapidly dividing

23. Which of the following sets of adverse effects is associated with estrogen-based therapies that prevent the return of breast cancer?

    A. Hot flashes, nausea, weight gain

    B. Nausea and vomiting, oral ulcerations, and pain

    C. Pain and cytopenias

    D. Vascular leak syndrome, decreased neutrophils, and lethargy

24. Which of the following is not a common complication of chemotherapy?

    A. Oral complications

    B. Nausea and vomiting

    C. Decreased immune function

    D. Enlarged lymph nodes

25. Leucovorin is a rescue drug for which chemotherapeutic agent(s)?

    A. Folic acid

    B. Methotrexate

    C. Cisplatin

    D. Alkylating agents

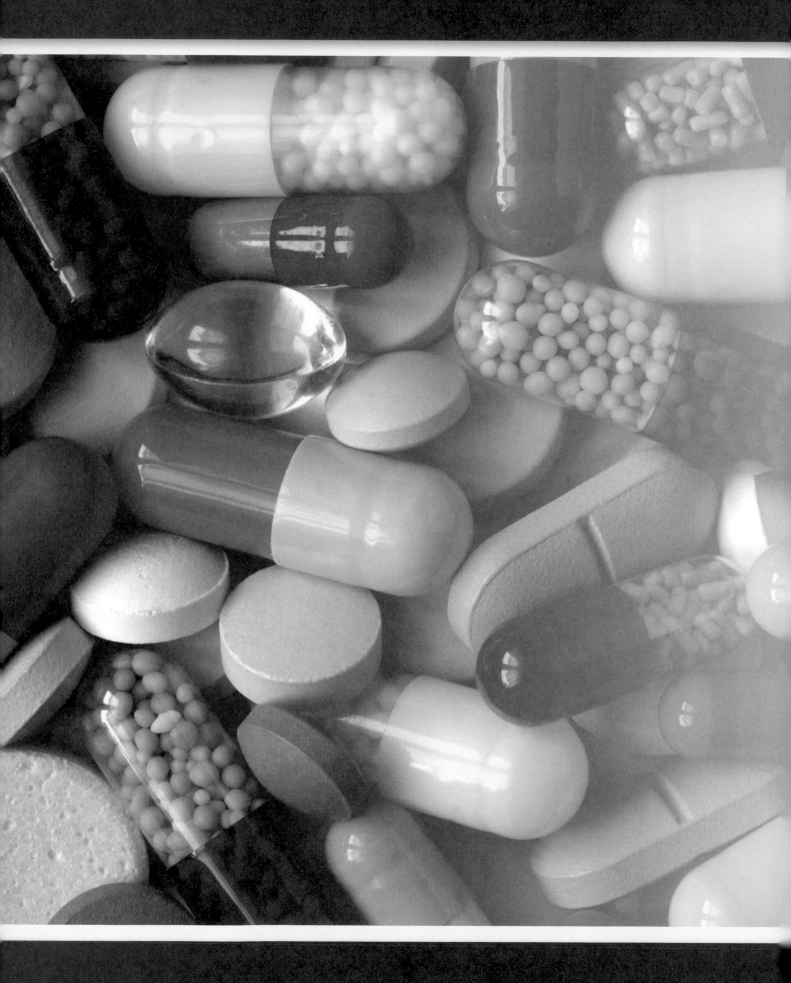

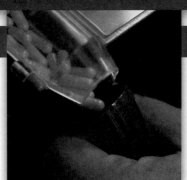

Labs for Sterile Compounding

OBJECTIVES

After reading this chapter, you will be able to:

- Demonstrate proper aseptic handwashing technique.
- Understand USP 797 requirements for compounding sterile products.
- Perform garbing procedures outlined in USP 797.
- Complete proper cleaning of a laminar airflow hood.
- Apply aseptic technique to the preparation of small- and large-volume parenteral products.
- Solve calculations relating to the preparation of small- and large-volume parenteral products.
- Apply aseptic technique to the preparation of sterile powder drug vials.
- Solve calculations relating to the preparation of sterile powder drug vials.
- Apply aseptic technique to the preparation of medication obtained from an ampule.
- Understand the role of vitamins and electrolytes in the human body.
- Compare and contrast enteral and parenteral nutrition.
- Recognize commonly used vitamins, herbs, nutritional products, and dietary supplements.
- Discuss supportive therapy in the treatment of poisoning.
- List the contents of a code cart and their uses.
- Describe the role of a pharmacy technician in the event of a bioterrorism attack.

KEY TERMS

Acidosis	Code cart	Enteral nutrition
Alkalosis	Complementary and	Fat-soluble vitamin
Bacteriostatic	alternative medicine	Garbing
Bioterrorism	(CAM)	Gastric lavage
Bioterrorism agent	Dehydration	Hyponatremia
Code Blue	Electrolyte	Jejunostomy tube

Macronutrient	Neonatal	Scoop method
Major contamination	Overnutrition	Undernutrition
Malnutrition	Parenteral nutrition	Vitamin
Micronutrient	Percutaneous	Water-soluble vitamin
Mineral	endoscopic	
Minor contamination	gastrostomy (PEG)	
Nasoenteric tube	tube	

Chapter Overview

Aseptic technique is an essential principle of infection control in the clinical setting. The proper use of aseptic technique in preparing sterile pharmaceutical products is a fundamental responsibility of a pharmacy technician, particularly in a hospital or institutional setting. Aseptic technique and sterile compounding require the removal or killing of all microorganisms from the hands of the technician completing the compounding and from the equipment and workspace used for compounding. These practices reduce the risk of infection for the patient receiving the prepared product.

In 2008, Chapter 797 of the United States Pharmacopaeia (USP 797) established enforceable guidelines regarding the compounding of sterile pharmaceutical products. USP 797 created practices that are recommended to be followed by every institution that handles or prepares sterile pharmaceutical products. Most state boards of pharmacy require full compliance with USP 797 or adhere to some of their minimum standards of practice for pharmaceutical compounding and sterile preparation. The requirements are stringent and numerous. In addition, each hospital or pharmacy setting will have site-specific training and policies directing sterile compounding. Pharmacy technicians should also be familiar with basic principles and instructions for personal practices relating to infection control and sterile compounding. This chapter reinforces the procedures for sterile compounding outlined in USP 797.

Lab: Aseptic Handwashing

First and foremost, aseptic technique requires proper handwashing. Handwashing is the simplest and most effective way to reduce the transmission of pathogens. Aseptic handwashing is essential to sterile compounding. Aseptic handwashing is more vigorous and comprehensive than basic handwashing, but the goal is the same: to eliminate disease-causing microorganisms from the skin and reduce the risk of contamination by touch, the most common source of contamination.

Aseptic handwashing procedures remove contamination from the fingertips to the elbows. A minimum of 30 seconds is required to complete proper aseptic handwashing procedures, but a thorough cleansing requires several minutes. For the first handwashing of the day prior to sterile preparation, it is recommended to wash hands from the tips of the fingers up to the elbows for two to four minutes. It is the hands that come in contact with the compounding products and equipment and they should be the cleanest part of the entire body.

Aseptic handwashing should be completed each time a technician enters the sterile compounding area, after eating, after using the restroom, after sneezing or coughing, after major contamination, or after touching anything that is not sterile. **Major contamination** is classified as a significant level of contamination and includes a needlestick or a spill of more than 5mL. **Minor contamination** is classified as a low level of contamination and includes the use of a calculator or pen, a small spill, or minor hand contamination such as adjusting eyeglasses or touching papers or medication labels. After minor contamination, repeating aseptic handwashing is not required; basic hand hygiene using sterile isopropyl alcohol is appropriate. In this lab, you will become familiar with the supplies and techniques used in aseptic handwashing. An instructor should watch you complete the steps to ensure compliance with proper technique and procedures.

USP 797 requires that the sink used for aseptic handwashing be designated for use only by pharmacy personnel who are involved in sterile compounding. The sink must be designed to minimize splashing to reduce contamination during subsequent handwashing procedures. The sink must have a gooseneck faucet and hot and cold running water. Preferably, the sink will have foot pedals to turn the water on and off.

Equipment Needed

- Sink suitable for aseptic handwashing
- Sterile surgical scrub sponge/brush containing antimicrobial solution
- Aseptic, lint-free paper towels

Steps

1. Remove all jewelry from the hands and arms. Nail polish and artificial nails should not be worn in the sterile compounding workspace. Roll up sleeves if necessary, exposing bare arms up to the elbows.

2. Squeeze the pre-packaged surgical sponge inside the package to activate the soap. Open the package and discard the wrapper. Do not set the sponge down.

In pharmacy practice, personal protective clothing, including hair covers, shoe covers, and a mask, should be put on prior to completing aseptic handwashing. For the purposes of this lab, you will simply demonstrate handwashing technique.

If you inadvertently drop the sponge or place it in the sink or on the counter, it must be discarded and you must begin the process of aseptic handwashing again.

3. Turn on the water and let it run until warm. Wet your hands and forearms. Use the nail pick provided with the sponge to clean under your fingernails. Discard the pick.

4. Wet the sponge and squeeze it several times until a rich, soapy lather appears.

Tip: If the sink you are using has foot pedal controls, you may turn the water off after step 4. If the sink has hand controls, let the water run during the entire handwashing procedure.

5. Use the brush side of the sponge to clean under the thumbnail of the first hand. When the thumbnail is clean, proceed to the index finger on the same hand and scrub under its nail with the brush. Continue to remaining fingers, moving from thumb to pinky, until each nail is clean.

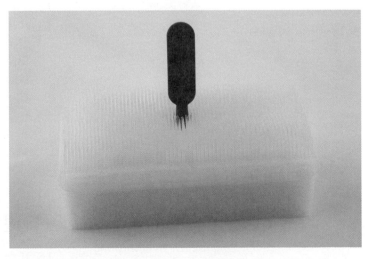

A disposable surgical scrub brush has a sponge on one side and a brush on the other. A nail pick is included to clean underneath the fingernails.

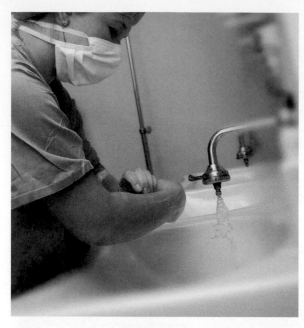

Wash all sides of each finger and the webbing between fingers.

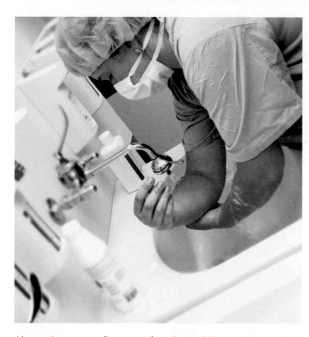

Always keep your fingers pointed up while washing and rinsing your hands to allow contamination to run down your arm, off your elbow, and into the sink.

 Do not apply lotion or any other materials to your hands after completing aseptic handwashing procedures. This results in contamination.

6. Switch to the opposite hand and clean under the nails with the scrub brush, beginning with the thumbnail.

7. Use the sponge to clean the fingers on the first hand. To begin, scrub the top, bottom, and two sides of the thumb. Clean the webbing between the thumb and index finger. Proceed to clean each finger and webbing in turn, taking care to scrub all sides of each finger.

8. Repeat step 7 on the opposite hand, cleaning all the fingers and webbing. Move from the thumb to the pinky.

Do not use the brush to clean the skin. This may cause damage to the skin or cause contaminated skin to flake off into the clean environment. Use only the sponge to clean the skin.

9. Use the sponge to wash the palm of the first hand. When the entire palm of the first hand is clean, clean the palm on the opposite hand.

10. Use the sponge to wash the back of the first hand. Repeat on opposite hand.

11. Use the sponge to clean the forearm of the first hand. Begin at the wrist and clean in a circular pattern around the forearm, winding toward the elbow. Stop cleansing at the elbow. Repeat this pattern on the opposite hand.

Because aseptic handwashing is designed to move contamination down the arm, from the fingers to the elbow, the fingers must always remain pointed up during handwashing and rinsing.

12. Throw the sponge away.

13. If the water is not on, turn it on with the foot pedals and let it run until warm. Rinse the hand and forearm of the first arm. Begin rinsing at the fingers, keeping the fingers pointed up through the entire rinse. The water should run down your elbow into the sink.

14. Repeat the rinsing process on the opposite hand. If the sink has foot pedals, turn off the water. If the sink has hand controls, continue to let the water run.

15. Use aseptic, lint-free towels to dry your hands. Discard the towels. Use new aseptic, lint-free towels to dry your forearms. Discard the towels.

16. If the sink has hand controls, use a new, aseptic lint-free towel to grab the handle of the faucet and turn off the water. Discard the towel.

Lab: Garbing According to USP 797 Requirements

Pharmacy technicians must wear an outer layer of sterile, lint-free clothing when compounding sterile products. Powder-free gloves must also be worn. These measures, governed by USP 797, maintain asepsis in the compounding environment and promote infection control. Along with hand hygiene, garbing is the first line of defense against contamination when compounding sterile products.

Garbing, or donning protective clothing, should be completed prior to handwashing, after you have entered the anteroom outside of the sterile workspace. In this lab, you will practice garbing according to USP 797 standards. You will complete an agar plate fingertip test at the end of the lab to verify asepsis.

Equipment Needed

- Instructions for agar plate fingertip test
- Shoe covers
- Hair cover
- Face mask
- Sterile gown
- Sterile, powder-free gloves
- Foamed 70 percent isopropyl alcohol
- Two agar plates
- Workspace that has been cleansed with 70 percent isopropyl alcohol

Steps

1. Read the instructions for the agar plate fingertip test. These are provided in a kit with the agar plates and will be provided by your instructor.
2. Remove all outerwear and jewelry, as directed by USP 797 requirements.
3. Wash hands with soap and water.
4. Place shoe covers over your shoes. Identify the longer end of the shoe cover and place it over the toes of the first shoe. Pull the shorter end of the cover over the heel of your shoe. Repeat on opposite shoe.
5. Place a hair cover over your hair. First, gather loose hair at the nape of your neck and tuck it inside the hair cover. Position the elastic against the back of your neck. Pull the hair cover over the front of your hair and place the elastic on your forehead. Tuck any loose hair inside the cover until no hair is exposed.
6. Place a face mask over your mouth and nose. Position the top of the mask on the bridge of the nose. If the face mask has elastic fasteners, tuck them behind your ears. If the face mask has strings, pull the top set of strings securely behind your head and tie them together. The strings should rest just above your ears. Tie the lower strings together at the back of your neck. Your nose, mouth, and chin should be covered by the face mask.
7. Don a sterile gown. Open the gown carefully. Do not let any portion of it touch the floor or any other contaminated surface. Ensure the gown is appropriately sized and secure it with the snaps, ties, or other closures.

Men with facial hair are required to cover beards and mustaches with hair covers before completing sterile compounding procedures.

USP 797 requirements do not specify what type of gown should be worn during sterile compounding. It may be a front- or back-closure gown. However, it must be well fitting and cover a majority of the body of the person performing the compounding.

Disposable gowns may be worn when compounding sterile products. If not visibly soiled or contaminated, the gown may be stored in the anteroom near the sterile workspace, turned inside out and hung in a low-traffic area, and then they may be reused for an entire shift. If non-disposable gowns are used, they should be laundered regularly and appropriately, according to policies for sterile use.

Sterile gloves will be labeled "Left" and "Right." Do not touch the outside of the gloves; the cuffs will be folded to allow you to grab the inside of the cuff and minimize contamination.

8. Practice hand hygiene according to your instructor's directions. Wash hands according to aseptic technique (outlined in the previous lab exercise). Alternatively, sanitize your hands with foamed alcohol. Dispense a small handful of foam into the palm of one hand. Rub your hands together and coat each finger, the palms, the back of the hands, and the wrists with alcohol.

9. After your hands are dry, open the outer wrapper of a pair of sterile gloves and drop the inner package on the sterile work surface or sterile field.

10. Grasp the inside of the cuff of one of the gloves and carefully pull it onto the opposite hand, up to the wrist. Pull the glove over the cuff of the gown. Pick up the second glove by sliding the fingers of the gloved hand under the cuff of the second glove. Be careful not to contaminate the gloved hand with the ungloved hand as the second glove is being put on.

11. Place the agar plates on the clean workspace. Remove the top of the first plate and press the gloved forefinger of your right hand onto the surface of the agar. Press the gloved thumb of your right hand onto a different section of the plate. Replace the cover on the agar plate.

12. Repeat step 11 with the second agar plate, using your gloved left hand.

13. Label the agar plates as directed and give them to your instructor.

14. Remove garb. Always remove protective clothing in the following order: gloves, gown, face mask, hair cover, and shoe covers. Discard items in the trash.

Agar plates will be incubated for 24 to 72 hours. After the incubation period, count the colony-forming units present on each plate. Each unit indicates microbial growth. The desired number of units is zero. Each plate with zero growth is a "negative" result. A "positive" result requires assessment and retraining of the garbing, hand-hygiene, and gloving procedures.

Lab: Cleaning a Horizontal Laminar Airflow Hood

A laminar airflow hood provides a constant flow of filtered air across a workspace and prevents the entry of contaminated air. The hooded workspace is used to prepare sterile compounded products. A horizontal laminar airflow hood contains a high-efficiency particulate air (HEPA) filter that removes 99.97 percent of all air particles that are 0.3 micron or larger in diameter.

The use of a laminar airflow hood does not guarantee sterility but the air out of the HEPA filter is sterile. Observance of aseptic technique is always required when performing sterile compounding procedures.

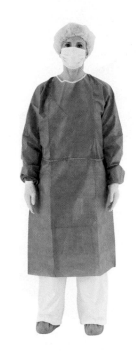

Laminar airflow hoods are available in several varieties, including horizontal airflow hoods and vertical airflow hoods, also called biological safety cabinets. Horizontal airflow hoods are the most frequently used, suitable for compounding a variety of sterile products. The HEPA filter is located across the back of the horizontal airflow hood; air blows from the filter, toward the worker, and out of the hood. Vertical laminar flow hoods are used for compounding chemotherapy products or working with other hazardous materials. Vertical hoods are also called biological hoods, radiological hoods, and chemo hoods. In vertical airflow hoods, air blows from the top of the hood down, protecting the worker from exposure to materials inside the hood. The hoods have pull-down, see-through Plexiglas fronts and are designed to prevent caustic materials such as drugs and gases from escaping from the

Proper garbing includes wearing shoe covers, hair covers, a face mask, a gown, and gloves.

hood. This protects the preparer of the medication or hazardous material. The use of any laminar flow hood requires specialized training and institution-specific policies and procedures. The horizontal airflow hood, used commonly in many pharmacy settings, is the focus of this lab exercise.

When working in a horizontal airflow hood, all work should be completed at least 6 inches from the outside edge of the hood to prevent room air from contaminating the materials inside the hood. A laminar flow hood should be left operating continuously. If it is turned off, the hood must be turned on and allowed to run for 30 minutes before use in order to establish sterile airflow. The hood must be cleaned prior to each use or after major contamination. The hood is always cleaned from back to front and top to bottom, moving away from the filter. A hood-cleaning log should be attached to the hood and completed each time the hood is cleaned. Regulatory agencies require the maintenance of cleaning logs for at least two years.

In this lab, you will learn the steps involved in cleaning a horizontal laminar flow hood and completing the cleaning log. An instructor should watch you complete the steps to ensure compliance with proper technique and procedures.

Equipment Needed

- A 250mL bottle of sterile water for irrigation
- A 250mL bottle of sterile 70 percent isopropyl alcohol
- Sterile gauze pads or other sterile, lint free, non-shedding towels or cleaning pads
- A horizontal laminar flow hood
- Hood-cleaning log sheet

Do not let anything come in contact with the HEPA filter at any time.

Once you reach the outer edge of the hood, the gauze is considered contaminated and should be discarded and replaced with clean, sterile gauze

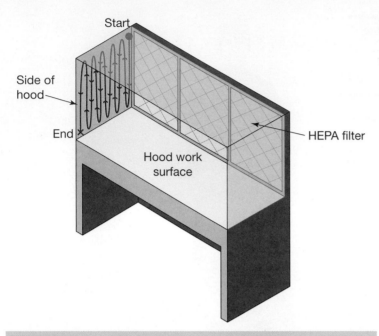

FIGURE 19.1 Clean the sides of a horizontal laminar flow hood from top to bottom and back to front, moving away from the filter.

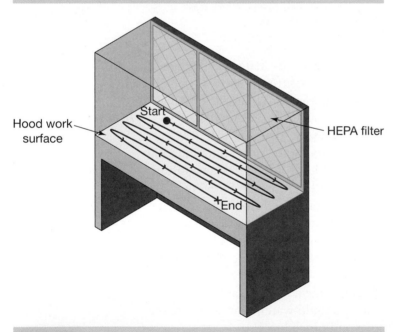

FIGURE 19.2 Clean the work surface of a horizontal laminar flow hood from back to front, moving away from the filter.

The hood should be cleaned with water first to remove any residue that is not soluble in alcohol.

Steps

1. Don appropriate personal protective clothing and gloves, as directed by your instructor.

2. Remove all objects from the hood.

3. Place a stack of sterile gauze pads at least 6 inches from the edge of the hood.

4. Wet the stack of gauze with water for irrigation. The pads should be lightly saturated, but not dripping with water.

5. Grab one-quarter of the gauze pads and clean the bar and hooks within the hood. Then clean the ceiling of the hood. Begin at the back corner and use sweeping side-to-side motions to wipe the ceiling. Overlap the motions, gradually moving from the back of the hood to the outer edge. When you reach the outer edge of the hood, discard the gauze.

6. Grab another one-quarter of the gauze pads and clean the sides of the hood. Begin in an interior upper corner and use overlapping up-and-down wipes to clean the side of the hood. Gradually move from the back of the hood to the outer edge **FIGURE 19.1**. When you reach the outer edge of the hood, discard the gauze.

7. Grab another one-quarter of the gauze pads and repeat step 6 on the opposite side of the hood.

8. Use the remaining one-quarter of gauze pads to clean the work surface **FIGURE 19.2**. Again, start at a back corner and use overlapping side-to-side wipes to clean the work surface. Gradually move from the back of the hood to the outer edge. When you reach the outer edge of the hood, discard the gauze.

9. Obtain a new stack of sterile gauze pads and soak them with 70 percent isopropyl alcohol. Complete steps 5 through 8 using the alcohol-soaked pads.

10. Complete the cleaning log attached to the hood **FIGURE 19.3**.

PHARMACY HOOD CLEANING LOG

Pharmacy_____   Month:_____

Hood #_____   Model#_____   Serial#_____

| DATE | First Shift | | | | | | Second Shift | | | | |
	Shift Start	Prior to Prep	30-min schedule	Spill	Initials	Shift Start	Prior to Prep	30-min schedule	Spill	Initials
1										
2										
3										
4										
5										
6										
7										
8										
9										
10										
11										
12										
13										
14										
15										
16										
17										
18										
19										
20										
21										
22										
23										
24										
25										
26										
27										
28										
29										
30										
31										

FIGURE 19.3 A cleaning log.

Lab: Preparing Large-Volume Parenteral Products

Pharmacy technicians in a hospital or institutional environment routinely handle and manipulate sterile products for administration to patients. This may include single doses of medication, dialysis solutions, fluid or electrolyte replacement, or parenteral nutrition products. In the previous lab exercises, you learned the basic principles of personal practices and cleaning procedures for working in a sterile environment. The remaining four labs apply those basic principles to the preparation of sterile products.

Large-volume parenterals (LVPs) are parenteral products that contain more than 100mL. The most common LVPs are 0.9 percent sodium chloride (normal saline), dextrose 5 percent in water (D_5W), dextrose 5 percent in normal saline, and lactated Ringer's solution. These solutions are often used as the base fluid for administering electrolytes or nutrients. They are usually administered through a main intravenous (IV) line.

In this lab, you will prepare a 25mEq dose of potassium chloride (KCl) in normal saline. You will complete all calculations associated with the preparation of the product and prepare the product for administration to a patient.

Equipment Needed

- Calculator
- 20mL bottle of potassium chloride, 2mEq/mL
- 1L IV bag of 0.9 percent sodium chloride solution for injection
- Sterile dispensing pin
- 20mL syringe
- 1-inch 21 gauge needle, without filter or vent
- Sharps container
- Trash container
- Three alcohol swabs

When working in a horizontal airflow hood, never place items in such a way as to obstruct airflow FIGURE 19.4. *All objects should have air flowing freely around them, without other objects or body parts blocking airflow from the filter to the outside of the hood. Never place equipment, supplies, or body parts between the filter and another object.*

Steps

1. Calculate the volume of KCl solution needed to provide the required dose of KCl. Start with this equation:

$$\frac{2mEq}{1mL} = \frac{25mEq}{xmL}$$

   Then cross-multiply and solve for *x*: *x* = 12.5mL.

2. Wash your hands, garb, glove, and clean the hood according to aseptic principles, as outlined in previous exercises.

3. Remove and discard the outer wrapping of the normal saline IV bag. Place the bag in the hood. Place all other equipment needed for compounding inside the hood, at least 6 inches from the outer edge. Use isopropyl alcohol 70 percent to clean all supplies placed in the hood. Place the sharps and trash containers on the floor next to the hood.

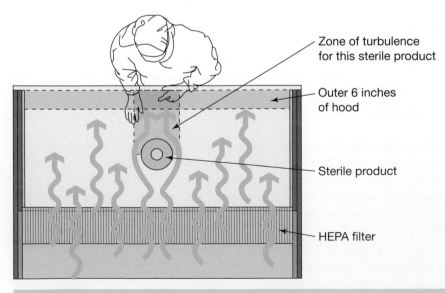

FIGURE 19.4 Do not place items inside the laminar flow hood in such a way that they block airflow from the filter.

4. Remove the metal cap from the bulk bottle of KCl. Lift up on the pull tab to remove it from the top of the bottle; then pull the tab straight down toward the bottom of the bottle. After it is removed, use the top as a tool to pry the metal ring off the top of the bottle. The rubber stopper should now be exposed.

5. Wipe the KCl bottle's rubber stopper with an alcohol swab. Place the swab to the side of the workspace in an area free from airflow obstruction.

The components of a syringe.

6. Remove and discard the wrapper on the sterile dispensing pin. Hold the top of the pin in one hand and remove the spike from the cap with the other hand.

7. Hold the bottle of KCl steady on the work surface of the hood with your non-dominant hand. Use your dominant hand to insert the pin into the bottle of KCl. Push the pin straight down into the bottle, through the rubber stopper.

8. Remove the cap from the top of the dispensing pin. Place the cap on the used alcohol swab.

9. Remove and discard the wrapping from the syringe. If the syringe has a cap over its hub, remove and discard the cap.

10. Attach the hub of the syringe to the open port on top of the dispensing pin.

Never lay an uncapped syringe on the work surface.

Do not touch or block airflow to the plunger shaft of the syringe, the hub of the syringe, the dispensing pin, or the neck of the vial.

---

11. Holding the bottle of KCl in your non-dominant hand, carefully invert the bottle. Use your dominant hand to pull down on the plunger until you obtain approximately 15mL of solution in the syringe (slightly more than the calculated amount that is required for this product).

There is no need to dispense air into the bottle of KCl because the dispensing pin includes a vent.

---

12. Gently tap the syringe reservoir with your palm or fingertips to force air bubbles toward the hub of the syringe. When all the air bubbles have moved toward the hub, push up on the plunger to expel the air. Move the plunger up until the desired volume is reached.

13. Invert the bottle of KCl and set it on the work surface. Grab the barrel of the syringe and gently twist counterclockwise to remove it from the dispensing pin. Do not interrupt airflow to critical areas of the syringe or bottle.

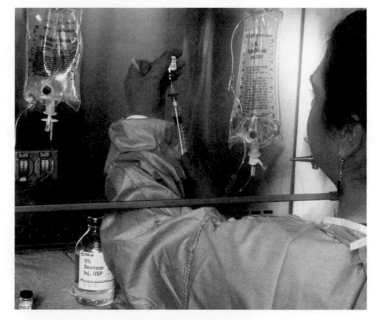

Hold the inverted bottle with your non-dominant hand and pull the plunger of the syringe with your dominant hand.

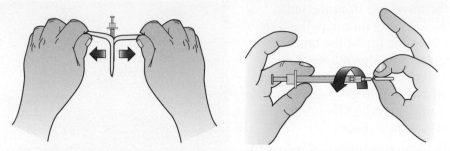

FIGURE 19.5 Do not remove the wrapper from the needle until it is attached to the syringe.

14. Using aseptic technique, attach the needle to the syringe. That is, while holding the syringe, carefully open the wrapper of the needle, peeling the wrapper back to expose the part of the needle that will be attached to the syringe. Hold the needle inside the wrapper and attach it to the hub of the syringe. Remove and discard the wrapper **FIGURE 19.5**. Leave the needle cap in place.

15. Place the syringe on the work surface, taking care not to obstruct airflow around the syringe or any other object inside the hood.

16. Replace the cap on the top of the dispensing pin with the cap that was placed on the alcohol swab.

17. Ask an instructor to verify the volume of KCl solution in your syringe.

18. Move the IV bag to a position where the injection port receives adequate, uninterrupted airflow. Clean the injection port with a new alcohol wipe. Discard the wipe.

19. Hold the syringe in your dominant hand. Carefully remove the cap of the needle and discard it. Hold the injection port with your non-dominant hand and insert the needle straight into the injection port.

20. Press the plunger of the syringe, dispensing the KCl solution from the syringe into the IV bag.

21. Hold the barrel of the syringe and remove the needle from the IV bag. Discard the syringe with the attached needle into the sharps container. Do not recap the needle.

22. Visually inspect the bag for precipitate formation or contamination. Gently squeeze the bag to check for leaks.

23. Discard any trash and clean the workspace. Remove personal protective clothing as outlined in previous exercises.

24. Present the final product to your instructor.

Potassium preparations must always be diluted in at least 100mL of base fluid and administered over an extended period of time. Potassium should never be administered via IV push, because of the risk of cardiotoxicity.

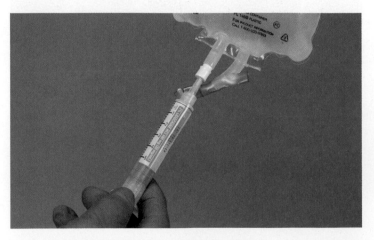

Insert the needle directly into the injection port.

Lab: Preparing Small-Volume Parenteral Products

Small-volume parenterals (SVPs) are products containing 100mL or less. The most common SVPs are administered via IV piggyback (IVPB), in which a small volume is attached to the main IV line and administered with the main IV fluid. The base solutions commonly used in SVPs include normal saline, D_5W, and 0.45 percent sodium chloride (½ normal saline).

In this lab, you will prepare two doses of metoclopramide: 10mg in 50mL D_5W and 7.5mg in 50mL D_5W. You will complete all calculations associated with the preparation of the products and prepare the products for administration to a patient.

Equipment Needed

- Calculator
- Two vials metoclopramide 10mg/2mL
- Two 50mL IVPB bags of D_5W with injection port
- Two regular needles, without filter or vent
- Two 5mL syringes
- Sharps container
- Trash container
- Four alcohol swabs

Steps

1. Calculate the volumes of metoclopramide solution needed to provide the required doses of metoclopramide. For dose 1, start with this equation:

$$\frac{10mg}{2mL} = \frac{10mg}{xmL}$$

    Then cross-multiply and solve for x: $x = 2mL$.

    For dose 2, start with this equation:

$$\frac{10mg}{2mL} = \frac{7.5mg}{xmL}$$

    Then cross-multiply and solve for x: $x = 1.5mL$.

2. Wash your hands, garb, glove, and clean the hood according to aseptic principles, as outlined in previous exercises.

3. Remove and discard the outer wrapping of the D_5W IV bags. Place the bags in the hood by dropping them into the sterile field so that the field is not touched with the outer liner and only the inner bag falls into the sterile field. Place all other equipment needed for compounding inside the hood, at least 6 inches from the outer edge. Clean all the vials and equipment with 70 percent isopropyl alcohol just prior to placing these products inside the hood. Place the sharps and trash containers on the floor next to the hood.

4. Remove and discard the cap from the metoclopramide vial. Clean the top of the vial with an alcohol swab. Place the swab to the side of the workspace in an area free from airflow obstruction.

5. Using aseptic technique, attach a needle to a syringe. Remove the cap and place it on the alcohol swab, with the open end of the cap toward the filter.

Review aseptic technique for attaching a needle to a syringe in "Lab: Preparing Large-Volume Parenteral Products" section.

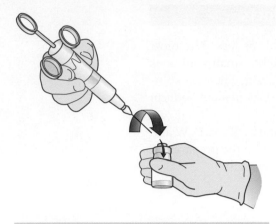

FIGURE 19.6 When inserting a needle into a vial, begin with the needle parallel to the work surface. Gently apply downward pressure to the needle as you rotate your arm up until the needle is perpendicular to the work surface.

6. Fill the syringe with an amount of air equal to the volume that will be withdrawn from the vial.

7. Hold the syringe between the thumb and forefinger of your dominant hand (similar to holding a dart or a pen). Securely hold the vial on the work surface with your non-dominant hand. With the bevel of the needle facing up, lay the tip of the needle against the center of the rubber stopper of the vial.

8. Insert the needle into the vial by gently pressing into the rubber stopper and simultaneously rotating your arm up until the needle is perpendicular to the top of the vial and the tip of the needle has passed through the rubber stopper **FIGURE 19.6**.

> Correct technique when inserting a needle into a vial prevents coring, or the breaking of small pieces of rubber into the vial. Correct technique requires that the bevel and the heel of the needle tip enter the rubber stopper in the same location.

9. Keep the syringe fully inserted into the vial and invert the vial. Hold the vial with your non-dominant hand and hold the syringe with your dominant hand.

10. Press the plunger to dispense the air in the syringe into the vial. This creates a positive-pressure environment inside the vial and assists in withdrawing the solution. A positive-pressure environment is one in which the pressure inside a system such as a vial of medication is greater than the pressure outside the system. Release the plunger and allow the syringe to fill with fluid.

11. Tap the syringe gently to move any air bubbles toward the hub of the syringe. Press the plunger to dispense the air bubbles back into the vial. Verify that the required amount of solution is in the reservoir of the syringe. If there is too much solution in the syringe, expel the excess solution into the vial. If there is not enough solution, withdraw the required amount from the vial, taking care to remove any excess air from the syringe before proceeding.

12. Invert the vial of metoclopramide, with the needle and syringe still inserted. Place the vial on the work surface and continue to hold it with your non-dominant hand. Hold the barrel of the syringe and gently remove the needle from the syringe by pulling it straight up out of the vial.

13. Carefully recap the needle. Be aware that recapping needles is dangerous and puts healthcare workers at risk for needlesticks. The **scoop method** is one of the most common methods for recapping syringes. This one-handed method begins with the cap on a flat surface. Hold the barrel of the syringe in your dominant hand and move the tip of the needle inside the cap. When most of the needle is inside the cap, lift the syringe, careful to lift the cap with the needle, and move it to an upright position. Use the non-dominant hand to snap the cap in place. Do not touch the needle to the work surface, your hands, or your fingers while recapping the needle.

Do not touch the plunger of the syringe at any time.

Never use two hands to recap a needle.

> Recapping a needle should be avoided if possible.

14. Repeat steps 4 through 13 with another syringe and needle to obtain the required volume of metoclopramide for the second preparation.

15. Place both filled syringes, with capped needles, on the work surface and ask an instructor to verify the volumes in each syringe.

16. Move the first IV bag to a position where the injection port receives adequate, uninterrupted airflow. Clean the injection port with a new alcohol swab. Place the swab to the side of the workspace, where it will receive uninterrupted airflow.

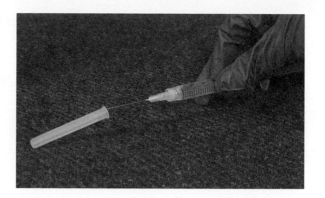

Use the scoop method to safely recap needles.

17. Hold the first syringe in your dominant hand. Carefully remove the cap of the needle and discard it. Hold the injection port with your non-dominant hand and insert the needle straight into the injection port.

18. Press the plunger of the syringe, dispensing the metoclopramide solution into the IV bag.

19. Hold the barrel of the syringe and remove the needle from the IV bag. Discard the syringe with the attached needle into the sharps container. Do not recap the needle.

20. Visually inspect the bag for precipitate formation or contamination. Gently squeeze the bag to check for leaks.

21. Repeat steps 16 through 20 for the second dose of metoclopramide.

22. Discard any trash and clean the workspace. Remove personal protective clothing as outlined in previous exercises.

23. Present the final product to your instructor.

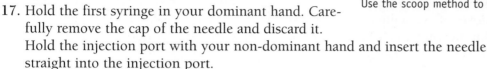

Lab: Preparing Sterile Powder for Injection

Some solutions for injection are supplied in liquid form from the manufacturer. Others are supplied as a dry powder and require reconstitution with an appropriate diluent prior to administration. Aseptic technique is essential for reconstituting sterile powders for injection.

Normal saline and sterile water for injection are the two most common diluents for reconstituting sterile powders for injection. Each of these diluents is available with or without preservatives to prevent the growth of bacteria within the vial. Diluents with preservatives are known as **bacteriostatic**. The most common preservatives are methylparaben and benzyl alcohol. Diluents without preservatives are often designated as preservative-free (PF); PF diluents are used in cases of **neonatal** administration, intrathecal administration (injection into a subarachnoid or subdural space), or upon the request of the physician.

In this lab, you will reconstitute sterile antibiotic powder and prepare two doses for injectable administration: ampicillin 450mg and ampicillin 375mg. You will complete all calculations associated with the preparation of the products and prepare the products for administration to a patient.

Equipment Needed

- Calculator
- 1g vial ampicillin powder for injection

- 10mL vial sterile water for injection
- 10mL syringe
- Two 5mL syringes
- Three regular needles, without filter or vent
- Vented needle
- Sharps container
- Three alcohol swabs

Steps

1. Calculate the volumes of ampicillin solution needed to provide the required doses of ampicillin. Once reconstituted, the final concentration of ampicillin solution will be 1g/10mL. For dose 1, start with this equation:

$$\frac{1,000mg}{10mL} = \frac{450mg}{xmL}$$

   Then cross-multiply and solve for x: $x = 4.5$mL.

   For dose 2, start with this equation:

$$\frac{1,000mg}{10mL} = \frac{375mg}{xmL}$$

   Then cross-multiply and solve for x: $x = 3.75$mL.

2. Wash your hands, garb, glove, and clean the hood according to aseptic principles, as outlined in previous exercises.

3. Remove and discard the cap from the sterile water vial. Clean the top of the vial with an alcohol swab. Place the swab to the side of the workspace in an area free from airflow obstruction.

4. Using aseptic technique, attach a needle to a 10mL syringe. Remove and discard the wrapper from the needle. Remove the needle cap and place it on the alcohol swab, with the open end facing the filter.

5. Fill the syringe with an amount of air equal to the volume that will be withdrawn from the vial.

6. Hold the syringe between the thumb and forefinger of your dominant hand (similar to holding a dart or a pen). Securely hold the vial on the work surface with your non-dominant hand. With the bevel of the needle facing up, lay the tip of the needle against the center of the rubber stopper of the vial.

7. Insert the needle into the vial by gently pressing into the rubber stopper and simultaneously rotating your arm up until the needle is perpendicular to the top of the vial and the tip of the needle has passed through the rubber stopper.

8. Keep the syringe fully inserted into the vial and invert the vial with your non-dominant hand.

9. Use your dominant hand to press the plunger of the syringe to dispense approximately half of the air in the syringe into the vial. This creates a positive-pressure environment inside the vial and assists in withdrawing the solution. Release the plunger and allow the syringe to fill with fluid. Add another small amount of air to the vial and allow the syringe to fill with more fluid. Repeat this milking technique until all of the air has been dispensed into the vial and the desired amount of fluid has been withdrawn.

10. Tap the syringe gently to move any air bubbles toward the hub of the syringe. Press the plunger to dispense the air bubbles back into the vial. Verify that the required amount of solution is in the reservoir of the syringe. If there is too much solution in the syringe, expel the excess solution into the vial. If there is not enough solution, withdraw the required amount from the vial, taking care to remove any excess air from the syringe before proceeding.

11. Invert the vial of diluent, with the needle and syringe still inserted. Place the vial on the work surface and hold it securely with your non-dominant hand. Hold the barrel of the syringe with your dominant hand and gently remove the syringe from the vial by pulling it straight up out of the vial.

12. Using the scoop method, carefully recap the needle.

13. Hold the syringe so the needle is pointing straight up. Then pull the plunger down approximately 0.5mm, withdrawing any fluid present in the needle into the syringe. Remove the regular needle and discard it.

14. Using aseptic technique, attach a vented needle to the syringe. Hold the syringe upright and push up on the plunger to remove any air from the reservoir of the syringe. Tap the barrel of the syringe to move air bubbles toward the hub of the syringe. Pull down on the plunger to remove any fluid from the needle. Gently push up on the plunger until the fluid enters the needle hub. This technique should remove all the air from the reservoir of the syringe.

15. Place the syringe, with capped vented needle, on the work surface. Ask an instructor to verify the volume of diluent in the syringe.

16. Remove the cap of the ampicillin vial. Pick up the syringe of diluent and remove the cap from the vented needle. Discard the cap.

17. Hold the ampicillin vial securely against the work surface with your non-dominant hand and hold the syringe directly above and perpendicular to the vial with your dominant hand. Apply direct downward pressure to insert the vented needle and its sheath through the rubber stopper of the vial.

Vented needles can only be used to inject diluent into a vial. They are not used to withdraw fluid.

---

18. Position the hub of the needle approximately ⅛-inch above the rubber stopper. Press the plunger of the syringe, releasing the diluent into the vial. There should be no pooling of fluid on top of the rubber stopper. If this happens, the needle was either inserted too far or not far enough into the rubber stopper. Ask your instructor for directions on how to proceed.

19. Hold the barrel of the syringe with your dominant hand and pull straight up to remove the needle from the vial. Discard the syringe and needle.

20. Shake the vial of ampicillin to dissolve the entire quantity of powder in the sterile water. Allow the vial to rest on the work surface until all foam or bubbles have disappeared.

21. Using aseptic technique, attach a regular needle to a 5mL syringe.

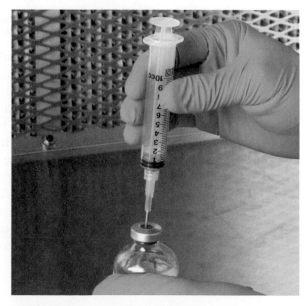

Vented needle.

22. Wipe the top of the vial of ampicillin solution with a new alcohol swab. Place the swab to the side of the workspace, so that the vial of drug receives unobstructed airflow.

23. Uncap the needle and place the cap on the alcohol swab. The open end of the cap should face the filter.

24. Insert the needle into the vial using appropriate technique to prevent coring. There is no need to add air to the vial because it was already vented when the diluent was added.

Review proper technique for inserting a needle into a vial of solution in the previous lab.

---

25. Invert the vial and withdraw the volume needed for the first dose of medication. Keep the tip of the needle covered by fluid in the vial to avoid drawing air into the syringe.

26. Remove any bubbles or air from the syringe. Tap the syringe gently to move any air bubbles toward the hub of the syringe. Press the plunger to dispense the air bubbles back into the vial. Verify that the required amount of solution is in the reservoir of the syringe. If there is too much solution in the syringe, expel the excess solution into the vial. If there is not enough solution, withdraw the required amount from the vial, taking care to remove any excess air from the syringe before proceeding.

27. Invert the vial with the syringe still attached. Place it on the work surface and hold it securely with your non-dominant hand. Hold the barrel of the syringe with your dominant hand and pull up to remove the needle from the vial. Carefully recap the needle using the scoop method.

28. Repeat steps 22 through 28 with the other needle and syringe to obtain the second dose of medication.

29. Place both needles, with capped syringes, on the work surface. Ask an instructor to verify your final products.

30. Discard any trash and clean the workspace. Remove personal protective clothing as outlined in previous exercises.

Lab: Using Ampules

Ampules are glass containers used to supply solutions of medication and usually contain no more than 2mL **FIGURE 19.7**. Drugs are often supplied in ampules instead of vials when the drug is incompatible with plastic, rubber, polyvinyl chloride (PVC), or any other component of a medication vial.

The ampule must be broken at its neck before solution can be withdrawn, and aseptic technique is essential to ensure that no contaminants are introduced into the ampule during or after opening. A filter needle must be used when withdrawing solution from an ampule to remove any fragments of glass, paint, or dust that may have entered the ampule. The filter needle must be removed and replaced with a new needle prior to the next manipulation. Once opened, an ampule is open to the air, so the contents can be immediately removed. Open ampules must be discarded in the sharps container because of the risks associated with broken glass.

Ampules and the Risk of Broken Glass

Opening a glass ampule produces shards of broken glass, most of which are not visible with the naked eye. Most reports estimate the presence of approximately 100 glass particles per 10mL ampule, and the particle count increases in proportion to the size of the ampule. These pieces of glass might contain bacteria, which emphasizes the importance of cleaning the outside of the ampule with alcohol before opening it. If these glass particles remain in the drug solution and are administered to the patient, they pose a risk of injury to blood vessels and tissues. Filter needles are an important step in preventing the parenteral injection of glass particles.

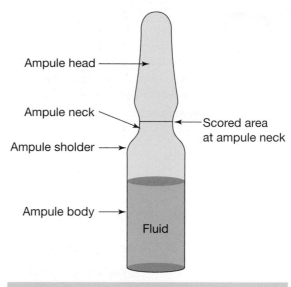

FIGURE 19.7 Components of an ampule.

In this lab, you will prepare two doses of IV medication available in an ampule: promethazine 25mg and promethazine 10mg. You will complete all calculations associated with the preparation of the products and prepare the products for administration to a patient.

Equipment Needed

- Calculator
- Ampule of promethazine 50mg/2mL
- 3mL syringe
- 1mL syringe
- Two filter needles
- Two regular needles, without filter or vent
- Four alcohol swabs
- Two 50mL IVPB bags of D$_5$W
- Trash container
- Sharps container

Steps

1. Calculate the volume of promethazine solution needed to provide the required dose. The concentration of promethazine provided in the ampule is 50mg/2mL. For dose 1, start with this equation:

$$\frac{50mg}{2mL} = \frac{25mg}{xmL}$$

Then cross-multiply and solve for x: x = 1mL.

For dose 2, start with this equation:

$$\frac{50mg}{2mL} = \frac{10mg}{xmL}$$

Then cross-multiply and solve for x: x = 0.4mL.

2. Wash your hands, garb, glove, and clean the hood according to aseptic principles, as outlined in previous exercises.

3. Gently tap or swirl the ampule to move fluid from the top of the ampule down into the body. Wipe the neck of the ampule with an alcohol swab.

Because of the risk of injury from broken glass when the ampule breaks, you should not hold the neck of the ampule.

4. Hold the body of the ampule with your non-dominant hand. Hold the head of the ampule with the thumb and index finger of your dominant hand. Quickly snap the head of the ampule back, snapping your wrist away from your body. Never break an ampule toward the HEPA filter.

5. Discard the head of the ampule in the sharps container. Place the body of the ampule on the work surface.

6. Open an alcohol swab and place it to the side of the workstation where it receives unobstructed airflow and thus does not contaminate the drug in the open ampule.

7. Using aseptic technique, attach a filter needle to a syringe. Remove the cap and place it on the alcohol swab with the open end of the cap facing the hood's filter.

8. Hold the barrel of the syringe with your dominant hand. Hold the ampule on the work surface with your non-dominant hand. Angle the ampule so the solution flows toward the neck of the ampule. Turn the syringe so the bevel of the needle faces down and insert the needle into the solution in the ampule.

9. Use your dominant hand to pull the plunger of the syringe back to slightly more than the desired volume of solution.

10. Remove the needle from the ampule and carefully recap the needle. Place the ampule on the work surface.

11. Hold the syringe upright and push up on the plunger to remove any air from the reservoir of the syringe. Tap the barrel of the syringe to move air bubbles toward the hub of the syringe. Pull down on the plunger to remove any fluid from the needle. Gently push up on the plunger until the fluid enters the needle hub. This technique should remove all the air from the reservoir of the syringe.

12. Insert the needle back into the ampule and expel any extra fluid from the syringe until the desired volume is obtained.

13. Carefully recap the needle using the scoop method. Remove the needle and discard it in the sharps container.

14. Using aseptic technique, attach a regular needle to the syringe.

15. Repeat steps 6 through 14 for the second dose of promethazine.

16. Place both syringes, with capped needles, on the work surface. Ask your instructor to check the volumes of promethazine in your syringes.

17. Move the first IV bag to a position where the injection port receives adequate, uninterrupted airflow. Clean the injection port with a new alcohol wipe. Place the wipe to the side of the workspace, where it will receive uninterrupted airflow.

18. Hold the first syringe in your dominant hand. Carefully remove the cap of the needle and discard it. Hold the injection port with your non-dominant hand and insert the needle straight into the injection port.

19. Press the plunger of the syringe, dispensing the promethazine solution into the IV bag.

20. Hold the barrel of the syringe and remove the needle from the IV bag. Discard the syringe with the attached needle into the sharps container. Do not recap the needle.

21. Visually inspect the bag for precipitate formation or contamination. Gently squeeze the bag to
check for leaks.

22. Repeat steps 17 through 21 for the second IVPB.

23. Discard any trash into the trash container and
clean the workspace. (Needles and syringes
should already have been placed into the sharps
container.) Remove personal protective clothing
as outlined in previous exercises.

24. Present the final product to your instructor.

Always use a puncture-proof sharps container when
disposing of used needles or syringes.

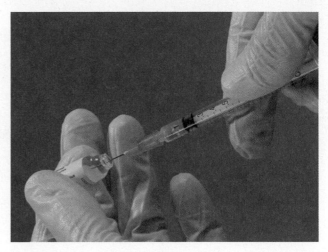

Tilt the ampule gently to move the solution toward the neck
of the ampule.

Drug Insights: Nutrition, Over-the-Counter Supplements, and Miscellaneous Topics

Nutritional assessment is critical to patient care. Classification of nutritional status
identifies patients who are overweight, obese, malnourished, undernourished, or at risk
for any nutritional disorder. Poor nutrition can complicate pharmacological treatment
plans because of poor nutrient intake, altered metabolism, or malabsorption disorders.
A comprehensive nutritional assessment includes a medical, surgical, lifestyle and
dietary history along with body measurements and laboratory tests.

Vital components of nutritional status are vitamins and minerals, electrolytes, and
fluid levels. The body uses vitamins and minerals to prevent disease and maintain
homeostasis, or equilibrium within the body. Electrolytes regulate the electrical activity within the body. Fluids levels of the body must be properly maintained to avoid
dehydration and fluid retention. These vitamins, minerals, electrolytes, and fluids are
obtained primarily from food, although some patients turn to nutritional supplements
and complementary and alternative medicines to achieve adequate intake. In a community setting, pharmacy technicians direct patients in finding the location of over-
the-counter (OTC) nutritional supplements and assist the pharmacist in evaluating
drug and food interactions with OTC products. In a hospital or institutional setting,
pharmacy technicians may prepare nutritional products for patients.

Additionally, pharmacy technicians play a vital role in emergency preparedness.
Whether timely attention is required in the case of a poisoning, or a patient needs
life-saving intervention, pharmacy technicians must remain vigilant and prepared to
act quickly and effectively. Pharmacy technicians must also be prepared in the event
of bioterrorism. Pharmacy technicians must understand the risks associated with
bioterrorism agents and how to manage the effects. In this way, pharmacy technicians
help to prepare pharmacies and the public to safely and calmly respond to a bioterrorism attack.

Nutrition

Inadequate nutrition contributes to poor outcomes of many disease states. Poor nutrition is also associated with the increased use of healthcare resources. Nutritional
interventions contribute to decreased lengths of hospital stays and reduced morbid-

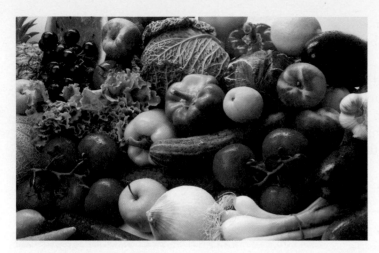

When a balanced diet cannot meet nutritional needs, supplements may be required.

ity (incidences of a particular disease) and mortality (death) associated with poor nutrition.

Malnutrition refers to any nutrition disorder and encompasses a variety of nutrition states. As many as 20 percent of hospitalized patients experience some form of malnutrition. **Overnutrition** describes excess nutrient intake and leads to weight gain and obesity. **Undernutrition** describes inadequate nutrient intake and leads to weight loss and altered organ function. Nutrition disorders, both overnutrition and undernutrition, can result from a variety of conditions, including medical, social, economical, and psychological factors. Substance abuse, fad diets, and eating disorders also contribute to nutritional deficiencies.

Nutritional Deficiencies and Malnutrition

Proper nutrition requires adequate levels of **micronutrients** (vitamins, minerals, and trace elements) and **macronutrients** (fats, carbohydrates, and proteins). Poor nutrition increases the risk for cancer, infections, and complications from surgery or other medical treatments. Wound healing time and mortality are increased across a range of diseases and conditions because of nutritional deficiencies. Nutritional deficiencies cause inadequate nutrient delivery, synthesis, and absorption, and lead to depletion of the body's nutrient stores, biochemical changes in the functioning of the body, physical manifestations of deficiency, and morbidity and mortality.

The goal of treatment of nutritional deficiencies is to replenish compromised nutrient stores, correct the deficiencies, and maintain healthy nutrition status. A healthy, balanced diet should be the cornerstone of correcting nutrient deficiencies, if possible. Supplementation may be used in patients who are unable to obtain adequate intake from food sources. Often, vitamins and minerals are absorbed more completely and efficiently from food than from supplements. A once-daily multivitamin containing no more than 100 percent of the recommended daily intake of micronutrients is sufficient for the majority of people. No benefit has been shown from patients self-medicating with high doses of single nutrients. Under medical guidance, high doses of vitamin C and vitamin D have been effective in anticancer and antimicrobial regimens, respectively. Patients should not attempt to replicate these regimens with OTC products without proper medical supervision. When macronutrient intake is needed, such as in cases of malnutrition, liquid supplementation or enteral or parenteral nutrition may be necessary. If patients are unable to achieve sufficient intake of proteins, fats, and carbohydrates through diet, nutrition supplementation can augment the caloric intake.

Enteral Nutrition

The gastrointestinal (GI) tract is an important part of the body's immune system. The GI tract destroys pathogens and toxins through chemical processes and physical barriers. The GI tract also efficiently absorbs the quantity and quality of nutrients needed by the body. When a patient cannot take nutrition by mouth, but the GI tract is functioning, enteral nutrition should be administered to the patient. **Enteral nutrition** is the delivery of food directly to the stomach or intestines through the mouth or a tube in the GI tract. Enteral nutrition is always preferred to parenteral nutrition because it is safer and less expensive to produce.

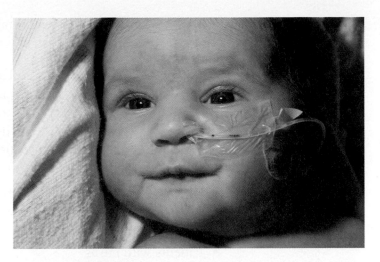

> Remember the adage: "If the gut works, use it."

Several types of tubes can be used for enteral feedings. A nasogastric tube is introduced into the nose and runs to the stomach. A **nasoenteric tube** is also introduced into the nose, but runs into the small intestine. Alternatively, a tube may be placed surgically through the abdomen and inserted directly into the stomach (gastrostomy tube) or the small intestine (**jejunostomy tube**). One type of gastrostomy

Tubes for enteral feeding can be used for pediatric and adult patients.

tube is a **percutaneous endoscopic gastrostomy (PEG) tube**, which is placed in the stomach during an endoscopic procedure. Enteral nutrition may be delivered to the stomach by a continuous or an intermittent infusion or bolus administration. Enteral nutrition should be delivered to the small intestine via continuous infusion.

Enteral nutrition should be used for patients who cannot or will not eat, but still possess a functioning GI tract. The composition of the nutritional product depends on the patient's individual needs, other disease states, and nutrient digestibility and absorption. Special enteral formulations are available for patients with specific disease states. Constipation is a common complication of enteral nutrition, so fiber should be added to the product, or constipation should be managed with pharmacological therapy as needed.

In some settings, pharmacy technicians are responsible for dispensing enteral nutrition products, while a nutrition or dietary department is responsible in other institutions. Home enteral feeding programs are increasing, and pharmacy technicians are involved in the preparation of products for delivery to patients. Pharmacy technicians must also be aware of enteral feedings because enteral nutrition can interfere with other medications. Also, medications for oral use can be crushed and administered through an enteral feeding tube in some cases. Enteric-coated or sustained-release

Table 19.1 Common Enteral Nutrition Products

Name	Characteristics/Uses
Fibersource HN, Jevity Plus, Probalance	High protein and fiber content; used for non-injured patients, including nursing-home patients
Fibersource, Jevity, Nutren, Ultracal	Provide complete, balanced nutrition; used for patients with intact GI tracts who are unable to eat
Isosource VHN, Promote, Replete	Used for patients with high nitrogen needs, including burn victims and trauma patients
Magnacal Renal, Nepro, Novasource Renal, Renalcal	Used for patient with renal failure or those receiving dialysis
Crucial, Impact, Impact Glutamine, Perative	High calorie and high protein content; used for immunocompromised and seriously ill patients
Choice DM, Glucerna, Resource Diabetic	Used for diabetic patients

products and sublingual or buccal tablets must never be crushed and administered through a tube.

Always verify the location of the enteral feeding tube before dispensing a medication intended for oral use.

Total Parenteral Nutrition

When a patient is unable to receive nutrition into the GI tract, **parenteral nutrition** may be supplied directly into a patient's vein. Total parenteral nutrition (TPN) should be considered for patients who cannot meet nutritional requirements through the GI tract. Parenteral nutrition is appropriate for the following patients:

- Patients with obstructions or tumors of the GI tract
- Patients with severe vomiting or diarrhea
- Patients with pancreatitis
- Patients with burns
- Patients with liver, respiratory, or organ failure
- Patients undergoing major GI surgery
- Patients with GI disease or conditions such as gallbladder disease, Crohn's disease, or inflammatory bowel disease
- Patients with anorexia nervosa who refuse to eat or to receive enteral nutrition

Patients with burns and patients with pancreatitis have increased nutritional requirements that may not be adequately met with a normal diet or enteral nutrition.

Patient age, disease state, and metabolic abnormalities must be considered before initiating TPN. Nutrition is not an emergency intervention in previously well-nourished patients. Because TPN is administered directly into a vein, the risk for infection is increased compared to enteral nutrition. TPN is administered through a peripheral line or a central line, depending on the anticipated duration of parenteral-nutrition treatment, metabolic complications, the risk for infection, and the severity of nutritional deficiencies. A continuous or intermittent infusion may be used to administer parenteral nutrition.

TPN contains macronutrients, micronutrients, and water. Each product is formulated according to the individual patient's nutritional needs. Patients receiving TPN are still at risk for nutritional deficiencies. Vitamin and trace element supplementations are essential for these patients. Each patient receiving TPN should be routinely assessed for dehydration, acid-base balance, lipid concentrations, hyperglycemia and hypoglycemia, decreased albumin, liver toxicity, and electrolyte imbalance.

Common trace elements in parenteral nutrition include chromium, copper, and manganese.

Common vitamins in parenteral nutrition include ascorbic acid, biotin, cyanocobalamin, ergocalciferol, folic acid, niacin, pyridoxine, retinol, riboflavin, thiamine, and tocopherol.

Pharmacy technicians are often responsible for preparing TPN products. They may also be responsible for reporting patient lab results to the pharmacist prior to administration.

Vitamins, Minerals, Fluids, and Electrolytes

Vitamins are organic molecules that regulate metabolic processes within the body. These processes support growth, homeostasis, and reproduction. Vitamins are classified as water-soluble or fat soluble. **Minerals** are inorganic substances that exist in body fluids and regulate homeostasis, or function as constituents of organic compounds. Vitamins (except for vitamins D and K) and minerals cannot be produced by the body in sufficient quantities for optimal growth and health. They must be obtained from food sources or supplementation. One-half of Americans consume a nutritional supplement on a daily basis, and vitamin and mineral supplements account for nearly $10 billion in sales revenue each year in the United States.

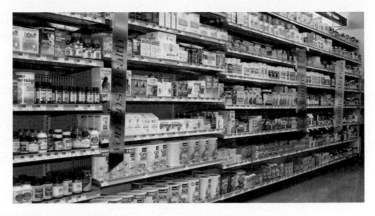

Vitamin supplements are a multibillion dollar industry.

Fluids are administered to the patient intravenously to treat different medical diagnoses and electrolyte deficiencies as well as dehydration. Electrolytes are replenished parenterally as well to treat electrolyte imbalances and various diseases that cause electrolyte deficiencies. Fluids and electrolytes can be given together in large-volume IVs. Small-volume IVs are used to replenish electrolytes quickly in some situations.

Water-Soluble Vitamins

Water-soluble vitamins are present in extracellular fluids and excreted by the kidneys. The body does not store water-soluble vitamins, so regular intake is required.

Vitamin C (ascorbic acid) is found in green, leafy vegetables, tomatoes, strawberries, kiwi, citrus fruits, and potatoes. Vitamin C is an antioxidant, promotes immune-system function, and possesses anti-inflammatory properties. Scurvy, a disorder that causes anemia, hemorrhages, spongy gums, and hardening of leg muscles, is caused by a vitamin C deficiency.

Vitamin B is a group of vitamins that contains several members:

- Vitamin B_1 (thiamine) is found in animal products such as liver, kidney, and pork; whole grains; peas; beans; wheat germ; and yeast. It supports carbohydrate metabolism, cardiac function, mental and cognitive proficiency, and energy production. A vitamin B_1 deficiency causes beriberi and leads to edema, cardiac abnormalities, weight loss, muscular dysfunction, and impaired sensory perception. Alcoholics frequently suffer from a thiamine deficiency.

- Vitamin B_2 (riboflavin) is found in meats, poultry, fish, dairy products, and green vegetables. It supports hair, skin, and nail growth. It also plays a small role in nerve function and in the production of red blood cells.

- Vitamin B_3 (nicotinic acid or niacin) is found in lean meats, fish, liver, poultry, grains, eggs, peanuts, and milk. It facilitates fat synthesis and protein metabolism. Niacin is used therapeutically to lower cholesterol levels. A niacin deficiency is known as pellagra and leads to diarrhea, depression, mental confusion, and dermatitis.

- Vitamin B_5 (pantothenic acid) is found in most vegetables, meat, fish, eggs, and yeast. In fact, pantothenic acid is found in at least small quantities in almost all foods. It supports growth, energy production, and normal physiological functioning. A pantothenic acid deficiency leads to fatigue, headache, sleepiness, nausea, muscle spasms, and decreased coordination.

- Vitamin B_6 (pyridoxine) is found in meats, cereals, lentils, nuts, legumes, milk, and egg yolks. It is found in virtually every food of plant and animal origin. It supports nerve growth and function. Pyridoxine is used therapeutically to treat alcoholics who have nerve damage and patients with pyridoxine deficiency as a result of isoniazid or hydralazine treatment.

- Vitamin B$_7$ (biotin) is also known as vitamin H. It is found in liver, yeast, eggs, most vegetables, bananas, mushrooms, peanuts, and milk. It supports fatty acid synthesis and carbohydrate, protein, and fat metabolism for energy production. It promotes healthy hair, skin, and nail growth, as well as nerve-tissue, bone-marrow, and sweat-gland formation. Biotin is found in many foods and can be recycled by the body, unlike most water-soluble vitamins. Biotin can also be produced by intestinal flora.

- Vitamin B$_9$ (folic acid or folate) is found in liver, lean beef, wheat, whole grains, eggs, fish, and fresh green vegetables. Folic acid works with vitamin B$_{12}$ to promote the growth of red blood cells, and can be used therapeutically to treat anemia. Folic acid is also responsible for fetal development in the first few weeks of pregnancy. Therefore, it is important that women of childbearing age who might become pregnant receive adequate intake of folic acid. Inadequate folic-acid intake during pregnancy is related to neural-tube birth defects. Depression is a symptom of folic-acid deficiency.

- Vitamin B$_{12}$ (cyanocobalamin) is found in animal tissues and dairy products. It is a co-factor that supports the production of red blood cells. Cyanocobalamin must work with the intrinsic factor in the stomach in order to exert its effect. A deficiency in either vitamin B$_{12}$ or the intrinsic factor leads to anemia. Cyanocobalamin is poorly absorbed from the GI tract, so intramuscular or intravenous administration is recommended for supplementation. If taken orally, cyanocobalamin supplements must be taken in extremely large quantities.

Vitamin B complexes and vitamin C are water soluble.

Many compounds that were once believed to be vitamins have be reclassified as other substances—hence the gaps in the numbering of B-complex vitamins.

What Would You Do?

Question: A young woman approaches your community pharmacy to obtain multiple bottles of B-complex vitamins. She reveals that she read information on the Internet claiming that taking high doses of vitamins could prevent disease. She intends to consume 10 times the recommended dose of vitamins to ensure that she receives adequate intake. What would you tell her?

Answer: Remind the patient that a standard daily multivitamin containing no more than 100 percent of the recommended daily intake is suitable for most people. Taking high doses of vitamins has not been shown to have a health benefit. If she is concerned about her health or nutrition status, encourage her to talk to a physician, nutritionist, or dietician. Encourage her to speak to the pharmacist to assess any possible drug or disease state interactions associated with the vitamins she intends to purchase. If a patient asks a specific question regarding vitamins, refer him or her to the pharmacist for counseling.

Fat-Soluble Vitamins

Fat-soluble vitamins are absorbed with the fats in the diet and are stored by the body, primarily in the liver. Deficiencies in fat-soluble vitamins occur after prolonged periods of decreased intake. Intake of fat-soluble vitamins should be monitored carefully by a prescriber, as an overdose is much easier with fat-soluble vitamins than with water-soluble vitamins.

Vitamin A, retinol, is found in liver, milk, eggs, and dairy products. The body can produce vitamin A from pigments and carotene present in many fruits and vegetables. Vitamin A supports normal growth, bone formation, reproduction, and repairing epithelial tissue. A vitamin A deficiency leads to keratomalacia, a softening of the cornea.

Vitamin D (D$_2$, ergocalciferol; D$_3$, cholecalciferol) is found in dairy products, eggs, and fish oils. It is formed in the skin following exposure to ultraviolet radiation. Calciferol, the active form of vitamin D, is formed from precursors D_2 and D_3 and transported to the blood stream. A vitamin D deficiency disrupts calcium-phosphate balance and inhibits healthy bone growth and formation. In children, vitamin D deficiency causes rickets, a disorder in which the bones of the legs and the spine become distorted. In adults, vitamin D deficiency causes osteomalacia, a condition in which the skeleton is weakened due to the demineralization of the bones.

Vitamin E (tocopherol) is a group of compounds found in soybeans, wheat germ, nuts, corn, butter, eggs, liver, and green vegetables. Vitamin E is an antioxidant and prevents cataracts, enhances immune response, prevents cardiovascular disease, and decreases the progression of dementia. An overdose of vitamin E can damage the heart.

Vitamin K (phytonadione) is found in liver, vegetable oils, spinach, kale, broccoli, and cauliflower. Vitamin K promotes blood clotting through the formation of thrombin in the liver. Vitamin K is used as an antidote to reverse overdoses of anticoagulants.

Vitamins A, D, E, and K are fat soluble.

Vitamin Deficiencies

Five primary vitamin deficiencies are seen in humans:

- Keratomalacia (vitamin A)
- Rickets (vitamin D)
- Beriberi (vitamin B_1)
- Pellagra (vitamin B_3)
- Scurvy (vitamin C)

The signs and symptoms of vitamin deficiencies can be reversed with supplementation of the deficient vitamin.

Minerals

Minerals account for approximately 4 percent of the weight of the human body, primarily due to the presence of calcium and phosphorous in the bones. Minerals are also present throughout the body as components of organic and inorganic compounds. Minerals maintain cell-membrane permeability, osmotic pressure, acid-base balance, and water balance. The most significant minerals required for the healthy functioning of the human body include calcium, phosphorous, and iron.

When a balanced diet fails to meet mineral requirements, supplementation may be necessary. Minerals may be supplemented as part of an oral multivitamin, or as a parenteral product, depending on the patient's disease state and ability to take nutrition by mouth. Minerals can be included in large-volume fluids, small-volume products, or parenteral nutritional.

Fluids

The human body is composed of roughly 50 percent water. Water is the primary element in all living cells, and the fluids that are outside the cells, such as lymph and plasma, are composed of high proportions of water.

The amount of water in the human body varies by age, disease state, gender, and body weight. There is an inverse relationship between fatty tissue and water, and overweight individuals have a smaller percentage of body water than lean, muscular individuals. Newborns have the highest percentage of body water: 75 percent or more.

The body loses water as it ages. The elderly generally have the lowest proportion of body water.

Water accounts for 50 to 60 percent of body weight for the average adult male and 45 to 50 percent of body weight for the average adult female.

Changes in the normal proportion of water in the body can lead to organ dysfunction, electrolyte imbalance, and cardiac and muscle irregularities. The proportion of body water can change because of certain medications, disease states, environmental conditions, exercise, or increased or decreased intake of fluid. **Dehydration**, or the loss of body water, can be caused by vomiting, diarrhea, edema, excessive sweating, significant weight loss, or large urine output. Dehydration can causes dry skin and mucous membranes, hypotension, tachycardia, and lowered body temperature. Chronic dehydration causes mental disturbances, headache, depression, and fatigue. A loss of 25 percent of body water can cause death.

The human body can survive several weeks without food, but only three days without water.

Sometimes referred to as water intoxication, drinking too much water in a short amount of time is as dangerous as dehydration. Large volumes of water cannot be quickly filtered by the kidneys, so the blood begins to absorb the water, leading to decreased concentrations of electrolytes in the blood. This sudden and severe drop in electrolyte concentration disrupts the body's normal electrophysiological processes and leads to water entering the brain and other organs. **Hyponatremia**, or a decreased concentration of sodium in the blood, is the most severe consequence of large water intake, and can lead to lethargy, confusion, seizures, coma, and death.

The average fluid requirement for an adult is 30 to 35mL/kg, or roughly 1,500mL every 24 hours. Fluid requirements may be increased in the case of fever, vomiting, increased urination, diarrhea, nasogastric suction, phototherapy, hyperventilation, excessive sweating, hyperthyroidism, diabetes insipidus, or other environmental or physiological factors. Likewise, fluid requirements may be decreased in the case of fluid overload, cardiac failure, decreased urination, high humidity, kidney failure, starvation, or a host of other conditions.

Fluids may be administered intravenously in patients who are unable to ingest enough water to meet their daily needs. Fluids may also be administered to correct electrolyte imbalances. Large-volume fluids may be administered that contain electrolytes, minerals, or medications. The administration of small volumes of fluids containing electrolytes are needed to quickly correct or replenish electrolytes.

Electrolytes

An electrolyte is a compound that exists as an ion when dissolved in water. Ions are electrically charged and possess either a positive charge (cation) or negative charge (anion). In healthcare, electrolytes are measured in milliequivalents (mEq), a relation of the molecular weight (that is, the mass of one molecule of a substance) to the charge of the ion. Electrolytes maintain homeostasis and coordinate the electrophysiological processes of the body.

Sodium (Na^+) is the primary cation present in the extracellular fluid or fluid outside of the cell. Sodium retains fluid in the body, generates nerve impulses, and regulates enzymatic activity. The kidneys maintain optimal sodium levels in the body. Sodium supplementation is not usually necessary because the average dietary intake is more than sufficient to meet physiological needs.

Potassium (K^+) is the primary cation present intracellularly or inside the cell. Potassium regulates nerve signaling and muscle function. Excess potassium leads to cardiac abnormalities. Potassium deficiencies may be seen in patients who take diuretics. Potassium supplementation can correct the deficiency.

Calcium (Ca^{2+}) functions in bone formation, muscle contraction, and blood coagulation. Calcium in the blood is attached to albumin, so low albumin levels can cause low calcium levels. Four calcium salts are available, each used for a different purpose:

- Calcium chloride—Calcium chloride regulates nerve and muscle activity. It is quickly absorbed into the bloodstream, so it is the calcium salt of choice in cardiac emergencies. It is only available in IV form.

- Calcium carbonate—Calcium carbonate is an antacid and sold OTC under many different names including TUMS. It can be used as a dietary supplement for individuals with a calcium deficiency. Calcium carbonate can only be taken by mouth.

- Calcium acetate—Calcium acetate binds to phosphorous more efficiently than other calcium salts and is used to treat hyperphosphatemia associated with end-stage renal disease. Calcium acetate can be administered orally or by injection.

- Calcium gluconate—Calcium gluconate regulates nerve, muscle, and cardiac function. It prevents calcium deficiencies in patients receiving parenteral nutrition. Calcium gluconate can be administered orally or by injection.

Hydrogen (H^+) determines the acid-base balance of body fluids. Normal blood pH is slightly alkalinic, with a pH of 7.4. **Acidosis** (a blood pH below 7.35) is a metabolic condition caused by the excessive loss of sodium or bicarbonate due to dehydration or starvation. In the respiratory system, acidosis causes increased carbon dioxide levels. **Alkalosis** (a blood pH above 7.45) is a metabolic condition caused by the excessive loss of potassium or chloride due to vomiting or diarrhea. Alkalosis causes hyperventilation and decreased carbon dioxide levels.

Signs and Symptoms of Fluid and Electrolyte Imbalances
The following are symptoms of fluid and electrolyte imbalances:

- Thirst
- Dry mouth
- Hypotension
- Decreased urine output
- Sunken eyes
- Weakness
- Fatigue
- Diminished reflexes
- Muscle cramps
- Tingling in extremities
- Confusion
- Shortness of breath
- Nausea and vomiting

Magnesium (Mg^{2+}) is a cation located inside cells and bones. It regulates enzymatic functions and controls nerve and muscle impulse generation. Magnesium can be lost from the body due to alcohol abuse, stress, or medications that increase magnesium excretion such as digoxin, estrogen, and diuretics.

Chloride (Cl^-) maintains homeostasis and acid-base balance. In parenteral nutrition, chloride ions should equal the concentration of sodium ions.

Imbalances in fluid and electrolyte concentrations can lead to a variety of signs and symptoms. Fluid and electrolyte replacement therapy can be used to replenish lost fluids and electrolytes or to maintain homeostasis.

Complementary and Alternative Supplements

Complementary and alternative medicine (CAM) encompasses diverse medical and healthcare systems, therapies, and products. CAM includes dietary supplements such as herbs, minerals, and botanical preparations. CAM therapies are often used concurrently with traditional medications and therapies. They may be used to treat chronic conditions, acute illnesses, pain, sleep disturbances, sexual dysfunction, and mental health, as well as a host of other diseases and conditions. Use of CAM crosses all gender, age, socioeconomic, educational, and racial lines. Many supporters of CAM feel that "natural" preparations, such as those derived from plants or other naturally occurring compounds, are safer than traditional pharmaceutical products. In general, CAM also encourages a philosophy of integrative and holistic treatment, which is often not the case in traditional medical specialties.

The use of dietary supplements is increasing because of healthcare costs and patient desire for autonomy. Pharmacists and pharmacy technicians should be educated in common dietary supplements in order to provide accurate evidence-based information to patients. Also, knowledge of potential drug-supplement interactions will help prevent potentially dangerous scenarios of unwanted effects. Pharmacists and technicians in every practice setting should be aware of supplement use:

Dietary Supplement and Health Education Act

As part of the Dietary Supplement and Health Education Act (DSHEA) of 1994, the FDA requires that all dietary supplements that make a disease-specific claim contain the following statement on the label: "This statement has not been evaluated by the Food and Drug Administration. This product is not intended to diagnose, treat, cure, or prevent any disease."

- Practitioners in compounding pharmacies must avoid duplicate therapy and potential interactions of drug products or inactive ingredients with dietary supplements.

- Practitioners in retail pharmacies must advise patients on selecting dietary supplements and counsel them on avoiding potential drug-supplement and food-supplement interactions.

- Practitioners in hospital settings must complete medication-reconciliation procedures that involve identifying every drug or supplement a patient is taking in order to minimize complications and maximize therapeutic benefit.

Common dietary supplements and their potential side effects and drug interactions are listed in **TABLE 19.2**.

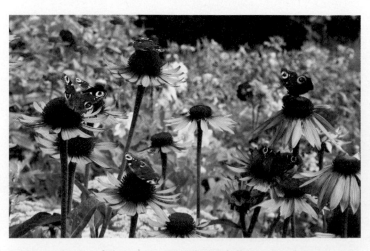

Echinacea is one of the most commonly used dietary supplements. It is derived from the purple coneflower.

Table 19.2 Common Dietary Supplements

Name	Intended Use	Side Effects/Safety	Drug Interactions
Black cohash	Symptoms of PMS and menopause	GI upset, weight gain, headache	None reported
Chondroitin	Osteoarthritis	None reported	NSAIDs, anticoagulants
Coenzyme Q10	Cardiovascular disease	Mild insomnia, elevated liver enzymes	HMG-CoA reductase inhibitors (statins)
Echinacea	Enhanced immune function	GI upset, tingling of the tongue, headache; May lead to immunosuppression with long-term use; should not be used in patients with autoimmune disorders	Econazole, immunosuppressants, cyclophosphamide
Evening primrose oil	Breast pain, symptoms of PMS and menopause	GI upset, headache	Phenothiazines, NSAIDs, anticoagulants, antiplatelet agents
Feverfew	Headache	GI upset, allergic reactions, antiplatelet effects, withdrawal symptoms	Anticoagulants and antiplatelet agents
Garlic	Hyperlipidemia, hypertension, diabetes mellitus	GI upset, bad breath, allergic reactions; caution when used with anticoagulants	May induce metabolism by cytochrome P450 enzymes
Ginger	Antiemetic	Weak antiplatelet effects	None reported
Ginkgo biloba	Alzheimer's disease and dementia, vascular disease	GI upset, headache, dizziness, allergic reactions; possible seizures or lowering of seizure threshold	Trazodone
Ginseng	Anemia, diabetes mellitus, insomnia, impotence, fever	Insomnia, headache, blood-pressure changes, anorexia, rash, vaginal bleeding	Corticosteroids, caffeine, psychotropic drugs
Glucosamine	Osteoarthritis	GI upset	NSAIDs, insulin, antidiabetic agents
Kava-kava	Muscle relaxant, anticonvulsant, sleep	Rash	Benzodiazepines, opioids, valerian
Licorice	Peptic ulcer disease	Pseudoaldosteronism, hypokalemia; caution for patients with renal or liver disease	ACE inhibitors, aspirin, diuretics, oral contraceptives, digoxin, corticosteroids, insulin, laxatives
Melatonin	Sleep disorders	Vivid dreams, drowsiness, GI upset, headache, irritability, breast enlargement, decreased sperm count in men	Antidepressants, antipsychotics, benzodiazepines, calcium channel blockers, beta blockers, anticoagulants, NSAIDs, corticosteroids, caffeine, tobacco, alcohol
Milk thistle	Liver disease and cirrhosis	Mild diarrhea	May inhibit metabolism by cytochrome P450 enzymes
Red yeast	Hypercholester-olemia (high cholesterol)	Should not be used in patients with liver disease	None reported
Saw palmetto	Benign prostatic hyperplasia	GI upset	Finasteride, antiplatelet agents, anticoagulants, oral contraceptives
St. John's wort	Depression	Insomnia, vivid dreams, restlessness, GI upset, fatigue, dry mouth, dizziness, headache; caution in patients with bipolar disorder or schizophrenia	May induce or inhibit metabolism by cytochrome P450 enzymes
Valerian	Sedative/hypnotic	Headache, excitability, insomnia; may induce uterine contractions in pregnant women	Opioids, barbiturates, benzodiazepines

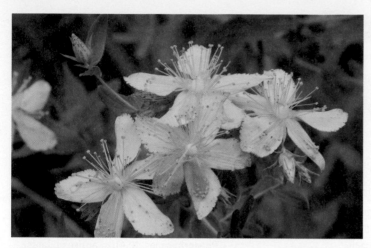

St. John's wort (*Hypercium perforatum*) is the source of a popular supplement that poses a risk for many drug interactions.

When patients inquire about dietary supplements, remind them that these supplements are not approved by the FDA and that data about their safety and effectiveness is limited. Encourage them to speak to the pharmacist, who can provide evidence-based drug information regarding safety, effectiveness, side effects, and drug interactions.

Recommend that all patients keep a list of all medications, vitamins, and supplements that they are taking. Tell them to keep this list with them at all times and share it with their physicians and pharmacist.

Safety is a primary concern related to the use of CAM supplements. These products are not approved as safe and effective by the U.S. Food and Drug Administration (FDA); therefore, no guarantees of a product's safety or effectiveness can be made. The FDA simply mandates that dietary supplements cannot claim to treat, prevent, or diagnose any disease or condition. Evidence from randomized, controlled clinical trials is limited for dietary supplements, and patients should be warned of the risks associated with taking dietary supplements.

Patients should be advised to keep a complete list of all the medications and dietary supplements they are taking, and to share the list with their physician and pharmacist. Pharmacy technicians can be supportive and nonjudgmental of consumers who ask for advice in selecting a dietary supplement. Respecting cultural or ideological differences facilitates trust between patients and the healthcare system. However, safety is paramount and must be considered first and foremost so that healthcare providers do no harm in treating their patients. The more open patients are about the drugs and supplements they are taking, the more effective healthcare providers can be at delivering safe, accurate health information.

Poisons

Poisoning is a common and potentially life-threatening condition. Unintentional poisonings occur most frequently among children under five years of age. Fatalities related to poisonings have decreased significantly since the 1970s, but poisonings are still a leading cause of hospitalization among preschool-aged children. Prescription and/or nonprescription medications are involved in more than half of the poisonings reported. Often, improper storage of drugs and hazardous chemicals can contribute to accidental poisonings. Repackaging medications from their original dispensed container, keeping drugs in containers without childproof lids, or keeping various hazardous chemicals such as antifreeze in common containers instead of safety locked containers can lead to accidental poisonings. Safe storage is imperative for preventing accidental poisoning.

Most poisonings can be managed at home with telephone support from a poison-control center. Less than 1 percent of poisonings are fatal. The most significant poisonings occur with drugs found in nearly every household. Iron tablets are a leading cause of death due to accidental poisoning; only a small amount of iron, available in supplements and multivitamins, can be fatal to a small child. Tricyclic antidepressants, including amitriptyline,

The availability of common OTC products in homes, such as cough and cold products, vitamins, and oral hygiene products, underscores the need for proper storage and child-resistant containers for all medications.

doxepin, imipramine, and nortriptyline, can cause heart arrhythmias, seizures, and shock in small children. Calcium channel blockers lead to heart failure and hypotension in children, and opiates cause decreased respiration. Aspirin poisoning causes tinnitus, nausea, and vomiting. Alcohol, present in many mouthwashes, can cause hypoglycemia, seizures, and coma.

Poisonings also occur among adults who mistake chemicals or other medications for another product. Occupational exposures to noxious chemicals are another cause of accidental poisoning, most often through skin contamination or inhalation.

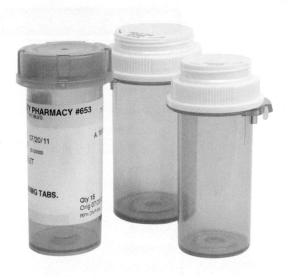

Elimination

Child-resistant caps can help prevent accidental poisonings.

Ingestion is the most common route of poisoning. Once the poison is in the GI tract, the body must rid itself of the chemical. Expulsion of the poison from the GI tract prevents systemic absorption. If the body does not induce vomiting on its own, vomiting can be induced with several cathartic agents to decrease the amount of time the poison is in the GI tract. Saline cathartics include magnesium sulfate and magnesium citrate. Sorbitol is a hyperosmotic cathartic. Another method of expulsion is **gastric lavage**, more commonly known as a stomach pump. It involves passing a tube through the mouth into the stomach, pumping in warm water or saline, and pumping out gastric fluids.

Instruct patients and consumers to store medications and household chemicals in containers with child-resistant closures and out of the reach of children at all times.

If the poison is corrosive or volatile, neither vomiting nor gastric lavage should be performed because of the risk of damage to the GI tract. Gastric lavage should not be performed if more than one hour has passed since the ingestion of the poison.

Teach patients the phone number for poison control: 1-800-222-1222.

Activated charcoal is a charcoal powder dispersed in water. It is often administered in emergency rooms to prevent the systemic absorption of poison from the GI tract. Activated charcoal should not be used for patients at risk for aspiration.

Antidotes

If the poison cannot be eliminated entirely from the GI tract, steps must be taken to decrease the effects of systemic absorption. Antidotes are administered, if available, to counteract the activity of the poison. Chelating agents, a type of antidote, bind to metal ions and remove them from the body. Antidotes are also used to reverse overdoses of medications, either from accidental administration or medical errors. Common antidotes, and the poisons or chemicals they reverse, are listed in **TABLE 19.3**.

Emergency Procedures

Life-saving interventions require quick thinking and efficient action to provide care and stabilize a patient in an emergency. Maintaining circulation and respiration are critical to life-support functions. Cardiac life support prevents death due to myocardial

Table 19.3	Common Antidotes
Generic Name	**Antidote For**
Acetylcysteine	Acetaminophen
Amyl nitrate	Cyanide
Deferoxamine	Iron
Digoxin Immune Fab	Digoxin, digitoxin
Edetate calcium disodium	Lead
Flumazenil	Benzodiazepines
Fomepizole	Ethylene glycol, methanol
Glucagon	Insulin
Naloxone	Opioids
Octreotide	Sulfonylureas
Vitamin K	Warfarin
Protamine sulfate	Heparin

infarction, ischemia, ventricular fibrillation, or other cardiac abnormalities. Emergency personnel must have the necessary drugs and equipment readily available at all times to perform these life-saving interventions.

Pharmacy technicians are often responsible for maintaining code carts in hospitals. A **code cart**, sometimes called a crash cart, is a cart that contains all the necessary drugs and equipment to provide life-saving care in an emergency. Most hospitals maintain an alert system to identify life-threatening emergencies and inform specially trained teams of healthcare workers that emergency care is needed. This is most commonly called a **Code Blue**. A properly stocked code cart must be available for every Code Blue alert. The recommended drugs for a code cart are listed in TABLE 19.4 .

Pharmacy technicians must routinely inspect code carts, replacing drugs or supplies that have been used, that have expired, or that will expire in the next one to two months. Logs must be maintained that account for every item in a code cart. Once filled, the contents of the cart are sealed inside bags with a safety seal or another device that will reveal proof of tampering, should it occur. Also, plastic breakaway locks must be placed on code carts so that medications or supplies cannot be inadvertently removed from a cart. Take care not to store lookalike or sound-alike medications next to each other in a code cart because they may be easily confused in an emergency. A pharmacist must ultimately verify the work of a pharmacy technician filling a code cart, but it is the pharmacy technician who is responsible for appropriate maintenance, record-keeping, and security of code carts to ensure emergency drugs and devices are available for use in life-saving scenarios.

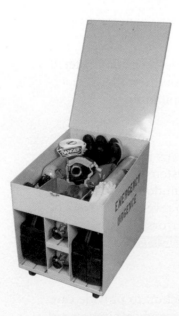

Pharmacy technicians are responsible for maintaining an adequate, in-date stock of drugs in code carts.

Bioterrorism

Bioterrorism is an attack, or threat of an attack, with bioterrorism agents as the weapon. A **bio-**

Table 19.4 Code Cart Recommended Contents

Generic Name	Brand Name	Use
Amiodarone	Cordarone	Ventricular fibrillation
Atropine	None	Bradycardia
Calcium chloride	None	Cardiac resuscitation
Dextrose 50 percent	None	Diabetic coma
Digoxin	Lanoxin	Suppresses atrioventricular nose conduction
Diltiazem	Cardizem	Atrial fibrillation or flutter, supraventricular tachycardiac
Dobutamine	Dobutrex	Increases heart rate or cardiac output
Dopamine	Intropin	Increases blood pressure
Epinephrine	Adrenalin	Cardiac stimulant
Etomidate	Amidate	Facilitate intubation
Flumazenil	Romazicon	Reverse benzodiazepine overdoses
Ibutilide	Corvert	Atrial fibrillation or flutter
Lidocaine	Xylocaine	Ventricular arrhythmias
Magnesium sulfate	None	Cardiac arrhythmias
Naloxone	Narcan	Reverse opioid overdoses
Nimodipine	Nimotop	Blood vessel spasm
Norepinephrine	Levophed	Increases blood pressure and coronary blood flow
Procainamide	Pronestyl	Cardiac arrhythmias
Vasopressin	Pitressin	Control bleeding
Verapamil	Isoptin	Atrial fibrillation or flutter

terrorism agent is an organism or toxin that can cause disease or death in humans, plants, or animals. Bioterrorism is used to incite terror and fear among masses of people. Once released, bioterrorism agents are difficult to control and contain. Although bioterrorism, in varied forms, has been used for thousands of years, bioterrorism moved to the forefront of Americans' minds after deadly terrorist acts in 2001, including the release of anthrax through the U.S. Postal Service. In response, the federal government and the Centers for Disease Control and Prevention (CDC) have categorized high-threat bioterrorism agents based on their ease of dissemination and transmission, potential for mortality, potential public-health impact, potential public panic and social disruption, and required action of public-health workers. The categories are listed as A, B, and C, with A identifying the most-threatening agents, and C identifying less-threatening agents. **TABLE 19.5** lists possible bioterrorism agents.

Category A and B agents require specialized training and public-health preparedness. In contrast, category C agents are emerging pathogens that are currently difficult to disseminate and, thus, pose a lower risk to public health. However, they have the same potential

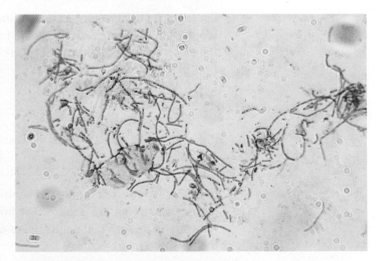

Bacillus anthracis, the bacteria that cause anthrax. Anthrax may be disseminated in forms for cutaneous, inhalation, or gastrointestinal exposure.

Table 19.5   Possible Bioterrorism Agents

Name	Category	Effects	Treatment
Anthrax	A	High mortality	Antibiotics
Botulism	A	Lethargy, acute respiratory distress, weakness, blurred vision, paralysis	Supportive care
Plague	A	Similar to community-acquired pneumonia	Antibiotics
Smallpox	A	Fever, headache, lesions	Supportive care
Tularemia	A	Influenza-like illness	Antibiotics
Viral hemorrhagic fever	A	Bleeding, fever, malaise, abdominal pain	Supportive care
Brucella	B	Fever, chills, malaise; low mortality	Antibiotics
Q fever	B	Flu- or pneumonia-like illness	Antibiotics
Ricin	B	Allergic-type reaction, fever, arthralgia, cough	Supportive care

for morbidity and mortality as category A and B agents if effectively disseminated. Category C agents include severe acute respiratory syndrome (SARS), tick-borne viruses, yellow fever, antimicrobial-resistant organisms, and rabies.

Some bioterrorism agents cause diseases that can be treated with antibiotics, antitoxins, or other antidotes. Others can be treated only with supportive care. Pharmacy technicians may be responsible in some settings for researching the availability of drugs or antidotes to be dispensed in the case of a bioterrorism attack. Pharmacy technicians will need to be educated in disease states associated with bioterrorism attacks to assist with identification, triage, dispensing, and patient education during a disease outbreak. Pharmacy technicians can also assist in the planning and implementation of local emergency-response plans. In the event of a bioterrorism attack, pharmacy technicians will be called upon to provide efficient, directed care that will calm, comfort, educate, and empower the public.

Tech Math Practice

Question: A physician orders ampicillin 175mg in 100mL normal saline IV, administered over 30 minutes every 6 hours for a pediatric patient who weighs 35 pounds. If the IV set delivers 10 drops/mL, what is the flow rate in mL/hr? What is the rate of flow in drops/min?

Answer: First, calculate the flow rate:

$$\frac{100mL}{0.5hr} = 200mL/hr$$

Next, calculate the drops per minute: $\frac{100mL}{0.5hr} \times \frac{10 \text{ Drops of IV Set}}{mL \text{ of IV Set}} \times \frac{1hr}{60min} = 33 \text{ drops/min.}$

Question: A physician orders sodium nitroprusside 50mg in 250mL D$_5$W for a pediatric patient who weighs 35 pounds. The initial dose is 1.5mcg/kg/min. What is the initial flow rate in mL/hr? If the nurse uses a microdrip set to deliver 60 drops/mL, what is the flow rate in drops/min?

Answer: First, calculate the patient's weight in kg:

$35lb \times {}^{1lb}\!/_{2.2kg} = 15.9kg$

Next, calculate the mg/min:

$15.9kg \times {}^{1.5mcg}\!/_{1kg/min} = {}^{23.85mcg}\!/_{min} = {}^{0.02385mg}\!/_{min}$

Next, calculate the flow rate in mL/hr:

${}^{0.02385mg}\!/_{min} \times {}^{250mL}\!/_{50mg} \times {}^{60min}\!/_{1hr} = 7.16mL/hr$, rounded to 7mL/hr.

Finally, calculate the flow rate in drops/min:

${}^{7mL}\!/_{1hr} \times {}^{60 \text{ drops of IV Set}}\!/_{mL \text{ of IV Set}} \times {}^{1hr}\!/_{60min} = 7$ drops/min

---

Question: **A patient is receiving chemotherapy with vincristine 0.3mg/m^2/day for 5 days. If he has a body surface area of 1.73m^2, what is the total dose for the 5-day regimen? If vincristine is available in a 1mg/mL solution in 2mL vials, how many vials will be needed for the total dose?**

Answer: First, calculate the dose:

$1.73m^2 \times {}^{0.3mg}\!/_{m^2/day} = {}^{0.519mg}\!/_{day} \times 5$ days $= 2.6mg$.

Next, determine how many vials you need:

$2.6mg \times {}^{1 \text{ vial}}\!/_{2mL} = 1.3$ vials.

Question: **A physician orders voriconazole for an adult patient weighing 65kg. The dose is 3mg/kg to be administered as an IV infusion over 90 minutes. The final concentration of the solution containing voriconazole is 5mg/mL. What is the flow rate in mL/hr?**

Answer: First, calculate the dose:

65 kg $\times {}^{3mg}\!/_{kg} = 195mg \times {}^{1mL}\!/_{5mg} = 39mL$.

Next, calculate the flow rate:

$39mL \div 1.5hr = 26mL/hr$.

Question: **Selenium 85 mcg/day is ordered to be added to an adult TPN. Selenium solution is available in 10mL vials containing 40mcg/mL. What volume of selenium solution is needed for compounding the TPN?**

Answer: Use the following equation:

$85mcg \times {}^{1mL}\!/_{40mcg} = 2.13mL$.

Chapter Summary

- Aseptic handwashing technique reduces the transmission of pathogens and contamination in the preparation of sterile products. The procedure moves contamination from the fingertips, down the arms, to the elbow. Aseptic handwashing should be completed each time a technician enters the sterile compounding area, after eating, after using the restroom, after sneezing or coughing, and after major contamination.

- Garbing according to USP 797 directives is the first layer of defense against contamination when compounding sterile products. Hair covers, shoe covers, a face mask, and a sterile, lint-free gown must be worn in the sterile compounding area. Sterile gloves must be worn over the cuffs of the gown.

- A horizontal laminar airflow hood prevents contaminated air from entering the sterile compounding workspace. The hood should be cleaned prior to each use and after major contamination. The hood should always be cleaned from back to front and top to bottom, moving contamination away from the air filter and out of the hood. Hood-cleaning logs must be maintained for two years.

- Large-volume parenteral products include medications, fluid or electrolyte replacement, dialysis fluids, and parenteral nutrition products.

- Small-volume parenteral products include medications or small volumes of fluid or electrolytes.

- Compounding large- and small-volume parenteral products requires adherence to aseptic technique. Never block the flow of air within the hood while compounding. Do not touch or block airflow to the plunger shaft of the syringe, the hub of the syringe, the dispensing pin, or the neck of a medication vial. Use proper technique when inserting needles into vials to prevent coring and contamination. Break ampules carefully and away from your body to prevent injury from broken glass. Use a filter needle to withdraw solution from an ampule.

- Poor nutrition contributes to poor health outcomes. Malnutrition, including overnutrition and undernutrition, results from a variety of medical, social, economical, and psychological factors. Nutrition should be assessed and deficiencies should be addressed to ensure the best possible health outcomes.

- Enteral nutrition is the delivery of food directly into the stomach or intestines. It may be delivered through the mouth or through a tube passed directly into the stomach or intestines. Enteral nutrition is always preferred to parenteral nutrition because of safety and cost concerns. Enteral nutrition is appropriate for patients who have a functioning gastrointestinal tract but cannot or will not eat. Constipation is the most common side effect of enteral nutrition.

- Parenteral nutrition is the delivery of food directly into a vein. Parenteral nutrition is appropriate when patients do not have a functioning GI tract or when patients experience severe vomiting and diarrhea or other disease states that increase their nutritional needs. Complications of parenteral nutrition include dehydration, acid-base imbalance, changes in blood-sugar concentrations, increased lipid concentrations, decreased albumin, liver toxicity, and electrolyte imbalances.

- Vitamins and minerals regulate metabolic processes in the body. Most vitamins and minerals cannot be produced by the body, so they must be consumed in the diet. When they cannot be consumed in sufficient quantities, supplements can be used to achieve the recommended daily intake. Vitamin deficiencies cause a variety of metabolic conditions, but can usually be corrected with supplementation of the deficient vitamin.

- The human body is roughly 50 percent water by weight. Changes in the normal proportion of water can lead to dehydration or hyponatremia, both of which can lead to organ dysfunction, altered mental status, and death in extreme cases.

- Electrolytes are charged particles that regulate electrophysiological processes within the body. Electrolytes also regulate homeostasis. The most common electrolytes include sodium, potassium, calcium, hydrogen, magnesium, and chloride.

- Complementary and alternative medicine includes the use of dietary supplements. These supplements are not regulated by the FDA and pose safety and quality concerns. Advise patients to inform their physician and pharmacist if they are taking over-the-counter supplements or medications.

- Accidental poisoning is a common cause of hospitalization in children. Accidental poisonings also occur in adults when chemicals or medications are mistaken for other products. All medications should be maintained in child-resistant containers out of the reach of children. Poisonings are treated by inducing vomiting or performing gastric lavage to rid the gastrointestinal tract of the poison. Antidotes are administered to counteract the effects of poisons that are absorbed into systemic circulation.

- Pharmacy technicians are responsible for maintaining code carts that are used during emergency life-saving interventions. Code carts should be routinely checked and restocked. Do not store lookalike, sound-alike medications near each other in a code cart.

- Pharmacy technicians will play a critical role in the event of a bioterrorism attack. Pharmacy technicians may be responsible for obtaining, storing, and dispensing antidotes to bioterrorism agents. Pharmacy technicians may also provide patient education and support before, during, or after an attack.

Learning Assessment Questions

1. When compounding sterile products, under what circumstance is it appropriate to cleanse your gloved hands with isopropyl alcohol instead of repeating aseptic handwashing?
   A. If you receive a needlestick
   B. If there is a spill of more than 5mL in the laminar flow hood
   C. If you adjust your eyeglasses while working in the laminar flow hood
   D. After you sneeze

2. According to USP 797, which of the following characteristics is not required for a sink in order for it to be used for aseptic handwashing?
   A. The sink must be accessible to all pharmacy personnel.
   B. The sink should have a gooseneck faucet.
   C. The sink should minimize splashing.
   D. The sink must have both hot and cold running water.

3. Which of the following is the correct principle for aseptic handwashing technique?
   A. Apply a sterile lotion to your hands after completing aseptic handwashing to minimize the risk of irritation from the soap.
   B. Use the brush side of the surgical sponge to provide a deep cleansing for the surface of the skin.
   C. Wash the palms of the hands first, because they are the most contaminated.
   D. Move contamination down the arm from the fingers to the elbows.

4. What is the correct order for donning personal protective clothing prior to compounding sterile products?
   A. Gloves, gown, hair cover, shoe covers, face mask
   B. Shoe covers, hair cover, face mask, gown, gloves
   C. Hair cover, face mask, gown, shoe covers, gloves
   D. Gown, shoe covers, gloves, face mask, hair cover

5. What is the purpose of the agar plate fingertip test?

    A. To verify the stability of compounded sterile products

    B. To test the activity of antibiotics

    C. To test the sterility of lab equipment

    D. To verify asepsis in the completion of garbing, hand hygiene, and gloving procedures

6. Which of the following statements is true regarding laminar airflow hoods?

    A. Horizontal airflow hoods must be cleaned weekly.

    B. Vertical airflow hoods blow air from the work surface up out of the hood to minimize the risk of contamination.

    C. Vertical airflow hoods are used to compound chemotherapy and other hazardous or cytotoxic products.

    D. Horizontal airflow hoods possess a filter that moves air from left to right across the hood.

7. What is the correct procedure for cleaning a horizontal airflow hood?

    A. Clean the hood from top to bottom, moving the contamination across the filter: ceiling, back, and work surface.

    B. Clean the hood from back to front and top to bottom, moving contamination away from the filter: ceiling, sides, and work surface.

    C. Clean the hood from right to left, moving contamination across the filter: right side, work surface, and left side.

    D. Clean the hood from front to back, moving contamination into the filter: work surface, sides, and ceiling.

8. A solution of 0.9 percent sodium chloride for injection is also known as what?

    A. Ringer's solution

    B. Surgical cleanser

    C. Salt water

    D. Normal saline

9. Which of the following is not a common base fluid for small-volume parenteral products?

    A. Lactated Ringer's solution

    B. 5 percent dextrose in water

    C. 0.45 percent sodium chloride

    D. 0.9 percent sodium chloride

10. How do you create a positive-pressure environment when withdrawing solution from a vial?

    A. Withdraw excess air into the syringe.

    B. Core the rubber stopper on top of the vial.

    C. Dispense air into the vial equal to half the volume of the solution you need to withdraw.

    D. Use a dispensing pin.

11. Which set of diluents is most commonly used for reconstituting sterile powder for injection?

    A. 5 percent dextrose and sterile water

    B. Normal saline and sterile water

    C. Lactated Ringer's and normal saline

    D. 10 percent dextrose and half normal saline

12. What is the proper technique for using a vented needle?

    A. Use a vented needle to inject diluent into a vial; never use a vented needle to withdraw fluid.

    B. Press the hub of the needle all the way to the rubber stopper to ensure a tight seal with the vented needle.

    C. To insert the needle into the vial, begin with the needle and syringe in a horizontal position and apply downward pressure as you rotate your wrist and bring the syringe to a vertical position.

    D. Take care to insert the needle, but not its sheath, completely through the rubber stopper.

13. Which of the following is not a risk associated with using an ampule?
    A. Broken glass can injure the technician completing compounding procedures.
    B. Particles of dust or other contaminants can fall into the drug solution.
    C. Fragments of glass can cause blood-vessel injury if administered to a patient.
    D. Filter needles should be used to administer drugs to a patient to remove any contaminants in the drug solution.

14. Which of the following routes of administration cannot be used to administer enteral nutrition?
    A. Intermittent infusion
    B. Continuous infusion
    C. Bolus administration
    D. IV push

15. What is the most common complication of enteral nutrition?
    A. Hypoglycemia
    B. Electrolyte imbalance
    C. Constipation
    D. Dehydration

16. Under what circumstances is total parenteral nutrition administration not indicated?
    A. A patient with Crohn's disease
    B. A patient with a functioning GI tract who cannot eat due to severe oral ulcers
    C. A patient with a bowel obstruction
    D. A patient who is vomiting repeatedly

17. Which vitamin can be produced by the body?
    A. Vitamin A
    B. Vitamin D
    C. Vitamin E
    D. Vitamin B_2

18. Which vitamin supplement cannot be administered orally?
    A. Cyanocobalamin
    B. Folate
    C. Retinol
    D. Ascorbic acid

19. A deficiency of which of the following vitamins is not usually seen in humans?
    A. C
    B. A
    C. B_7
    D. B_1

20. What is the most severe complication of drinking too much water?
    A. Diarrhea
    B. Hyponatremia
    C. Increased urine output
    D. Cardiac arrhythmias

21. Which calcium salt can only be administered orally?
    A. Calcium acetate
    B. Calcium chloride
    C. Calcium gluconate
    D. Calcium carbonate

22. Which regulation mandates labeling on dietary supplements?
    A. USP 797
    B. DSHEA
    C. CAM
    D. ISMP

23. Which of the following agents is considered a hyperosmotic cathartic?
    A. Sorbitol
    B. Romazicon
    C. Magnesium sulfate
    D. Activated charcoal

24. Which of the following pairs of lookalike, sound-alike drugs should be present in a code cart?
    A. Amiodarone-Amantadine
    B. Digoxin-Digibind
    C. Epinephrine-Ephedrine
    D. Dopamine-Dobutamine

25. Which of the following is not classified as a category A bioterrorism agent?
    A. Anthrax
    B. Botulism
    C. Plague
    D. SARS

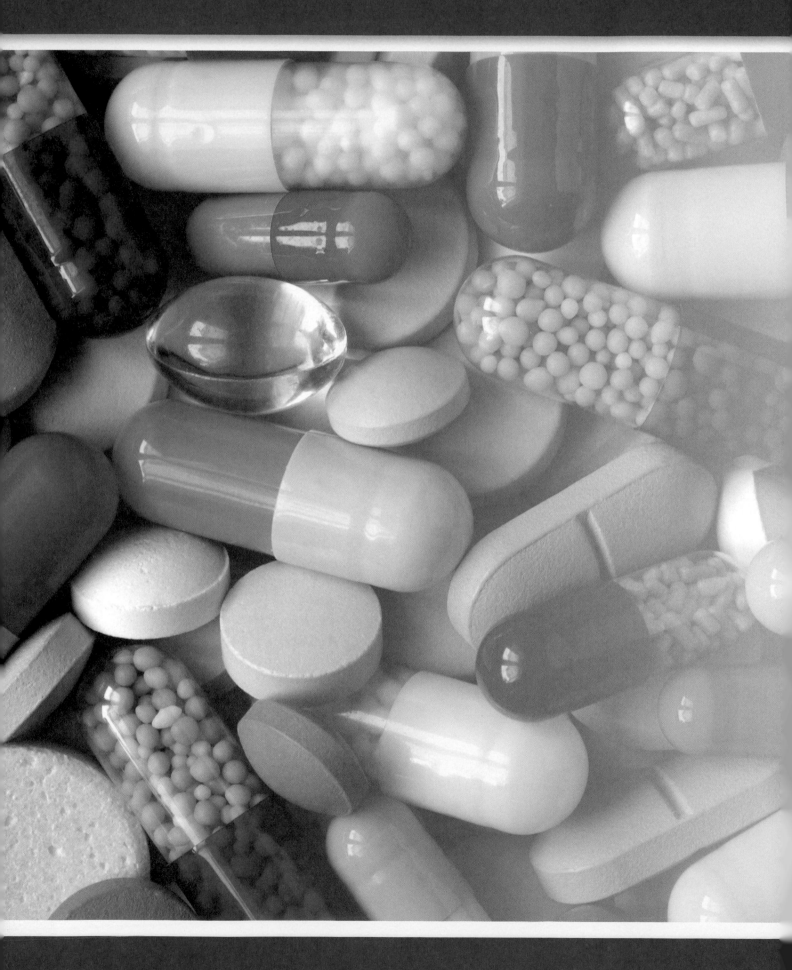

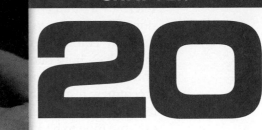
Your Future as a Pharmacy Technician

OBJECTIVES

After reading this chapter, you will be able to:

- Compare and contrast various work environments.
- Develop a professional image.
- Describe the processes and requirements for licensure, certification, and registration.
- Compare the formats and criteria of the PTCB and ICPT exams.
- Understand the importance of involvement in professional organizations.
- Complete a resume and cover letter.
- Execute a job search and prepare for an interview.
- Understand and display ethical behavior.
- Solve ethical dilemmas.
- Identify trends for the future of the pharmacy profession.
- Begin your career as a pharmacy technician.

KEY TERMS

Certification
Certified pharmacy
   technician (CPhT)
Cover letter
Duties
Ethical dilemma
Ethical distress
Ethical issue
Ethical problem
Group morality

Institute for Certification
   of Pharmacy
   Technicians (ICPT)
Licensure
Locus-of-authority
   problem
Morality
Moral judgment
Paraprofessional
Pharmacy Technician

Certification Board
   (PTCB)
Professional
Professional
   stewardship
Registration
Resume
Values

Chapter Overview

There are a number of diverse sites and environments in which to practice the profession of pharmacy. With different job functions and duties required at each practice site, there are countless opportunities for pharmacy technicians to continually challenge themselves, both personally and professionally. With the growing and changing needs of health care delivery, pharmacy technicians will be asked to establish new roles and accept new responsibilities in patient care. Pharmacy technicians will need to be flexible and willing to learn new skills as the profession of pharmacy evolves. This is an exciting time to be a pharmacy technician, and the future holds limitless prospects for technicians to gain varied experience in many dimensions of pharmacy practice.

Work Environments

The role of the pharmacy technician has evolved over the years from a clerk who only assisted the pharmacist with menial tasks to a technician who assisted in preparing prescriptions. Now, technicians are taking on more professional and administrative tasks and receiving more personal responsibility and self-direction to practice as pharmacy technicians. This expansion of accountability enables the pharmacist to spend more time in direct clinical-care activities rather than supervising technician activities. The evolution of the role of the pharmacy technician somewhat mimics the evolution of the pharmacist.

Most pharmacy technicians work in patient-care settings under the supervision of a pharmacist. They assist the pharmacist with pharmacy activities that do not require the clinical judgment of a pharmacist. Pharmacy technicians may also work in less patient-centered work environments, including managed-care organizations, mail-order pharmacies, long-term care facilities, hospice, drug- and poison-information centers, academia, home healthcare, professional organizations, and the pharmaceutical industry.

In most work environments, the technician is accountable to the supervising pharmacist. Ultimately, the supervising pharmacist is accountable, by law, for the tasks and activities conducted in the pharmacy. In general, pharmacy technicians receive and process prescriptions or medication orders, collect and communicate patient-related data, maintain inventory and record keeping, update patient information, and communicate with third-party payers for product coverage. In many settings, pharmacy technicians are increasingly responsible for clarifying prescriptions and medication orders with physicians, monitoring patient data, purchasing and controlling inventory, supervising technician staff, improving medication safety, and preventing medication errors. This expansion of duties has also precipitated growth in training and certification programs. While training, education, and certification requirements vary according to state, several national pharmacy organizations support the national standardization of pharmacy-technician requirements to reduce the variability in technician qualifications and experience.

Professionalism

A pharmacy technician is considered a **paraprofessional**, or someone who is trained to assist a professional. A **professional**, such as a pharmacist, is someone with recognized training or expertise in a specific field. A professional is expected to act with autonomy, use his or her knowledge and skills to benefit others, and adhere to an ethical code of conduct.

As the role of the pharmacy technician expands, so does the view of the technician as a professional. Once merely clerical assistants to pharmacists, pharmacy technicians must now maintain a level of personal integrity and professionalism to represent the profession of pharmacy in a positive manner. Developing a professional image involves exhibiting professional behaviors, a positive attitude, and a professional appearance.

Actions

Establishing a rapport with coworkers and patients is the first step in behaving like a professional. Be respectful, courteous, and willing to listen to others. Always address others with proper titles and respectful salutations.

Communication is an integral component of a professional image. Be clear, concise, and accurate in all types of communication. Do not use foul language or inappropriate nonverbal gestures. Personal conversations at work can be distracting and do not foster a professional image. Always maintain patient confidentiality in all communication.

Attitude

Being cheerful and displaying a positive, helpful attitude shows a willingness to work with others and an eagerness to learn. Willingness to learn new skills and take on new responsibilities is essential to cultivating a professional image.

Preserving tact and a positive demeanor across all situations also fosters a professional image. Maintaining composure, even in stressful situations, will allow the pharmacy technician to be seen as a leader and role model for other technicians.

Appearance

Personal appearance complements professional actions and attitudes. Dressing in a manner that is appropriate for your workplace and maintaining a suitable physical appearance displays self-control and competence. Alert and well-groomed employees are able to perform their best. In general, conservative dress is appropriate for work environments. Adhere to organizational guidelines for facial hair, head coverings, tattoos, piercings, and other adornments.

Certification, Licensure, and Registration

One component of professionalism is specialized education and training. To that end, pharmacy technicians are increasingly asked to obtain specialized experience or credentials, including licensure, registration, or certification.

Licensure is the granting of a license by a state in order to work in a particular profession. Licensure may require successful completion of an exam or specialized training. A license is renewable if the license holder demonstrates continued competence within the profession and remains up to date on current knowledge. A license is a legal requirement for practicing a profession. Currently, a license is not required for pharmacy technicians in all states.

Registration means that an individual must log his or her identity with a state organization before practicing a profession. Simply, a pharmacy technician may be asked to give his or her name, address, and place of employment to the board of pharmacy in his or her state. In many states, no education or training is required for registration, but certification may be in some states. Registration allows state boards of pharmacy to track individuals with a history of criminal misconduct, especially crimes related to drug diversion.

Certification is approval by a nongovernment agency asserting that an individual has met specific training or educational requirements. Certification is not mandatory, from a legal sense, in order to practice a profession. However, some states now require certification for pharmacy technicians. Certification through a national examination is not state-specific and is transferrable to other states. Currently, the two most widely recognized examinations are the Pharmacy Technician Certification Examination (PTCE) and the Exam for Certification of Pharmacy Technicians (ExCPT). Upon passing either exam, a technician is credentialed as a **certified pharmacy technician (CPhT)**.

PTCE

In 1995, the **Pharmacy Technician Certification Board (PTCB)** was created through a joint effort by the American Pharmacists Association, the Illinois Council of Health-System Pharmacists, and the Michigan Pharmacists Association. The mission of the PTCB is to establish and maintain national criteria for pharmacy-technician certification and recertification. PTCB created the PTCE, which candidates must pass in order to receive the title of CPhT.

To be eligible for the PTCE, individuals must have completed high school or received a GED (or the foreign equivalent) and cannot have a felony conviction. The PTCB evaluates the basic knowledge and skills necessary for competent practice as a pharmacy technician. No previous training or education is required for the PTCE, but formal training and education does assist a candidate in preparing for and passing the exam.

The PTCE is administered in a multiple-choice, computer-based format. Study materials are available from several sources. The pharmacy technician seeking certification is responsible for exam preparation; there is no guarantee that purchasing these training materials will produce a passing grade on the PTCE. The content of the exam consists of three general categories, outlined in TABLE 20.1: assisting the pharmacist in serving patients, maintaining medication and inventory-control systems, and participating in the administration and management of pharmacy practice.

Table 20.1   Exam Content of the PTCE

Category	Activities Evaluated	Portion of Exam
Assisting the pharmacist in serving patients	Receiving prescriptions or medication orders Collecting and communicating patient-specific data Assessing prescriptions or medication orders for completeness, accuracy, authenticity, legality, and reimbursement eligibility Processing a prescription or medication order Compounding a prescription or medication order Providing prescriptions or medication to patients or patient representatives Directing patients or patient representatives to the pharmacist for counseling	66 percent
Maintaining medication and inventory-control systems	Identifying pharmaceuticals, durable and non-durable medical equipment, devices, and supplies to be ordered Removing from inventory expired, discontinued, slow-moving, or overstocked pharmaceuticals and supplies Performing required inventories and maintaining associated records	22 percent
Participating in the administration and management of pharmacy practice	Coordinating written, electronic, and oral communication throughout the practice setting Updating and maintaining patient information Using and maintaining automated and point-of-care dispensing technology Communicating with third-party payers to determine or verify coverage for products or services	12 percent

ExCPT

The **Institute for Certification of Pharmacy Technicians (ICPT)** is part of the National Healthcareer Association. The mission of the ICPT is to recognize pharmacy technicians who have acquired the skills necessary for safe, accurate, and efficient practice. The ICPT promotes standards of excellence for pharmacy technicians. The ICPT created and administers the ExCPT in order to certify pharmacy technicians who have achieved a minimum level of competence in the practice of pharmacy. Candidates must pass the ExCPT in order to receive the title of CPhT.

Like the PTCE, to be eligible for the ExCPT, individuals must have completed high school or received a GED (or the foreign equivalent) and cannot have a felony conviction. No previous training or education is required for the exam, but formal training and education does assist a candidate in preparing for and passing the exam.

Also like the PTCE, the ExCPT is administered in a multiple-choice, computer-based format. Study materials are available from several sources. The content of the exam consists of three general categories, outlined in TABLE 20.2 : regulations and technician duties, drugs and drug products, and the dispensing process.

Recertification Requirements

Recertification is required every two years by both the PTCB and the ICPT. Recertification requires at least 20 hours of approved continuing education, at least one hour of which must be in pharmacy law. Continuing education is readily available through employers, professional organizations, journals, and Web sites. Much of it is available free of charge.

Table 20.2   Exam Content of the ExCPT

Category	Topics Evaluated	Portion of Exam
Regulations and technician duties	Role of pharmacists and pharmacy technicians, technician functions, prescription-department layout and workflow, pharmacy security, inventory control, and identifying expired products Controlled substances, schedules and regulations, refills, filing, prescription transfers, and Schedule V sales Federal privacy act, generic substitution, professionals with prescribing authority, child-resistant packaging, role of government agencies, manufacturer drug-package labeling, and OTC package labeling	25 percent
Drugs and drug products	Major drug classes, dosage forms, OTC products, and NDC numbers Brand and generic names, basic mechanisms of action and drug classifications, primary indications, and common adverse reactions, interactions, and contraindications	23 percent
Dispensing process	Information required on a valid prescription, telephones and faxed prescriptions, refill requirements, patient information, and interpreting prescribers' directions for prescription labels Avoiding errors, checking prescriptions, automated dispensing systems, preparing prescriptions and data entry, labeling prescriptions, patient records, packaging and storage, and managed-care prescriptions Conversions, systems of measurement, calculations for dispensing and compounding, calculating dosages and administration rates for IVs, and business calculations Drug distribution in hospitals and nursing homes, repackaging medications, prescription compliance aids, aseptic technique, procedures for chemotherapy, routes of administration for parenteral products, sterile products, maintaining a sterile environment, and compounding and labeling sterile product prescriptions	52 percent

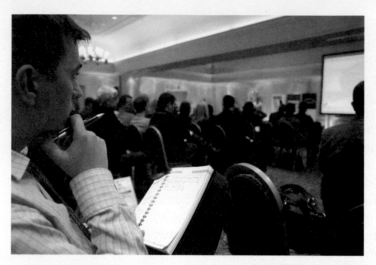

Continuing education is available via seminars, workshops, and online study.

Regulations and requirements affecting certification, recertification, licensure, and registration vary by state. It is the responsibility of the pharmacy technician to stay up to date on current requirements. Some states require completion of an education curriculum or a minimum number of hours of experiential education prior to practicing as a pharmacy technician.

> Review the requirements of the state board of pharmacy in the jurisdiction in which you wish to practice to confirm the requirements for education, training, certification, licensure, and registration.

Education, training, and licensing requirements for pharmacy technicians underscore the ideal that pharmacy is a competency-based profession. These requirements ensure that all practitioners in the profession maintain proficiency, continue professional development, and enhance their careers. The consistency and quality-assurance fundamental to the credentialing requirements promote a standard of care determined by the needs of the patients.

Professional Organizations

Being an active professional and promoting professional stewardship compels participation in a professional organization. **Professional stewardship** involves promoting professional standards, enhancing individual performance, and identifying individuals with outstanding commitment to the profession of pharmacy. Pharmacy technicians should work together to shape the future of the profession. Organizations exist on local, state, and national levels that make the views of pharmacy technicians heard by decision-makers and, thereby, effect change.

Network with other pharmacy technicians and professional organizations to discuss issues facing the profession of pharmacy and pharmacy technicians. Take ownership of your profession and advance principles that are important to you.

National Professional Organizations

- American Association of Pharmacy Technicians (www.pharmacytechnician.com)
- American Society of Health-System Pharmacists, Pharmacy Technicians (http://www.ashp.org/menu/InformationFor/Technicians.aspx)
- American Society of Health-System Pharmacists, Advisory Group (www.ashp.org)
- National Association of State Boards of Pharmacy (www.nabp.net)
- National Pharmacy Technician Association (www.pharmacytechnician.org)
- Pharmacy Technician Certification Board (www.ptcb.org)
- Pharmacy Technician Educators Council (www.rxptec.org)

Effective Job Searches

Searching for a job can be a daunting task, but it becomes more manageable when broken down into clear-cut steps. Job hunts can lead to opportunities to grow as a professional, to network with other people in your profession, and to ensure that you are a good fit for an employer and the employer is a good fit for you.

Identify Your Strengths

Start your job search by identifying your strengths. First, understand that your talents are enduring and unique. Your greatest room for growth and success are in areas of your greatest strengths.

You know that a pharmacy technician must meet certain requirements, and pharmacies need technicians to fulfill certain roles and duties, regardless of personal strengths or weaknesses. However, knowing yourself well will enable you to conduct an effective job search and develop a career plan.

Three basic work-related skill sets needed for any job include the following:

- Self-management skills—These include accepting supervision and direction, being honest, being punctual, being a hard worker, and working well with others.
- Job-related skills—These are activities at which you must be proficient in order to complete a certain job. These will vary by job, but examples of job-related skills required for many pharmacy technicians include receiving prescriptions or medication orders, contacting prescribers, processing insurance-coverage claims, stocking medications, dispensing medications, and communicating with patients.
- Transferable skills—These are not necessarily related to your job function, but do come in handy at work. These include skills such as the ability to speak in public, exceptional writing skills, the ability to operate complex types of equipment or machinery, being detail-oriented, negotiating, being a good listener, creating new ideas, motivating others, delegating responsibilities, and mediating problems.

Identify your own skills and preferences and emphasize these in your job search. With a variety of practice sites available for pharmacy technicians, you do not need to work in a job that does not maximize your strengths. If you enjoy research and compiling data regarding drug use, a job in drug information may be for you. If you enjoy interacting with the public, a community pharmacy practice may suit you best. If you enjoy compounding or preparing intravenous preparations, a home infusion pharmacy may offer the best job opportunity for you.

Career Goals

After you have identified your strengths, define your career goals. Start by clarifying your ideal job. Consider what makes a job satisfying for you. It may be the challenges inherent to the job itself, the coworkers and staff at the facility, a schedule that allows you a work-life balance, or the financial compensation and benefits provided. When defining your career goals, consider the following:

- First, identify what skills you want to use in your job. Also, note what special skills or expertise you have that can help you in a job. A hobby or family experience may be just the skill for which a particular employer is searching.

- Name the type of people with whom you want to work. Do you prefer working with geriatric patients or pediatric patients? Do you prefer laid-back coworkers or aggressive, competitive coworkers?

- Describe your ideal work environment. Do you prefer an office environment or a research and development laboratory? Do you prefer a quiet, low-volume pharmacy or a busy, high-volume mail-order pharmacy?

- Define where you want to work. Does it need to be near your home or near a childcare facility? Are you willing to move or commute for a new job? Is transportation a consideration?

- Calculate how much money you need to make. Consider the costs of commuting, buying clothes or supplies for a job, or obtaining insurance coverage. Also consider the total compensation package, including salary, benefits, educational assistance, childcare resources, and training.

- Clarify how much autonomy and responsibility you desire. Do you prefer to work independently or as part of a group? Are you willing to supervise or manage other workers? Do you like being in charge of projects?

- Finally, decide what is most important to you. Do you want to climb a corporate ladder, help patients, improve the healthcare system, educate the public, or simply have a fulfilling work-life balance?

Ask pharmacists in different practice settings about the different skills required for pharmacy technicians to determine what type of work interests you.

By enumerating the qualities you seek in an ideal job, you can effectively set a job objective. You may find that your ideal job is in a field that you have not yet considered. If you have trouble identifying personal skills or job-related characteristics, talk to your friends and family who know you, your likes and dislikes, and your strengths and weaknesses. Also talk to other pharmacy professionals to learn about different practice settings and the skills required in each. Further, career counselors who can assist you in refining your job search and career goals are available at many schools, as well as through employment associations or professional organizations.

Finding the right job for you is not only possible, but likely. Most pharmacy technicians report a high level of job satisfaction and career commitment. Career turnover for pharmacy technicians is low.

Resume

A **resume** is an essential tool for promoting your educational and professional experience to obtain a job. A basic, simple resume should offer a summary of the skills and knowledge you will bring to a job. Every resume should follow a standard format and should be as short as possible, without omitting valuable information. Try to limit your resume to one page; it should never be more than two pages. Keep in mind a manager may receive many resumes but only have time to interview a handful of candidates. Consider brevity and relevance to highlight points that must stand out.

A resume is a marketing tool that you use to sell yourself to employers.

Volunteer work in a healthcare setting may be a nice addition to the professional experience section of a resume. It shows that your scope of healthcare work expands outside of the pharmacy itself.

Resume-writing services are available, but writing your resume yourself forces you to examine your experience yourself and evaluate what skills you wish to highlight. Regardless of who writes your resume, it should be error-free. Always have a trusted friend or colleague review your resume for grammar and spelling mistakes. A resume should always be presented on high-quality, conservative paper. Unusual colors and textures portray an unprofessional image. For the same reason, use traditional font styles and sizes in your resume. Refrain from using colored text in your resume. Often, you will be applying for a job online. Make sure you submit online resumes in accepted file formats. If you must copy and paste a resume into a text box, do not simply use the copy and paste function of your computer. This will result in formatting loss and an unprofessional looking document. Instead, save an edited text version of your resume for cases that require such a submission type.

While your resume should highlight your qualifications and expertise, do not overstate your experience. Be honest with how much experience you have or what tasks you have completed in previous jobs. Be positive and emphasize your accomplishments, while also being humble. A resume should not include your faults or failures. Finally, be specific. Where possible, use numbers, percentages, or dollar amounts to define your experience.

Use action words and phrases to describe duties and accomplishments in your resume and cover letter. TABLE 20.3 contains some examples.

Most resumes are completed in chronological order, with the most relevant education and experience listed first. This format is appropriate for most job seekers with experience in one primary education or occupational field. For those changing careers or with limited experience, a skills resume may be more appropriate. Examples of sections that should be included in a chronological resume include the following:

- Heading—Give your full name, address (to protect your identity, providing only your city and state is acceptable), and contact information. Use an appropriate e-mail address for professional contacts.

Table 20.3 Action Words and Phrases

Achieved	Acted	Administered	Advanced
Advised	Analyzed	Arranged	Assessed
Authored	Automated	Built	Coached
Communicated	Composed	Conceptualized	Conducted
Consulted	Contained	Contracted	Controlled
Coordinated	Created	Cut	Decreased
Demonstrated	Designed	Developed	Directed
Eliminated	Established	Evaluated	Expanded
Facilitated	Focused	Headed up	Identified
Implemented	Improved	Increased	Influenced
Initiated	Innovated	Instituted	Introduced
Led	Maintained	Managed	Negotiated
Operated	Organized	Performed	Planned
Prepared	Produced	Promoted	Provided
Published	Reduced	Reported	Researched
Restructured	Reversed	Saved	Scheduled
Solved	Streamlined	Taught	Trained
Trimmed	Wrote		

- Objective—This is an optional section of the resume in which you can describe the type of job you are seeking. Tailor the objective to the job for which you are applying.

- Education and training—List formal training and education you have had or are currently taking related to the job you are seeking. You may include your GPA if it will help sell your experience, as well as special honors or accomplishments you received as part of your education. List certifications, registrations, and licensures that are applicable to the job.

- Previous experience—In reverse chronological order, list previous jobs, the job title, dates of employment, and your responsibilities. Do not include jobs that are irrelevant or unimpressive to a potential employer. Do list accomplishments, advancements, and promotions.

- Skills and affiliations—List special skills that you have, such as experience with specialized software or equipment. Also list any professional memberships that you have.

- References—Do not list references on your resume. You may wish to include "References available upon request" at the bottom of your resume, but if employers want to speak to references, they will, regardless of whether or not you place them on your resume.

Following is a sample chronological resume:

Mary Jones
1234 Center Avenue
My City, VA 23800
804-555-5555
MJones@mail.org

Objective: To obtain employment as a pharmacy technician that will allow me to use my skills in dispensing and compounding medications, evaluating patient profiles, and completing third-party billing.

Education:
Diploma from Pharmacy Technician's College, Park Place, VA
May 2010
GPA 3.4

Certification:
National Pharmacy Technician Certification Exam
July 2010

Experience:
Customer Service Associate, Big City Drug Store
June 2008–present
Duties included operating cash register, stocking inventory, and customer service.
Cashier, My Town Grocery
May 2006–June 2008
Duties included operating cash register and customer service.

Skills:
Proficient in third-party billing procedures
Knowledgeable in PharmMaster software
Mastery of aseptic technique

References: Available upon request

When preparing a resume for the professional with multiple jobs, education, and training, it would be prudent to format the resume with two columns to shorten the length of the resume and provide all of the information in an easy-to-read document.

Remember to ask people ahead of time if they are willing to serve as employment references for you.

Examples of sections that should be included in a skills resume include the following:

- Heading—Give your full name, address, and contact information. Use an appropriate e-mail address for professional contacts.
- Objective—This is an optional section of the resume in which you can describe the type of job you are seeking. Tailor the objective to the job for which you are applying.
- Areas of experience—Emphasize each area of strength rather than job titles or dates. Skills might include management, communication, administration, leadership, public speaking, fundraising, or marketing.
- Employment—Briefly list your employment history and dates.
- References—Do not list references on your resume. You may wish to include "References available upon request" at the bottom of your resume, but if employers want to speak to references, they will, regardless of whether or not you place them on your resume.

Following is a sample skills resume:

Sam Davis
876 Fillmore Street
My City, VA 23800
804-555-5555
SamDavisCPhT@mymail.com

Objective: To obtain employment as a pharmacy technician in a growing organization that will allow me to use my interpersonal, organizational, and communication skills.

Education:
Diploma from Pharmacy Technician's College, Park Place, VA
May 2008
GPA 3.5

Certification:
National Pharmacy Technician Certification Exam
July 2008

Management:
Supervise a team of 15 pharmacy technicians.
Complete scheduling duties and personnel support.
Order supplies and equipment.
Established new policies and procedures for maintaining inventory.

Communication:
Evaluate employees yearly for job performance and satisfaction.
Conduct monthly staff meetings with pharmacy technicians and pharmacists.
Treat patients, coworkers, and superiors with respect and compassion.
Establish a rapport with coworkers and well as other departments.
Act as a liaison between pharmacists and nurses.

(continues)

Staff Training:
Conducted quarterly inservices for pharmacy technicians and nurses on new drugs, supplies, and equipment.
Developed employee-training manuals and guidelines for patient profile review.
Created hospital-wide employee-training procedures for obtaining drug information.

Employment:
Senior Pharmacy Technician, HealthLife Hospital, Place Town, VA, 2009–present
Pharmacy Technician, MidAtlantic Hospital, Place Town, VA, 2008–2009

References: Available upon request

Resume Tips

- Write it yourself
- Make it free of errors
- Have it proofread
- Have it proofread again by another professional
- Apply a professional and conservative presentation
- Be honest and positive
- Cite specific examples
- Use action words

A curriculum vita, or CV, is a detailed summary of academic and work history. It is usually longer than a resume and provides history of all research and publication experience. CVs are often used in academic and scientific communities instead of resumes.

Cover Letter

A **cover letter** accompanies a resume when you contact a potential employer regarding a job. If you are presenting your resume in person, the cover letter should be printed on the same high-quality paper as the resume, and both the cover letter and resume should be enclosed in an envelope addressed to a specific person. When electronically submitting the cover letter and resume, be certain to use proper writing etiquette and spelling, and to adhere to deadlines for job postings. Include the name and job title of the person to whom the letter and resume are being sent. Make the letter personal and specific for the job. The cover letter should connect with the person reading the letter and tell them that something exceptional (your resume) follows.

Like resumes, cover letters highlight your qualifications and call attention to your experience. A cover letter should be no more than one page long and should be completed in a professional, conservative style. Like the resume, the cover letter should be brief but specific, free from errors, and positive. The sections of a standard cover letter include the following:

- Date—Include the current date in either the upper-left or upper-right corner.
- Employer's contact information—Include the name, title, and position of the person to whom the letter is addressed. Include the company and full address.
- Salutation—Use the name of the person to whom the letter is addressed instead of "Dear Sir or Madam" or "To Whom It May Concern." Be professional and use the person's title and last name.

- First paragraph—Explain why you are writing and what position you are seeking. Mention how you learned of the position. If you have a personal connection with the company or the person hiring, explain it here.

- Second paragraph—List why you are interested in the position and the organization. Use specific facts to show that you have researched the company and indicate why you would make a good addition to their team.

- Third paragraph—Refer to your enclosed resume. Explain specific items or highlight key accomplishments.

- Fourth paragraph—Indicate that you would like to schedule an interview or discuss the job opportunity further. Provide your contact information again. Thank the reader for his or her time.

- Closing and signature—Use a professional close to the letter such as "Sincerely" and sign the letter using blue or black ink.

Following is a sample cover letter:

July 1, 2010
Mark Johns, Pharm.D.
Pharmacy Manager, Main Street Apothecary
1800 Main Street
Anytown, GA 30060

Dear Dr. Johns:

I am interested in applying for the pharmacy-technician position open at your pharmacy, which was recently advertised in the *Marietta Daily Journal*. My family has been a long-time customer of your store and has been pleased with the level of care and service provided.

I am familiar with your pharmacy's innovative medication therapy management practices, and would welcome the opportunity to be involved in such proactive patient care. My education and work experience have prepared me for the challenges of community pharmacy practice, including a college GPA of 3.7 and recognition on the Health Sciences Honor Roll, three years of experience as a pharmacy technician in a pharmacy that filled 750 prescriptions per day, and elective training in communicating with patients. I recently passed the National Pharmacy Technician Certification Examination and I am an active member of the Georgia Chapter of the National Pharmacy Technician Association.

My enclosed resume details my education and work history. As you can see, I have a history of reliability as a pharmacy technician and many years of customer-service experience. I was also honored as "Technician of the Year" by my previous employer.

I would enjoy the opportunity to discuss how my skills and background would benefit Main Street Apothecary. I will contact you next week to schedule an interview. Or, you may contact me at PharmTech@mail.com or 678-555-5555.

Sincerely,

Leigh Adams

Interview

If a successful cover letter and resume have piqued an employer's interest, you will be asked to interview in person. Begin preparing for the interview as much in advance as possible; sloppy and hasty preparation and presentation translates to sloppy and hasty workmanship in the eyes of the employer. First, find out as much about the company as you can and the position for which you are applying. (This should have been completed, at least in part, when writing your cover letter.) It is helpful to visit the site beforehand. If it is a pharmacy, grab a merchandise cart and pretend to be shopping. Details about the company can provide topics for questions during the interview and allow you to discern whether the employer is a good fit for your career goals. Also, determine the codes of dress and behavior at the specific company so you can act accordingly during your interview.

Practice your interview skills with a friend, colleague, or career counselor. Engage in role playing to practice answering basic interview questions. Be prepared to take a dose calculations test and to demonstrate professional pharmacy skills. Also, develop a list of questions that you want to ask the employer. Remember, the interview is as much a process for you to learn about the employer as for the employer to learn about you.

Prior to an interview, prepare yourself for answering questions about your work experience and goals for your career and this specific position. Think about how you would answer to represent yourself positively as a strong employee compared with others who may interview. Practice your answers with a colleague or friend to ensure you sound confident and can explain your experience and specific job functions you have performed. Consider their feedback and re-answer questions that do not positively reflect your abilities and the type of individual you are. Be ready when you walk into the interview and prepare yourself to calmly and confidently answer other questions for which you may not have prepared. Following are several examples of questions an interviewer may ask you. Review these questions and prepare answers in advance of the interview. Doing so will make sure you appear confident and prepared, and not flustered or inconsistent.

- **Tell me about yourself.** Talk about yourself in a professional and positive way.
- **Why did you apply for this job?** Give truthful answers and insight as to why you have applied for this position.
- **What interests you about this job?** Provide specific aspects of the position that interest you and why.
- **What are your qualifications?** Cite your experience and training or certifications that prove you meet the qualifications identified in the job description or those that may add to your viability as a candidate for this position.
- **What did you like most/least about your previous job?** Answer this question honestly to provide insight in what you are looking for in a position and why you left your previous job.
- **Why did you leave your previous job?** Be honest. If you were fired from your last position, let them know. Explain what you could and will do differently in the future.
- **Where do you see yourself in five years? Where do you see yourself in 10 years?** Include your personal-growth goals as well as your professional-development and position goals. The hiring party is interested in what your long-term goals are and how those fit in with the goals of the organization.
- **Explain the gaps in your education/employment.** Succinctly explain what you did during the gaps in education, training, and employment.
- **Describe a time when you had difficulty communicating in the workplace.** This is an opportunity to make a negative communication encounter serve as a growth opportunity for you professionally. Explain the situation, what you learned from it, and how you will communicate differently in such situations in the future.
- **Describe a rule you have found difficult to follow.** State the rule and state clearly why this rule is difficult for you to follow.

- **What are your weaknesses?** Be prepared for this question and answer confidently.

- **Are you willing to work overtime? Weekends?** Be honest about your scheduling hurdles and your availability.

- **What are your hobbies?** State clearly your hobbies and outside interests.

- **Why did you choose this occupation?** Respond to this question with a heartfelt answer, specific to you and this occupation.

- **Why did you choose your school?** This is a very straightforward question that only requires you to share the reasons why you chose the school where you studied.

- **Does your GPA in school reflect your work ability?** This is a personal question that only you can answer. Be sure to know your GPA and answer how you think it reflects your work ability.

- **Name things that you learned in school that you would use in this job.** This is a great question to really reveal things you have learned in your training and how you would apply them to this specific job. Be prepared to answer this type of question.

- **What was your favorite subject in school? Why?** Pinpoint the subject you liked the most and consider why you liked it before the interview so you are ready to answer this type of question.

- **What have you learned from your mistakes?** This is a very popular question and enables the interviewer to assess whether you acknowledge making mistakes and how you learn from those mistakes and prevent them in the future. Be ready for this question and be truthful about the types of mistakes you have made. Also be truthful about what you have learned from them and carried on with you in your professional endeavors.

- **Have you ever gone out of your way to help a patient?** Answer this question with a yes or no and explain your answer.

- **What motivates you?** This is crucial for aligning the right person for a position with the right fit. Carefully answer this question, sharing the things that truly motivate you to work well in the job for which you are applying.

- **What are your future educational goals?** This question addresses your professional goals and long-term plans. Think about this prior to the interview and answer honestly and with confidence.

The interview is the employer's chance to learn about you and your chance to learn about the job.

- **What was the hardest decision you have ever made?** Be prepared for this question and answer it with some thought.

- **Why should I hire you?** Explain fully to the employer why you are the person who should be hired for this job. Have confidence, be honest, and base your answer on your life and professional experiences. This is your chance to give your complete and solid input on why you are the best employee for this position.

The most important question an employer can ask is "Why should I hire you?" Prepare a confident answer that highlights your experience and expertise without being aggressive or showing off.

Following are several questions for you to ask the interviewer:

- How many employees does the company/department have?

- What are the company's plans for growth or expansion?
- Does the pharmacy function separately from other departments?
- How important is the pharmacy department to senior management?
- What is the supervisor's management style?
- How long has the position been open?
- Why is the position open?
- How many employees have been promoted from this position?
- What are the most important duties of this position?
- What do you expect an employee to accomplish?
- How long will it take to make a hiring decision?

At least one day prior to the scheduled interview, confirm the date, time, and location with the potential employer. Obtain directions or instructions for parking, if necessary. The night before the interview, get plenty of sleep.

Dress appropriately for your interview. Although your work attire may allow for more casual dress or a uniform, business dress is appropriate for a job interview. Bring extra copies of your resume to the interview, as well as the names and contact information of people who have agreed to serve as your references. Arrive at the interview 10 to 15 minutes early and be courteous to those you meet. Remember, your interview starts when you enter the building, not when you meet the interviewer. Do not sit in the lobby and chat on your phone or text friends while waiting. The easiest way to accomplish this is by leaving your phone at home or in your car as there should be no reason you will need it during your interview.

Dressing for an interview includes proper grooming and hygiene. Remember, even the smallest things can make a big impression. Shine your shoes, trim your nails, do not wear perfume or cologne, and style your hair to make a positive impression.

Greet the interviewer by name and introduce yourself. Shake hands firmly and professionally. Remain standing until invited to sit down. When you sit, do not slouch, but maintain good posture.

During the interview, speak clearly and confidently. Make eye contact with the interviewer. Remain poised but enthusiastic about the job. Answer questions briefly, while presenting relevant skills. You may want to bring a small bottle of water with you as dry mouth is a common nervous reaction, but no other food or drink is appropriate, including candy and gum. Do not exaggerate, but do not be modest, either, when addressing your previous experience. Do not criticize former employers, coworkers, or working conditions. Avoid discussing salary requirements until the interviewer raises the subject.

At the end of the interview, thank the interviewer for his or her time, as well as the opportunity to learn about the organization. Always follow the interview with a thank-you note within 24 hours. In an age of electronic communication, an e-mail is acceptable, but a hand-written note will stand out. Also, follow up with a phone call a few days later, offering to

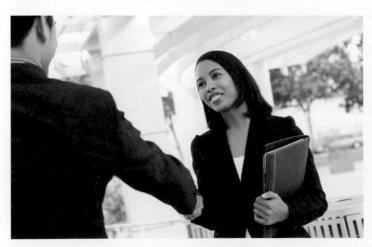

Present a professional image during an interview.

provide additional information or answer additional questions. Be persistent, but not aggressive. If you do not get the job, be courteous and thankful, and ask the employer to keep your resume on file for future jobs.

Interview Tips

- Confirm the appointment.
- Dress and groom professionally.
- Speak clearly and confidently.
- Thank the interviewer.
- Follow up.

Following is a sample thank-you note:

May 13, 2010

Dear Dr. Smith,

Thank you for meeting with me yesterday and discussing the pharmacy-technician position open at TriCity Hospital.

I appreciate the information you provided about the organization and the pharmacy department. I was impressed with the technology available in the hospital. I was also pleased to learn about the opportunities for growth that are present within the organization.

Working with a well-respected organization such as yours appeals to me as I start my career as a pharmacy technician.

Thank you for your consideration. I look forward to hearing from you soon.

Sincerely,

John Q. Anderson

Ethics in Pharmacy Practice

Every society establishes guidelines—spoken and unspoken, written and unwritten—that enable people to coexist peacefully and with a sense of **morality**. Fostering morality helps to ensure a high quality of life for each individual within a society, as well as the community at large.

The concept of morality encompasses values and duties. **Values** are qualities that embody a fulfilled and meaningful life. Objects, relationships, or experiences that have value—that is, things that society holds dear or of which we think highly—are important aspects of living together peacefully. **Duties** are actions in which individuals or societies engage to ensure peace and harmony. Duties may be either self-imposed or imposed by others, such as laws and regulations.

Morality, values, and duties are part of the human condition and may be learned from family and friends, mentors and community leaders, religious and cultural teachings, school and work acquaintances, and various forms of media. It is the responsibility of every individual to internalize and personalize this input to grow into a person who respects the moral values and duties of society.

Personal morality is the set of values and duties an individual recognizes. This personal set of beliefs may come from family traditions, customs, laws, or personal beliefs. Recognizing the personal morality of others is important for healthcare providers. Respect for others' beliefs and customs encourages communication between patient and provider, ultimately ensuring improved health outcomes.

Societal morality is larger than personal morality and consists of the shared values and duties among members of a community. These moral common denominators may be based in culture, ethnicity, or geographic customs and beliefs. Often, personal morality and societal morality are at odds. Specifically, in healthcare, debates concerning abortion, physician-assisted suicide, and the overall status of the healthcare system place groups and individuals on opposite sides of the moral spectrum, without either party being right or wrong.

Group morality refers to the shared values and duties of a subgroup of society, such as a church or religious organization or a profession. As a group, healthcare providers have specific values and duties that they must uphold and a standard of conduct and professional behavior to which they must adhere. Some of these practice standards are imposed by federal and state laws, while others are imposed by society's beliefs about what constitutes satisfactory care. Again, group morality may conflict with personal morality when decisions or actions are in conflict with personal beliefs or customs. In the healthcare professions, limited protections of personal morality exist to ensure that practitioners are not forced to engage in behavior that violates their personal morality.

Moral conflicts arise during the course of every personal and professional journey. Ethics are the methods or guidelines for approaching moral situations. The term ethics refers to a systematic discipline that calls for reflection on behavior, customs, and traditions when a moral decision is unclear. Analyzing the situation and arriving at a conclusion is called making a **moral judgment**. In order to make an effective moral judgment, an individual must first obtain all the facts surrounding the situation or question, be impartial, and generalize his or her conclusion to affect everyone in a similar situation.

An **ethical issue** is a situation with moral challenges. An ethical issue does not necessarily require action; it is merely a situation in which two sides of opposing moral opinion are present. As mentioned earlier, ethical issues facing healthcare include universal access to healthcare, abortion rights, and euthanasia. Often, these topics do not require an individual practitioner to take a certain action, but they are topics that are divisive and debated frequently.

Conversely, an **ethical problem** is a situation with moral challenges, and possibly negative implications, that does require action. There are three types of ethical problems:

- Ethical distress—An **ethical distress** is a challenge to maintain integrity or the integrity of the profession.
- Ethical dilemma—An **ethical dilemma** requires an individual or group to choose between two distinct judgments.
- Locus-of-authority problem—A **locus-of-authority problem** is a challenge about who should make a decision in a given situation.

Ethical Distress

An ethical distress focuses on an individual and the challenge he or she faces when prevented from doing what is right. Organizational policies or traditional practice roles may prevent a pharmacy technician from providing the best care to patients. The barrier may not always be easy to identify, and it may be that the situation is new or complex. Emotions and feelings are psychological responses to an ethical distress. These internal responses signal a threat to personal or professional integrity. Character traits such as compassion, caring, competence, and courage are resources for analyzing and resolving an ethical distress.

Ethical Dilemma

For a person who wishes to uphold high standards of moral behavior, an ethical dilemma poses a difficult choice and requires a judgment before engaging in an action. An ethical dilemma offers two distinct courses of action, both of which could be morally correct, but both of which are mutually exclusive. Ethical dilemmas may involve conflicting character traits or ethical conduct. A pharmacy technician may be required to choose between maintaining patient confidentiality and sharing information with a caregiver that you feel is in the best interest of the patient. Or, a pharmacy technician may need to choose between following organizational policies regarding dispensing certain medications and providing a treatment that would relieve a patient's pain or suffering.

Consider an elderly patient at your busy community pharmacy. He shops at your pharmacy frequently and you enjoy chatting with him when he drops off or picks up new medications. He has impaired eyesight and hearing, so when he picks up his medications, you often read the prescription labels and directions to him. Sometimes, he enjoys sharing stories of his grandchildren with you. This often takes you away from other pharmacy duties, and your coworkers have complained that you are socializing with customers and not finishing your own work. When you do not take the time to talk to the patient the next time he comes in to the pharmacy, you feel guilty. Your pharmacy is understaffed and fills a large volume of prescriptions daily. But, you feel it is important to spend time with the patients, ensuring that their questions are answered and they are comfortable with their medications. You also feel it is important for patients to have a comfortable and friendly relationship with the pharmacy staff. In this situation, you may wish to advise the patient to come to the pharmacy during a slower time of the day, so that you may provide him the attention that he deserves without compromising your workflow or placing undue stress on your coworkers.

Locus-of-Authority Problem

A locus-of-authority problem relates to who has the authority and ability to make a moral decision. Sometimes, the agent charged with ultimate authority is unclear. In healthcare, it may be the health professional himself or herself, the department supervisor, an administrator or manager, or the government or a regulatory agency. A locus-of-authority problem might also be present in the case of elderly patients or patients with mental disabilities. In these cases, other caregivers, family members, or healthcare providers may attempt to make decisions for the patient, and it may be unclear if the patient possesses his or her own decision-making skills.

Authority in ethical decision making comes from professional expertise, traditional roles, institutional arrangements and policies, and experience. When the decision maker is clearly identified, the course of action is determined by his or her decision. When ambiguity exists, an ethical problem calls for analysis of the situation regarding who should make the ultimate decision.

Consider a patient presenting a prescription for a narcotic. This person is well known in the community, and you have heard rumors that she is addicted to pain killers. Filling the prescription would maintain your obligations to your employer but could be harmful to your customer. But refusing to fill the prescription would embarrass the patient and endanger patient confidentiality, especially if you spread rumors with other pharmacy staff. You must uphold legal and appropriate dispensing of medications, while acknowledging the importance of confidentiality and maintaining truth and accuracy. In this situation, you would ask the pharmacist for assistance in determining the next course of action, which may include contacting the physician.

Suppose the policy at the community pharmacy where you work is to charge patients a fee for custom compounding of medications. You know one patient is facing a financial hardship, and that he will not be able to afford his medication if the extra fee is included. If the fee were to be waived, he could pay for his much-needed drugs. While you may feel responsible for making a decision on whether or not to charge the patient the extra fee, you, as the pharmacy technician, do not have the authority to make financial or billing decisions. You must adhere to the organizational policies and procedures as they pertain to dispensing, compounding, and charging patients. However, you may refer the case to a manager or supervisor who does possess the authority to alter practices in special circumstances. You may wish to communicate to the patient that you will assist him in contacting the supervisor or manager who can help find affordable options for obtaining his medications.

Solving Ethical Problems

The practice of pharmacy requires ethics and professional responsibility. Many healthcare- and medication-related decisions are intertwined with public and private life. The role of technology, rising healthcare costs, access to the healthcare system, the definition of life, genetic engineering, biotechnology, and assisted suicide are just a few of the countless ethical problems facing healthcare today. Translating beliefs and values into actions is difficult, and not all decisions can be generalized to all members of society. The responsibility to act in a moral way and to use sound ethical reasoning in the pharmacy profession requires self-confidence, self-determination, compassion, justice, experience, and practical wisdom.

An ethical problem requires making a choice between two morally correct choices, both of which cannot be followed at the same time. When faced with an ethical problem in your personal and professional life, a decision-making process can aid in analyzing and resolving it in an organized, objective manner.

The first step is to gather all information relevant to the ethical problem. Close attention to detail is essential for preventing rushes to judgment or arriving at false conclusions. From a healthcare perspective, fact-finding includes four major categories of questions:

- Clinical indications—Understanding the clinical indications helps to identify the diagnosis and prognosis, the medical treatments available, the patient's medical history, and the treatment needed to provide comfort and relieve suffering.

- Patient preferences—Identifying patient preferences clarifies the needs and wants of the patient and verifies that he or she is competent to make such decisions.

- Quality of life—Quality of life addresses the patient's beliefs and values about what is important in life and evaluates whether those beliefs and values are being upheld.

- Contextual factors—Contextual factors influencing an ethical problem include institutional policies and procedures that influence what can be done, legal issues that affect the outcome, and resource limitations, including financial resources, that can hinder the provision of services.

The next step is to identify the type of ethical problem: ethical distress, ethical dilemma, or locus-of-authority problem. Once identified, analyze the possible alternatives to an ethical choice. Use your imagination to outline possible scenarios and their outcomes. Confer with colleagues and gather opinions about available strategies. Diligently search for options to guarantee that no moral wrong goes unchecked.

Next, complete the chosen course of action. Some moral decisions are relatively straightforward. In healthcare, however, some are very literally life-and-death decisions. Professionals must have the courage and strength to complete the chosen action, even if there are repercussions.

Finally, evaluate the process, decision, and outcome. A retrospective examination of the ethical problem solving provides answers to several questions:

- What did you do well and why?
- What were the greatest challenges of the situation?
- How can you apply this experience to other experiences?
- Who was the most helpful in this situation?
- What did the patient or his or her caregivers say about the course of action and the outcome?
- Most importantly, what did you learn?

Reviewing the answers to these questions will help you grow as an ethical professional, and ease the process of moral decision making in the future. Strive always to maintain your integrity, compassion, and courage in your future as a pharmacy technician, upholding beliefs and values that ensure patient safety, respect, and health.

> **What Would You Do?**
>
> Question: A patient presents a prescription for emergency contraception. The prescription is legal and valid, and the patient meets the age requirement for OTC dispensing in your state. Based on your religious beliefs, you do not support the use of emergency contraceptives. How do you handle the situation?
>
> Answer: As a healthcare professional, you cannot prevent a patient from receiving medication ordered by a legal, valid prescription based on your beliefs. In this situation, you may ask another technician or pharmacist to fill the prescription in your place, removing yourself from the situation. If that option is not available to you, you must remember that you represent the pharmacy, and the best course of action would be to fill the prescription, knowing that the pharmacist ultimately will verify it and take responsibility for dispensing the emergency contraception. Another alternative, although not desirable as you want to maintain the patient's business in the pharmacy, is to direct the patient to another pharmacy that will dispense the contraception. The bottom line: Although you may not wish to be involved in the process of dispensing emergency contraception, you must either prepare the prescription for filling and dispensing or provide the patient an alternative means for obtaining the medication without impressing your personal beliefs on the patient. If you are not able to do this in your current pharmacy practice setting, it is best to seek other employment.

The Future of Pharmacy Practice

As you prepare for your future as a pharmacy technician, ask yourself, "What are technicians doing now, and what could they be doing tomorrow?" Many of the issues facing the healthcare system today will shape the pharmacy practice of tomorrow. With challenges facing the pharmacy workforce, medical innovation, healthcare costs, and future drug development, pharmacies are asked to provide more clinical services with fewer resources.

Workforce

Pharmacy manpower expectations may fluctuate while, at the same time, prescription volume is increasing. Additionally, the services provided by pharmacy personnel are expected to grow. Plus, an increased focus on patient safety and medication-error prevention calls for all pharmacists and pharmacy technicians to work harder and under more scrutiny than they have before.

Pharmacists are increasingly participating in patient-care activities and decreasing the time spent on dispensing duties. Thus, pharmacy technicians are asked to take on more responsibility and handle duties once assigned to pharmacists. This expanded use of the pharmacy technician will increase productivity, improve patient care, manage risk, and enhance drug-distribution systems.

The demand for pharmacy technicians is expected to increase by 31 percent between 2008 and 2018.

To enable them to take on more responsibility, increased training and education programs will be available for pharmacy technicians. Pharmacy technicians of the future will likely be able to specialize in specific areas of pharmacy practice such as vaccinations, wellness, IV preparation, or geriatrics. This larger knowledge base will allow pharmacy technicians to fill a larger number of roles in traditional pharmacy operations. In the future, highly skilled pharmacy technicians will likely be part of an integrated, multidisciplinary healthcare team.

Changes in the landscape of the pharmacy workforce will also open new avenues for employment in nontraditional practice sites, including mail-order pharmacies, managed-care organizations, and home healthcare. Pharmacy technicians with specialized training or formal education may also be able to take on more clinical responsibility.

Innovation

Today, many pharmacies employ automated processes to dispense medications, decreasing the need for pharmacists and pharmacy technicians to simply count pills. Similarly, electronic entry of medication orders decreases the need for prescription processing in some settings. These changes enable pharmacists and pharmacy technicians to focus less on clerical and dispensing duties and more on patient care.

By embracing technology and learning new skills, pharmacy technicians will be able to assist in expanding counseling, disease-state management, immunization, and education programs. Technology is also decreasing medication errors and reducing risk in drug distribution.

Costs

Healthcare costs continue to rise in the United States, and the government programs that provide healthcare coverage for the elderly, the poor, and the disabled are expected to more than double their expenditures in the next decade. Likewise, private-sector healthcare providers are passing costs to consumers in the form of higher insurance premiums and out-of-pocket costs. Healthcare reimbursement is decreasing, while demand for services is increasing.

Pharmacy technicians will need to be knowledgeable about government and private healthcare insurance plans and prescription-assistance programs to help people obtain the care they need. Pharmacists, pharmacy technicians, and patients will have to work together with physicians and healthcare providers to determine the most affordable and cost-effective options for medications.

 As a pharmacy technician, you must remain up to date on healthcare funding regulations, third-party payer policies and procedures, and assistance programs that can help people afford their medications.

Drug Development

The pace of innovation in drugs and delivery systems is increasing. Novel routes of application such as ocular inserts, and innovative drug designs such as monoclonal antibodies have opened opportunities for research, development, and training. Biotechnology and genetic engineering is an area of drug development that will receive increased attention in the future. As new dosage forms, delivery systems, and drug targets are identified, pharmacists and pharmacy technicians must adapt to the changing environment. Pharmacy technicians will be asked to understand and dispense new drugs and new dosage forms. Pharmacy is a profession of continuous change and learning.

Pharmacy is moving from a product-focused profession to a patient-focused profession, and pharmacy technicians are an integral part of that transformation. The expansion of pharmacy services will lead to improved patient care and advanced career opportunities for pharmacy technicians.

> *Pharmacy is an ever-changing field, and pharmacy technicians must never stop learning.*

Next Steps

After the didactic learning is completed in a pharmacy-technician curriculum, an externship offers practical experience in a real-world pharmacy setting. You will work with practicing pharmacists and pharmacy technicians to gain hands-on experience in assisting and supporting pharmacists, answering patient questions, and completing administrative duties. Use the externship experience to strengthen your skills and expand your professional network.

After the Externship

Most pharmacy-technician curricula that include an externship program do so at the end of the program. Once you have successfully completed the externship and your preceptors, or supervisors during the externship, ensure competency and proficiency with required skills and activities, your formal training to become a pharmacy technician is finished. You may be required to submit a formal report or project, depending on your program requirements. You will receive a diploma from your program and you are ready to begin your career as a pharmacy technician. Check with your state board of pharmacy for any licensing, certification, or registration requirements.

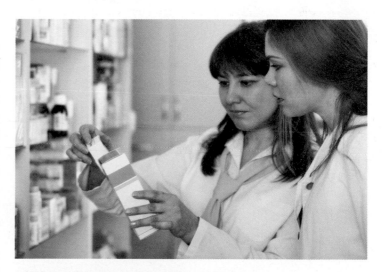

Ask plenty of questions during your externship.

Applying for Certification, Registration, and Licensure

Check with your state board of pharmacy or the National Association of Boards of Pharmacy to determine the requirements for certification, registration, and licensure. Often, the requirements are extensive, with state boards requiring documentation of education, examination scores, and a background check. Most states charge a fee to apply for licensure or to register. Pharmacy-technician licenses and registrations are not transferrable from state to state. Conversely, certification as a CPhT is transferrable

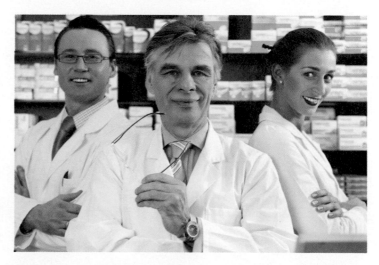

A career as a pharmacy technician offers exciting and rewarding challenges as part of the healthcare team.

and is not state specific. The fees required to take either the PTCE or ExCPT may be reimbursed by your employer.

More than 80 percent of jurisdictions require either licensure, certification, or registration of pharmacy technicians.

WRAP UP

Chapter Summary

- Pharmacy technicians take on more responsibility and autonomy than ever before.

- Pharmacy technicians are developing new skills that will offer limitless career opportunities.

- A pharmacy technician is a paraprofessional. As such, pharmacy technicians are expected to conduct themselves with a professional image, which includes exhibiting professional behavior, a positive attitude, and professional appearance.

- Pharmacy technicians are expected to obtain specialized training and education. The requirements vary by state, but this may include licensure, registration, or certification. To become a certified pharmacy technician, one must pass either the PTCE or the ExCPT.

- Participation in a professional organization is one way to actively promote standards of excellence in pharmacy. Professional organizations offer the opportunity for pharmacy technicians to work together to shape the future of their profession.

- To begin a job search, first identify your strengths. Skill sets that you already have or enjoy offer the best opportunities for growth in a new career. Next, establish career goals to clarify what type of job would be the best for you. Define the type of coworkers, the environment, the schedule, the responsibilities, and the compensation desired in a new job.

- A resume is a tool for promoting your work and educational experience to potential employers. A resume should always be completed in a conservative, professional style and be free of errors. A resume should emphasize your qualifications and experience, and minimize your failures or faults.

- A cover letter accompanies a resume when applying for a job and is another summary of your experience and qualifications. The cover letter should be personal and specific for the job.

- Successful interviews require professional attire and appearance, speaking clearly and confidently, and following up after the interview. Prepare answers to basic interview questions prior to the interview. Also, prepare questions to ask the interviewer about the job or organization.

- Healthcare frequently presents situations with moral challenges. By applying ethics, moral judgments can be made to address these challenges. An ethical issue is a situation that does not necessarily require action. In contrast, an ethical problem does require action. A step-by-step approach to the decision-making process requires gathering all the facts, assessing possible outcomes, completing the action, and evaluating the outcome. Ethical decision making will help pharmacy technicians maintain integrity, compassion, and courage in their careers.

- Many changes are taking place in healthcare. Dynamic changes in the pharmacy workforce, technology and innovation, healthcare costs, and drug development are expanding the role of the pharmacy technician. Pharmacy is moving from a product-focused profession to a patient-focused one, and these new paradigms will offer advanced career opportunities for pharmacy technicians.

- Once the formal educational program and experiential learning are complete, new pharmacy technicians are ready to begin exciting careers in healthcare. Pharmacy technicians must contact local state boards of pharmacy to learn the requirements for licensure, registration, and certification.

Learning Assessment Questions

1. Which of the following is not a requirement for developing a professional image?

   A. Exhibiting professional behaviors

   B. Showing a positive attitude

   C. Obtaining licensure in your state

   D. Displaying a professional appearance

2. What two organizations are responsible for certifying pharmacy technicians?

    A. PTCB and ICPT

    B. APhA and NAPB

    C. GED and CPhT

    D. NHA and ASHP

3. What are the two primary prerequisites for eligibility to take a pharmacy technician certification exam?

    A. 600 hours of externship experience and a GED

    B. A high-school diploma or equivalent and no felony convictions

    C. Two years of experience as a pharmacy technician and state registration

    D. Membership in the NPTA and 20 hours of continuing education

4. How often is recertification required for certified pharmacy technicians?

    A. Recertification is not required

    B. Whenever you have completed 20 hours of continuing education

    C. Every four years

    D. Every two years

5. Which of the following are required of professional stewardship?

    A. Exhibiting low career turnover and high job satisfaction

    B. Promoting professional standards and enhancing individual performance

    C. Membership in the NPTA and two years of experience as a pharmacy technician

    D. Volunteering for a professional organization and obtaining certification

6. Which of the following skill sets are important to define prior to beginning a job search?

    A. Management style, education level, and salary

    B. Communication and professionalism

    C. Moral duties and values

    D. Self management, job-related skills, and transferable skills

7. What are the two standard formats for resumes?

    A. Educational and occupational

    B. Chronological and skills

    C. Curriculum vitae and cover letter

    D. Experiential and referential

8. A standard cover letter should not include which of the following?

    A. How you heard about the position

    B. Your complete contact information

    C. The reasons you disliked your last job

    D. Facts about the company to which you are applying

9. Which of the following is not appropriate for a professional interview?

    A. Dressing in scrubs if you will be allowed to do so on the job

    B. Bringing an extra copy of your resume

    C. Providing the names and contact information for your references

    D. Following up with a hand-written thank-you note

10. Which of the following is not a type of ethical problem?

    A. An ethical distress

    B. A moral judgment

    C. An ethical dilemma

    D. A locus-of-authority problem

Appendix A: Abbreviations Used in Medical Prescriptions

Key

Official Do-Not-Use list in the United States required by Joint Commission
Not recommended for use by other organizations

Abbreviation	Latin	Meaning	Possible confusion
aa	ana	of each	
ad	ad	up to	
a.c.	ante cibum	before meals	
a.d.	auris dextra	right ear	"a" can be mistaken as an "o" which could read "o.d.", meaning right eye
ad lib.	ad libitum	use as much as one desires; freely	
admov.	admove	apply	
agit	agita	stir/shake	
alt. h.	alternis horis	every other hour	
a.m.	ante meridiem	morning, before noon	
amp		ampule	
amt		amount	
aq	aqua	water	
a.l., a.s.	auris laeva, auris sinistra	left ear	"a" can be mistaken as an "o" which could read "o.s." or "o.l.", meaning left eye
A.T.C.		around the clock	
a.u.	auris utraque	both ears	"a" can be mistaken as an "o" which could read "o.u.", meaning both eyes
bis	bis	twice	
b.d./b.i.d.	bis in die	twice daily	
B.M.		bowel movement	
BNF		British National Formulary	

Abbreviation	Latin	Meaning	Possible confusion
bol.	bolus	as a large single dose (usually intravenously)	
B.S.		blood sugar	
B.S.A.		body surface areas	
b.t.		bedtime	mistaken for "b.i.d", meaning twice daily
BUCC	bucca	inside cheek	
cap., caps.	capsula	capsule	
c, c.	cum	with (usually written with a bar on top of the "c")	
cib.	cibus	food	
cc	cum cibo	with food, (but also cubic centimetre)	mistaken for "U", meaning units; also has an ambiguous meaning; use "mL" or "milliliters"
cf		with food	
comp.		compound	
cr., crm		cream	
CST		Continue same treatment	
D5W		dextrose 5% solution (sometimes written as D_5W)	
D5NS		dextrose 5% in normal saline (0.9%)	
D.A.W.		dispense as written (i.e., no generic substitution)	
dc, D/C, disc		discontinue or discharge	ambiguous meaning
dieb. alt.	diebus alternis	every other day	
dil.		dilute	
disp.		dispersible or dispense	
div.		divide	
d.t.d.	dentur tales doses	give of such doses	
D.W.		distilled water	
elix.		elixir	
e.m.p.	ex modo prescripto	as directed	
emuls.	emulsum	emulsion	
et	et	and	
eod		every other day	
ex aq	ex aqua	in water	
fl., fld.		fluid	
ft.	fiat	make; let it be made	
g		gram	
gr		grain	
gtt(s)	gutta(e)	drop(s)	
H		hypodermic	

Abbreviation	Latin	Meaning	Possible confusion
h, hr	hora	hour	
h.s.	hora somni	at bedtime	
h.s		hour sleep or half-strength	ambiguous meaning
ID		intradermal	
IJ, inj	injectio	injection	mistaken for "IV", meaning intravenously
IM		intramuscular (with respect to injections)	
IN		intranasal	mistaken for "IM", meaning intramuscular, or "IV", meaning intravenously
IP		intraperitoneal	
IU		international unit	mistaken for "IV" or "10", spell out "international unit"
IV		intravenous	
IVP		intravenous push	
IVPB		intravenous piggyback	
L.A.S.		label as such	
LCD		coal tar solution	
lin	linimentum	Liniment	
liq	liquor	Solution	
lot.		Lotion	
mane	mane	in the morning	
M.	misce	Mix	
m, min	minimum	a minimum	
mcg		microgram	
m.d.u.	more dicto utendus	to be used as directed	
mEq		milliequivalent	
mg		milligram	
MgSO4		magnesium sulfate	may be confused with "MSO4", spell out "magnesium sulfate"
mist.	mistura	mix	
mitte	mitte	send	
mL		millilitre	
MS		morphine sulfate or magnesium sulfate	can mean either morphine sulfate or magnesium sulfate, spell out either
MSO4		morphine sulfate	may be confused with "MgSO4", spell out "morphine sulfate"
nebul	nebula	a spray	
N.M.T.		not more than	
noct.	nocte	at night	

Abbreviation	Latin	Meaning	Possible confusion
non rep.	non repetatur	no repeats	
NS		normal saline (0.9%)	
1/2NS		half normal saline (0.45%)	
N.T.E.		not to exceed	
o_2		both eyes, sometimes written as o$_2$	
od	omne in die	every day/once daily (preferred to qd in the UK)	
od	oculus dexter	right eye	"o" can be mistaken as an "a" which could read "a.d.", meaning right ear, confusion with omne in die
om	omne mane	every morning	
on	omne nocte	every night	
o.p.d.		once per day	
o.s.	oculus sinister	left eye	"o" can be mistaken as an "a" which could read "a.s.", meaning left ear
o.u.	oculus uterque	both eyes	"o" can be mistaken as an "a" which could read "a.u.", meaning both ears
oz		ounce	
per	Per	by or through	
p.c.	post cibum	after meals	
pig./pigm.	pigmentum	paint	
p.m.	post meridiem	evening or afternoon	
p.o.	per os	by mouth or orally	
p.r.	per rectum	by rectum	
PRN, prn	pro re nata	as needed	
pulv.	Pulvis	Powder	
PV	per vaginam	via the vagina	
q	Quaque	Every	
q.a.d.	quoque alternis die	every other day	
q.a.m.	quaque die ante meridiem	every day before noon	
q.d.s.	quater die sumendus	four times a day	can be mistaken for "qd" (every day)
q.p.m.	quaque die post meridiem	every day after noon	
q.h.	quaque hora	every hour	
q.h.s.	quaque hora somni	every night at bedtime	
q.1h, q.1°	quaque 1 hora	every 1 hour; (can replace "1" with other numbers)	

Abbreviation	Latin	Meaning	Possible confusion
q.d., q1d	quaque die	every day	mistaken for "QOD" or "qds", spell out "every day" or "daily"
q.i.d.	quattuor in die	four times a day	
q4PM		at 4pm	mistaken to mean every four hours
q.o.d.		every other day	mistaken for "QD", spell out "every other day"
qqh	quater quaque hora	every four hours	
q.s.	quantum sufficiat	a sufficient quantity	
QWK		every week	
R		rectal	
rep., rept.	repetatur	repeats	
RL, R/L		Ringer's lactate	
s	sine	without (usually written with a bar on top of the "s")	
s.a.	secundum artum	use your judgement	
SC, subc, subcut, subq, SQ		subcutaneous	"SC" can be mistaken for "SL", meaning sublingual; "SQ" can be mistaken for "5Q" meaning five every dose
sig		write on label	
SL		sublingually, under the tongue	
sol	solutio	solution	
s.o.s., si op. sit	si opus sit	if there is a need	
ss	semis	one half or sliding scale	ambiguous meaning; mistaken for "55" or "1/2"
SSI, SSRI		sliding scale insulin or sliding scale regular insulin	mistaken to mean "strong solution of iodine" or "selective serotonin reuptake inhibitor"
stat	statim	immediately	
supp	suppositorium	suppository	
susp		suspension	
syr	syrupus	syrup	
tab	tabella	tablet	
tal., t	talus	Such	
tbsp		tablespoon	
troche	trochiscus	Lozenge	
t.d.s.	ter die sumendum	three times a day	
t.i.d.	ter in die	three times a day	

Abbreviation	Latin	Meaning	Possible confusion
t.i.w.		three times a week	mistaken for twice a week
top.		Topical	
T.P.N.		total parenteral nutrition	
tr, tinc., tinct.		Tincture	
tsp		Teaspoon	
U		Unit	mistaken for a "4", "0" or "c", spell out "unit"
μg		Microgram	mistaken for "mg", meaning milligram
u.d., ut. dict.	ut dictum	as directed	
ung.	unguentum	Ointment	
U.S.P.		United States Pharmacopoeia	
vag		vaginally	
w		with	
wf		with food (with meals)	
w/o		without	
X		times	
Y.O.		years old	

Reproduced from Wikipedia, the free encyclopedia at http://en.wikipedia.org/wiki/List_of_abbreviations_used_in_medical_prescriptions, accessed on September 9, 2011.

Appendix B: Answer Key

CHAPTER 1

1. B	6. A	11. C	16. B
2. C	7. C	12. A	17. B
3. C	8. B	13. C	18. B
4. C	9. D	14. C	19. B
5. B	10. C	15. A	20. B

CHAPTER 2

1. C	6. D	11. B	16. D
2. A	7. D	12. D	17. A
3. A	8. C	13. D	18. C
4. A	9. A	14. B	19. B
5. B	10. A	15. A	20. A

CHAPTER 3

1. B	6. B	11. A	16. A
2. B	7. C	12. D	17. A
3. C	8. B	13. B	18. C
4. C	9. A	14. C	19. D
5. B	10. B	15. C	20. C

CHAPTER 4

1. D	6. B	11. D	16. A
2. A	7. B	12. B	17. A
3. A	8. C	13. D	18. C
4. B	9. A	14. B	19. D
5. A	10. D	15. D	20. A

CHAPTER 5

1. A	7. C	13. C	19. C
2. D	8. A	14. C	20. A
3. C	9. C	15. B	21. A
4. B	10. B	16. C	22. C
5. D	11. C	17. A	23. A
6. A	12. A	18. B	24. C

CHAPTER 6

1. C	6. D	11. B	16. C
2. C	7. A	12. A	17. B
3. D	8. B	13. D	18. D
4. C	9. D	14. A	19. B
5. B	10. A	15. B	20. C

CHAPTER 7

1. C	6. B	11. B	16. B
2. D	7. A	12. C	17. D
3. C	8. B	13. B	18. B
4. B	9. B	14. A	19. A
5. A	10. B	15. B	20. A

CHAPTER 8

1. B	7. C	12. B	17. D
2. A	8. C	13. D	18. A
3. B	9. B	14. D	19. B
4. B	10. D	15. B	20. C
5. B	11. A	16. A	21. B
6. C			

CHAPTER 9

1. B	6. C	11. B	16. B
2. A	7. D	12. A	17. A
3. D	8. D	13. C	18. D
4. C	9. A	14. B	19. A
5. D	10. B	15. C	20. D

CHAPTER 10

1. A	6. A	11. A	16. A
2. A	7. B	12. B	17. B
3. D	8. A	13. D	18. A
4. B	9. C	14. C	19. C
5. C	10. C	15. D	20. D

CHAPTER 11

1. D	6. A	11. B	16. A
2. A	7. C	12. D	17. B
3. C	8. B	13. A	18. D
4. A	9. A	14. B	19. C
5. D	10. D	15. D	20. B

CHAPTER 12

1. A	6. A	11. A	16. D
2. D	7. C	12. D	17. A
3. C	8. D	13. B	18. B
4. C	9. B	14. C	19. C
5. D	10. C	15. C	20. A

CHAPTER 13

1. C	6. A	11. D	16. A
2. A	7. D	12. A	17. C
3. B	8. C	13. A	18. A
4. A	9. A	14. B	19. D
5. B	10. A	15. C	

CHAPTER 14

1. C	8. C	14. B	20. A
2. A	9. A	15. D	21. B
3. B	10. D	16. C	22. B
4. C	11. A	17. C	23. A
5. A	12. C	18. A	24. C
6. C	13. D	19. B	25. C
7. B			

CHAPTER 15

1. C	6. C	11. B	16. A
2. D	7. D	12. A	17. D
3. B	8. D	13. C	18. D
4. A	9. A	14. C	19. A
5. A	10. B	15. C	20. C

CHAPTER 16

1. B	6. C	11. D	16. D
2. A	7. A	12. B	17. C
3. D	8. D	13. D	18. A
4. A	9. B	14. D	19. D
5. B	10. C	15. A	20. D

CHAPTER 17

1. B	6. D	11. A	16. D
2. C	7. B	12. B	17. A
3. A	8. A	13. D	18. C
4. D	9. D	14. C	19. A
5. A	10. A	15. B	20. C

CHAPTER 18

1. D	8. B	14. B	20. B
2. B	9. B	15. B	21. A
3. D	10. C	16. A	22. B
4. B	11. D	17. D	23. A
5. D	12. A	18. A	24. D
6. B	13. A	19. C	25. B
7. D			

CHAPTER 19

1. C	8. D	14. D	20. B
2. A	9. A	15. C	21. D
3. D	10. C	16. B	22. B
4. B	11. B	17. B	23. A
5. D	12. A	18. A	24. D
6. C	13. D	19. C	25. D
7. B			

CHAPTER 20

1. C	4. D	7. B	9. A
2. A	5. B	8. C	10. B
3. B	6. D		

Glossary

A

Absence seizure—A type of seizure characterized by a brief episode of staring, with no convulsions. Absence seizures, formerly called petit mal seizures, can include changes in muscle activity.

Absorption—The process by which a medication enters or passes through natural body barriers.

Abuse—Healthcare provider practices that are inconsistent with sound fiscal, business and medical practices that will result in unnecessary costs or financial loss.

Accuracy—How well a measurement represents the true value.

Acetylcholine—A neurotransmitter that has stimulating effects and plays a role in Parkinson's disease.

Acidic solution—A solution with a pH value less than 7.

Acidosis—A metabolic condition in which the pH of the blood is below 7.35.

Acne—Inflammation of the skin due to overactivity of hormones on the skin's oil glands.

Acne vulgaris—Lesions on the skin that result from overactive and infected sebaceous glands.

Acquired immune deficiency syndrome (AIDS)—The lack of specific immune cells which prevent disease.

Actinic keratosis—A precancerous condition characterized by scaly skin lesions. Caused by overexposure to the sun.

Active immunity—Provides memory for the immune system. Active immunity allows the immune system to initiate a quick response to a pathogen on subsequent exposures. It is obtained from previous infections or vaccinations.

Active ingredient—The pharmacologically active component of a drug that exerts the desired therapeutic effect.

Actuation—The act of releasing medication from a metered-dose inhaler while taking a slow, deep breath.

Acute pain—The type of pain experienced when an injury occurs, such as a burn or a cut. It is easy to manage, usually lasting for only a short period of time.

Adaptive immune system—The part of the immune system that mounts a specific defense toward invading organisms. The adaptive immune system includes cell-mediated immunity and humoral immunity.

Addiction—The perceived need to use a drug to attain physical and psychological effects.

Addison's disease—A disease that results from a deficiency of corticosteroids caused by damage to the adrenal cortex.

Addition—The process of adding numbers together to find their sum.

Additives—Inert ingredients that may be needed for a successful preparation of the dosage form.

Adjunctive therapy—A drug or therapy that is added to existing therapy.

Admitting order—An order that is written by a physician when a patient is admitted to the hospital.

Admixture—Made by adding small volumes of one or more drugs or solutions to a large volume of fluid.

Adrenal gland—A gland located directly above the kidneys. The adrenal gland is composed of two layers of tissue: the medulla and the cortex.

Adrenocorticotropic hormone (ACTH)—A hormone produced by the pituitary that stimulates the release of cortisol from the adrenal cortex.

Adsorption stage—The stage in virus reproduction in which the virus attaches to a potential host cell.

Adulteration—The preparation and storage of a medication that can lead to contamination/impurity, falsification of contents, or loss of potency.

Aerobic—Living in the presence of oxygen.

Aerosol—A spray that contains very fine liquid or solid drug particles in a gas propellant that is packaged under pressure.

Afferent system—A division of the peripheral nervous system, including all nerves and sense organs that send information to the central nervous system.

Affinity—The strength, or how tightly a drug binds to its receptor.

Agonist—A drug that binds to a cell receptor and may trigger a response.

AIDS-defining illness (ADI)—The group of diseases used to diagnose AIDS.

Alchemy—The theory that combining elements of chemistry, metallurgy, physics, and medicine with astrology and spiritualism could turn metals into gold.

Alcoholic solution—An alcohol-based solution.

Alcoholism—A condition also described as alcohol dependence that makes those affected unable to stop consuming alcohol. Those afflicted with this condition show signs of physical addiction.

Algae—A group of organisms that do not cause human disease, some of which are beneficial to the practice of pharmacy.

Algorithm—A flowchart of drug-treatment choices for a specific disease.

Alkaline solution—A solution with a pH value greater than 7.

Alkalosis—A metabolic condition in which the pH of the blood is greater than 7.45.

Allergen—Any substance that elicits an allergic reaction.

Allergic reaction—A local or general response of the immune system to an antigen.

Allergy—An immune response that occurs in response to a foreign substance.

Alligation—A method of solving problems for a specific concentration by mixing or combining components of two different concentrations of the same substance.

Alveolar wall—A wall that separates the alveoli in the lungs.

Alveoli—Tiny, delicate air sacs in the lungs where the gas-blood exchange occurs.

Alzheimer's disease (AD)—A degenerative disorder of the brain that leads to loss of brain function, resulting in memory impairment and the loss of judgment, decision-making ability, and speech.

Ampule—A glass container with a single dose of active ingredient.

Anaerobic—Living outside the presence of oxygen.

Analgesics—Drugs that decrease, control, or block pain.

Anaphylactic reaction—A severe allergic response to an allergen. This can be an immediate, life-threatening reaction that involves respiratory distress (difficulty breathing) followed by shock.

Anaphylaxis—An extreme, often life-threatening, allergic reaction.

Androgens—Male hormones produced by the testes.

Anemia—A decrease in the number of red blood cells.

Anesthetics—Drugs that prevent signals from going to or returning from the brain.

Angina pectoris—Chest pain caused by a decreased oxygen supply to the heart. A sign of ischemic heart disease. also referred to as angina.

Antagonist—A drug that blocks the action of the natural chemical messengers found in the body.

Antecubital area—The area in front of the elbow. Veins in this area are often used for IV administration of drugs.

Anti-anxiety agent—A drug used to treat anxiety.

Antibody—An immunoglobulin made in response to an antigen. It neutralizes the effect of the antigen.

Anticipatory compounding—A compounded preparation prepared in anticipation of a prescription.

Anticonvulsants—The drugs of choice for seizure control. Also known as antiepileptic drugs.

Antidepressant—A drug used to treat depression.

Antifungal—Describes drugs that kill fungus.

Antigen—A molecule that stimulates an immune response.

Antihistamines—Drugs that block the activity of H_1 receptors.

Antineoplastic drug—A drug used to treat cancer.

Antipsychotic—A drug used to treat psychiatric diseases.

Antipyretic—A drug that reduces fever.

Antiretroviral—Describes drugs that prevent retrovirus replication.

Antiseptic—A substance that inhibits the growth of infection-causing microorganisms.

Antitussives—Medications that suppress or reduce the frequency of coughing.

Antiviral—Describes drugs that prevent virus replication.

Apocrine sweat glands—Sweat glands that produce sweat containing organic material.

Apothecary—A Latin term for pharmacist; it is also a shop where drugs are sold.

Aqueous solution—A water-based solution.

Aqueous suspension—A suspension that contains medications distributed in water.

Aromatic water—A solution of water that contains oil or other volatile substances.

Arrhythmia—Variation in the heart's normal rate and/or rhythm.

Arthritis—Inflammation of one or more joints that can result in pain, stiffness, and limited movement.

Asepsis—The absence of infection-causing microorganisms.

Aseptic technique—The procedure by which sterile products are prepared to avoid contamination.

Aspiration—Inhalation of fluids from the mouth and throat.

Assembly stage—The stage in virus reproduction in which viral parts are assembled.

Assault—Threatening another with bodily harm.

Asthma—A chronic inflammatory airway disease in which the muscles around the bronchioles contract, narrowing the air passages so that air cannot be inhaled properly.

Ataxia—Irregular muscle movements or incoordination.

Atherosclerosis—The narrowing of arteries caused by the buildup of cholesterol deposits.

Atonic seizure—A type of seizure that begins with a sudden loss of muscle strength. Also known as drop attacks.

Attention-deficit/hyperactivity disorder (ADHD)—A disorder characterized by a persistent pattern of frequent, severe inattention and/or hyperactivity or impulsivity.

Aura—Unusual visual or sound sensations that precede a seizure.

Autoclave—A machine that generates heat and pressure to sterilize objects.

Autonomic nervous system (ANS)—The nerve system that controls organs and body systems automatically, such as maintaining heart rate.

Autoimmune disease—An illness in which the body's tissues are attacked by their own immune system. The antibodies in the blood target the body's own tissues.

Average wholesale price (AWP)—The average drug price charged by a wholesaler.

B

Bacteria—Microorganisms that can be harmful or beneficial to humans.

Bactericidal antibiotic—An antibiotic that kills bacteria.

Bacteriostatic—A diluent that contains a preservative to prevent the growth of bacteria.

Bacteriostatic antibiotic—An antibiotic that stops the growth of bacteria.

Basal cell carcinoma—A slow-growing skin tumor that rarely metastasizes.

Battery—Causing physical harm to another person.

B-cell—A lymphocyte that secretes pathogen-specific antibodies to neutralize pathogens.

Benign tumor—A tumor that is not harmful, progressive, or recurrent.

Benzodiazepines—A class of drugs prescribed for treatment of anxiety and insomnia.

Beta-blocker—A drug that blocks a beta receptor. These drugs are frequently prescribed for hypertension. Also called beta-blocking drug.

Beyond-use date—The date on which the compounded preparation expires or after which it should not be used. It is based on the date on which the preparation was compounded, not the date on which it was dispensed.

Binders—Promotes the adhesion of active and inactive ingredients in tablets.

Bioavailability—The degree to which a drug is available to the site of action to produce the desired effect.

Bioequivalent—A term used when two drugs have similar bioavailability when given in the same dosage form and dose.

Biologic response modifier—A therapeutic agent that enhances the body's own immune activity.

Biopharmaceutical—A drug that is produced from recombinant DNA technology.

Bioterrorism—The attack, or threat of an attack, with a bioterrorism agent as the weapon.

Bioterrorism agent—An organism or toxin that can cause disease or death in humans, plants, or animals.

Bipolar disorder—A disease noted by mood swings between mania and depression.

Black-box warning—A statement on the patient package insert that alerts prescribers to serious or even life threatening adverse reactions from a drug.

Blending—The process of combining two substances.

Body-surface area (BSA)—A representation of a person's weight and height relative to each other.

Bolus dose—Administration of a drug intravenously all at once or over a short period of time.

Brand name—The proprietary name under which a manufacturer markets a drug; it is also referred to as the trade name.

Broken contract—The simplest form of torts; a broken promise to do or not do an act.

Bronchitis—Inflammation of the lining of the bronchial airways, which leads to obstruction of airflow upon exhalation.

Bronchospasm—Spasmodic contraction of the bronchial smooth muscles.

Buccal—An oral route of administration in which the medication is placed between the cheek and gum.

Bursitis—Inflammation of a bursa, which is a small, fluid-filled sac that acts as a cushion between a bone and muscles, tendons, or skin.

C

Calcitonin—Hormone produced in the thyroid gland that is involved in the regulation of calcium levels. It inhibits the resorption of calcium from the bone and kidney.

Cancer—A group of diseases characterized by uncontrolled cellular growth, local tissue invasion, and distant metastases.

Candidiasis—An infection of the skin caused by *Candida albicans*.

Caplet—A hybrid of a tablet and capsule.

Capsid—The structure that protects a virion.

Capsule—A solid dosage form that uses a hard or soft gelatin shell.

Capture—An adjudication of a third-party claim that results in a payment.

Carbuncle—A group of infected hair follicles.

Carcinogen—A substance that causes cancer.

Cardiac cycle—The set of coordinated events that occurs during one beat of the heart. It involves electrical activation of the atria and ventricles, contraction and relaxation of the atria and ventricles, closing and opening of cardiac valves, and filling and emptying of atria and ventricles.

Cardiac output—The amount of blood pumped by the heart in one minute; the product of stroke volume and heart rate; a determinant of blood pressure.

Cart-fill list—A list that has unit-dose profiles for all patients.

Cartilaginous joint—A type of joint in which the cartilage between the bones holds the bones together to make a joint.

Cash price—The price of a prescription that a patient will pay if he does not have insurance coverage or chooses not to file a third-party claim.

Catheter-associated urinary tract infection (CAUTI)—An infection that occurs when bacteria enter the urinary tract through a catheter.

Ceiling effect—The effect that occurs when increases in the dose of the drug have no further effect on the body above a particular dosage level.

Cell-mediated immunity—The component of the adaptive immune system controlled by T-cells.

Cellulitis—A bacterial skin infection.

Central line-associated bloodstream infection (CLABSI)—An infection that occurs when an infection-causing agent enters the bloodstream through a central line, which is a tube placed in a large vein in the neck, chest, or arm to administer fluids, blood, or medications.

Central nervous system (CNS)—All the nerves in the brain and spinal cord.

Cerebrospinal fluid—The fluid that fills the spaces in the brain and spinal cord, maintaining normal pressure, acting as a lubricant, and cushioning shocks.

Certification—Approval by a nongovernmental agency asserting that an individual has met specific training or educational requirements.

Certified pharmacy technician (CPhT)—A pharmacy technician who has passed either the PTCE or the ExCPT.

Cerumen—Earwax; a wax-like substance produced by apocrine glands in the ear canal.

Chain pharmacy—A retail pharmacy that consists of many pharmacies located nationally or regionally; most decisions are made at the corporate level.

Chart—A hospital record that contains physician's notes, medication orders, nurses' notes, medication administration records, and lab results for an individual patient.

Chelation—The process of removing heavy metals from the blood.

Chemical name—The name that describes the chemical structure of a drug.

Chemokine coreceptor inhibitor—A class of drugs that bind with the chemokine coreceptor cavities, thus inhibiting the entry of HIV-1 into host cells and thereby assisting in the treatment of HIV infection.

Chemoreceptor trigger zone (CTZ)—A chemosensory organ in the brain that stimulates nausea and vomiting.

Chemosensory organ—A structure that receives input relating to the perception of chemicals.

Chewable tablet—A solid dosage form that is designed to be chewed.

Child-resistant container—A medication container with a lid that cannot be opened by 80 percent of children younger than five years old, but can be opened by 90 percent of adults.

Chlamydia—A sexually transmitted disease caused by an infection of the bacterium *Chlamydia trachomatis*.

Cholesterol—A fatty substance found in animal tissues; used as a building block for many chemicals and hormones in the body.

Chronic bronchitis—Inflammation of the lining of the bronchial airways, which leads to obstruction of airflow upon exhalation.

Chronic malignant pain—The same as chronic pain, except the cause is known to be from cancer.

Chronic obstructive pulmonary disease (COPD)—A disease where there is less oxygen available or the amount of surface area for the exchange of oxygen and carbon dioxide is reduced.

Chronic pain—Pain that generally lasts more than three months and is not caused by a malignant disease such as cancer.

Class II balance—An electronic balance that has a digital readout of the weight. No weights are used with this balance.

Class III balance—A two-pan torsion balance that is used to weigh small amounts of material. It uses counterbalance to determine the weight of the substance being measured. It uses special weights in a range of milligrams and grams.

Cloning—The duplication of a bacterium.

Closed-system transfer device—A packaging system for small-volume parenteral systems that minimizes preparation time and workload, decreases costs and drug wastage, and reduces the possibility of contamination.

Clostridium difficile (C. diff) infection—An infection of the gastrointestinal tract that occurs after prolonged antibiotic use or after exposure to contaminated surfaces, objects, or body parts.

Code Blue—An alert used in many hospitals to signal a life-threatening emergency.

Code cart—A cart that contains drugs and equipment needed to provide life-saving care in an emergency situation.

Co-insurance—A plan in which the patient must pay a certain percentage of the cost for medical care or for a prescription.

Comminution—The process of reducing solid substances to small fragments such as powders.

Complementary and alternative medicine (CAM)—A medical practice that encompasses diverse healthcare systems, therapies, and products. CAM includes dietary supplements and botanical preparations and are often used concurrently with traditional medications and therapies.

Component—Any ingredient that is used in the compounding of a drug product. A component might not appear on the labeling of the product.

Compounded preparations—Medications prepared from bulk ingredients.

Compounded sterile product (CSP)—A sterile product that is prepared outside of a manufacturing facility.

Compounding—The preparation of a drug product pursuant to a prescription or medication order. It involves mixing ingredients, substances, elements, or parts to make the pharmaceutical compound.

Compounding log—A compounding log is like the master control record, but is specific for each individual prescription. It contains all the calculations necessary to make the preparation, as well as listing the equipment the technician will need when preparing the compound. It contains the same information as the master control record, but also includes the date of compounding and assigned lot number, as well as the manufacturer, NDC number, and expiration date of each ingredient.

Compounding pharmacy—A specialized pharmacy wherein the pharmacist mixes medications that are customized specifically for the unique healthcare needs of the patient.

Common denominator—A number into which both denominators of two fractions can divide evenly.

Concentration—The amount of active substance or drug in a total quantity.

Concretion—The process of becoming harder or more solid.

Condoms—A barrier device used during sexual intercourse to prevent pregnancy and the spread of sexually transmitted diseases.

Conjunctivitis—Inflammation of the outer membrane of the eye.

Constipation—The decreased frequency of bowel movements or difficulty defecating.

Contamination—The presence of microorganisms or chemicals on or near a structure, area, person, or object.

Continuation order—An order written by a physician that indicates that medication should be continued as previously ordered; similar to a refill.

Continuous infusion—A type of IV administration in which the drug is placed in a large volume of fluid and continuously dripped into a vein.

Contraindication—A drug, disease, or symptom for which a drug is not indicated or will cause harm.

Control group—The group in a clinical trial that receives an inactive substance or a standard treatment for a particular disease or illness.

Controlled-release—Dosage forms that regulate the rate of release of the active ingredient.

Controlled substance—Any schedule drug with the potential for abuse.

Controlled-substance schedules (CI, CII, CIII, CIV, CV)—Controlled substances are ranked into numbered categories based on their addiction and abuse potential, with CI drugs being the most addictive and having the greatest potential for abuse.

Convulsion—An involuntary contraction and relaxation of the muscles, which causes the body to shake rapidly and uncontrollably.

Co-pay—The amount of money a patient must pay for a prescription or doctor's visit before insurance coverage benefits.

Cortex—Located in the adrenal gland, it is a tissue that synthesizes three hormones: corticosteroids (glucocorticoids and mineralocorticoids), androgens, and estrogens.

Corticosteroid—A hormone produced by the cortex of the adrenal gland.

Corticotropin releasing factor (CRF)—A factor produced by the hypothalamus that stimulates the pituitary to produce ACTH.

Cortisol—A steroid produced in the adrenal gland and released from the cortex when a person is under stress.

Cover letter—A letter that accompanies a resume as part of a job application, highlights qualifications, and directs readers to your resume.

Crash carts—Critical-care medications that are brought to the patient's bedside for immediate administration.

Cream—A semisolid dosage form that is an O/W emulsion because it contains a small amount of oil dispersed in water.

Credit card—A form of payment that is a type of loan that is paid off at the end of the month or accrues a finance charge.

Cretinism—A condition caused by hypothyroidism that can cause severe mental retardation.

Crohn's disease—Widespread inflammation and lesions throughout the GI tract.

Cross-multiplication—The multiplication of the numerator of the first fraction by the denominator of the second fraction and the multiplication of the denominator of the first fraction by the numerator of the second fraction.

Crushing—The act of pulling down on the syringe plunger several times to expel fluid and air bubbles.

Cushing disease—A disease that results from the release of too much ACTH from the pituitary.

Cyclooxygenase I (COX-1)—An enzyme in the synovial fluid that converts arachadonic acid to prostaglandin, resulting in pain and inflammation associated with arthritis. COX-1 enzymes maintain the normal lining of the stomach and are involved in kidney and platelet function.

Cyclooxygenase II (COX-2)—An enzyme in the synovial fluid that converts arachadonic acid to prostaglandin, resulting in pain and inflammation associated with arthritis. COX-2 enzymes are present at the sites of inflammation.

Cystic fibrosis (CF)—A disease that involves the gastrointestinal and pulmonary systems.

Cystitis—A urinary tract infection that occurs in the bladder.

Cytopenia—A decrease in any type of blood cell.

Cytotoxic drug—Any drug that has a toxic effect on cells.

D

Days' supply—The length of time that a dispensed medication will last.

Debit card—A form of payment in which the cost of the purchase is automatically deducted from the user's bank account.

Decimal number—A number written using base 10; a number containing a decimal point.

Decongestants—A drug that causes the mucous membranes to shrink, allowing the nasal passages to drain.

Deductible—The amount that must be paid by the insured before the insurance company will consider paying.

Deep vein thrombosis—A blood clot in a vein deep within the body, usually occurring in the legs.

Defendant—The party being sued.

Dehydration—The loss of body water.

Delayed-release—The drug is administered over an extended period of time.

Deltoid—The muscle of the upper arm. The deltoid is an injection site for IM administration.

Denominator—The number below the line in a fraction. The denominator indicates the number of equal parts into which a whole is divided.

Deoxyribonucleic acid (DNA)—A complex, helically shaped molecule that carries the genetic code for an individual.

Depot—An injectable in which the release and duration of action of the drug is prolonged.

Depression—A mental-health disorder that may be accompanied by feelings of hopelessness, low self-worth, and loss of interest, along with many other symptoms.

Dermatitis—Any redness or inflammation of the skin; a non-specific term used to describe skin conditions of unknown origin; also called eczema.

Dermis—The second layer of skin, underneath the epidermis; the layer of skin responsible for sensory input.

Destructive agent—A drug that destroys or kills abnormal and sometimes normal cells.

Diabetes mellitus—A chronic metabolic disorder caused by a deficiency of insulin.

Diagnostic agent—Any drug that is used diagnostically.

Dialysis—A process that filters waste products from the blood when the kidneys are not able to do so.

Diarrhea—An increased frequency and decreased consistency of fecal matter.

Diastole—Relaxation of the heart muscles during the cardiac cycle.

Dietary supplement—A vitamin, mineral, or herbal product.

Difference—An amount obtained when subtracting numbers.

Diluent powder—An inactive substance that is added to an active ingredient in compounding of a tablet or capsule.

Diluents—Additives used to increase the bulk weight or volume of a dosage form.

Dilution—The process of adding a diluent or inactive ingredient to a substance to make it less concentrated.

Diplopia—The perception of two images of a single object. Also referred to as double vision.

Director of pharmacy—The pharmacist responsible for all of the hospital's pharmacy services.

Direct price cost—The cost of a drug from the manufacturer.

Discount—A percentage off the original price.

Discrimination—Preferential treatment or mistreatment of persons based on several factors, including age, religion, sexual orientation, race, national origin, and disability.

Disease-modifying antirheumatic drugs (DMARDs)—A class of drugs used early in the treatment of rheumatoid arthritis to prevent irreversible damage to the joints and minimize toxicities associated with NSAIDs. They have no immediate analgesic effects, but over time can control symptoms and have been shown to delay and possibly stop progression of the disease.

Disinfectant—A chemical that destroys microorganisms on objects or surfaces.

Disintegration—The decomposition of a drug or tablet.

Dispersion—A liquid in which the medication is not dissolved, but distributed throughout the vehicle.

Dissolution—The dissolving of drug particles.

Diuretic—A drug that increases the amount of urine excreted.

Division—The operation inverse to multiplication. The process of dividing numbers to find the quotient.

Dopamine—A neurotransmitter that plays a role in Parkinson's disease.

Dosage—The determination and regulation of the size, frequency, and number of doses. The dosage is the entire regimen or schedule of doses. The entire regimen or schedule of doses.

Dosage form—A system, device, or physical form of a dose by which the drug is delivered or administered to the body.

Dose—The amount of drug administered.

Dose-response curve—A curve that defines the relationship between the dose of the drug and the response or effect of the drug at that dose.

Double-blind trial—A trial in which neither the participants nor those who are running the study know who is receiving a placebo and who is receiving the experimental treatment.

Drug abuse—Use of a drug for purposes other than that for which it was prescribed or in amounts other than that which was prescribed.

Drug allergy—A hypersensitivity to a drug, which may cause symptoms such as itching, rash, or hives.

Drug dependence—The body needs the drug to function normally. Abrupt discontinuation of the drug will lead to withdrawal symptoms.

Drug diversion—Use of a prescription drug for purposes other than that for which it was originally prescribed.

Drug Enforcement Administration (DEA)—The U.S. government agency responsible for regulating the sale and use of scheduled drugs.

Drug Facts and Comparisons—A drug reference source.

Drug side effect—Any effect a drug can routinely cause as part of its method of action, such as upset stomach or constipation.

Drug-treatment pathway—A flowchart for the treatment of a specific disease.

Drug-utilization review (DUR)—The process used by a pharmacist to compare an existing treatment to a new treatment.

Duration of action—The length of time that a drug exerts its therapeutic effect.

Duties—Actions in which individuals or societies engage to ensure peace and harmony.

Dwarfism—A condition caused by hypothyroidism that can cause a child's growth to be stunted.

Dyskinesia—Diminished voluntary movement.

E

Eccrine sweat glands—Sweat glands that produce sweat containing water and salt.

Eczema—Any redness or inflammation of the skin; a non-specific term used to describe skin conditions of unknown origin; also called dermatitis.

Efferent system—A division of the peripheral nervous system that sends signals from the central nervous system to body organs or systems.

Efficacy—The ability of a drug to produce a predictable effect in controlling or curing an illness in the body.

Electrolyte—A fluid containing a dissolved mineral salt.

Electronic medication administration record (eMAR)—An electronic medication administration record. Often used in hospitals to electronically document all medication-related actions.

Elimination—The removal of the drug from the body.

Elixir—A clear, sweet solution that contains dissolved medication in a base of water and ethanol (hydroalcoholic).

Emesis—The expulsion of gastric contents through the mouth; also called vomiting.

Emollients—Topical preparations that are used on the skin to restore moisture and hydration.

Empathy—The ability to recognize and try to feel what another person feels.

Emphysema—An irreversible lung disease characterized by destruction of the alveoli.

Empirical treatment—The use of a broad-spectrum antibiotic to fight multiple types of bacteria.

Emulsifying agent—An ingredient used to bind together substances that normally do not mix.

Emulsion—A mixture of two substances that are unblendable. One substance is dispersed in the other.

Endocrine system—A body system composed of the thyroid, hypothalamus, pituitary, parathyroid, adrenal, pineal body, ovaries, and testes. The pancreas is also part of the endocrine system.

Enteral feeding—Feeding through a tube instead of normal swallowing.

Enteral nutrition—The delivery of food directly into the stomach or intestines, either through the mouth or a tube in the gastrointestinal tract.

Enteric-coated—A coating that is designed to resist degradation in the acidic pH of the stomach.

Envelope—The coating on the outside of some viruses.

Enzymes—Substances produced by living organisms, which are often proteins. They act as catalysts in biochemical reactions.

Epidermis—The outermost layer of the skin.

Epididymitis—A painful condition of the ducts attached to the testicles that may lead to infertility if left untreated.

Epilepsy—A neurological condition that is also known as a seizure disorder. It is characterized by sudden and recurring seizures.

Epiphyseal fusion—Fusion of the epiphyseal plates at the ends of long bones.

E-prescribing—The electronic transmission of prescription information.

Equal Employment Opportunity Commission (EEOC)—The agency in the United States that enforces Equal Employment Opportunity laws.

Equal Employment Opportunity (EEO) laws—Federal Equal Employment Opportunity laws prohibit preferential treatment or mistreatment of persons based on several factors, including age, religion, sexual orientation, race, national origin, and disability.

Erectile dysfunction—Also known as impotence. The inability to achieve or maintain an erection.

Erosions—Superficial degradations of the GI mucosa.

Erythema—Redness of the skin.

Estrogen—A sex hormone secreted by the ovaries that stimulates the development of breasts and genitals, produces endometrial growth, increases cervical mucus, and regulates the menstrual cycle.

Ethical dilemma—An ethical problem that requires an individual or group to choose between two distinct courses of action.

Ethical distress—An ethical problem that poses a challenge to maintain the integrity of an individual or profession.

Ethical issue—A situation with moral challenges that does not necessarily require action.

Ethical problem—A situation with moral challenges that does require action; includes ethical distress, ethical dilemmas, and locus-of-authority problems.

Ethics—A system of moral standards of conduct and behavior for a person, group, or profession.

Eukaryotic organisms—Microorganisms with specific center structures that can be seen with an electron microscope. Animal cells, including human cells, are eukaryotic cells.

Excipients—Inactive substances used as carriers for the active ingredient.

Excitatory impulse—Uncontrollable firing of neurons that can lead to a seizure.

Exophthalmos—Bulging of the eye.

Expectorants—A drug that decreases the viscosity of mucus, enabling the patient to get rid of the secretions when coughing.

Expiration date—The date after which a manufactured product should no longer be used.

Extemporaneous compounding—The compounding of two or more ingredients in a non-sterile environment. Also called non-sterile compounding.

Extended-release—Dosage forms that release the medication at a constant rate for a prolonged period so that the frequency of dosing is less than that of immediate-release dosage forms.

Extract—A powder or solid derived from animal or plant sources in which all or most of the solvent has been evaporated.

Extra-dose error—When a patient receives more doses than were actually prescribed.

Extrapyramidal symptom (EPS)—A symptom that derives from the extrapyramidal pathways in the nervous system.

Extreme obesity—A BMI of 40 or greater.

F

Factor—One of two or more numbers that, when multiplied together, produce a product.

Fat-soluble vitamin—A vitamin that is absorbed by the body with dietary fats. Examples include vitamins A, D, E, and K.

Federal upper limit (FUL)—The ceiling or highest price the federal government pays to pharmacists for the prescription drugs they dispense to Medicaid beneficiaries.

Fee for service—A payment plan in which the patient pays the provider for each service separately.

Fiber—An indigestible portion of plant-based foods.

Fibrous joint—Bone surfaces are joined together by fibrous connective tissue.

Film-coated—A thin outer layer of a polymer that is used to coat a tablet.

First-pass effect—The extent to which a drug bypasses the gastrointestinal tract and is metabolized by the liver before it even enters the bloodstream.

First-pass metabolism—The phenomenon by which a large fraction of active drug is lost through metabolism by the liver, so that only a small fraction of active drug reaches systemic circulation.

Flex card—A medical credit card that is used for prescription co-pays and some OTC medications.

Floor stock—Medications and supplies that are kept on hand and stored on the floor.

Folliculitis—Inflammation of a hair follicle.

Food and Drug Administration (FDA)—The U.S. governmental regulatory agency whose purpose is to ensure the safety and efficacy of all food and drugs currently on the market.

Forceps—Instruments used to pick up and transfer pharmaceutical weights.

Formulary—A list of pre-approved drugs that can be ordered, stocked, and administered at a given facility; also a term used by insurance companies for what medications they will pay for.

Fractions—A way of representing a part of a whole.

Franchise pharmacy—A small chain of community pharmacies that have the right to use the name of a company and market a company's goods or services within a certain territory or location.

Fraud—An intentional act of deception, misrepresentation or concealment by a person that could result in an unauthorized medical benefit to that or another person.

Front-end merchandise—Nonprescription merchandise that is sold in the front of the store.

Fungus—A group of eukaryotic organisms, some of which cause disease in humans.

Furuncle—An infection of the sebaceous gland and hair follicle; more commonly known as a boil.

Fusion inhibitors—These drugs prevent the original HIV from entering the human immune cell.

G

Gamma-aminobutyric acid (GABA)—A neurotransmitter found in the nervous system. The presence of GABA in the synapse of the nerve pathway prevents the rapid transmission of nerve signals, thus decreasing the symptoms of anxiety.

Garbing—Donning protective clothing.

Gastric emptying time—The time it takes for food to pass through the stomach.

Gastric lavage—A method used to eliminate poisons from the stomach. More commonly known as a stomach pump.

Gastritis—Widespread inflammation of the lining of the stomach.

Gastroenteritis—An inflammation of the gastrointestinal tract.

Gastroesophageal reflux disease (GERD)—The abnormal reflux of stomach contents into the esophagus; commonly referred to as heartburn.

Gastrointestinal (GI) system—An integrated group of glands and organs that digest and absorb food.

Gastroparesis—Delayed gastric emptying.

Gastrostomy tube—A plastic tube that is inserted directly into the stomach through the abdomen that can be used for feeding or administered medications.

Gel—A semisolid dosage form that contains ultrafine solid particles in liquid.

General anesthesia—The terminology for when a patient is placed in a reversible unconscious state in which there is no response to painful stimuli.

General anxiety disease (GAD)—Long-term feelings of excessive worry and anxiety that may be accompanied by physical symptoms. Generally, there is not a specific cause for the GAD diagnosis.

Generic name—The non-proprietary name of a drug.

Genital herpes—A sexually transmitted disease caused by the herpes simplex virus type 1 (HSV-1) or type 2 (HSV-2).

Germ theory of disease—The idea that microorganisms cause disease.

Gingival hyperplasia—Overgrowth of the gum tissue.

Glaucoma—An eye disease characterized by increased ocular pressure.

Glucocorticoids—Hormones involved in the metabolism of lipids, carbohydrates, and proteins.

Gluconeogenesis—The conversion of fatty acids and protein to glucose.

Glutamate—An excitatory neurotransmitter that plays a role in the pathogenesis of seizures.

Gluteus maximus—The muscle of the buttocks. The gluteus maximus is an injection site for IM administration.

Glycosuria—The presence of glucose in the urine.

Goiter—An enlargement or swelling of the thyroid gland.

Gonorrhea—A sexually transmitted disease caused by an infection of the bacterium *Neisseria gonorrhoeae*.

Good manufacturing practices (GMPs)—FDA guidelines designed to guarantee the delivery of safe and effective products to the patient.

Gouty arthritis—A disease that results from a buildup of uric acid. It leads to the formation of tophi, which deposit in tissues, especially joints, and result in joint inflammation.

Graduated cylinders—Instruments used to measure liquids.

Granules—Larger than powders, granules are wetted, allowed to dry, and ground into coarse, irregularly shaped pieces.

Graves' disease—An autoimmune disorder in which the body makes antibodies to TSH receptors.

Group morality—The shared values and duties of a subgroup of society.

Group purchasing organization (GPO)—A group of pharmacies that work together to negotiate a discount for high-volume purchases.

Growth hormone (GH)—A hormone secreted by the pituitary that promotes growth in the body.

Growth hormone releasing factor (GHRH)—Accelerates the secretion of growth hormone from the pituitary gland.

Gynecomastia—Enlargement of the gland tissue of the male breast.

H

Half-life—The amount of time it takes for the plasma concentration of the drug to decrease by 50%.

Hand hygiene—The use of alcohol-based hand sanitizers to cleanse hands and control the spread of infection.

Handwashing—The use of soap and water to cleanse hands and control the spread of infection.

Healthcare-associated infection (HAI)—An infection that occurs during the course of medical care; also known as a nosocomial infection.

Healthcare spending account—An account that can be used to cover medical and prescription co-pays or expenses not covered under medical insurance.

Health insurance—Coverage of medical costs such as doctors visits, laboratory costs, and hospitalization.

Health Insurance Portability and Accountability Act (HIPAA)—An act enacted "to improve portability and continuity of health insurance coverage in the group and individual markets, to combat waste, fraud, and abuse in health insurance and healthcare delivery, to promote the use of medical savings accounts, to improve access to long-term care services and coverage, to simplify the administration of health insurance, and for other purposes."

Health-maintenance organization (HMO)—A type of healthcare plan that provides care that is focused on keeping patients healthy or managing chronic diseases in an effort to decrease hospitalizations and emergency-room visits.

Heart failure—A syndrome in which the heart cannot pump enough blood to meet the needs of the body.

Helminths—A group of organisms, commonly called worms, which cause disease in humans.

Hematocrit—The portion of red blood cells in the blood.

Hemoglobin—The concentration of iron-containing protein in the blood.

Hepatitis—A viral infection of the liver that causes the liver to become swollen and tender.

Hirsutism—Excessive growth of thick dark hair in areas where there is minimal hair growth.

Histamine—The chemical released or produced by the body as an immune response during an allergic reaction.

Home healthcare—The delivery of medical, nursing, and pharmaceutical services to patients at home.

Home infusion pharmacy—A pharmacy that provides intravenous medications and supplies needed for their administration to patients who are home bound.

Homeostasis—The balance of the body with respect to fluid levels, pH, osmotic pressure, and concentrations of various substances.

Homogenous—Evenly distributed.

Hormones—Chemical messengers that regulate mood, growth and development, tissue function, metabolism, sexual function, and reproduction.

Hospital—A complex organization with many departments, all working together to provide emergency, medical, trauma, and surgical care to the community.

Hospital pharmacy—An institutional pharmacy that dispenses drugs and provides drug information to inpatients and healthcare professionals in the hospital.

Human-failure error—An individual, performance-related medication error.

Human immunodeficiency virus (HIV)—The virus(s) that cause AIDS.

Humoral immunity—The component of the adaptive immune system controlled by B-cells.

Hydroalcoholic solution—A water- and alcohol-based solution.

Hydrolysis—A chemical reaction with water.

Hyperglycemia—High blood glucose levels.

Hyperosmotic—A solution that has a higher osmolarity than another solution.

Hypertension—A systolic blood pressure over 140mm Hg and/or a diastolic blood pressure over 90mm Hg.

Hyperthyroidism—A condition caused by oversecretion of hormones from the thyroid gland.

Hypertonic—A solution that has a lower osmotic pressure than another solution.

Hypnotic drug—A drug that induces sleep.

Hypodermis—The innermost layer of skin; also known as subcutaneous tissue.

Hypoglycemia—A deficiency of glucose in the bloodstream.

Hyponatremia—A decreased concentration of sodium in the blood.

Hypo-osmotic—A solution that has a lower osmolarity than another solution.

Hypothalamus—An area of the brain that produces hormones that control body temperature, moods, sex drive, and release of hormones.

Hypothyroidism—A condition that occurs when the thyroid gland is not able to produce and secrete sufficient levels of T_3 and T_4.

Hypotonic—A solution that has a lower osmotic pressure than another solution.

I

Idiosyncratic reaction—An allergic reaction that is unusual or unexpected and unrelated to the dose of the drug.

Immediate-release—The medication is released within a short period of time after the drug is taken.

Immunocompromised—Having a compromised or impaired immune system; often from illness or treatment.

Immunoglobulin E—Antibodies found in the lungs, skin, and mucous membranes.

Immunomodulatory agent—A drug that alters the immune response by preventing it from producing antibodies that would recognize and react with an antigen. A drug that may suppress or stimulate the immune system response.

Immunosuppressant—A drug or radioactive agent that suppresses the immune response.

Impetigo—A superficial, contagious, bacterial skin infection.

Impotence—Also known as erectile dysfunction. The inability to achieve or maintain an erection.

Improper fraction—A fraction with a value equal to or greater than 1.

Incontinence—The inability to control bladder or bowel function.

Independent pharmacy—A community pharmacy that is owned and operated by one pharmacist or a group of pharmacists.

Indication—When a drug is given according to its labeling and is known to be beneficial for a specific disease, symptom, or condition.

Indigent—Having no money to pay for healthcare.

Induction—The process by which other drugs enhance the metabolism of a drug by inducing the enzyme responsible for the metabolism of that drug, resulting in a decreased pharmacologic response to the other drug.

Induration—A circular area of hardened tissue at the site of PPD injection.

Inert ingredient—Also called an inactive ingredient. An inert ingredient has little or no therapeutic or treatment value.

Infarction—The destruction of heart tissue due to a sudden decrease in blood supply to the cardiac tissue.

Inflammatory bowel disease (IBD)—An inflammatory condition of the GI tract that includes Crohn's disease and ulcerative colitis.

Infusion—A type of IV administration in which the drug is infused over a specified period of time.

Inhalation—The act of breathing in.

Inhibition—The process by which other drugs decrease the metabolism of another drug by competitive or complete inhibition of the enzyme responsible for the metabolism of that drug, resulting in an increased pharmacologic response to the other drug.

Inhibitors—Chemical substances that prevent or block the action of another substance.

Inhibitory impulse—An impulse that prevents a neuron from firing.

Innate immune system—The part of the immune system that mounts a nonspecific defense against invading organisms. The innate immune system includes monocytes, macrophages, neutrophils, basophils, mast cells, eosinophils, and natural killer cells.

Inscription—The part of a prescription that provides the name, strength, dosage form, and quantity of medication ordered.

Insomnia—The inability to fall asleep or to stay asleep.

Institute for Certification of Pharmacy Technicians (ICPT)—A pharmacist-run organization that recognizes pharmacy technicians who have acquired the skills necessary for safe, accurate, and efficient practice. The ICPT administers the ExCPT.

Institute for Safe Medication Practices (ISMP)—An organization that monitors medication errors and makes recommendations on how to prevent them.

Institutional pharmacy—A facility organized under a corporate structure that provides pharmaceutical care to an institutional facility or organized healthcare system.

Insulin—A hormone that regulates carbohydrate and fat metabolism.

Integrase inhibitor—The mode of drug action that blocks the integrase enzyme in viral replication.

Interferon—A substance sent out by a human cell infected with a virus.

Intermittent infusion—A type of IV administration in which the drug is placed in an intermediate volume of fluid and infused over a specified period of time at regularly spaced intervals.

Intradermal—A route of administration by which a parenteral medication is injected into the skin.

Intramuscular—A route of administration by which a parenteral medication is injected into a muscle.

Intravenous—A route of administration by which a parenteral solution is administered into a vein.

Inventory—The entire stock of products on hand for sale.

Inventory value—The total value of drugs and merchandise.

Investigational drug—A drug that is currently in human testing, prior to being sent to the FDA for approval.

Investigational New Drug (IND) application—The plan submitted to the FDA that the manufacturer or sponsor develops for testing the drug in humans.

Ions—A charged atom or molecule.

Irrigating solution—A solution that is used for cleansing an area of the body.

Irritable bowel syndrome (IBS)—A syndrome that includes chronic abdominal pain and altered bowel habits.

Ischemic heart disease—A condition in which the muscle of the heart receives a decreased supply of blood.

Isomer—Compounds that have different structures, but contain the same number and type of atoms. Isomers are often distinguished by dextro, or right, and levo, or left.

Iso-osmotic—A solution that has the same number of particles dissolved in solution as blood.

Isotonic—A solution with the same osmotic pressure as blood.

Isotope—A form of a chemical element that contains the same number of protons as the regular element, but a different number of neutrons.

IV admixture service—A central pharmacy service that prepares parenteral medications in a sterile environment.

IV piggyback (IVPB)—A small-volume parenteral product that is added to a running IV line and infused over a short time.

IV push—The IV administration of a drug over a short period of time; also called a bolus.

IV set—A sterile, disposable device used to administer IV medications or fluids from an IV container or reservoir.

J

Jejunostomy tube—A tube used for enteral nutrition that is surgically placed through the abdomen and enters the small intestine.

Joint—The place where two or more bones meet.

K

Keratoacanthoma—An epithelial tumor caused by repeated exposure to UV radiation.

Keratococonjunctivitis—Chronic dry eye.

Ketoacidosis—A complication of diabetes that occurs when the body cannot utilize glucose because there isn't enough (or any) insulin.

L

Large-volume parenteral (LVP)—A product for parenteral administration that contains more than 100mL.

Law—A rule of conduct or procedure established to represent the minimum level of acceptable standards.

Legend drugs—Drugs that require a prescription because they are not considered safe for use without medical supervision.

Legibility—The readability of handwriting or print.

Levigation—The process of grinding a solid into powder. Typically used during the preparation of an ointment.

Libel—Written communication of false statements against another individual.

Libido—Sexual drive.

Licensure—The granting of a license by a state in order for an individual to work in a certain profession.

Loading dose—The amount of drug that is required to quickly bring serum concentrations of the drug to a therapeutic level.

Local anesthesia—The terminology for when a drug is used to cause reversible loss of feeling in a specific area of the body.

Local effect—The effect of the drug is confined to one area or organ of the body.

Locus-of-authority problem—An ethical problem that poses a challenge about who should make a decision.

Long-term care facility—An institution that provides a broad range of services for patients requiring a longer length of stay. These facilities may include nursing homes or assisted-living facilities.

Long-term care pharmacy—A pharmacy that is owned by or contracts with a long-term–care facility to provide prescription medications to the residents of that facility.

Look-alike sound-alike—Describes drug names that are often confused due to similar-looking or similar-sounding names.

Lotion—An O/W emulsion that contains insoluble dispersed solids or immiscible liquids.

Lozenges—Also known as troches or pastilles, hard, oval, or discoid solid dosage forms with a drug contained in a flavored sugar base.

Lymph—A type of interstitial fluid, which bathes tissue in the body.

Lymphadenopathy—Enlarged lymph nodes.

Lymphatic system—Part of the immune system. The lymphatic system includes a network of vessels that carry lymph, the lymph nodes, and the lymphoid organs.

Lymphocyte—A white blood cell.

M

Macronutrient—Nutrition components such as fats, carbohydrates, and proteins.

Mail-order pharmacy—A centralized pharmacy operation that dispenses a large number of prescriptions; prescriptions are delivered in the mail.

Maintenance dose—The amount of drug given at a particular frequency to maintain therapeutic levels.

Major contamination—A significant level of contamination. Includes a needlestick or a spill of more than 5mL.

Malaria—An infection of the blood caused by the parasite *Plasmodium spp*.

Malignant tumor—An invasive or progressive tumor.

Malnutrition—Any disorder of nutrition status.

Malpractice—Negligence in meeting the standard of care.

Managed-care organization—An organization that controls the financing and delivery of healthcare services for those who are involved in a specific healthcare plan; it is designed to control costs by keeping patients healthy.

Manufactured products—Products that are manufactured by a pharmaceutical company.

Markup—The amount added to the cost of a particular product to cover overhead and profit.

Mast cells—Cells rich in histamine and heparin that can be profound throughout the body.

Master control record—The instructions or recipe for making a compounded preparation. It lists the name, strength, ingredients, dosage form, quantities, mixing instructions, and beyond-use date.

Material safety data sheet (MSDS)—Contains important information on the properties of chemicals, including flammability, safe use, and procedures for responding to accidental ingestion. It should be filed for all bulk ingredients or drug substances.

Medicaid—A state program for low-income residents, including uninsured pregnant women.

Medical error—Any action, inaction, or decision that contributes to an unintended consequence in healthcare.

Medicare—A federal program for seniors, the disabled, and dialysis patients.

Medication administration record (MAR)—A manual or electronic patient-specific record that includes the names of all drugs the patient receives, doses, routes and times of administration, start and stop dates, and any special instructions.

Medication error—An event that leads to inappropriate medication use or patient harm.

Medication Error Reporting Program (MERP)—A medication error–reporting system for healthcare providers. Supported by the USP and ISMP.

Medication order—A prescription for a medication written in a hospital setting.

Medication profile—A list of all the medications a patient receives.

MEDMARX—An Internet-based medication error–reporting system for hospitals and healthcare providers. Supported by the USP.

Medulla—A layer of tissue located in the adrenal gland that synthesizes and secretes the catecholamines, epinephrine, and norepinephrine.

MedWatch—The FDA adverse drug event–reporting system for healthcare providers, patients, and consumers.

Melanoma—A highly malignant skin cancer.

Meninges—Coverings for the brain and spinal cord, primarily for protection.

Meniscus—The concave shape of the liquid; the level at the bottom at which liquids are measured.

Menopause—The point at which menstrual cycles end, representing the end of a woman's fertility.

Menstrual cycle—A series of changes a woman's body goes through to prepare for a possible pregnancy.

Metabolic pathway—The sequence of steps by which a drug is converted to its metabolite.

Metabolism—The process by which the body breaks down medications to active or inactive substances.

Metabolite—The byproduct or the substance into which a drug is converted when it is metabolized.

Metastasis—The spread of cancerous cells from the primary site to distant sites to form new tumors.

Metered dose inhaler (MDI)—A device that delivers a fine mist of medication to reach the innermost parts of the lungs using compressed gas.

Micronutrient—Nutrition components such as vitamins, minerals, and trace elements.

Mineral—An inorganic substance that is present in body fluids to regulate homeostasis and act as constituents of organic molecules.

Mineralocorticoids—Hormones that regulate the secretion of water and sodium by the kidney.

Minor contamination—A low level of contamination. Includes the use of a calculator or pen, a small spill, or minor hand contamination.

Misbranding—Labeling of a product that is false or misleading.

Mitotic spindle fibers—Fibers that separate strands of DNA during replication.

Mixed analgesic—A combination of a narcotic and non-narcotic analgesic.

Mixed number—A number that contains both whole numbers and fractions.

Mold—Fungi that exist in a multicellular filamentous arrangement.

Monoamine oxidase inhibitor (MAOI) drug—A drug that prevents an enzyme or oxidase from destroying a specific neurotransmitter. MAOI drugs are usually prescribed for depression.

Monoclonal antibody—An antibody produced in a laboratory from clones of B-cells that target a specific antigen.

Monograph—A format for drug information.

Mood-stabilizing agent—A drug prescribed to stabilize a patient between the states of mania and depression.

Morality—The process of understanding relationships between people and how people can live together peacefully. Morality includes duties and values.

Moral judgment—The process of analyzing a moral situation and arriving at a conclusion.

Mortar and pestle—Compounding equipment used to crush solids and for grinding and mixing.

Multidrug-resistant tuberculosis (MDR-TB)—A strain of TB that is resistant to many currently used drugs.

Multiplication—The process of multiplying numbers to find their product.

Muscle relaxants—A diverse group of drugs approved by the FDA to treat spasticity caused by neurological disorders or for musculoskeletal conditions.

Mutagen—A substance that causes a genetic mutation.

Myocardial infarction (MI)—A heart attack. Occurs after a prolonged period of decreased oxygen supply to the muscles of the heart.

Myoclonic seizure—A type of seizure characterized by sudden, brief muscle jerks or twitching on both sides of the body.

Myxedema—A severe case of hypothyroidism that can lead to coma.

N

Naked virus—A virus with no envelope.

Nasal—Pertaining to the nose.

Nasoenteric tube—A tube used for enteral nutrition that is passed through the nose and runs to the small intestine.

Nasogastric tube—A plastic tube that is inserted through the nose, past the throat, and directly into the stomach. Used for feeding patients unable to take nutrition by mouth.

National Association of Boards of Pharmacy (NABP)—The professional association that helps to develop uniform standards for all state boards of pharmacy.

National Drug Code (NDC)—The Federal identification number for each drug.

Nausea—The feeling of imminent vomiting.

Nebulizer—A device used to administer inhaled medications using airflow to create a fine mist.

Needle—The component that is attached to a syringe that delivers medication.

Needle gauge—The size of the hole in a needle.

Needle length—The length of a needle.

Negative feedback mechanism—A mechanism that is the primary regulatory mechanism used to maintain homeostasis.

Negligence—Conduct that falls below the standards of behavior established by law.

Neonatal—Of or relating to the newborn infant especially the first four weeks after birth.

Neoplasm—A tumor.

Neoplastic disease—A disease defined by the growth of tumors.

Nephrotoxicity—Damage to the kidney.

Neuromuscular blocker—A drug that blocks the neurotransmitter in the muscle system.

Neurons—The building block of the brain that serves as the basic unit of information processing.

Neurotransmitters—Chemicals released at many of the nerve endings.

Neutropenia—A decrease in the number of white blood cells.

Noncompliance—Failure to adhere to the prescribed drug regimen.

Non-nucleoside reverse transcriptase inhibitors (NNRTIs)—A drug with a mechanism of action that prevents the formation of the DNA copy of a virus by blocking a non-nucleoside.

Non-sterile compounding—The compounding of two or more ingredients in a non-sterile environment.

Nonsteroidal anti-inflammatory drugs (NSAIDs)—First-line drugs used to reduce inflammation, pain, and swelling associated with arthritis.

Non-verbal communication—Communication through wordless messages.

Norepinephrine—A neurotransmitter found in the nervous system that enables nerve signals to travel up or down the spinal cord.

Nosocomial infection—An infection that occurs during the course of medical care; also known as a healthcare-associated infection.

NR notation—The notation on a prescription that means "no refill."

Nuclear pharmacy—A specialized pharmacy that promotes health through the safe and effective use of radioactive drugs for diagnosis and therapy.

Nucleoside reverse transcriptase inhibitors (NRTIs)—A drug with a mechanism action that prevents the formation of the DNA copy of a virus by blocking a nucleoside.

Nucleotide reverse transcriptase inhibitors (NtRTIs)—A drug with a mechanism of action that prevents the formation of the DNA copy of a virus by blocking a nucleotide.

Number—A quantity or amount that is made up of one or more numerals.

Numerator—The number above the fraction line. The numerator indicates the number of parts out of the whole.

Nutritional support—Artificial feeding for people who cannot get enough nourishment by eating or drinking.

Nystagmus—Involuntary movement of the eyeballs.

O

Obesity—A BMI of 30 or greater.

Obsessive-compulsive disorder (OCD)—A mental-health disease characterized by repetitive actions.

Oil-in-water (O/W) emulsion—An emulsion that contains a small amount of oil dispersed in water.

Ointment—A semisolid dosage form that is applied externally to the skin or mucous membranes. An ointment is an example of a W/O emulsion because it contains a small amount of water dispersed throughout oil.

Oleaginous—A greasy or oily base used for compounding of suppositories.

Omission error—When a prescribed dose is not administered.

Online adjudication—Using wireless technology to process a prescription claim.

Open-ended question—A question that requires the patient to answer with a complete sentence, not just a yes- or no-type answer.

Ophthalmic—Pertaining to the eye.

Opiate—A narcotic alkaloid found in opium or a semi-synthetic derivative of the alkaloid.

Opioid—Drugs made from the opium poppy, such as morphine or codeine.

Opium poppy—A plant cultivated for use in manufacturing opium and related drugs.

Oral candidiasis—A type of fungal infection commonly caused by use of corticosteroid inhalers.

Oral disintegrating tablet (ODT)—A solid dosage form designed to dissolve in the mouth.

Orange Book—The official government source comparing generic drugs.

Order—A prescription that is issued and dispensed in an institutional setting.

Organizational-failure error—When institutional policies or procedures lead to a medication error.

Orphan drug—A drug that is developed by a drug company specifically for a rare disease or condition. Drugs that have been designated orphan drugs follow a different approval process with the Food and Drug Administration (FDA).

Orthostatic hypertension—An increase in blood pressure when moving to an upright position.

Osmolarity—The number of particles dissolved in solution.

Osmotic pressure—The pressure required to maintain equilibrium between two solutions.

Osteoarthritis—A degenerative joint disease that affects the cartilage.

Otalgia—Ear pain.

Otic—Pertaining to the ear.

Ototoxicity—Damage to the organs of hearing.

Ovaries—Female organs responsible for hormones that regulate the menstrual cycle and pregnancy.

Overhead—The cost of doing business. Overhead takes into account salaries, cost of equipment, operating expenses, and rent.

Overnutrition—A nutrition disorder that is characterized by excess nutrient intake; leads to overweight and obesity.

Overweight—A BMI of 25 or greater.

Over-the-counter (OTC) drugs—Drugs that can be legally obtained without a prescription and are generally safe for use without medical supervision.

P

Pancreas—A glandular organ below and behind the stomach that secretes pancreatic juice and insulin.

Panic attack—An extreme type of anxiety. A panic attack has a specific starting point and ending point, and usually involves an overwhelming feeling of fear or apprehension.

Panic disorder—A particular type of anxiety characterized by life-threatening fear.

Paraprofessional—Someone who is trained to assist a professional.

Parasympathetic nervous system—A division of the autonomic nervous system that functions to return the system to a normal, resting state.

Parathyroid gland—The gland that produces parathyroid hormone.

Parenteral—A route of administration by which the medication is administered by a needle or catheter into one or more layers of the skin.

Parenteral nutrition—The delivery of nutrition directly to a vein.

Parenteral product—A product intended for administration by injection either through the skin or via another external barrier.

Parenteral solution—A sterile solution that is administered by a needle or catheter into one or more layers of the skin.

Paresthesias—Sensation of numbness or tingling on the skin.

Parkinson's disease (PD)—A motor-system disorder caused primarily by progressive degeneration of dopamine-containing neurons in the substantia nigra.

Partial seizure—A type of seizure that is centered in a specific area of the brain, but can progress to other areas of the brain.

Passive immunity—The acquisition of antibodies without the immune system mounting a response; the transfer of antibodies across the placenta to a fetus or through breast milk to an infant.

Paste—A semisolid dosage form that contains more solid material and a lesser amount of liquid base than a solid.

Pathogens—Microorganisms that cause disease.

Patient identifier—Any information that can identify a patient, such as his or her address, social security number, or date of birth.

Pediculosis—An infestation of lice.

Pelvic inflammatory disease (PID)—An infection of the uterus, fallopian tubes, or other reproductive organs that causes symptoms such as lower abdominal pain.

Penetration stage—The stage in virus reproduction in which the host cell's outer wall is penetrated.

Peptic ulcer—Damage that extends deep into the mucosal lining of the GI system.

Peptic ulcer disease (PUD)—The frequent recurrence of peptic ulcers.

Percentage error—The maximum potential error multiplied by 100 and divided by the quantity desired.

Percentages—A ratio used to express the number of parts of 100.

Percussion—A type of therapy used for CF patients that involves a tapping movement to induce cough and expectoration of sputum.

Percutaneous absorption—Absorption through the skin.

Percutaneous endoscopic gastrostomy (PEG) tube—A tube used for enteral nutrition that is endoscopically placed through the abdomen into the stomach.

Perioperative—The period of time during and around a surgical procedure.

Peripheral nervous system (PNS)—All the nerves in the body except those in the central nervous system, which is composed of the brain and the spinal cord.

Permeability—The ease with which a liquid or gas is able to pass through a membrane.

Peroral (PO)—Commonly referred to as the oral route. A route of administration in which the drug is administered orally through the mouth and swallowed to reach the stomach.

Perpetual log book—Also called a perpetual inventory record, a book used for recording all narcotics that are withdrawn and added to the narcotic floor stock. This is the official record for all Schedule II substances that are kept in the narcotic cabinet.

Personal digital assistant (PDA)—An electronic piece of equipment that can transmit information. In the pharmacy, this may be health-related information, drug orders and prescriptions.

Pharmaceutical Compounding Centers of America (PCCA)—An organization that is a source for obtaining ingredients. It provides information and research on compatibility and stability.

Pharmacist—A licensed professional trained to prepare and dispense medications, provide drug information, and monitor response to therapy.

Pharmacodynamic agent—Any drug that alters bodily functions.

Pharmacodynamics—The effects that a drug has on the body.

Pharmacognosy—The study of the medicinal properties of natural products from plant and animal sources and minerals.

Pharmacology—The study of drugs, their properties, and their mechanisms of action.

Pharmacy benefit manager (PBM)—The company responsible for administering prescription drug benefits and pharmacy reimbursement on behalf of the insurance company.

Pharmacy technician—A paraprofessional who can assist in all daily activities, under the direct supervision of a licensed pharmacist, that do not require the professional judgment of a pharmacist.

Pharmacy Technician Certification Board (PTCB)—The organization that establishes and maintains national criteria for pharmacy technician certification and recertification. The PTCB administers the PTCE.

Pharyngitis—Inflammation of the pharynx.

Photosensitivity—An abnormal sensitivity to light.

Physical dependence—Physical dependence to a drug occurs when physical symptoms of withdrawal, such as sweating, racing heart, and difficulty, breathing present when the use of the drug is stopped.

Pill tile—A slab used for mixing medicines with a spatula.

Pineal body—A gland that produces and secretes melatonin, a hormone that regulates the circadian cycle.

Pipette—A long, thin tube with a suction device used to transfer volumes less than 1.5mL.

Pituitary gland—A gland that produces hormones that affect the activity of other endocrine glands and specific organs of the body.

Placebo—An inert compound that has no pharmacological effect.

Plaintiff—The person or party filing a case.

Pneumonia—A lung infection caused by organisms that grow in the lower respiratory tract.

Point-of-service (POS) plan—A type of managed healthcare plan that is a hybrid of an HMO and a PPO. It is called as a point-of-service plan because each time a member seeks medical care, he or she must decide which option—HMO or PPO—to choose.

Polydypsia—Excessive thirst.

Polypharmacy—Concurrent use of multiple medications.

Polyuria—Increased urination.

Posting—The process of reconciling the invoice and updating the inventory in the database.

Posttraumatic stress disorder (PTSD)—A disorder commonly seen in patients after a trauma, either physical or emotional. PTSD is often seen in returning combat military personnel or patients who have experienced severe emotional or physical trauma.

Postural hypotension—A decrease in blood pressure that occurs when a person rises from a prone position.

Powder—Finely ground mixtures of dry drugs and inactive ingredients that can be used topically or internally.

Precision—How well a series of measurements can be reproduced; how close the measurements are to each other.

Preferred provider organization (PPO)—A type of managed healthcare plan that is similar to an HMO in that it has a preferred provider network, but patients do not need to see a primary care physician for a referral to a specialist.

Prehypertension—A systolic blood pressure between 120 and 139mm Hg and/or a diastolic blood pressure between 80 and 89mm Hg.

Prescribing error—Any occurrence in the prescribing decision or prescription-writing process that leads to reduced effectiveness of therapy or an increased risk of harm.

Prescription—A written or verbal order for a specific medication, to be dispensed to a patient by a licensed pharmacist.

Preservatives—Substances that prevent or minimize the growth of bacteria or other microorganisms in the dosage form.

Priapism—A persistent erection that is usually painful.

Primary care physician—A type of doctor who serves a gatekeeper to control access to healthcare and costs.

Primary generalized seizure—A seizure that involves both sides of the brain and has no local origin.

Prime—The process by which air and debris are removed from tubing prior to IV administration to the patient.

Prime-vendor purchasing—A type of purchasing system in which an exclusive agreement is made by a pharmacy to purchase a specified percentage or dollar amount from the vendor.

Probiotics—Agents that restore normal microbial flora in the GI tract.

Prodrug—An inactive form of a drug that is metabolized in the body to the active metabolite.

Product—An amount obtained when multiplying numbers.

Professional—Someone with recognized training or expertise in a field. A professional is expected to act with autonomy, use his or her knowledge and skills to benefit others, and adhere to an ethical code of conduct.

Professional standard—Reference point or norm by which quality of a product or the performance of a professional is measured.

Professional stewardship—Promoting professional standards, enhancing individual performance, and identifying individuals with outstanding commitment to one's profession.

Progesterone—A sex hormone secreted by the ovaries that prepares the uterus for implantation of the fertilized ovum. It also stimulates the development of ducts and glands of the breasts to prepare for lactation.

Progestin—A synthetic form of progesterone.

Prokaryotic organisms—Microorganisms, including most bacteria, without any specific center structures, including no specific nucleus

Proper fraction—A fraction whose value is less than 1.

Prophylactic agent—Any drug that prevents a disease or illness from occurring.

Prophylaxis—The treatment given before an event or exposure to prevent a disease or symptom.

Proportion—An equation that states two ratios that are equal.

Protease inhibitors (PIs)—A mode of drug action that prevents the production of protease enzymes in a new virus.

Protist—A single-celled organism of the kingdom Protista; includes protozoa.

Protozoa—A group of living organisms that cause disease in humans.

Pruritis—Intense itching.

Psychiatrist—A medical doctor, with additional training, who specializes in treating patients with mental-health diseases.

Psychological dependence—Psychological dependence to a drug occurs when psychological symptoms, such as irritability, inability to sleep, or depression, present when the use of the drug is stopped.

Psychomotor—Movement or muscular activity that is associated with mental processes.

Psychosis—Describes mental illnesses that dramatically interfere with a person's ability to function normally. Symptoms of psychosis include personality changes, impaired function, and a distorted sense of reality.

Psychotherapy—Personal counseling by a mental-health professional such as a psychotherapist or psychiatrist.

Pulmonary embolism (PE)—A blood clot that travels to the lungs and blocks the pulmonary artery.

Pulverization—The process of reducing the particle size of a solid by mixing or dissolving the solid in a substance in which it is soluble, such as alcohol.

Purchasing—Ordering of products for use or sale by the pharmacy.

Pyelonephritis—A urinary tract infection that occurs in the kidney.

Pyrogens—Substances produced in response to bacterial or viral infections that stimulate the release of prostaglandins, which causes the body to produce a fever.

Q

Quotient—An amount obtained when dividing numbers.

QT interval—The time it takes for an electrical signal in the heart to travel through the ventricles. If the QT interval is increasing, the ventricles are not pumping rapidly enough to maintain adequate blood flow.

R

Ratio—The relationship between two like quantities.

Ratio strength—The concentration of weak solutions.

Receptor—A protein on the surface of the cell or within the cell that binds with specific molecules, producing some effect within the cell.

Reconstitution—The addition of a diluent to a powder vial.

Receipt—Proof of purchase.

Receiving—The receipt of products from a wholesaler or warehouse.

Reconstitute—To add water or other fluid to a dry powder, making it into a liquid dosage form.

Rectal—Pertaining to the rectum.

Red Book—A pharmacy reference book that also contains drug prices.

Registration—Logging your identity with a state organization before practicing a profession.

Regulation—A written rule or established guideline that exists to carry out a federal or state law.

Release stage—The stage in virus reproduction in which a new virus is released.

Renal (urinary) system—An organ system that consists of the kidneys, ureters, bladder, and urethra, which are all part of the urinary tract.

Replication—The process by which DNA makes an exact copy of itself.

Rescue drug—Drugs that are administered as antidotes to chemotherapy drugs. Rescue drugs decrease the risk of side effects and toxicities associated with chemotherapy.

Resorption—Destruction or loss of the elements of bone.

Respiratory distress syndrome—A syndrome that occurs in newborns because of inadequate production of surfactant.

Resume—A summary of work experience and education that you will bring to a job.

Retail pharmacy—Any independent, chain, or franchise pharmacy that dispenses prescription drugs to outpatients; also known as a community pharmacy.

Retinopathy—A disorder characterized by damage to the blood vessels of the retina.

Retrovirus—A virus that can copy its own genetic material, which is in the form of RNA, onto the host cell's DNA by using a special enzyme called reverse transcriptase.

Reuptake inhibitor drug—A drug with a mode of action that prevents the reuptake of something, usually a neurotransmitter.

Rheumatoid arthritis—An autoimmune disease in which the body's immune system attacks its own connective tissue.

Rhinitis—Stuffy nose.

Rhinitis medicamentosa—Rebound nasal congestion due to the extended use of topical nasal decongestants.

Rhinorrhea—Runny nose.

Ribonucleic acid (RNA)—One of the three major macromolecules (along with DNA and proteins) that are essential for all known forms of life.

Ring—A dosage form inserted vaginally for administering hormones used for birth control.

Ringworm—A tinea infection; often characterized by a red ring-like lesion on the skin.

Route of administration—How the medication is to be administered.

Rx—Rx is derived from a Latin term meaning "take thou," means "recipe" or "prescription," and appears on prescriptions before the drug being prescribed. It is also commonly used to refer to a prescription.

S

Schizophrenia—A common psychiatric disease where symptoms can include auditory or visual hallucinations.

Scoop method—A one-handed technique for recapping a needle that reduces the risk of injury or needlestick.

Sebaceous glands—Glands contained in the skin that produce sebum.

Sebum—An oily substance produced by the sebaceous glands that lubricates and moisturizes the skin.

Seizure—Abnormal electrical discharges in the brain caused by sudden, excessive firing of a small number of neurons.

Selective serotonin reuptake inhibitor (SSRI) drug—A type of drug that prevents serotonin from being removed at certain nerve endings. SSRI drugs are commonly prescribed for depression.

Semi-synthetic drug—A drug that contains a combination of artificially created molecules and natural molecules.

Sense organs—Human organs that support the senses, such as the ears, eyes, and nose.

Sensitivity—Awareness of and respect for the feelings of others.

Sentinel event—An unanticipated event that results in death or serious injury to a patient, or has the potential to do so.

Serotonin—A neurotransmitter found in the nervous system that enables nerve signals to travel up or down the spinal cord.

Serotonin and norepinephrine reuptake inhibitor (SNRI) drug. A drug class whose mechanism of action is to prevent the reuptake of norepinephrine and serotonin.

Serotonin syndrome—A condition in which the patient has too much serotonin. It can be caused by combining SSRIs or SNRIs.

Sexual harassment—Defined by the United States Supreme Court as the creation of an unpleasant or uncomfortable work environment through sexual action, innuendo, or related means.

Sexually transmitted disease (STD)—Any disease that can be transmitted by sexual intercourse.

Side effect—The effect of a drug in addition to its intended effect.

Sifting—A process used to combine powders using a sieve.

Sig—Derived from a Latin term. It indicates that patient directions follow.

Signa—The part of the prescription that provides directions for use to be included on the label.

Sinus rhythm—The normal beating of the heart.

Slander—Verbal communication of false statements against another individual.

Small-volume parenteral (SVP)—A product for parenteral administration that contains less than 100mL.

Solute—The medication that is dissolved in a liquid vehicle (solvent).

Solution—An evenly distributed mixture of one or more dissolved medications in a liquid vehicle.

Solvent—The liquid vehicle in which a solute or medication is dissolved.

Somatic nervous system—A division of the efferent portion of the peripheral nervous system. The somatic nervous system carries signals to and from skeletal muscles.

Somnolence—Drowsiness.

Spacer—A device used with an MDI to decrease the amount of medication deposited in the back of the throat.

Spansule—Capsules that are filled with granules that dissolve at different rates, in effect causing a sustained release of the active ingredients.

Spatulas—Tools used for preparing ointments and creams or to transfer ingredients to weighing pans.

Spatulation—A method of blending ingredients into a homogenous mixture by scraping and smoothing them with a spatula on an ointment slab.

Specific gravity—The density of a solid or liquid compared to the density of water.

Specificity—The property of a receptor site that allows it to bind with a chemical messenger.

Spirit—An alcoholic or hydroalcoholic solution that contains volatile, aromatic ingredients.

Spray—A container that has a valve assembly unit that contains various bases, such as alcohol or water, in a pump-type dispenser.

Sprinkles—Similar to spansules but unique in that they are designed to be pulled apart and the contents sprinkled onto food, making it easier to administer the medication.

Stable angina—Chest pain induced by exercise or exertion; episodes are predictable and usually relieved with rest.

Standard of care—The level of performance that is expected of a healthcare worker in carrying out his or her professional duties.

State boards of pharmacy—Regulatory bodies that oversee pharmacy activities in each individual state.

Stat order—A medication order that is to be filled and sent to the floor immediately.

Status epilepticus—Continuous tonic-clonic seizures that last at least 30 minutes.

Sterile compounding—Compounding of medications, such as parenterals or ophthalmic preparations, that must be free from microorganisms or particulate matter. Usually done in a hospital pharmacy.

Sterilization—Any process that destroys infection-causing microorganisms.

Stratum corneum—The outermost layer of the epidermis; the layer of skin that is exposed to the environment.

Stroke—A period of decreased oxygen supply to the brain.

Subcutaneous—A route of administration by which a parenteral medication is injected under the skin.

Subcutaneous tissue—The innermost layer of skin; also known as the hypodermis.

Sublingual—An oral route of administration in which medication is placed under the tongue.

Substantia nigra—A layer of gray substance in the brain that is involved in Parkinson's disease.

Substrate—The substance on which an enzyme reacts.

Subtraction—The process of subtracting numbers to find their difference.

Sugar-coated—A coating made of sugar that is used to protect medication and improve the appearance and flavor of a tablet.

Sum—An amount obtained when adding numbers.

Suppository—A semisolid dosage form that is designed for insertion into the rectum, vagina, or urethra.

Surgical site infections (SSIs)—Infections that occur after surgery, in the part of the body where the surgery took place.

Suspension—A mixture of undissolved, very fine, solid particles distributed through a gas, liquid, or solid.

Sustained-release—Dosage forms that allow the frequency of dosing of a medication to be reduced compared to that of immediate-release dosage forms.

Sweat glands—Glands contained in the skin that produce sweat to cool the body and rid the body of organic material.

Sympathetic nervous system—Used to stimulate the body for vigorous activity, stressful situations, and emergencies.

Synergism—When two substances (drugs) have a better effect together than alone.

Synovial joint—A joint in which the bone is covered by cartilage and connected by a fibrous connective tissue capsule lined with synovial membrane.

Synthesis stage—The stage in virus reproduction in which the virus controls the cell's mechanism, thus beginning the production of new virus components.

Synthesized drug—A drug created in the laboratory to mimic the pharmacologic actions of a naturally occurring drug.

Synthetic drug—A drug that is created artificially and that has a specific mechanism of action that results in a specific pharmacologic effect.

Syphilis—A sexually transmitted disease caused by an infection of the bacterium *Treponema pallidum*.

Syringe—A calibrated medical instrument that is used to accurately draw up, measure, or deliver medication to a patient.

Syrup—A sugar-based solution that may be medicated or non-medicated. Syrups mask the taste of the drug.

Systemic effect—When the effect of a drug is on the entire body.

Systole—Contraction of the heart muscles during a cardiac cycle.

T

Tablet—A solid dosage form produced by compression that is composed of one or more active ingredients and one or more inert substances.

Tardive dyskinesia—A set of involuntary repetitive body movements.

Target—The tissue or organ that a hormone affects.

T-cell—A type of lymphocyte that binds to the surface of cells that display antigens and triggers an immune response.

Technical-failure error—Environmental, location, or equipment factors that lead to a medication error.

Teratogen—A substance that interferes with normal fetal development.

Testes—Male sex glands that produce testosterone.

Testosterone—The male hormone produced by the testes that is responsible for male characteristics and sperm production, red blood cell production, libido, and fat distribution.

Therapeutic agent—Any drug that relieves symptoms of a disease, stops or delays disease, or maintains health.

Therapeutic effect—The desired effect of a drug on the body, either to treat a disease or to relieve symptoms.

Therapeutic window—A range of serum concentrations at which a drug is most effective with minimal toxicity.

Third-party adjudication—The process through which an insurance company makes a decision regarding coverage and payment for prescriptions.

Thrombus—A blood clot transported within the blood.

Thyroglobulin—An iodine-containing protein of the thyroid gland.

Thyroid gland—A gland that secretes hormones that stimulate metabolic activity, growth, and the activity of the nervous system.

Thyroid-stimulating hormone (TSH)—Hormone that stimulates the thyroid to produce T_3 and T_4.

Thyroxine (T_4)—Hormone produced in the thyroid gland that stimulates metabolic activity, growth, and the activity of the nervous system.

Tiered co-pay—A differential pricing system in which the patient pays a lower co-pay for a generic or preferred brand and a higher co-pay for a nonpreferred brand.

Tincture—An alcoholic or hydroalcoholic solution that contains plant extracts.

Tolerance—The decrease in the pharmacological response to a drug that occurs with continued administration.

Tonic-clonic seizure—A type of seizure characterized by body rigidity followed by muscle jerks.

Tophi—Tiny crystals of urate that deposit in tissues, especially joints.

Topical—Application of a drug to the surface of the skin or mucous membranes.

Tort—A legal term for a lawsuit of personal injury that one citizen commits against another.

Total parenteral nutrition (TPN)—A parenteral solution that is specially formulated to provide nutrition for a patient who is unable to eat. A TPN will often contain protein, carbohydrates, lipids, vitamins, electrolytes, and vitamins.

Total parenteral nutrition (TPN) service—A service in the hospital that specializes in the preparation of TPNs. The service may consist of a dietician, physician, pharmacist, and nurse.

Transcription—The process by which a strand of RNA is made that corresponds to a strand of DNA.

Transdermal—A dosage form in which the medication is in a patch to be applied to the skin.

Transient ischemic attack (TIA)—Short periods of interrupted oxygen supply to the brain.

Transit time—The time it takes for food to pass through the GI tract.

Translation—The process by which ribosomes read the nucleotide sequence from RNA and assemble proteins.

Tricyclic antidepressant (TCA) drug—A class of drugs prescribed primarily for depression.

Triiodothyronine (T_3)—Hormone produced in the thyroid gland that stimulates metabolic activity, growth, and the activity of the nervous system.

Triptans—A class of drugs that constrict the overly relaxed blood vessels in the head and are used to treat migraine and cluster headaches.

Triturate—To break and grind into a fine powder.

Trituration—The process of grinding a substance into fine particles, usually with a mortar and pestle.

Tuberculosis (TB)—A lung disease caused by *Mycobacterium tuberculosis*.

Tumbling—The process of combining powders by placing them in a bag and shaking it.

Tumor necrosis factor (TNF)—A pro-inflammatory cytokine present in the synovium of patients with rheumatoid arthritis.

Twilight sleep—A shortened, altered state of consciousness with short-term memory loss.

Tyramine—A chemical compound that is present in many different foods, including aged cheese, pickled fish, some wines, many meat products, and broad beans.

U

Ulcerative colitis (UC)—Inflammation of the mucosa and submucosa of the colon and rectum.

Uncoating stage—The stage in virus reproduction in which the virus frees its core of either DNA or RNA.

Undernutrition—A nutrition disorder that is characterized by inadequate nutrient intake; leads to weight loss and altered organ function.

Unit dose—An individually prepackaged medication for a specific patient for a single administration.

Unit-dose profile—A patient-specific profile that includes the name, strength, formulation, and route and time of administration for each medication.

United States Pharmacopeia (USP)—A non-governmental, independent scientific organization that sets standards for all over-the-counter and prescription medications and other healthcare products manufactured or sold in the United States.

Unstable angina—Pain that occurs with increasing frequency and diminished response to treatment; may signal an oncoming myocardial infarction.

Urea—A chemical compound found in the urine that is formed from the breakdown of proteins.

Urethral—Pertaining to the urethra.

Urethritis—A urinary tract infection that occurs in the urethra.

Urinary tract infection (UTI)—A bacterial or fungal infection of any part of the urinary tract.

USP 797—USP's requirements for the stability and sterility of compounded sterile products, published in the National Formulary.

USP-NF—A compendium containing standards set by the USP for medicines, dosage forms, drug substances, excipients, dietary supplements, inert ingredients, and medical devices.

V

Vaccine—A biological preparation that improves immunity to a particular disease by invoking an immune response.

Vaginal—Pertaining to the vagina.

Values—The qualities that embody a fulfilled or meaningful life.

Variant angina—Chest pain caused by coronary artery spasm; episodes are unpredictable and are not stress-induced.

Vastus lateralis—The muscle at the top of the leg. The vastus lateralis is an injection site for IM administration in infants and children.

Ventilator-associated pneumonia (VAP)—An infection of the lung that develops while a patient is on a ventilator.

Verbal communication—Communication of a message using words.

Vertigo—A type of dizziness in which an individual feels a sense of motion even when still.

Virilization—Development of male characteristics in a female.

Virion—A fully formed virus.

Virus—A microorganism, some of which attack humans, which are unable to live without a living host.

Vitamin—An organic molecule that regulates metabolic processes.

Volume of distribution—The relationship between the blood concentration obtained and the dose of the drug.

Vomiting—The expulsion of gastric contents through the mouth; also called emesis.

W

Want book—A log or notebook for pharmacy personnel to write in medications or items that are low in stock and need to be re-ordered.

Waste—Overutilization of services or other practices that result in the misuse of resources.

Water-in-oil (W/O) emulsion—An emulsion that contains a small amount of water dispersed in oil.

Water-soluble vitamin—A vitamin that is not stored by the body, but is present in extracellular fluid and excreted by the kidney. Examples are vitamin B complexes and vitamin C.

Whole numbers—Counting numbers (0, 1, 2, …).

Wholesale acquisition cost (WAC)—The drug cost from the wholesale drug distributor.

Wholesaler purchasing—A purchasing system that allows numerous products from multiple brand and generic manufacturers to be purchased from one source.

Worker's compensation—A type of insurance coverage that covers medical care and compensation for employees who are injured on the job.

World Health Organization (WHO)—The public-health division of the United Nations.

Wrong-dosage form error—When the dose is not administered by the intended route.

Wrong-dose error—When the dose administered is not the intended dose.

Wrong-time error—When the dose is given at the wrong time.

Y

Yeast—Fungi that exist in unicellular form.

References

Chapter 1 References

American Association of Colleges of Pharmacy. (2011). Doctor of Pharmacy (Pharm.D.) Degree. *American Association of Colleges of Pharmacy*. Retrieved February 28, 2011, from http://www.aacp.org/resources/student/pharmacyforyou/documents/pharmd.pdf.

American Association of Pharmacy Technicians. (2009). Mission Statement. *AAPT*. Retrieved February 28, 2011, from http://www.pharmacytechnician.com/displaycommon.cfm?an=2.

American Heart Association. (2011). Managed Health Care Plans. American Heart Association. Retrieved February 28, 2011, from http://www.americanheart.org/presenter.jhtml?identifier=4663.

American Pharmacists Association. (n.d.). Getting Your License. *Pharmacist.com*. Retrieved February 28, 2011, from http://www.pharmacist.com/AM/Template.cfm?Section=Career_Resources&Template=/CM/ContentDisplay.cfm&ContentID=11570.

Armitstead, J.A. (2006). The Role of Pharmacists in the Hospital Setting. *American Society of Health-System Pharmacists*. Retrieved February 28, 2011, from http://www.ashp.org/s_ashp/docs/files/HospitalPharmacy.pdf.

Berenguer B., La Casa, C., De la Matta, M.J., and Martín-Calero, M.J. (2004). Pharmaceutical Care: Past, Present and Future. *Current Pharmaceutical Design*, *10*(31), 3931–46.

Blouin, R.A. (2007). Report of the AACP Educating Clinical Scientists Task Force. *American Journal of Pharmaceutical Education*, *71*(4), 1–11. Retrieved February 28, 2011, from http://www.ajpe.org/aj7105/aj7105S05/aj7105S05.pdf.

Duke University Libraries. (2008). Medicine and Madison Avenue–Duke Libraries. *Duke University Libraries*. Retrieved February 28, 2011, from http://library.duke.edu/digitalcollections/mma/timeline.html.

Eurek, S.E. (2003). Hatch-Waxman Reform and Accelerated Market Entry of Generic Drugs: Is Faster Necessarily Better? *Duke Law & Technology Review*. Retrieved February 28, 2011, from http://www.law.duke.edu/journals/dltr/articles/2003dltr0018.html.

Ganz, M. (2004). The Medicare Prescription Drug, Improvement, & Modernization Act of 2003: Are We Playing The Lottery With Healthcare Reform? *Duke Law & Technology Review*. Retrieved February 28, 2011, from http://www.law.duke.edu/journals/dltr/articles/2004dltr0011.html.

Greenberg, R.B. (1988). The Prescription Drug Marketing Act of 1987. *American Journal of Health-System Pharmacy*, *45*(10), 2118–2126. Retrieved February 28, 2011, from http://www.ajhp.org/content/45/10/2118.abstract.

Harris, M.A., and Parascondola, J. (1992). Images of Hospital Pharmacy in America. *American Journal of Hospital Pharmacy*. Retrieved February 28, 2011, from http://www.nlm.nih.gov/hmd/pdf/images.pdf.

Health Guide USA. (2009). Pharmacist Working Conditions. *Health Guide USA*. Retrieved February 28, 2011, from http://www.healthguideusa.org/careers/pharmacist_working_conditions.htm.

The Health Strategies Consultancy LLC. (2005, March). Follow the Pill: Understanding the U.S. Commercial Pharmaceutical Supply Chain. *Kaiser Family Foundation*. Retrieved February 28, 2011, from http://www.kff.org/rxdrugs/upload/Follow-The-Pill-Understanding-the-U-S-Commercial-Pharmaceutical-Supply-Chain-Report.pdf.

Holland, R.W., and Nimmo, C.M. (1999). Transitions, Part 1: Beyond Pharmaceutical Care [Abstract]. *American Journal of Health-System Pharmacy*, *56*(17),1758–64. Retrieved February 28, 2011, from http://www.ajhp.org/content/56/17/1758.abstract.

Kalman, S.H. (2005). American Pharmacists Association Foundation: A Catalyst for Change. *Journal of the American Pharmacists Association,* *45*(6), 663–669.

Megill, M. (2000). Heart Failure. *Dartmouth Medicine*, 35–37. Retrieved February 28, 2011, from http://dartmed.dartmouth.edu/fall00/pdf/Heart_Failure.pdf.

Millis, J.S. (1976). Looking Ahead—The Report of the Study Commission on Pharmacy. *American Journal of Health-System Pharmacy,* *33*(2), 134–8. Retrieved February 28, 2011, from http://www.ajhp.org/content/33/2/134.abstract.

National Association of Boards of Pharmacy. (2005). NABP/ASCP Joint Report: Model Rules for Long-Term Care Pharmacy Practice. *National Association of Boards of Pharmacy*. Retrieved February 28, 2011, from http://www.nabp.net/assets/NABP%20ASCP%20 Report%20on%20Long%20Term%20Care.pdf.

National Institutes of Health. (2009). Greek Medicine. *National Library of Medicine–National Institutes of Health*. Retrieved February 28, 2011, from http:// www.nlm.nih.gov/hmd/greek/index.html.

National Institutes of Health. (2009). Greek Medicine: Galen. *National Library of Medicine–National Institutes of Health*. Retrieved February 28, 2011, from http:// www.nlm.nih.gov/hmd/greek/greek_galen.html.

National Institutes of Health. (2002). Greek Medicine: Hippocrates: The Oath. *National Library of Medicine–National Institutes of Health*. Retrieved February 28, 2011, from http://www.nlm.nih.gov/hmd/greek/ greek_oath.html.

National Institutes of Health. (2009). Greek Medicine: Other Greek Physicians: Dioscorides. *National Library of Medicine—National Institutes of Health*. Retrieved February 28, 2011, from http://www.nlm.nih.gov/ hmd/greek/greek_dioscorides.html.

National Library of Medicine. (2004). Pure Food and Drug Act (1906). United States Statutes at Large (59th Cong., Sess. I, Chp. 3915, p. 768–772; cited as 34 U.S. Stats. 768). In *Medicine in the Americas: Historical Works*. Retrieved February 28, 2011, from http:// www.ncbi.nlm.nih.gov/books/NBK22116/.

Needful Provision, Inc. (n.d.). History of Plant Usage. *Needful Provision, Inc.* Retrieved February 28, 2011, from http://www.needfulprovision.org/vssr/usagehistory.php/.

Pharmacy Technician Certification Board. (2011). PTCB Mission Vision Statement. *Pharmacy Technician Certification Board*. Retrieved February 28, 2011, from https:// www.ptcb.org//AM/Template.cfm?Section=Home1.

Pharmacy Technician.net. (n.d.). Pharmacy Technician Certification and Licensing Requirements by State. *Pharmacy Technician.net*. Retrieved February 28, 2011, from http://www.pharmacy-technician.net/ state-licensing-requirements.

Society of Disabled Pharmacists. (2011). Jobs for Disabled Pharmacists. *Society of Disabled Pharmacists*. Retrieved February 28, 2011, from http://www. disabledpharmacists.org/2011/02/jobs-for-disabledpharmacists.html.

State of New Jersey Department of Health and Senior Services. (2011).Types of Licensed Facilities and Services. *State of New Jersey Department of Health and Senior Services*. Retrieved February 28, 2011, from http://www.nj.gov/health/healthfacilities/types. shtml#LTCHS.

United States Department of Labor. (2011). National Drug Code Directory. *U.S. Food and Drug Administration Home Page*. Retrieved February 28, 2011,

from http://www.fda.gov/Drugs/InformationOnDrugs/ ucm142438.htm.

United States of America, Consumer Product Safety Commission. (1970). *Poison Prevention Packaging Act*. Retrieved February 28, 2011, from http://www.cpsc.gov/ businfo/pppa.pdf.

U.S. Department of Health and Human Services. (n.d.). Health Information Privacy. *U.S. Department of Health and Human Services*. Retrieved February 28, 2011, from http://www.hhs.gov/ocr/privacy/.

U.S. Department of Justice Drug Enforcement Administration Office of Diversion Control. (2005). Drug Scheduling Actions—Implementation of the Anabolic Steroid Control Act of 2004. *U.S. Department of Justice Drug Enforcement Administration Office of Diversion Control*. Retrieved February 28, 2011, from http:// www.deadiversion.usdoj.gov/fed_regs/rules/2005/ fr1216.htm.

U.S. Department of Justice Drug Enforcement Administration Office of Diversion Control. (2006). General Information Regarding the Combat Methamphetamine Epidemic Act of 2005. *U.S. Department of Justice Drug Enforcement Administration Office of Diversion Control*. Retrieved February 28, 2011, from http://www.deadiversion.usdoj.gov/meth/cma2005_general_info.pdf.

U.S. Drug Enforcement Administration. (n.d.). DEA History Book, 1970–1975. *The United States Department of Justice*. Retrieved February 28, 2011, from http:// www.justice.gov/dea/pubs/history/deahistory_01. htm.

U.S. Drug Enforcement Administration. (n.d.). DEA Mission Statement. *U.S. Drug Enforcement Administration*. Retrieved February 28, 2011, from http://www.justice. gov/dea/agency/mission.htm.

U.S. Food and Drug Administration. (2009). Full Text of FDAMA Law. *U.S. Food and Drug Administration*. Retrieved February 28, 2011, from http://www.fda. gov/RegulatoryInformation/Legislation/FederalFoodDrugandCosmeticActFDCAct/SignificantAmendmentstotheFDCAct/FDAMA/FullTextofFDAMAlaw/ default.htm.

U.S. Food and Drug Administration. (2009). The 1938 Food, Drug, and Cosmetic Act. *U.S. Food and Drug Administration*. Retrieved February 28, 2011, from http://www.fda.gov/AboutFDA/WhatWeDo/History/ ProductRegulation/ucm132818.htm.

U.S. Food and Drug Administration. (2010). How Is FDA Organized? *U.S. Food and Drug Administration*. Retrieved February 28, 2011, from http://www.fda.gov/ AboutFDA/Transparency/Basics/ucm194884.htm.

U.S. Food and Drug Administration. (2010). Prescription Drug Marketing Act of 1987. *U.S. Food and Drug Administration*. Retrieved February 28, 2011, from http://www.fda.gov/RegulatoryInformation/Legislation/FederalFoodDrugandCosmeticActFDCAct/ SignificantAmendmentstotheFDCAct/Prescription-DrugMarketingActof1987/default.htm.

U.S. Food and Drug Administration. (2010). What Does FDA Do? *U.S. Food and Drug Administration.* Retrieved February 28, 2011, http://www.fda.gov/AboutFDA/ Transparency/Basics/ucm194877.htm.

U.S. Food and Drug Administration. (2011). Centers and Offices. *U.S. Food and Drug Administration.* Retrieved February 28, 2011, from http://www.fda.gov/ AboutFDA/CentersOffices/default.htm.

U.S. Pharmacopeia. (2011). About USP. *U.S. Pharmacopeia.* Retrieved February 28, 2011, from http://www. usp.org/aboutUSP/.

US PharmD. (n.d.). Pharmacy Technician General Career Information—Pharmacist Technician Requirements. *US PharmD.* Retrieved February 28, 2011, from http:// www.uspharmd.com/technician/pharmacy_techni-cian/.

Chapter 2 References

Ament, P.W., Bertolino, J.G., and Liszewski, J.L. (March 15, 2000). Clinically Significant Drug Interactions. *American Academy of Family Physicians.* Retrieved March 4, 2011, from http://www.aafp.org/afp/20000315/1745. html.

American Pregnancy Association. (2006, June). FDA Drug Category Ratings. *American Pregnancy Association.* Retrieved March 4, 2011, from http://www.american-pregnancy.org/pregnancyhealth/fdadrugratings.html.

Atkinson, A.J., Daniels, C.E., and Dedrick, R. (2001). *Principles of Clinical Pharmacology.* San Diego, CA: Academic Press.

ClinicalTrials.gov. (September 7, 2007). Understanding Clinical Trials. *ClinicalTrials.gov.* Retrieved March 4, 2011, from http://clinicaltrials.gov/ct2/info/under-stand.

DiPiro, J.T., Talbert, R.L., and Yee, G.C. (2008). Pharma-cotherapy: A Pathophysiologic Approach. New York, NY: McGraw-Hill Medical.

Fox, L.M., (2006). The Science and Practice of Pharmacy, 21st Edition. *The American Journal of Pharmaceutical Education, 70*(3), 71.

National Library of Medicine. (2004). Pure Food and Drug Act (1906). United States Statutes at Large (59th Cong., Sess. I, Chp. 3915, p. 768–772; cited as 34 U.S. Stats. 768). In *Medicine in the Americas: Historical Works.* Retrieved February 28, 2011, from http:// www.ncbi.nlm.nih.gov/books/NBK22116/.

Nobelprize.org. (2011). Marie Curie–Biography. *Nobelprize.org.* Retrieved March 4, 2011 from http:// nobelprize.org/nobel_prizes/physics/laureates/1903/ marie-curie-bio.html.

Patrick, G.L., Spencer, J. (2009). *An Introduction to Medicinal Chemistry.* New York, NY: Oxford University Press.

PBS.org. (1998). A Science Odyssey: Banting and Best Isolate Insulin. *PBS: Public Broadcasting Service.* Retrieved March 4, 2011 from http://www.pbs.org/wgbh/ aso/databank/entries/dm22in.html.

PBS.org. (1998). A Science Odyssey: Fleming Discovers Penicillin. *PBS: Public Broadcasting Service.* Retrieved March 4, 2011, from http://www.pbs.org/wgbh/aso/ databank/entries/dm28pe.html.

Rates, S.M. (2001). Plants as Sources of Drugs. *Toxicon, 39,* 603–613.

Riedel, S. (2005). Edward Jenner and the History of Small-pox and Vaccination. *Baylor University Medical Center Proceedings.* Retrieved March 4, 2011, from http:// www.ncbi.nlm.nih.gov/pmc/articles/PMC1200696/.

Scheindlin, S. (2001). A Brief History of Pharmacology. *Modern Drug Discovery, 4*(5), 87–88. Retrieved March 4, 2011, from http://pubs.acs.org/subscribe/journals/ mdd/v04/i05/html/05timeline.html.

U.S. Food and Drug Administration. (2002). Is It a Cosmetic, a Drug, or Both? (Or Is It Soap?). *U.S. Food and Drug Administration.* Retrieved March 8, 2011, from http://www.fda.gov/cosmetics/guidancecompli-anceregulatoryinformation/ucm074201.htm.

U.S Food and Drug Administration. (2009). The 1938 Food, Drug, and Cosmetic Act. *U.S. Food and Drug Administration.* Retrieved February 28, 2011, from http://www.fda.gov/AboutFDA/WhatWeDo/History/ ProductRegulation/ucm132818.htm.

U.S. Food and Drug Administration. (2010). The FDA's Drug Review Process: Ensuring Drugs Are Safe and Effective. *U.S. Food and Drug Administration.* Retrieved March 4, 2011, from http://www.fda.gov/drugs/re-sourcesforyou/consumers/ucm143534.htm.

U.S. Food and Drug Administration. (2011). National Drug Code Directory. *U.S. Food and Drug Administration.* Retrieved March 4, 2011, from http://www.fda. gov/Drugs/InformationOnDrugs/ucm142438.htm.

U.S. Food and Drug Administration. (2011). The FDA's Drug Review Process: Ensuring Drugs Are Safe and Effective. *U.S. Food and Drug Administration.* Retrieved March 4, 2011, from http://www.fda.gov/downloads/ Drugs/DevelopmentApprovalProcess/UCM071436. pdf.

U.S. Pharmacopeia. (2011). Revisions and Commentary. *U.S. Pharmacopeia.* Retrieved March 4, 2011, from http://www.usp.org/USPNF/revisions/.

UW Drug Information Center. (2011). FDA Pregnancy Categories. University of Washington. Retrieved March 4, 2011, from http://depts.washington.edu/ druginfo/Formulary/Pregnancy.pdf.

Chapter 3 References

Ansel, H.C. and M.J. Stoklosa. (2001). *Pharmaceutical Calculations, 11th ed.* Philadelphia: Lippincott, Williams & Wilkins.

Chapter 4 References

Allen, L.V., Popovich, N.G., and Ansel, H.C. (2010). *Ansel's Pharmaceutical Dosage Forms and Drug Delivery System* (9th ed.). Philadelphia, PA: Lippincott, Williams & Wilkins.

Ansel, H.C. and Stoklosa, M.J. (2001). *Pharmaceutical Calculations* (11th ed.). Philadelphia, PA: Lippincott, Williams & Wilkins.

Atkinson, A.J., Daniels, C.E., and Dedrick, R. (2001). *Principles in Clinical Pharmacology*. San Diego, CA: Academic Press.

DiPiro, J.T., Talbert, R.L., and Yee, G.C. (2008). *Pharmacotherapy: A Pathophysiologic Approach*. New York, NY: McGraw-Hill Medical.

Duke Clinical Research Institute. (2010). Beers Criteria (Medication List). Retrieved March 28, 2011, from https://www.dcri.org/trial-participation/the-beers-list.

Fox, L.M. (2006). The Science and Practice of Pharmacy, 21st Edition. *The American Journal of Pharmaceutical Education, 70*(3), 71.

Institute for Safe Medication Practices. (2010). ISMP's List of Error-Prone Abbreviations, Symbols, and Dose Designations. Retrieved March 28, 2011, from http://www.ismp.org/tools/errorproneabbreviations.pdf.

Patrick, G.L., Spencer, J. (2009). *An Introduction to Medicinal Chemistry*. New York, NY: Oxford University Press.

U.S. National Library of Medicine National Institutes of Health. (2008). How to Use Vaginal Tablets, Suppositories, and Creams. Retrieved March 28, 2011, from http://www.nlm.nih.gov/medlineplus/druginfo/meds/a608033.html.

U.S. National Library of Medicine National Institutes of Health. (2011). Metered Dose Inhaler Series. Retrieved March 28, 2011, from http://www.nlm.nih.gov/medlineplus/ency/presentations/100200_1.htm.

The United States Pharmacopeial Convention. (2009). Pharmaceutical Dosage Forms. Retrieved March 29, 2011, from http://www.usp.org/pdf/EN/USPNF/pharmaceuticalDosageForms.pdf.

Chapter 5 References

Ansel, H.C. and Stoklosa, M.J. (2001). *Pharmaceutical Calculations* (11th ed.). Philadelphia, PA: Lippincott Williams & Wilkins.

Ballington, D.A. and Green, T.W. (2010). *Pharmacy Calculations for Technicians: Succeeding in Pharmacy Math* (4th ed.). St. Paul, MN: Paradigm Publishing.

Bregman, A. (2005). Alligation Alternate and the Composition of Medicines: Arithmetic and Medicine in Early Modern Europe. *Medical History, 49*(3), 299–320.

The Institute for Safe Medication Practices. (2010). *ISMP's List of Error-Prone Abbreviations, Symbols, and Dose Designations*. Retrieved March 1, 2011, from http://www.ismp.org/Tools/errorproneabbreviations.pdf.

Lacy, C.F., et al., eds. (2009). *Drug Information Handbook*. Washington, DC: American Pharmacists Association.

Thompson, J.E. (1998). *A Practical Guide to Contemporary Pharmacy Practice*. Baltimore, MD: Williams & Wilkins.

Chapter 6 References

Agency for Healthcare Research and Quality. (2000). 20 Tips to Help Prevent Medical Errors. *Agency for Healthcare Research and Quality*. Retrieved March 8, 2011, from http://www.ahrq.gov/consumer/20tips.pdf.

American Academy of Pediatrics. (January 17, 2008). *American Academy of Pediatrics Urges Caution in Use of Over-the-Counter Cough and Cold Medicines*. [Press release]. Retrieved March 10, 2011, from http://www.aap.org/advocacy/releases/jan08coughandcold.htm.

Ballington, D.A. and Anderson, R.J. (2010). *Pharmacy Practice for Technicians: Mastering Community and Hospital Competencies* (4th ed.). St. Paul, MN: Paradigm Publishing.

Ballington, D.A. and Laughlin, M.M. (2010). *Pharmacology for Technicians: Understanding Drugs and Their Uses* (4th ed.). St. Paul, MN: Paradigm Publishing.

Bartholow, M. (2010). Top 200 Prescription Drugs of 2009. *Pharmacy Times*. Retrieved March 5, 2011, from http://www.pharmacytimes.com/issue/pharmacy/2010/May2010/RxFocusTopDrugs-0510.

Basco, W.T., Ebeling, M., Hulsey, T.C., and Simpson, K. (2010). Using Pharmacy Data to Screen for Look-Alike, Sound-Alike Substitution Errors in Pediatric Prescriptions. *Academic Pediatrics, 10*(4), 233–237.

Berardi, R.R., et al., eds. (2002). *Handbook of Nonprescription Drugs: An Interactive Approach to Self-Care* (13th ed.), Washington, DC: American Pharmaceutical Association.

Boh, L.E., ed. (2001). *Pharmacy Practice Manual: A Guide to the Clinical Experience* (2nd ed.). Baltimore, MD: Lippincott Williams & Wilkins.

Centers for Disease Control and Prevention. (2010). Medication Safety Basics. *Centers for Disease Control and*

Prevention. Retrieved March 8, 2011, from http://www. cdc.gov/MedicationSafety/basics.html.

Committee on Identifying and Preventing Medication Errors. (2007). *Preventing Medication Errors.* Ed. P. Aspden, J. Wolcott, J.L. Bootman, and L.R. Cronenwett. Washington, DC: National Academies Press.

Darker, I.T., et al. (2011). The Influence of "Tall Man" Lettering on Errors of Visual Perception in the Recognition of Written Drug Names. *Ergonomics, 54*(1), 21–33.

Dean, B., Barber, N., and Schachter, M. (2000). What is a Prescribing Error? *Quality in Health Care, 9,* 232–237.

Dipiro, J.T., et al., eds. (2008). *Pharmacotherapy: A Pathophysiologic Approach* (7th ed.). New York, NY: McGraw-Hill Medical.

Filik, R., et al. (2006). Labeling of Medicines and Patient Safety: Evaluating Methods of Reducing Drug Name Confusion. *Human Factors, 48*(1), 39–47.

Gibson, J.L. (2006). Lessons Learned from a Student-Initiated Antibiotic Awareness Program. *American Journal Health-System Pharmacy, 63*(17), 1590–1592.

Gibson, J.L. (2006). Infants and Over-the-Counter Cold Medications: Risky Business. *Virginia Pharmacist, 90*(2), 5.

Graham, A.S. (2008). Prescribing Errors. *California Journal of Health-System Pharmacy*, March/April, 5–15.

IMS Institute for Healthcare Informatics. (2011). The Use of Medicines in the United States: 2010. April, 1–37.

Institute for Safe Medication Practices. (2010). ISMP's List of Confused Drug Names. *Institute for Safe Medication Practices.* Retrieved March 5, 2011, from http://www. ismp.org/tools/confuseddrugnames.pdf.

Institute for Safe Medication Practices. (2010). ISMP's List of Error-Prone Abbreviations, Symbols, and Dose Designations. *Institute for Safe Medication Practices.* Retrieved March 1, 2011 from http://www.ismp.org/ Tools/errorproneabbreviations.pdf.

James, K.L., et al. (2009). Incidence, Type and Causes of Dispensing Errors: A Review of the Literature. *The International Journal of Pharmacy Practice, 17*(1), 9–30.

Knudsen, P., et al. (2007). Preventing Medication Errors in Community Pharmacy: Root-Cause Analysis of Transcription Errors. *Quality and Safety in Health Care, 16,* 2285–2290.

Kohn, L.T., Corrigan, J.M., and Donaldson, M.S., eds. (2000). *To Err Is Human.* Washington, DC: National Academy Press.

Lacy, C.F., et al., eds. (2009). *Drug Information Handbook* (18th ed.). Hudson, OH: Lexi-Comp.

McCarthy, R.L. and Schafermeyer, K.W. (2001). *Introduction to Health Care Delivery: A Primer for Pharmacists* (2nd ed.). Gaithersburg, MD: Aspen Publishers.

McCoy, L.K. (2005). Look-Alike, Sound-Alike Drugs Review: Include Look-Alike Packaging as an Additional Safety Check. *Joint Commission Journal on Quality and Patient Safety, 31*(1), 47–53.

National Coordinating Council for Medication Error Reporting and Prevention. About Medication Errors. *National Coordinating Council for Medication Error Reporting and Prevention.* Retrieved March 5, 2011, from http://www.nccmerp.org/aboutMedErrors.html.

National Coordinating Council for Medication Error Reporting and Prevention. Consumer Information for Safe Medication Use. *National Coordinating Council for Medication Error Reporting and Prevention.* Retrieved March 5, 2011, from http://www.nccmerp.org/consumerInfo.html.

National Coordinating Council for Medication Error Reporting and Prevention. Report a Medication Error. *National Coordinating Council for Medication Error Reporting and Prevention.* Retrieved March 5, 2011, from http://www.nccmerp.org/reportMedError.html.

Ogu, C.C. and Maxa, J.L. (2000). Drug Interactions Due to Cytochrome P450. *BUMC Proceedings* (Vol. 13, pp. 421–423).

Pushkin, R., et al. (2010). Improving the Reporting of Adverse Drug Reactions in the Hospital Setting. *Postgrad Med, 122*(6), 154–164.

Santell, J.P., et al. (2005). MedMarx Data Report. USP Center for the Advancement of Patient Safety.

Starlin, R., ed. (2005). *Infectious Diseases Subspecialty Consult.* Philadelphia, PA: Lippincott Williams & Wilkins.

U.S. Food and Drug Administration. (2008). Public Health Advisory: FDA Recommends that Over-the-Counter (OTC) Cough and Cold Products Not Be Used for Infants and Children Under 2 Years of Age. *U.S. Food and Drug Administration.* Retrieved March 10, 2011, from http://www.fda.gov/Drugs/DrugSafety/PostmarketDrugSafetyInformationforPatientsandProviders/ DrugSafetyInformationforHeathcareProfessionals/ PublicHealthAdvisories/ucm051137.htm.

U.S. Food and Drug Administration. (2010). Medication Errors. *U.S. Food and Drug Administration.* Retrieved March 6, 2011, from http://www.fda.gov/drugs/drugsafety/medicationerrors/default.htm.

U.S. Food and Drug Administration. (2011). Unapproved Prescription Cough, Cold, and Allergy Products. *U.S. Food and Drug Administration.* Retrieved March 10, 2011, from http://www.fda.gov/Drugs/ GuidanceComplianceRegulatoryInformation/EnforcementActivitiesbyFDA/SelectedEnforcementActionsonUnapprovedDrugs/ucm245106.htm.

U.S. Food and Drug Administration. (2011). Regulation of Nonprescription Products. *U.S. Food and Drug Administration.* Retrieved May 22, 2011, from http://www.fda.gov/aboutfda/centersoffices/cder/ucm093452.htm.

World Health Organization. (2007). Look-Alike, Sound-Alike Medication Names. *World Health Organization.* Retrieved March 5, 2011, from http://gis.emro.who.int/HealthSystemObservatory/PDF/Patient%20Safety/PS-Solution1.pdf.

Weingart, S.N., et al. (2000). Epidemiology of Medical Error. *BMJ, 320,* 774–777.

Chapter 7 References

Drug Facts and Comparisons 2011 (Bound). *Wolters Kluwer Health.* Retrieved March 3, 2011, from http://www.factsandcomparisons.com/drug-facts-and-comparisons-bound.asp.

Facts & Comparisons eAnswers. *Wolters Kluwer Health.* Retrieved March 1, 2011, from http://www.factsandcomparisons.com/facts-comparisons-Online.aspx.

Micromedex Gateway. *Thomson Reuters.* Retrieved March 15, 2011, from https://www.thomsonhc.com/micromedex2/librarian/ssl/true.

Red Book: Pharmacy's Fundamental Reference. *RAmEx Ars Medica.* Retrieved March 3, 2011, from http://www.ramex.com/title.asp?id=1144.

Chapter 8 References

U.S Equal Opportunity Commission. 2010. Facts About Sexual Harassment. *U.S. Equal Opportunity Commission.* Retrieved May 11, 2011, from http://www.eeoc.gov/eeoc/publications/fs-sex.cfm.

U.S. Equal Opportunity Commission. 2010. Federal Laws Prohibiting Job Discrimination Questions And Answers. *U.S. Equal Opportunity Commission.* Retrieved May 11, 2011, from http://www.eeoc.gov/facts/qanda.html.

U.S. Senate. *Health Insurance Portability and Accountability Act of 1996.* 104th Congress, P.L. 104-191. *Institute for Health Freedom.* Accessed May 7, 2011, from http://www.forhealthfreedom.org/BackgroundResearchData/HIPAA_Law.pdf.

Chapter 9 References

Ballington, D. and Laughlin, M. (2010). *Pharmacology for Technicians* (4th ed.). St. Paul, MN: Paradigm Publishing.

MA Pharm. (2010). Parts of a Written Prescription. *MA Pharm.* Retrieved May 5, 2011 from www.mapharm.com/prescr_parts.htm.

Rankin, E. (2000). *Quick Reference for Psychopharmacology.* Albany, NY: Delmar.

Chapter 10 References

Allen, L.V., Popovich, N.G., and Ansel, H.C. (2010). *Ansel's Pharmaceutical Dosage Forms and Drug Delivery System* (9th ed.). Philadelphia, PA: Lippincott Williams & Wilkins.

Ansel, H.C. and Stoklosa, M.J. (2001). *Pharmaceutical Calculations* (11th ed.). Philadelphia, PA: Lippincott Williams & Wilkins.

Atkinson, A.J., Daniels, C.E., and Dedrick, R. (2001). *Principles in Clinical Pharmacology.* San Diego, CA: Academic Press.

DiPiro, J.T., Talbert, R.L., and Yee, G.C. (2008). *Pharmacotherapy: A Pathophysiologic Approach.* New York, NY: McGraw-Hill Medical.

Epilepsy Foundation. (2011). Prolonged or Serial Seizures (Status Epilepticus). *Epilepsy Foundation.* Retrieved March 28, 2011, from http://www.epilepsyfoundation.org/about/types/types/statusepilepticus.cfm.

Fox, L.M. (2006). The Science and Practice of Pharmacy, 21st Edition. *The American Journal of Pharmaceutical Education, 70*(3), 71.

National Institute of Mental Health. (2010). Attention Deficit Hyperactivity Disorder (ADHD). *National Institute of Mental Health.* Retrieved April 1, 2011, from http://www.nimh.nih.gov/health/publications/attention-deficit-hyperactivity-disorder/complete-index.shtml.

National Institute of Neurological Disorders and Stroke. (2011). What is Parkinson's Disease? *National Institute of Neurological Disorders and Stroke.* Retrieved April 1, 2011 from http://www.ninds.nih.gov/disorders/parkinsons_disease/parkinsons_disease.htm.

Okie, S. (2006). ADHD in Adults. *New England Journal of Medicine, 354,* 2637.

U.S. National Library of Medicine National Institutes of Health. (2011). Alzheimer's Disease. *PubMed Health.* Retrieved April 2, 2011, from http://www.ncbi.nlm.nih.gov/pubmedhealth/PMH0001767.

U.S. National Library of Medicine National Institutes of Health. (2011). Central Nervous System. *Medline Plus.* Retrieved April 1, 2011, from http://www.nlm.nih.gov/medlineplus/ency/article/002311.htm.

U.S. National Library of Medicine National Institutes of Health. (2008). Seizures. *Medline Plus.* Retrieved April 2, 2011, from http://www.nlm.nih.gov/medlineplus/ency/article/003200.htm.

U.S. National Library of Medicine National Institutes of Health. (2008). Convulsions. *Medline Plus.* Retrieved April 2, 2011, from http://www.nlm.nih.gov/medlineplus/ency/article/000021.htm.

The United States Pharmacopeial Convention. (2009). Pharmaceutical Dosage Forms. *U.S. Pharmacopeia.* Retrieved March 29, 2011, from http://www.usp.org/pdf/EN/USPNF/pharmaceuticalDosageForms.pdf.

Chapter 11 References

AHFS Drug Information. (2009). Bethesda, MD: American Society of Health-System Pharmacists, Inc.

Ansel, H.C. and Stoklosa, M.J. (2001). *Pharmaceutical Calculations* (11th ed.). Philadelphia, PA: Lippincott Williams & Wilkins.

Atkinson, A.J., Daniels, C.E., and Dedrick, R. (2001). *Principles in Clinical Pharmacology.* San Diego, CA: Academic Press.

COPD International. (2008). Chronic Bronchitis. *COPD International.* Retrieved May 24, 2011, from http://www.copd-international.com/bronchitis.htm.

Centers for Medicare and Medicaid Services. (2008). What Is Medicaid? *Medicare.gov.* Retrieved July 17, 2011, from http://www.medicare.gov/publications/pubs/pdf/11306.pdf.

Centers for Medicare and Medicaid Services. (2008). What Is Medicare? *Medicare.gov.* Retrieved July 17, 2011, from http://www.medicare.gov/publications/pubs/pdf/11306.pdf.

DiPiro, J.T., Talbert, R.L., and Yee, G.C. (2008). *Pharmacotherapy: A Pathophysiologic Approach.* New York, NY: McGraw-Hill Medical.

Drug Facts and Comparisons (63rd ed.). (2008). St. Louis, MO: Wolters Kluwer Health.

Fauci, A.S., Braunwald, E., Kasper, D., et al. (2005). *Harrison's Principles of Internal Medicine* (16th ed.). New York, NY: McGraw-Hill Companies, Inc.

Federal Trade Commission. (2005). Pharmacy Benefit Managers: Ownership of Mail-Order Pharmacies. *Federal Trade Commission.* Retrieved May 20, 2011, from http://www.ftc.gov/reports/pharmbenefit05/050906pharmbenefitrpt.pdf.

Lacher, B.E. (2008). *Pharmaceutical Calculations for the Pharmacy Technician.* Baltimore, MD: Lippincott Williams &Wilkins.

Lacy, C.F., et al., eds. (2009). *Drug Information Handbook.* Washington, DC: American Pharmacists Association.

MedicineNet.com. (n.d.). Emphysema. *MedicineNet.com.* Retrieved May 20, 2011, from http://www.medicinenet.com/emphysema/article.htm.

MedicineNet.com. (n.d.). Pneumonia. *MedicineNet.com.* Retrieved May 20, 2011, from http://www.medicinenet.com/pneumonia/article.htm.

New York State Department of Health. (2007). Tuberculosis. *New York State Department of Health.* Retrieved May 20, 2011, from http://www.health.state.ny.us/diseases/communicable/tuberculosis/fact_sheet.htm.

Stedman's Concise Medical Dictionary for Health Professionals (3rd ed.). (1997). Baltimore, MD: Lippincott Williams & Wilkins.

Thompson, J.E. (1998). *A Practical Guide to Contemporary Pharmacy Practice.* Baltimore, MD: Williams & Wilkins.

U.S. Department of Health and Human Services National Institutes of Health. (2009). What Is Cystic Fibrosis? *U.S. Department of Health and Human Services National Institutes of Health.* Retrieved May 24, 2011, from http://www.nhlbi.nih.gov/health/dci/Diseases/cf/cf_what.html.

U.S. Department of Health and Human Services National Institutes of Health. (2009). What Is Respiratory Distress Syndrome? *U.S. Department of Health and Human Services National Institutes of Health.* Retrieved May 24, 2011, from http://www.nhlbi.nih.gov/health/dci/Diseases/rds/rds_whatis.html.

U.S. Department of Health and Human Services Health Resources and Services Administration. (n.d.). Glossary of Pharmacy Related Terms. *U.S. Department of Health and Human Services.* Retrieved July 17, 2011, from http://www.hrsa.gov/opa/glossary.htm.

U.S. Department of Justice Drug Enforcement Administration Office of Diversion Control. (n.d.). Pharmacist's Manual. *U.S. Department of Justice Drug Enforcement Administration Office of Diversion Control.* Retrieved May 31, 2011, from http://www.deadiversion.usdoj.gov/pubs/manuals/pharm2/pharm_manual.htm.

U.S. Drug Enforcement Administration. (n.d.). Drug Scheduling. *U.S. Drug Enforcement Administration.* Retrieved July 17, 2011, from http://www.justice.gov/dea/pubs/scheduling.html.

U.S. Food and Drug Administration. (2009). Claims That Can Be Made for Conventional Foods and Dietary Supplements. *U.S. Food and Drug Administration.* Retrieved May 31, 2011, from http://www.fda.gov/Food/LabelingNutrition/LabelClaims/ucm111447.htm.

U.S. Food and Drug Administration. (2009). Overview of Dietary Supplements. *U.S. Food and Drug Administration.* Retrieved July 17, 2011, from http://www.fda.gov/Food/DietarySupplements/ConsumerInformation/ucm110417.htm#what.

U.S. National Library of Medicine National Institutes of Health. (2011). Health Insurance. *MedlinePlus.* Retrieved May 24, 2011, from http://www.nlm.nih.gov/medlineplus/healthinsurance.html.

Chapter 12 References

Agur, A.M.R. and Lee, M.J. (1999). *Grant's Atlas of Anatomy.* Philadelphia, PA: Lippincott Williams & Wilkins.

Ansel, H.C. and Stoklosa, M.J. (2001). *Pharmaceutical Calculations* (11th ed.). Philadelphia, PA: Lippincott Williams & Wilkins.

Ballington, D.A. and Anderson, R.J. (2010). *Pharmacy Practice for Technicians: Mastering Community and*

Hospital Competencies (4th ed.). St. Paul, MN: Paradigm Publishing.

Ballington, D.A. and Laughlin, M.M. (2010). *Pharmacology for Technicians: Understanding Drugs and Their Uses* (4th ed.). St. Paul, MN: Paradigm Publishing.

Berardi, R.R., et al. (eds.). (2002). *Handbook of Nonprescription Drugs: An Interactive Approach to Self-Care* (13th ed.). Washington, DC: American Pharmaceutical Association.

Bickley, L.S. and Szilagyi, P.G. (eds.). *Bates' Guide to Physical Examination and History Taking* (8th ed.). Philadelphia, PA: Lippincott Williams & Wilkins.

Centers for Medicare & Medicaid Services. (2010). *2010 CMS Statistics. CMS Pub. No. 03501.* Washington, DC: U.S. Department of Health and Human Services.

Centers for Medicare & Medicaid Services. (2011). *Prescription Drug Benefit Manual (2006).* Retrieved July 30, 2011 from https://www.cms.gov/PrescriptionDrugCovContra/Downloads/PDBManual_Chapter9_FWA.pdf.

Dipiro, J.T., et al., eds. (2008). *Pharmacotherapy: A Pathophysiologic Approach* (7th ed.). New York, NY: McGraw-Hill Medical.

Greenwald, D.A. (2004). Aging, the Gastrointestinal Tract, and Risk of Acid-Related Disease. *The American Journal of Medicine, 117*(5), s8–13.

Lacy, C.F., et al., eds. (2009). *Drug Information Handbook.* Washington, DC: American Pharmacists Association.

McCarthy, R.L. and Schafermeyer, K.W. (2001). *Introduction to Health Care Delivery: A Primer for Pharmacists* (2nd ed.). Gaithersburg, MD: Aspen Publishers, Inc.

Rhoades, R. and Pflanzer, R. (2003). *Human Physiology* (4th ed.). Pacific Grove, CA: Thomson Learning.

Sparks, J. and McCartney, L. (2010). *Pharmacy Labs for Technicians: Building Skills in Pharmacy Practice.* St. Paul, MN: Paradigm Publishing.

Chapter 13 References

AHFS Drug Information. (2009). Bethesda, MD: American Society of Health-System Pharmacists, Inc.

Allen, L.V., Popovich, N.G., and Ansel, H.C. (2010). *Ansel's Pharmaceutical Dosage Forms and Drug Delivery System* (9th ed.). Philadelphia, PA: Lippincott Williams & Wilkins.

Allen, L.V. (2002). *The Art, Science, and Technology of Pharmaceutical Compounding* (2nd ed.). Washington, DC: APhA Publications.

Ansel, H.C. and Stoklosa, M.J. (2001). *Pharmaceutical Calculations* (11th ed.). Philadelphia, PA: Lippincott Williams & Wilkins.

Atkinson, A.J., Daniels, C.E., and Dedrick, R. (2001). *Principles in Clinical Pharmacology.* San Diego, CA: Academic Press.

Ballington D.A. and Anderson, R.J. (2010). *Pharmacy Practice for Technicians.* St. Paul, MN: Paradigm Publishing, Inc.

DiPiro, J.T., Talbert, R.L., and Yee, G.C. (2008). *Pharmacotherapy: A Pathophysiologic Approach.* New York, NY: McGraw-Hill Medical.

Drug Facts and Comparisons (63rd ed.). (2008). St. Louis, MO: Wolters Kluwer Health.

Fauci, A.S., Braunwald, E., Kasper, D., et al. (2005). *Harrison's Principles of Internal Medicine* (16th ed.). New York, NY: McGraw-Hill Medical.

Gupta, K. et al. (2001).Increasing Antimicrobial Resistance and the Management of Uncomplicated Community-Acquired Urinary Tract Infections. *Annals of Internal Medicine, 135*(1), 41–50.

International Academy of Compounding Pharmacists. (n.d.). Welcome. *International Academy of Compounding Pharmacists.* Retrieved April 8, 2011, from http://www.iacprx.org/site/PageServer?pagename=home_page.

Knottnerus, B.J., *et al.* (2008). Fosfomycin Tromethamine as Second Agent for the Treatment of Acute, Uncomplicated Urinary Tract Infections in Adult Female Patients in The Netherlands? *The Journal of Antimicrobial Chemotherapy, 62*(2), 356–359.

Lacher, B.E. (2008). *Pharmaceutical Calculations for the Pharmacy technician.* Baltimore, MD: Lippincott Williams & Wilkins.

Lacy, C.F., *et al.*, eds. (2009). *Drug Information Handbook.* Washington, DC: American Pharmacists Association.

Remington, J.P., and Beringer, P. (2006). *Remington: The Science and Practice of Pharmacy* (21st ed.). Baltimore, MD: Lippincott Williams & Wilkins.

The Renal Association. (n.d.). CKD Stages. *The Renal Association.* Retrieved April 8, 2011, from http://www.renal.org/whatwedo/InformationResources/CKDeGUIDE/CKDstages.aspx.

Stedman's Concise Medical Dictionary for Health Professionals (3rd ed.). (1997). Baltimore, MD: Lippincott Williams & Wilkins.

Thompson, J.E. (1998). *A Practical Guide to Contemporary Pharmacy Practice.* Baltimore, MD: Williams & Wilkins.

U.S. Food and Drug Administration. (2008). Good Manufacturing Practice (GMP) Guidelines/Inspection Checklist. *U.S. Food and Drug Administration.* Retrieved April 8, 2011, from http://www.fda.gov/cosmetics/guidancecomplianceregulatoryinformation/goodmanufacturingpracticegmpguidelinesinspectionchecklist/default.htm.

U.S. Pharmacopeia. (2008). USP Compounding Backgrounder. *U.S. Pharmacopeia*. Retrieved April 8, 2011, from http://www.usp.org/pdf/EN/aboutUSP/pressRoom/compoundingBackgrounder.pdf.

U.S. Pharmacopeia <795>. (n.d.). Pharmaceutical Compounding-Nonsterile Preparations. *U.S. Pharmacopeia*. Retrieved April 7, 2011 from http://www.pharmacopeia.cn/v29240/usp29nf24s0_c795.html.

U.S. Pharmacopeia <1075>. (n.d.). Good Compounding Practices. *U.S. Pharmacopeia*. Retrieved April 7, 2011 from http://www.pharmacopeia.cn/v29240/usp-29nf24s0_c1075.html#usp29nf24s0_c1075.

The United States Pharmacopeial Convention. (2009). Pharmaceutical Dosage Forms. *U.S. Pharmacopeia*. Retrieved March 29, 2011, from http://www.usp.org/pdf/EN/USPNF/pharmaceuticalDosageForms.pdf.

Wagenlehner, F.M., *et al.* (2009). An Update on Uncomplicated Urinary Tract Infections in Women. *Current Opinion in Urology, 19*(4), 368–374.

Chapter 14 References

Agur, A.M.R. and Lee, M.J. (1999). *Grant's Atlas of Anatomy*. Philadelphia, PA: Lippincott Williams & Wilkins.

Ansel, H.C., Allen, L.V., and Popovich, N.G. (1999). *Pharmaceutical Dosage Forms and Drug Delivery Systems* (7th ed.). Philadelphia, PA: Lippincott Williams & Wilkins.

Ansel, H.C. and Stoklosa, M.J. (2001). *Pharmaceutical Calculations* (11th ed.). Philadelphia, PA: Lippincott Williams & Wilkins.

Ballington, D.A. and Anderson, R.J. (2010). *Pharmacy Practice for Technicians: Mastering Community and Hospital Competencies* (4th ed.). St. Paul, MN: Paradigm Publishing.

Ballington, D.A. and Laughlin, M.M. (2010). *Pharmacology for Technicians: Understanding Drugs and Their Uses* (4th ed.). St. Paul, MN: Paradigm Publishing.

Dipiro, J.T., et al., eds. (2008). *Pharmacotherapy: A Pathophysiologic Approach* (7th ed.). New York, NY: McGraw-Hill Medical.

GlaxoSmithKline: Augmentin (amoxicillin/clavulanate potassium) Powder for Oral Suspension and Chewable Tablets: Prescribing Information. (2009). Research Triangle Park, NC: GlaxoSmithKline.

Lacy, C.F., et al., eds. (2009). *Drug Information Handbook*. Washington, DC: American Pharmacists Association.

Rhoades, R. and Pflanzer, R. (2003). *Human Physiology* (4th ed.). Pacific Grove, CA: Thomson Learning.

Sparks, J. and McCartney, L. (2010). *Pharmacy Labs for Technicians: Building Skills in Pharmacy Practice*. St. Paul, MN: Paradigm Publishing.

Thompson, J.E. (1998). *A Practical Guide to Contemporary Pharmacy Practice*. Baltimore, MD: Lippincott Williams & Wilkins.

Zentz, L.C. (2010). *Math for Pharmacy Technicians*. Sudbury, MA: Jones and Bartlett Publishers.

Chapter 15 References

American Society of Health-System Pharmacists, Inc. (2009). *AHFS Drug Information*. Bethesda, MD: American Society of Health-System Pharmacists, Inc.

Ansel, H.C. and Stoklosa, M.J. (2001). *Pharmaceutical Calculations* (11th ed.). Philadelphia, PA: Lippincott, Williams & Wilkins.

Atkinson, A.J., Daniels, C.E., and Dedrick, R. (2001). *Principles in Clinical Pharmacology*. San Diego, CA: Academic Press.

DiPiro, J.T., Talbert, R.L., and Yee, G.C. (2008). *Pharmacotherapy: A Pathophysiologic Approach*. New York, NY: McGraw-Hill Medical.

Eustice, C. (2003). The Facts of DMARDs. *About.com*. Retrieved April 15, 2011, from http://arthritis.about.com/cs/dmards/a/diseasemodifier.htm.

Eustice, C. (2009). Cyclooxygenase: COX-1 and COX-2 Explained: What You Need to Know About Cyclooxygenase. *About.com*. Retrieved April 15, 2011, from http://osteoarthritis.about.com/od/osteoarthritismedications/a/cyclooxygenase.htm.

Fauci, A.S., Braunwald, E., Kasper, D., et al. (2005). *Harrison's Principles of Internal Medicine* (16th ed.). New York, NY: McGraw-Hill Medical.

KidsHealth.org (n.d.). Bones, Muscles, and Joints: The Musculoskeletal System. *KidsHealth*. Retrieved April 15, 2011, from http://kidshealth.org/parent/general/body_basics/bones_muscles_joints.html#.

Lacher, B.E. (2008). *Pharmaceutical Calculations for the Pharmacy Technician*. Baltimore, MD: Lippincott, Williams &Wilkins.

Lacy, C.F., et al., eds. (2009). *Drug Information Handbook*. Washington, DC: American Pharmacists Association.

National Institute of Arthritis and Musculoskeletal and Skin Diseases, National Institutes of Health. Bursitis and Tendonitis. *National Institute of Arthritis and Musculoskeletal and Skin Diseases*. Retrieved April 12, 2011, from http://www.niams.nih.gov/Health_Info/Bursitis/default.asp.

National Institute of Arthritis and Musculoskeletal and Skin Diseases, National Institutes of Health. What is Osteoarthritis? *National Institute of Arthritis and Musculoskeletal and Skin Diseases*. Retrieved April 12, 2011, from http://www.niams.nih.gov/Health_Info/Osteoarthritis/osteoarthritis_ff.pdf.

Stedman's Concise Medical Dictionary for Health Professionals (3rd ed.). (1997). Baltimore, MD: Lippincott Williams & Wilkins.

Thompson, J.E. (1998). *A Practical Guide to Contemporary Pharmacy Practice*. Baltimore, MD: Williams & Wilkins.

U.S. Food and Drug Administration. (2008). Good Manufacturing Practice (GMP) Guidelines/Inspection Checklist. *U.S. Food and Drug Administration*. Retrieved April 15, 2011, from http://www.fda.gov/cosmetics/guidancecomplianceregulatoryinformation/goodmanufacturingpracticegmpguidelinesinspectionchecklist/default.htm.

U.S. Food and Drug Administration. (2011). Medication Guides. *U.S. Food and Drug Administration*. Retrieved April 15, 2011, from http://www.fda.gov/Drugs/DrugSafety/ucm085729.htm.

U.S. National Library of Medicine National Institutes of Health. (2007). Comparing Muscle Relaxants. Retrieved April 17, 2011, from http://www.ncbi.nlm.nih.gov/books/NBK1597/.

U.S. Pharmacopeia <1146>. (n.d.). Packaging Practice-Repackaging A Single Solid Oral Drug Product Into A Unit-Dose Container. *U.S. Pharmacopeia*. Retrieved May 7, 2011, from http://www.pharmacopeia.cn/v29240/usp29nf24s0_c1146.html#usp29nf24s0_c1146.

Wolters Kluwer Health. (2010). *Drug Facts and Comparisons. Pocket Version*. St. Louis, MO: Wolters Kluwer Health.

Chapter 16 References

About.com. (2008). Cortisol and Stress: How to Stay Healthy. *About.com*. Retrieved April 25, 2011, from http://stress.about.com/od/stresshealth/a/cortisol.htm.

American Society of Health-System Pharmacists, Inc. (2009). *AHFS Drug Information*. Bethesda: American Society of Health-System Pharmacists, Inc.

Ansel, H.C. and Stoklosa, M.J. (2001). *Pharmaceutical Calculations* (11th ed.). Philadelphia, PA: Lippincott Williams & Wilkins.

Atkinson, A.J., Daniels, C.E., and Dedrick, R. (2001). *Principles in Clinical Pharmacology*. San Diego, CA: Academic Press.

Centers for Disease Control and Prevention. (2010). Genital Herpes-CDC Fact Sheet. *Centers for Disease Control and Prevention*. Retrieved April 25, 2011, from http://www.cdc.gov/std/Herpes/STDFact-Herpes.htm.

Centers for Disease Control and Prevention. (2010). Syphilis-CDC Fact Sheet. *Centers for Disease Control and Prevention*. Retrieved April 25, 2011, from http://www.cdc.gov/std/syphilis/STDFact-Syphilis.htm.

Centers for Disease Control and Prevention. (2011). Chlamydia-CDC Fact Sheet. *Centers for Disease Control and Prevention*. Retrieved April 25, 2011, from http://www.cdc.gov/STD/chlamydia/STDFact-Chlamydia.htm.

Centers for Disease Control and Prevention. (2011). Gonorrhea-CDC Fact Sheet. *Centers for Disease Control and Prevention*. Retrieved April 25, 2011, from http://www.cdc.gov/std/gonorrhea/STDFact-gonorrhea.htm.

Centers for Disease Control and Prevention. (2011). Nationally Notifiable Infectious Conditions. *Centers for Disease Control and Prevention*. Retrieved April 25, 2011, from http://www.cdc.gov/osels/ph_surveillance/nndss/phs/infdis2011.htm.

DiPiro, J.T., Talbert, R.L., and Yee, G.C. (2008). *Pharmacotherapy: A Pathophysiologic Approach*. New York, NY: McGraw-Hill Medical.

Drug Facts and Comparisons, 63rd ed. (2008). St. Louis, MO: Wolters Kluwer Health.

emedicinehealth. (2010). Anatomy of the Endocrine System. *emedicinehealth*. Retrieved April 25, 2011, from http://www.emedicinehealth.com/anatomy_of_the_endocrine_system/article_em.htm.

Fauci, A.S., Braunwald, E., Kasper, D., et al. (2005). *Harrison's Principles of Internal Medicine* (16th ed.). New York, NY: McGraw-Hill Companies, Inc.

Grajower, M.M., Holcombe, J.H., Harris, W.C., and Sangiago, O.M. (2003). How Long Should Insulin Be Used Once a Vial Is Started? *American Diabetes Association*. Retrieved August 4, 2011, from http://care.diabetesjournals.org/content/26/9/2665.full.

Hatcher, R.A., Trussel, J., Nelson, A. (2004). *Contraceptive Technology 18th ed*. New York, New York: Ardent Media, Inc.

KidsHealth.org. (n.d.). Growth Problems. *KidsHealth.org*. Retrieved April 25, 2011, from http://kidshealth.org/teen/diseases_conditions/growth/growth_hormone.html.

Lacher, B.E. (2008). *Pharmaceutical Calculations for the Pharmacy Technician*. Baltimore, MD: Lippincott Williams &Wilkins.

Lacy, C.F., et al., eds. (2009). *Drug Information Handbook*. Washington, DC: American Pharmacists Association.

The Magic Foundation. (2011). Growth Hormone Deficiency in Children. *The Magic Foundation*. Retrieved April 25, 2011, from http://www.magicfoundation.org/www/docs/108/growth_hormone_deficiency_in_children.

Mayo Clinic. (2010). Hyperthyroidism (Overactive Thyroid). *Mayo Clinic*. Retrieved April 12, 2011, from http://www.mayoclinic.com/health/hyperthyroidism/DS00344/DSECTION=symptoms.

Mayo Clinic. (2010). Hypothyroidism (Underactive Thyroid). *Mayo Clinic*. Retrieved April 12, 2011, from http://www.mayoclinic.com/health/hypothyroidism/DS00353/DSECTION=symptoms.

Stedman's Concise Medical Dictionary for Health Professionals (3rd ed.). (1997). Baltimore, MD: Lippincott Williams & Wilkins.

Thompson, J.E. (1998). *A Practical Guide to Contemporary Pharmacy Practice*. Baltimore, MD: Williams & Wilkins.

U.S. Food and Drug Administration. (2008). Good Manufacturing Practice (GMP) Guidelines/Inspection Checklist. *U.S. Food and Drug Administration*. Retrieved April 15, 2011, from http://www.fda.gov/cosmetics/guidancecomplianceregulatoryinformation/goodmanufacturingpracticegmpguidelinesinspectionchecklist/default.htm.

U.S. Food and Drug Administration. (2011). Medication Guides. *U.S. Food and Drug Administration*. Retrieved April 15, 2011, from http://www.fda.gov/Drugs/DrugSafety/ucm085729.htm.

U.S. National Library of Medicine National Institutes of Health. (2009). Addison's Disease. *MedLine Plus*. Retrieved April 25, 2011, from http://www.nlm.nih.gov/medlineplus/ency/article/000378.htm.

U.S. National Library of Medicine National Institutes of Health. (2009). Cushing's Disease. *MedLine Plus*. Retrieved April 25, 2011, from http://www.nlm.nih.gov/medlineplus/ency/article/000348.htm.

Chapter 17 References

Agur, A.M.R. and Lee, M.J. (1999). *Grant's Atlas of Anatomy*. Philadelphia, PA: Lippincott Williams & Wilkins.

Ansel, H.C., Allen, L.V., and Popovich, N.G. (1999). *Pharmaceutical Dosage Forms and Drug Delivery Systems* (7th ed.). Philadelphia, PA: Lippincott Williams & Wilkins.

Ansel, H.C. and Stoklosa, M.J. (2001). *Pharmaceutical Calculations* (11th ed.). Philadelphia, PA: Lippincott Williams & Wilkins.

Ballington, D.A. and Anderson, R.J. (2010). *Pharmacy Practice for Technicians: Mastering Community and Hospital Competencies* (4th ed.). St. Paul, MN: Paradigm Publishing.

Ballington, D.A. and Laughlin, M.M. (2010). *Pharmacology for Technicians: Understanding Drugs and Their Uses* (4th ed.). St. Paul, MN: Paradigm Publishing.

Berardi, R.R., et al., eds. (2010). *Handbook of Nonprescription Drugs: An Interactive Approach to Self-Care* (13th ed.). Washington, DC: American Pharmacists Association.

Bickley, L.S. (2003). *Bates' Guide to Physical Examination and History Taking* (8th ed.). Philadelphia, PA: Lippincott Williams & Wilkins.

Centers for Disease Control and Prevention. (2011). Healthcare-Associated Infections. *Centers for Disease Control and Prevention*. Retrieved March 22, 2011, from http://www.cdc.gov/hai.

Dipiro, J.T., et al., eds. (2008). *Pharmacotherapy: A Pathophysiologic Approach* (7th ed.). New York, NY: McGraw-Hill Medical.

Gould, C.V., et al. (2010). Guideline for Prevention of Catheter-Associated Urinary Tract Infections 2009. *Infection Control and Hospital Epidemiology, 31*(4), 319–326.

Hidron, A.I., et al. (2008). Antimicrobioal-Resistant Pathogens Associated with Healthcare-Associated Infections: Annual Summary of Data Reported to the National Healthcare Safety Network at the Centers for Disease Control and Prevention, 2006–2007. *Infection Control and Hospital Epidemiology, 29*(11), 996–1011.

Institute for Healthcare Improvement. Protecting 5 Millions Lives Campaign. *Institute for Healthcare Improvement*. Retrieved March 22, 2011, from http://www.ihi.org/IHI/Programs/Campaign/.

Kienle, P.C. (2007). Understanding Beyond-Use Dating for Compounded Sterile Preparations. *Pharmacy Purchasing and Products*, March: 2–5.

Klevens, R.M., et al. (2007). Estimating Health Care-Associated Infections and Deaths in U.S. Hospitals, 2002. *Public Health Reports, 122*, 160–166.

Koenig, S.M. and Truwit, J.D. (2006). Ventilator-Associated Pneumonia: Diagnosis, Treatment, and Prevention. *Clinical Microbiology Reviews, 19*(4), 637–657.

Lacy, C.F., et al., eds. (2009). *Drug Information Handbook*. Washington, DC: American Pharmacists Association.

Lee, L.D. (2010). Compliant Compounding: Meeting USP 797 Pharmacy Regulations. *Health Facilities Management*, February.

Murray, P.R., et al. (2002). *Medical Microbiology* (4th ed.). St. Louis, MO: Mosby.

Nichols, R.L. (2001). Preventing Surgical Site Infections: A Surgeon's Perspective. *Emerging Infectious Diseases, 7*(2), 220–224.

Pittet, D., et al. (2008). Infection Control as a Major World Health Organization Priority for Developing Countries. *Journal of Hospital Infection, 68*, 285–292.

Saint, S., et al. (2009). Catheter-Associated Urinary Tract Infection and the Medicare Rule Changes. *Annals of Internal Medicine, 150*(12), 877–884.

Scott, R.D. (2009). The Direct Medical Costs of Healthcare-Associated Infections in U.S. Hospitals and the Benefits of Prevention. *Centers for Disease Control and Prevention*. Retrieved March 22, 2011, from http://www.cdc.gov/ncidod/dhqp/pdf/Scott_CostPaper.pdf.

Thompson, J.E. (1998). *A Practical Guide to Contemporary Pharmacy Practice*. Baltimore, MD: Lippincott, Williams & Wilkins.

U.S. National Library of Medicine, National Institutes of Health. Infection Control. *Medline Plus*. Retrieved March 22, 2011, from http://www.nlm.nih.gov/medlineplus/infectioncontrol.html.

Wilson, J.A., et al. (2007). Uniform: An Evidence Review of the Microbiological Significance of Uniforms and Uniform Policy in the Prevention and Control of Healthcare-Associated Infections. Report to the Department of Health (England). *Journal of Hospital Infection, 66*(4), 301–307.

World Health Organization. (2011). Infection Control. *World Health Organization*. Retrieved March 22, 2011, from http://www.who.int/topics/infection_control/en.

Chapter 18 References

Agur, A.M.R. and Lee, M.J. (1999). *Grant's Atlas of Anatomy*. Philadelphia, PA: Lippincott, Williams & Wilkins.

Ansel, H.C., Allen, L.V., and Popovich, N.G. (1999). *Pharmaceutical Dosage Forms and Drug Delivery Systems* (7th ed.). Philadelphia, PA: Lippincott, Williams & Wilkins.

Ansel, H.C. and Stoklosa, M.J. (2001). *Pharmaceutical Calculations* (11th ed.). Philadelphia, PA: Lippincott, Williams & Wilkins.

Ballington, D.A. and Anderson, R.J. (2010). *Pharmacy Practice for Technicians: Mastering Community and Hospital Competencies* (4th ed.). St. Paul, MN: Paradigm Publishing.

Ballington, D.A. and Laughlin, M.M. (2010). *Pharmacology for Technicians: Understanding Drugs and Their Uses* (4th ed.). St. Paul, MN: Paradigm Publishing.

Chung, C.H. (2008). Managing Premedications and the Risk for Reactions to Infusional Monoclonal Antibody Therapy. *The Oncologist, 13*(6), 725–732.

Dipiro, J.T., et al., eds. (2008). *Pharmacotherapy: A Pathophysiologic Approach* (7th ed.). New York, NY: McGraw-Hill Medical.

Lacy, C.F., et al., eds. (2009). *Drug Information Handbook*. Washington, DC: American Pharmacists Association.

McCartney, L. (2011). *Sterile Compounding and Aseptic Technique: Concepts, Training, and Assessment for Pharmacy Technicians*. St. Paul, MN: Paradigm Publishing.

Murray, P.R., et al. (2002). *Medical Microbiology* (4th ed.). St. Louis, MO: Mosby.

Rhoades, R. and Pflanzer, R. (2003). *Human Physiology* (4th ed.). Pacific Grove, CA: Thomson Learning.

Shargel, L. and Yu, A.B.C. (1999). *Applied Biopharmaceutics and Pharmacokinetics* (4th ed.). New York, NY: McGraw-Hill.

Thompson, J.E. (1998). *A Practical Guide to Contemporary Pharmacy Practice*. Baltimore, MD: Lippincott, Williams & Wilkins.

Chapter 19

Agur, A.M.R. and Lee, M.J. (1999). *Grant's Atlas of Anatomy*. Philadelphia, PA: Lippincott, Williams & Wilkins.

Ansel, H.C., Allen, L.V., and Popovich, N.G. (1999). *Pharmaceutical Dosage Forms and Drug Delivery Systems* (7th ed.). Philadelphia, PA: Lippincott, Williams & Wilkins.

Ansel, H.C. and Stoklosa, M.J. (2001). *Pharmaceutical Calculations* (11th ed.). Philadelphia, PA: Lippincott, Williams & Wilkins.

Ballington, D.A. and Anderson, R.J. (2010). *Pharmacy Practice for Technicians: Mastering Community and Hospital Competencies* (4th ed.). St. Paul, MN: Paradigm Publishing.

Ballington, D.A. and Laughlin, M.M. (2010). *Pharmacology for Technicians: Understanding Drugs and Their Uses* (4th ed.). St. Paul, MN: Paradigm Publishing.

Dipiro, J.T., et al., eds. (2008). *Pharmacotherapy: A Pathophysiologic Approach* (7th ed.). New York, NY: McGraw-Hill Medical.

Lacy, C.F., et al., eds. (2009). *Drug Information Handbook*. Washington, DC: American Pharmacists Association.

Lee, J.W. (2010). Fluid and Electrolyte Disturbances in Critically Ill Patients. *Electrolyte Blood Press, 8*(2), 72–81.

Livingston, A., Seamons, C., and Dalton, T. (2000). If the Gut Works, Use It. *Nurse Manage, 31*(5), 39–42.

McCartney, L. (2011). *Sterile Compounding and Aseptic Technique: Concepts, Training, and Assessment for Pharmacy Technicians*. St. Paul, MN: Paradigm Publishing.

Misita, C.P., Boosinger, A.B., and Kendrach, M.G. (2003). Bioterrorism Websites for Pharmacists. *The Annals of Pharmacotherapy, 37*(1), 132–5.

Rhinehart, E. and Friedman, M.M. (1999). *Infection Control in Home Care*. Gaithersburg, MD: Aspen Publishers.

Rhoades, R. and Pflanzer, R. (2003). *Human Physiology* (4th ed.). Pacific Grove, CA: Thomson Learning.

Sabon, R.L., et al. (1989). Glass particle contamination: influence of aspiration methods and ampule type. *Anesthesiology, 70*(5), 859–62.

Simmons, H. (2008). Personnel Hygiene and Gowning Requirements: How the Changes to USP <797> Will

Affect Your Practice. *Pharmacy Purchasing & Products*, January, 8–9.

Sparks, J. and McCartney, L. (2010). *Pharmacy Labs for Technicians: Building Skills in Pharmacy Practice*. St. Paul, MN: Paradigm Publishing.

Teeter, D. and Terriff, C. (2002). Implementing a Bioterrorism Response Plan in Your Pharmacy. *Journal of the American Pharmaceutical Association, 42*(5 Suppl 1), S52–3.

Terriff, C.M., et al. "Emergency Preparedness: Identification and Management of Biological Exposures." By J. DiPiro. 2008. *Pharmacotherapy: A Pathophysiologic Approach*. McGraw-Hill. Retrieved April 9, 2011 from http://highered.mcgraw-hill.com/sites/dl/free/007147899x/603552/Pharmacotherapy_chap011.pdf.

Terriff, C.M., Schwartz, M.D., and Lomaestro, B.M. (2003). Bioterrorism: Pivotal Clinical Issues. Consensus Review of the Society of Infectious Diseases Pharmacists. *Pharmacotherapy, 23*(3), 274–90.

Thompson, J.E. (1998). *A Practical Guide to Contemporary Pharmacy Practice*. Baltimore, MD: Lippincott. Williams & Wilkins.

University of Maryland Medical Center. (2011). Black Cohash. *University of Maryland Medical Center*. Retrieved April 2, 2011, from http://www.umm.edu/altmed/articles/black-cohosh-000226.htm.

University of Maryland Medical Center. (2011). Echinacea. *University of Maryland Medical Center*. Retrieved April 2, 2011, from http://www.umm.edu/altmed/articles/echinacea-000239.htm.

University of Maryland Medical Center. (2011). Evening Primrose Oil. *University of Maryland Medical Center*. Retrieved April 2, 2011, from http://www.umm.edu/altmed/articles/evening-primrose-000242.htm.

University of Maryland Medical Center. (2011). Feverfew. *University of Maryland Medical Center*. Retrieved April 2, 2011 from http://www.umm.edu/altmed/articles/feverfew-000243.htm.

University of Maryland Medical Center. (2011). Glucosamine. *University of Maryland Medical Center*. Retrieved April 2, 2011, from http://www.umm.edu/altmed/articles/glucosamine-000306.htm.

University of Maryland Medical Center. (2011). Licorice. *University of Maryland Medical Center*. Retrieved April 2, 2011, from http://www.umm.edu/altmed/articles/licorice-000917.htm.

University of Maryland Medical Center. (2011). Melatonin. *University of Maryland Medical Center*. Retrieved April 2, 2011, from http://www.umm.edu/altmed/articles/melatonin-000315.htm.

University of Maryland Medical Center. (2011). Saw Palmetto. *University of Maryland Medical Center*. Retrieved April 2, 2011, from http://www.umm.edu/altmed/articles/saw-palmetto-000272.htm.

University of Maryland Medical Center. (2011). St. John's Wort. *University of Maryland Medical Center*. Retrieved April 2, 2011, from http://www.umm.edu/altmed/articles/st-johns-000276.htm.

Waller, D.G. and George, C.F. (1986). Ampoules, infusions, and filters. *British Medical Journal, 292*, 714–5.

Chapter 20

Albanese, N.P. and Rouse, M.J. (2010). Scope of Contemporary Pharmacy Practice: Roles, Responsibilities, and Functions of Pharmacists and Pharmacy Technicians. *Journal of the American Pharmacists Association, 50*(2), e35–69.

Allen, J.G. (2000). *The Complete Q & A Job Interview Book* (3rd ed.). New York, NY: John Wiley & Sons.

Allen, J.G. (1995). *The Resume Makeover*. New York, NY: John Wiley & Sons.

Ballington, D.A. and Anderson, R.J. (2010). *Pharmacy Practice for Technicians: Mastering Community and Hospital Competencies* (4th ed.). St. Paul, MN: Paradigm Publishing.

Boh, L.E., ed. (2001). *Pharmacy Practice Manual* (2nd ed.). Baltimore, MD: Lippincott, Williams & Wilkins.

Buckingham, M. and Clifton, D.O. (2001). *Now, Discover Your Strengths*. New York, NY: The Free Press.

Chaar, B.B., Brien, J., and Krass, I. (2009). Professional Ethics in Pharmacy Practice: Developing a Psychometric Measure of Moral Reasoning. *Pharmacy World & Science, 31*(4), 439–49.

Desselle, S.P. (2003). Job Turnover Intentions Among Certified Pharmacy Technicians. *Journal of the American Pharmacists Association, 45*(6), 676–83.

Desselle, S.P. (2003). Survey of Certified Pharmacy Technicians in the United States: a Quality-of-Worklife Study. *Journal of the American Pharmacists Association, 45*(4), 458–65.

Desselle, S.P. and Holmes, E.R. (2003). Structural Model of Certified Pharmacy Technicians' Job Satisfaction. *Journal of the American Pharmacists Association, 47*(1), 58–72.

Dessing, R.P. (2000). Ethics Applied to Pharmacy Practice. *Pharmacy World & Science, 22*(1), 10–16.

Dessing, R.P. and Flameling, J. (2003). Ethics in Pharmacy: a New Definition of Responsibility. *Pharmacy World & Science, 25*(1), 3–10.

Farr, J.M. (1997). *How to Get a Job Now!* Indianapolis, IN: JIST Works, Inc.

Farr, J.M. (2005). *The Quick Resume and Cover Letter Book* (3rd ed.). Indianapolis, IN: JIST Works, Inc.

Friesner, D.L. and Scott, D.M. (2010). Identifying Characteristics That Allow Pharmacy Technicians to Assume

Unconventional Roles in the Pharmacy. *Journal of the American Pharmacists Association, 50*(6), 686–97.

Fung, S.M., et al. (2003). Nontraditional Roles for Certified Pharmacy Technicians in a Pharmaceutical Company. *Journal of the American Pharmacists Association, 46*(4), 507–10.

Keresztes, J.M. (2010). Education … A Must in All Levels of Pharmacy Practice. *The Annals of Pharmacotherapy, 44*(11), 1826–8.

Latif, D.A. (2000). Ethical Cognition and Selection-Socialization in Retail Pharmacy. *Journal of Business Ethics, 25*(4), 343–57.

Maddux, M.S., Dong, B.J., Miller, W.A., et al. (2000). 1997–1999 ACCP Clinical Practice Affairs Subcommittee A. A Vision of Pharmacy's Future Roles, Responsibilities, and Manpower Needs in the United States. *Pharmacotherapy, 20*(8), 991–1020.

McCarthy, R.L. and Schafermeyer, K.W. (2001). *Introduction to Health Care Delivery*. Gaithersburg, MD: Aspen Publication.

Muenzen, P.M., et al. (2003). Updating the Pharmacy Technician Certification Examination: A Practice Analysis Study. *Journal of the American Pharmacists Association, 46*(1), e1–6.

Purtilo, R. (1999). *Ethical Dimensions in the Health Professions* (3rd ed.). Philadelphia, PA: Saunders.

Rosenberg, A.D. and Hizer, D. (2003). *The Resume Handbook* (4th ed.). Avon, MA: Adams Media Corporation.

Wick, J.Y. (2008). Using Pharmacy Technicians to Enhance Clinical and Operational Capabilities. *The Consultant Pharmacist, 23*(6), 447–58.

Worthen, D.B. (2001). *Proctor & Gamble's Pharmacist's Handbook* (2nd ed.). Boca Raton, FL: CRC Press, LLC.

Index

Figures and tables are indicated with f and t following the page number.

Milliequivalents, 115, 118
Milrinone, 388
Mineralocorticoids, 461
Minerals, 561, 562, 565, 567. *See also* Supplements
Minor contamination, 542–543
Misbranding, 47
Misoprostol (Cytotec), 329, 420
Mitotic spindle fibers, 532
Mixed analgesics, 418–419
Mixed numbers, 63, 63*f*
Mobic (meloxicam), 421
Mobility, 521
Modes of action. *See* Mechanisms of action
Moist-heat sterilization, 478
Mold, 475
Monoamine oxidase inhibitors. *See* MAOIs
Monobactams, 164, 164*t*
Monoclonal antibodies (MABs), 524–526, 526*t*
Monographs, 54
Monophasic contraceptives, 456
Mood-stabilizing agents, 246
Morality, 599–600
Moral judgments, 600
Morphine, 214, 217, 220, 458
Mortar and pestles, 355, 358, 359
MPJE (Multistate Pharmacy Jurisprudence Exam), 12
MSDSs (material safety data sheets), 353
Mucolytics, 304
Mucomyst (acetylcysteine), 304, 305
Multidrug-resistant tuberculosis (MDR-TB), 306
Multiplication (mathematical operation), 61–62, 62*t*.
    See also Mathematical calculations
  cross-multiplication, 121–122, 121*f*
  of decimals, 69, 69*f*
  of fractions, 66–67
Multistate Pharmacy Jurisprudence Exam (MPJE), 12
Multivitamins. *See* Vitamins
Muscle pain and diseases, 414–423
  function and physiology, 415, 415*f*
  inflammation and swelling, 417–419
  relaxants, 414, 416–417
Muscle relaxants, 414, 416–417
Mutagens, 518
Myocardial infarction (MI), 384, 392
Myoclonic seizures, 270, 272, 273, 274
Myxedema, 451

N

NABP. *See* National Association of Boards of Pharmacy
Nabumetone (Relafen), 421
Naked viruses, 192
Naltrexone (ReVia), 251
NAPLEX. *See* North American Pharmacist Licensure
    Exam
Naproxen sodium, 421
Narcotics. *See* Controlled substances

Nasal corticosteroids, 310, 310*t*
Nasal decongestants, 307, 308–309, 308–309*t*
Nasal route of administration, 103
Nasoenteric tubes, 563
Nasogastric tubes, 372, 563
National Association of Boards of Pharmacy (NABP),
    12, 18, 25–26, 605
National Drug Codes (NDCs), 21, 52, 52*f*, 155, 157,
    186
National Formulary (NF). *See United States
    Pharmacopeia-National Formulary* (USP-NF)
National Healthcare Safety Network (NHSN), 481
National Pharmacy Technician Association (NPTA), 28
National Quality Forum, 152, 153–154
Nausea, 331, 332*t*
NDAs. *See* New Drug Applications
NDCs. *See* National Drug Codes
Nebulizers, 301, 305
Needles, 516, 516*f*, 552, 552*f*, 554, 554*f*
Negative feedback mechanisms, 450
Negligence, 27
Neonatal, 555
Neoplasms, 529–530
Neoplastic disease. *See* Cancer
Nephropathy, 463
Nephrotoxicity, 167, 169
Neptazane (methazolamide), 364
Nervous system. *See also* Central nervous system (CNS)
  autonomic, 215–216, 216*f*
  blood-brain barrrier and, 39
  disorders of, 268–280
  drug effects and, 216–217
  neurotransmitters and, 215–217, 215*f*
  overview, 214–216, 268, 269*f*
  parasympathetic, 216, 216*f*
  somatic, 216
  sympathetic, 215–216, 216*f*
Neuromuscular blockers, 217, 219, 219*t*
Neurons, 269, 275
Neurontin (gabapentin), 272
Neurotransmitters
  Alzheimer's disease and, 279, 280
  anxiety disorders and, 249
  bipolar disorder and, 246
  COPD and, 304
  depression and, 241, 242, 243, 245
  muscle relaxants and, 416, 417
  nausea and vomiting and, 331
  nervous system and, 215–217, 215*f*
  neuromuscular blockers and, 217
  Parkinson's disease and, 275, 276, 277–278
  schizophrenia, 247
  seizures and, 269, 271
  weight loss and, 338
Neutropenia, 527
New Drug Applications (NDAs), 19, 20, 22, 23, 46–48

Credits

Chapter 11

Page 288 © Comstock/Thinkstock; **page 291** © Radius Images/Alamy Images; **page 295** © Benis Arapovic/ShutterStock, Inc.; **page 301** © Jones and Bartlett Publishers. Courtesy of MIEMSS; **page 301** Courtesy of Rhonda Beck; **page 306** © Medical-on-Line/Alamy Images; **page 307** © aceshot1/ShutterStock, Inc.

Chapter 12

Page 320 © Jeniicorv8/Dreamstime.com; **page 323** © Mangostock/Dreamstime.com; **page 324** © Tom Tracy Photography/Alamy Images; **page 325** © Jupiterimages/Comstock/Thinkstock; **page 327** © Ronald Sumners/ShutterStock, Inc.; **page 335** © S.White/Fotolia; **page 337** © Monkey Business Images/ShutterStock, Inc.; **page 340** © Dmitry Knorre/Fotolia.

Chapter 13

Page 350 © Robert Kneschke/ShutterStock, Inc.; **page 354** © Photodisc; **page 355** Courtesy of Fulcrum Inc, The TORBAL Scales company; **page 355** Courtesy of Fulcrum Inc, The TORBAL Scales company; **page 355** © AbleStock; **page 356** © Carlos Davila/Alamy Images; **page 358** © Photodisc; **page 359** © Lisa F. Young/ShutterStock; **page 360** © BSIP SA/Alamy Images

Chapter 14

Page 372 © Sandra van der Steen/Fotolia; **page 373** © Olivier/Fotolia; **page 378** Fahrner78/Dreamstime.com; **page 380** Lisa F. Young/ShutterStock.

Chapter 15

Page 409 © Biomedical Communications/Custom Medical Stock Photo; **page 410** Courtesy McKesson Corporation; **page 411** © Barbara J. Petrick/ShutterStock, Inc.; **page 412** © Alain Daussin/Getty Images; **page 413** Courtesy of Omnicell, Inc.

Chapter 16

Page 432 © Javier Larrea/age fotostock; **page 434** © Senior Airman S.I. Fielder/US Air Force; **page 440** © Aleksandrs Jermakovichs/ShutterStock; **page 456** © LiquidLibrary; **page 465** © Dynamic Graphics/Thinkstock.

Chapter 17

Page 472 © David Joel/age fotostock; **page 473** Courtesy of Dr. Wood/US Department of Agriculture; **page 474 (top)** Courtesy of Dr. Fred Murphy/Center for Disease Control; **page 474 (bottom)** © Valentyn Volkov/ShutterStock, Inc.; **page 475 (top)** Courtesy of John Pitt of CSIRO Food Science, Australia; **page 475 (bottom)** © Dubults/Fotolia; **page 476** © AbleStock; **page 478** © Chris Pole/ShutterStock, Inc.; **page 479 (top)** © Cupertino/ShutterStock, Inc.; **page 479 (bottom)** © AbleStock; **page 480** © Mikhail Olykainen/ShutterStock, Inc.; **page 483** © Blaj Gabriel/ShutterStock, Inc.; **page 486** © Amy Walters/Fotolia; **page 487** © jelena zaric/Fotolia; **page 488** © Suzanne Tucker/ShutterStock, Inc.; **page 489** © Chubykin Arkady/ShutterStock, Inc.; **page 491** © Levent Konuk/ShutterStock, Inc.; **page 492** © carroteater/ShutterStock, Inc.; **page 493** © F.C.G./ShutterStock, Inc.; **page 494** © Carolina K. Smith, MD/Fotolia; **page 496** © pzRomashka/ShutterStock, Inc.

Chapter 18

Page 508 © Deborah Aronds/ShutterStock, Inc.; **page 510** © Photodisc/Getty Images; **page 513** © Jones & Bartlett Learning. Courtesy of MIEMSS; **page 533** © NREY/ShutterStock, Inc.

Chapter 19

Page 543 © Henry Adams/Fotolia; **page 544 (top)** © Digital Vision/Thinkstock; **page 544 (bottom)** © Photodisc/Thinkstock; **page 547** © Ambrophoto/ShutterStock, Inc.; **page 551** © Mira/Alamy Images; **page 557** Courtesy of Baxa Corporation; **page 562** © Tomo Jesenicnik/Fotolia; **page 563** © Rickís Photography/ShutterStock, Inc.; **page 565** © Jones & Bartlett Learning. Photographed by Kimberly Potvin; **page 570** © Irene Teesalu/Fotolia; **page 571** © LianeM/ShutterStock, Inc.; **page 573** © Melinda Fawver/ShutterStock, Inc.; **page 574** © AbleStock; **page 575** © Carolina K. Smith, MD/ShutterStock, Inc.

Chapter 20

Page 589 © shock/Fotolia; **page 598** © Stephen Coburn/ShutterStock, Inc.; **page 605** © Lena Sergeeva/ShutterStock, Inc.; **page 605** © Kzenon/ShutterStock, Inc.